FOUNDATIONS OF LOW VISION:
CLINICAL AND FUNCTIONAL PERSPECTIVES

**Anne L. Corn
and
Alan J. Koenig,
Editors**

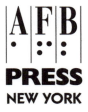

PRESS
NEW YORK

Printed in the United States of America

2000 Reprinting

Library of Congress Cataloging-in-Publication Data

Foundations of low vision / Anne L. Corn and Alan J. Koenig, editors.
    p. cm.
    Includes bibliographical references (p.   ) and index.
    ISBN 0-89128-941-0 (alk. paper)

    1. Low vision.   I. Corn, Anne Lesley.   II. Koenig, J., 1954–

RE91.F64   1996
617.7'12--dc20
                       96-30666

CONTENTS

PART THREE Functional Perspectives

PART FOUR Changing Perspectives

FOREWORD

It is often said in the field of blindness and visual impairment that no two people see exactly alike. Those of us who work in the field emphasize this point to convey both the variability of visual impairments and the importance of paying attention to the individual's needs and abilities in delivering services. Nevertheless, the point bears continued repeating, and rarely has it been expressed as well as it has been by the authors and editors of *Foundations of Low Vision: Clinical and Functional Perspectives.*

Although volumes have been written about visual impairment and its implications, clinical measures expressed in numbers such as 20/200 have often been used to define the impact of impaired vision on an adult or child. However, we all know that what one person sees with 20/200 vision may be entirely different from what another person with the same measurement sees. In its careful examination of the experience of low vision and its emphasis on the functional dimensions of visual impairment, *Foundations of Low Vision* does all of us a service by helping us see what low vision really means to the person who lives with it. This important new text provides a solid base on which professionals who either work or plan to be working with people with low vision can build effective ways of understanding and meeting their needs. Here, in one source, practitioners of the key disciplines in the field, whether they be educators, rehabilitators, clinicians, orientation and mobility instructors, administrators, or planners, will find the significant issues and strategic considerations they need to confront in order to provide services in a successful and satisfying way.

By publishing this comprehensive text, which we believe readers will find an essential handbook on how to work with people with low vision, the American Foundation for the Blind has continued its commitment to improve the quality of life of persons who are visually impaired. By promoting an understanding of the various aspects of low vision and helping professionals learn more effective ways of delivering important services, *Foundations of Low Vision* marks another milestone in the literature of the field.

Carl R. Augusto
President
American Foundation
for the Blind

PREFACE

This book marks an important milestone in the development of low vision rehabilitation as a distinct discipline. It demonstrates the importance of teamwork among professionals from different backgrounds so that the client's functional abilities are optimized.

For too long, low vision care has lingered in a no-man's-land between eye care for sighted individuals and services for persons who are blind. In recent years, however, the black-and-white dichotomy between the needs of those who are "legally sighted" and those who are "legally blind" has been replaced by a continuous gray scale with black and white as end points. Service delivery for the low vision population needs to borrow from both ends of the spectrum, but it also has its own distinct set of skills and knowledge.

The recorded history of care for blind persons goes back at least seven centuries to 1260 when the *Hôpital des Quinze-Vingts* was established in Paris to take care of soldiers who were blinded as hostages during the Crusades. The concept of low vision care is much younger. It was only half a century ago that the concept that sight could be "saved" by not using it was abandoned. It was only two decades ago that the World Health Organization (WHO) threw out the old dichotomy of "legally sighted" versus "legally blind" and defined various ranges of vision loss instead. This was done in the ninth revision of WHO's *International Classification of Diseases* (ICD-9, 1977), which is also the basis for the official classification used in the United States, issued by the National Center for Health Statistics (the *International Classification of Diseases, 9th Revision, Clinical Modification,* or ICD-9-CM, issued in 1978 and revised annually). (An example of the use of these ranges is shown in a table in Chapter 1 of this book.)

In ICD-9-CM, the level of vision loss previously identified as "legal blindness" is now identified as "severe vision loss." This is more than just a change of words; it signifies a change in attitudes. The old term was based on a dichotomous view of vision loss and thus supported the concept of a dichotomy in service delivery. The new term is based on a continuous scale of ranges of vision loss and thus promotes a continuum of service delivery and smoothly integrated teamwork. Use of the old term should be avoided by all who deal with patients and clients with low vision. To call a person with severe vision loss "legally blind" is as preposterous as calling a person with a severe illness "legally dead."

In the past, eye care professionals have taken care of those who are sighted. Their solutions (eyeglasses, contact lenses) required very little instruction for use. In the past, schools for blind students provided educational services but, since their residents had lost all eyesight, the need for continuing eye care was minimal. This dichotomous approach resulted in a lack of contact between those trained in the health care system and those trained in the educational system. We now realize that all patients with low vision have some eye disorder that warrants periodic eye examinations. They also have vision that can benefit from the use of optical and nonoptical devices. The proper use of those devices is not always obvious, so patients need education about how to use them and about possible adaptations in home, school, or workplace.

This continuum of service delivery is best expressed through the terms promoted by WHO's *International Classification of Impairments, Disabilities and Handicaps* (ICIDH, 1980, a companion volume to ICD-9). These concepts, which apply to any kind of functional loss (hearing, musculoskeletal, and so on), are shown in a sidebar in this book's opening chapter. Unfortunately, they have not yet received the same attention from rehabilitation workers in this country as they have from audiences in other parts of the world. Clients are not adequately served if any of the necessary interventions are skipped, yet it is clear that no single individual can be expected to provide the whole spectrum of services. Success-

ful rehabilitation, therefore, must be based on teamwork among different professionals. This, in turn, requires communication and a common understanding of each other's terminology and goals. The first chapter of this book discusses the confusion and miscommunication that can arise from inconsistent terminology.

Foundations of Low Vision describes various perspectives on vision loss, recognizing that the unifying link among these perspectives is not found in the various professionals, but rather in the functional needs of the client. To work as a team, clinicians need to understand the educational perspective, while educators need to understand the clinical perspective. A well-known parable describes how five blind men, working in isolation, could not reach consensus on how to describe an elephant. May this book show how much more effective their efforts could have been had they worked and communicated as one low vision rehabilitation team.

August Colenbrander, M.D.
Director, Low Vision Services
California Pacific Medical Center

INTRODUCTION

Foundations of Low Vision: Clinical and Functional Perspectives is a general text about low vision, written for practicing professionals and soon-to-be professionals who will provide educational, rehabilitation, and clinical services to people with low vision. The editors hope that it will also be of value to individuals with congenital or acquired low vision and that those who have low vision will find that the challenges and successes they experience are appropriately and respectfully portrayed.

The term *perspectives* was chosen as a unifying theme for this text. It exemplifies the following concepts:

- This book is for professionals in various disciplines, each of which has its own and shared perspectives with other disciplines.

- Low vision services are not based solely on a clear-cut science; rather, service providers combine the tools of the discipline with their perspectives to develop high-quality services.

- No two persons with low vision experience low vision the same way. Each brings to the experience a medical and personal history that influences the development of his or her personal perspectives about low vision.

Throughout this text, the reader will also note the focus on the functional uses of low vision. The contributing authors, experts on low vision, were asked not to write a review of the academic literature or research but to use their personal and professional expertise to help the reader learn how children and adults with low vision learn to function with their visual abilities and to keep in perspective the extent to which low vision is or is not an efficient sensory channel. The themes of perspectives and functionality are emphasized in this book to provide the reader with a real-life sense of what low vision is, what the needs of people with low vision are, and what the effective delivery of low vision services entails.

The text is divided into four parts: Personal and Professional Perspectives, Clinical Perspectives, Functional Perspectives, and Changing Perspectives. In Personal and Professional Perspectives, the reader is introduced to low vision as a life condition and as a professional discipline.

- Chapter 1 presents definitions, the use of terminology, demographics, and the make-up of professional teams. The reader is asked to consider whether the use of terms to describe the population of persons with low vision has helped or hindered the availability of services.

- Chapter 2 discusses personal perspectives on low vision, including a consideration of experiences that people with low vision share and the myths and misconceptions of normally sighted persons about low vision, and helps the reader understand what it means to grow up with or to acquire low vision. The ways in which professionals can help visually impaired adults and children address feelings about low vision and the attitudes of normally sighted people toward them are also examined.

◆ Chapter 3 speaks to the options that persons with low vision have in their daily lives and how people can take control of their lives and their visual environments.

◆ Chapter 4 presents the issues and dimensions of literacy for persons with low vision, including the unique aspects of defining literacy for this population and the ways in which professionals can ensure that appropriate literacy skills are gained. It emphasizes the importance of literacy for the success of children and adults in school and employment, as well as in everyday activities.

In Clinical Perspectives, the reader learns about the visual system and the medical and optical aspects of providing specialized clinical services to persons with low vision. Throughout this section, the authors have striven to describe how such diverse topics as organic structures, optics, genes, and devices relate to the daily functioning of people with low vision.

◆ Chapter 5 uses an anatomy and physiology lesson to convey, in functional terms, how the experience of sight occurs and brings richness to life.

◆ Chapter 6, on the causes and functional implications of visual impairments, focuses on the visual effects of various conditions.

◆ Chapter 7 introduces basic principles of optics and low vision devices. By stressing how and why optical devices are produced and the wide variety of optical and other devices that are available, it helps demonstrate the "match" that must be made among the individual, the device, and the task for visual efficiency to develop.

◆ Chapter 8 describes the procedures of the clinical low vision evaluation and what this evaluation can accomplish and distinguishes it from the examination used by general eye care providers.

In Functional Perspectives, the reader learns how educational and rehabilitation services help people with low vision become visually efficient and place functional limitations in perspective with their life's goals.

◆ Chapter 9 discusses the roles and functions of teachers of students with visual impairments who provide low vision services through school systems. It describes functional vision assessments and provides guidance for preparing instructional programs based on such assessments.

◆ Chapter 10 covers the visual functioning of children with low vision and additional severe disabilities, including how visual functioning is assessed and how this information is used to enhance children's functional use of vision.

◆ Chapter 11 presents a comprehensive and systematic approach to selecting learning and literacy media for students with visual impairments, a process called a "learning media assessment."

◆ Chapter 12 discusses factors that influence reading with low vision and specific instructional strategies and guidelines for teaching reading and writing skills to ensure that students with low vision develop solid and meaningful literacy skills.

◆ Chapter 13 provides information on orientation and mobility (O&M) for children and adults with low vision, including the use of functional vision assessments for mobility and travel, environmental cues, and how O&M instructors can foster new skills, such as the use of visual landmarks and of optical devices.

◆ Chapter 14 explores the experiences of working-age adults with congenital or acquired low vision, discussing their personal and social needs, and describes the role of rehabilitation teaching and other services from which adults with low vision may benefit as they work to develop skills for independent living.

◆ Chapter 15 discusses how rehabilitation services can help adults with low vision determine career goals, develop job-seeking skills, and acquire adaptive tools and skills for obtaining employment. It also covers legislation related to rehabilitation and the practices of rehabilitation counselors who work with individuals with low vision.

◆ Chapter 16 presents basic information on promoting the independence of older adults with low vision, discussing changes in the visual system that come with the aging process, functional vision assessments as well as clinical low vision evaluations for older persons, and environmental modifications and techniques to facilitate independent living.

Changing Perspectives contains two chapters:

◆ Chapter 17 describes the evolution of low vision services, including the history of interdisciplinary professional development, philosophical changes, and improvement in clinical knowledge.

◆ Chapter 18 revisits the lives of children and adults featured in the vignettes in various chapters and explores trends in technology and service delivery from a futuristic perspective. It postulates what may happen to individuals from the vignettes and considers important directions for professional activity.

The chapters all follow a pattern. Each begins with a vignette of a person or persons with low vision that introduces the reader to several concepts that are included in the chapter. Although the characters in the vignettes are fictitious, their experiences are based on the real lives of the many persons with low vision with whom the authors are acquainted. The reader is encouraged to consider how the information in a chapter relates to the vignette of the person's life. Authors were asked to include in the text of their chapters information that a new professional would need to begin to carry out his or her responsibilities.

Each chapter concludes with suggested activities and From Your Perspective. The activities are designed to present experiences related to the content of the chapter and promote involvement in community services and interactions with children or adults who have low vision. From Your Perspective asks the reader to reflect on the vignette and the content of the chapter and to think deeply about and respond to a philosophical query and its implications for individuals with low vision.

This book provides a compendium of perspectives about low vision that should be of use to a wide range of readers, from professionals who work with children or adults with low vision to persons with low vision or those who have relatives with low vision to individuals who are conducting research or who are intellectually curious about the topic. Its goal is to help the reader develop an understanding of low vision, a flexible approach to meeting the needs of individuals, and a belief that people with low vision can have a good quality of life.

THE CONTRIBUTORS

Anne L. Corn, Ed.D., is Professor of Special Education and Ophthalmology at Vanderbilt University, Nashville, Tennessee, where she is also coordinator of the teacher preparation program in visual disability at Peabody College. The winner in 1994 of the AER [Association for Education and Rehabilitation of the Blind and Visually Impaired] Division 7 (Low Vision) Award for Contributions to Literature and Research and in 1990 of the Distinguished Service Award, Low Vision Section of the American Optometric Association, she is the author of numerous books, articles, and other publications and a frequent speaker at national and international conferences. Dr. Corn is past president of the Division on Visual Handicaps of the Council for Exceptional Children and past chair of AER's Division 17 (Personnel Preparation).

Alan J. Koenig, Ed.D., is Associate Professor in the Division of Educational Psychology and Leadership at Texas Tech University in Lubbock, where he coordinates the teacher preparation program in visual impairment. A leading researcher on the selection of appropriate literacy media for students with visual impairments, he is co-author of *Foundations of Braille Literacy, Learning Media Assessment of Students with Visual Impairments: A Resource Guide for Teachers,* and *New Programmed Instruction in Braille.* Dr. Koenig is also co-editor of the *Special Issue on Literacy* of the *Journal of Visual Impairment & Blindness* and past president of the Division on Visual Handicaps of the Council for Exceptional Children.

Chapter Authors

Virginia E. Bishop, Ph.D., is a private consultant in special education and an adjunct faculty member at the University of Texas at Austin and Peabody College, Vanderbilt University, Nashville, Tennessee.

Jane N. Erin, Ph.D., is Associate Professor in the Department of Special Education and Rehabilitation at the University of Arizona, Tucson.

Duane R. Geruschat, Ph.D., is Director of Educational Support at the Maryland School for the Blind, Baltimore.

Gregory L. Goodrich, Ph.D., is Supervisory Research Psychologist, Psychology Service and Western Blind Rehabilitation Center, U.S. Department of Veterans Affairs Palo Alto Health Care System, Palo Alto, California, and Assistant Clinical Professor at the School of Optometry at the University of California at Berkeley.

Gaylen Kapperman, Ed.D., is Professor and Coordinator of Programs in Vision at Northern Illinois University, DeKalb.

Patricia J. Koenig, M.A., is Project Director and Instructor, Programs in Vision, Faculty of Special

Education, at Northern Illinois University, DeKalb.

J. Elton Moore, Ed.D., is Director of the Rehabilitation Research and Training Center on Blindness and Low Vision at Mississippi State University, Mississippi State.

Beth Paul was, at the time of writing, National Program Associate at the American Foundation for the Blind in New York City.

Evelyn J. Rex, Ph.D., is Professor Emeritae of Special Education at Illinois State University in Normal and Coordinator, Project ABLE, of the American Foundation for the Blind.

Sharon Zell Sacks, Ph.D., is Professor in the Division of Special Education and Rehabilitative Services at San Jose State University, San Jose, California.

Audrey J. Smith, Ph.D., is Director of the Institute for the Visually Impaired at the Pennsylvania College of Optometry in Philadelphia.

Virginia M. Sowell, Ph.D., is Associate Provost and Professor of Special Education at Texas Tech University in Lubbock.

Marjorie E. Ward, Ph.D., is Associate Professor in the College of Education at Ohio State University, Columbus.

Gale R. Watson, M.Ed., is Research Health Scientist in the U.S. Department of Veterans Affairs,

Decatur, Georgia, and Adjunct Professor at the Pennsylvania College of Optometry in Philadelphia and at Emory University and Georgia State University, Atlanta.

Mark E. Wilkinson, O.D., is Optometric Director in the Vision Rehabilitation Institute at the Genesis Medical Center in Davenport, Iowa, and Optometric Consultant at the Iowa Braille and Sight Saving School's Low Vision Clinic, Vinton.

Karen E. Wolffe, Ph.D., is a career counselor and a private consultant in Austin, Texas.

George J. Zimmerman, Ph.D., is Associate Professor and Chair and Coordinator of the Vision Studies Program of the Department of Instruction and Learning at the University of Pittsburgh, Pittsburgh, Pennsylvania.

Sidebar Authors

August Colenbrander, M.D., is Director of Low Vision Services, Program Coordinator of the Ophthalmology Matching Program, and a full-time faculty member of the Department of Ophthalmology at the California Pacific Medical Center as well as Clinical Scientist at the Smith-Kettlewell Eye Research Institute, San Francisco.

Judy C. Matsuoka, M.S.Ed., is Instructor in the Department of Rehabilitation at the University of Arkansas at Little Rock.

PART ONE

Personal and Professional Perspectives

CHAPTER 1

Perspectives on Low Vision

Anne L. Corn and Alan J. Koenig

VIGNETTE

Carol, an experienced journalist, has written a variety of stories associated with human services, from childhood nutrition to new living options for elderly people to the opening of new rehabilitation centers for persons with traumatic head injury. While on assignment to cover the winter Olympics in Lillehammer, Norway, Carol was watching an ice-skating event when the announcer commented that the mother of one ice skater was legally blind. As the camera focused on this woman, who was seated in the arena, Carol noticed that the mother was watching television up close to see her daughter skating. Puzzled and intrigued, Carol decided to do a story about people who are legally blind.

Within weeks, Carol had spoken with people from the American Council of the Blind, the American Foundation for the Blind (AFB), the National Federation of the Blind, and several schools for blind children. Although she asked similar questions about blindness and described what she saw on television to everyone she interviewed, Carol found that some professionals thought that legal blindness is not a useful term and that each spoke about people with useful vision who nevertheless met the definition of legal blindness. Some professionals commented that the current term was *low vision* but could not really define it; others said that people with useful vision are visually impaired but should not be considered blind. They all said that their schools or organizations served "these" people, who were not "really" blind.

Carol wanted a good slant to her story but could not see how she could write about such an ill-defined group of people. She thought that describing how people "who could see a little" could improve the quality of their lives and would be interesting, but she wondered whether she should get her information from organizations "for the blind." Finally, Carol decided to go to the library to find a text on the subject. She came upon *Low Vision: The Reference* (Goodrich & Jose, 1993), which lists 4,600 references about people with visual problems who are not totally blind. How could she digest it all? She needed one text to explain what people with low vision see and how they receive help, adjust to their impairments, and improve the quality of their lives. Furthermore, she realized that she would also need to speak directly to a number of people with low vision to get some idea of the wide variety of experiences associated with low vision.

INTRODUCTION

In the vignette that opens this chapter, a journalist who was attempting to learn about people with low vision discovered that people are not just blind or normally sighted and that sometimes people who are called "blind" can see. She also found that there is a rich literature about the problems of people who are "in the middle" between normal sightedness and blindness. Most important, however, she decided that to understand how people with low vision function and how they can get on with their lives, she would have to ask individuals with low vision themselves.

This chapter is an introduction to the issues faced by persons with low vision and the professionals who provide educational, rehabilitation, and clinical low vision services to them. It addresses the functional use of vision in relation to the definitions and the demographics of the population involved, the roles of professionals on a low vision team, and the services available for children and adults with low vision.

DEFINITIONS

A Definition of Low Vision

In the opening vignette, the mother of an ice skater wanted to see her daughter perform in the rink. Other people with normal vision who were watching the performance could see the skater with or without their standard eyeglasses (or binoculars). However, this woman with low vision needed to enhance her functional vision to see her daughter well enough to derive pleasure and gain information from the visual experience. Therefore, to gain access to the action in the rink, she used a television set that allowed her to move as close as necessary to view the image.

People with low vision may frequently need to make such adjustments in their viewing of objects. For them, a discrepancy exists between what they want to do with vision and what others with standard corrective lenses are able to do. However, persons with low vision can use devices, techniques, or modifications of the environment to increase the visual information they receive and to complete tasks more efficiently. They may also become expert at reading environmental cues that become more significant for them than for those with normal vision.

This book uses the following definition of a

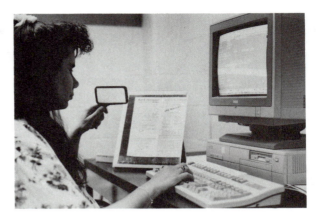

With the use of adaptive devices and techniques and environmental modifications, individuals with low vision can undertake tasks that are otherwise difficult, pursue activities and interests, and achieve educational and employment goals.

person with low vision: *a person who has difficulty accomplishing visual tasks, even with prescribed corrective lenses, but who can enhance his or her ability to accomplish these tasks with the use of compensatory visual strategies, low vision and other devices, and environmental modifications.* This definition, which encompasses a complex set of variables, provides a foundation for the remainder of the book.

Confusion over Terminology

Although many professionals and people with visual impairments use the term *low vision*, various definitions of the term exist. To date, there is no commonly accepted or legal definition of low vision. Services for those who have low vision emerged from services for those who are blind, and it is the term *blind* from which definitions of low vision have evolved.

Until the 20th century, people without sight were generally called "blind"; it was rare that one would come across information or references pertaining to persons with poor vision. In the 20th century, several countries, as well as the World Health Organization (WHO), began to use the term *legal blindness*, rather than *blindness*, and their various definitions tended to encompass different levels of visual impairment—even though most people think of a blind person as one who is completely without sight. Herein lies a dilemma: Can a person be blind and see?

How a society defines the physical characteristics of a group of people has the power to influence the sense of self and societal, legal, and personal identity of members of the group. In this regard, one may say that people are "blinded by definition." That is, persons with low vision who have been told over and over again that they are blind, even "legally blind," without an explanation of the term, may come to believe that their vision is so impaired that it is "as if" they are blind or severely visually impaired. However, these persons may include those who can read regular print (with or without optical devices), play ball, and drive motor vehicles, as well as those who can use vision only for such tasks as becoming oriented to an open door, finding a child who is wearing a red shirt, or using their visual perception of large objects to avoid bumps. Professionals in the field of visual impairment know that the terms *blind* and *legally blind* leave much room for interpreting the amount of vision a person has and how the person functions with that vision. Nevertheless, people who are told that they are legally blind may incorporate that term into their self-image and beliefs about the extent to which vision is available or unavailable, usable or unusable (see Chapter 2 for a further discussion of the general perceptions of low vision and their impact and the psychological implications of low vision).

The following two examples illustrate this point. One describes a person for whom the term *blindness* defines an emotional identity; the other describes someone whose feelings of identity are relatively unaffected by the application of the term. These examples present two perspectives on how individuals may perceive their visual impairments, even when the clinical measures of their vision are similar. (The reader is cautioned against concluding that developing one's identity either as a person with low vision or as a person who is blind has a higher value.)

For several years, Mr. Brown told people that his wife was blind and made several references to his wife's "blindness." When an eye care professional who knew Mr. Brown finally met Mrs. Brown, he observed that she had a significant amount of usable vision for locating a chair, establishing eye contact, and signing her name in a guest book. Mrs. Brown referred to herself as blind and believed that her vision was so impaired that she could do little with it. Mrs. Brown's blindness was significant in her life, and she discussed her condition and its implications during the first 15 minutes of meeting any person.

Tom believed that he had vision problems but was certainly not blind. He felt no shame about the term *legal blindness,* and being able to do many tasks visually had convinced him that it was just a term that allowed him to obtain financial assistance for hiring readers while he attended college. He also thought that the term was confusing because his acquaintances knew he obviously could see. When a representative of the state's commission for the blind visited Tom's college campus, he told several professors that Tom was blind. When Tom's professors contacted him with great concern and asked if he was losing his vision, Tom decided that he should meet with the commission's representative. At that meeting, the representative told Tom, "You're a blind student, and the sooner you stop denying your blindness, the better off you will be." Twenty-five years later, Tom still believes he has vision problems but that he is not blind.

Legal Blindness

Many persons with low vision do not know the origin of the term *legal blindness.* When they are told they are legally blind, they are given no explanation of why they are classified that way or what relationship the term has to their functional vision—that is, to their visual skills and abilities and the way in which they use them. In 1934, during the Great Depression, the U.S. government asked the American Medical Association

(AMA) to formulate a definition of blindness that could be used to determine which people were in need of special care because of their visual impairments (Koestler, 1976). The AMA arrived at the following definition, whose wording was later incorporated into the Social Security Act of 1935:

> central visual acuity of 20/200 or less in the better eye with corrective glasses or central visual acuity of more than 20/200 if there is a visual field defect in which the peripheral field is contracted to such an extent that the widest diameter of the visual field subtends an angular distance no greater than 20 degrees in the better eye. (Koestler, 1976, p. 45)

According to this definition, individuals can be considered legally blind for two reasons: limitations in their visual acuity or in their visual field. The majority are those whose *visual acuity is 20/200 or less*; that is, they must be 20 feet (the first number) or closer to an object, using their best conventional correction (eyeglasses or contact lenses), to be able to recognize details, such as a face, that people with standard visual acuity (20/20) can recognize at 200 feet (the second number). (The acuity measure is not a fraction, nor does it constitute a percentage of normal vision.) Others are considered legally blind because the *extent of their visual field is 20 degrees or less,* regardless of their visual acuity; that is, they can detect objects only within a field of 20 degrees or less (A. Colenbrander, personal communication, August 1995). (The normal field of vision for both eyes extends 90 degrees to either side of center, making a total visual field of approximately 180 degrees.) Chapters 6 and 8 give additional information on these topics.

However, the definition does not take into account other aspects of vision, such as tolerance of light or contrast sensitivity, which may have a significant impact on the individual's ability to use vision. It also does not relate to visual functioning, although it implies that there is a general degree of limitation—a person with 20/200 acuity would not be able to read the line on an eye chart representing 20/70 or 20/30 acuity. That is, the

definition does not imply that a person will or will not be able to catch a ball, visually recognize a friend in a store, or use vision when clearing dishes off a table. In short, a wide range of visual abilities will be exhibited by persons classified as legally blind, and the clinical measures used to define that term make no allowance for that reality.

For example, on a standard Snellen eye chart used to measure visual acuity, there are no measures between 20/100 and 20/200. One line with two letters on it represents the 20/100 measure. If a person is unable to read that line, the next option is to read the 20/200 line. Although special charts have been designed to measure the visual acuity of people with low vision (see Chapter 8), most general eye care specialists do not include such charts in their examination procedures or ask an individual to walk toward the chart to vary the size of the image. As a result, people with visual acuities of 20/125, 20/150, or other measures between 20/100 and 20/200 are said to have 20/200 visual acuity and thereby are categorized as legally blind. This label may not present difficulties for a person who is functionally unable to do the tasks of a person with better visual acuities and who can benefit from services and equipment available to those who are legally blind. However, it can pose a problem for persons who live in states where 20/125 vision may be required to take a driver's test or for children who may be psychologically affected by being considered blind by teachers and relatives. Because the results of tests using a standard eye chart are generally accepted, these people are indeed legally "blinded" by definition.

Since definitions of blindness vary from country to country, a person may be considered legally blind in one nation but be categorized as "legally sighted" after crossing the border into the next. The authors' primary objection to the definition of legal blindness used in the United States is that it is an arbitrary clinical standard that was developed over 60 years ago, when there was little information about how people use vision for performing various tasks. Thus, the authors contend that functional definitions of visual impairment—the extent to which one can use vision to complete activities—rather than clinical definitions should be used to determine who is eligible for services.

Partial Sight

The term *partially sighted* came into vogue in the mid-20th century. In academic circles, it was applied to persons with a best-corrected visual acuity in the better eye of 20/70 to 20/200. However, it was generally used to refer to any person who could use vision, and often the cutoff for legal blindness was not considered a criterion for judging who was considered partially sighted. Many professionals and consumers would further delineate partially sighted people as "high partials" and "low partials" to indicate whether they were functioning with a substantial or a minimal amount of usable vision, without relying wholly on the tactile and auditory senses. The term *partially sighted* is still in professional use today, for example, in such names as the Center for the Partially Sighted, but the term *low vision* is more common.

Functional Blindness

The term *functionally blind* is sometimes used, mostly by educational agencies, to indicate children with or without usable vision who could benefit from instruction in braille reading and writing. One could infer that children who are not included in this category are functionally sighted and would use print as a primary reading and writing medium. Therefore, such a definition provides a direct link between the characteristics of students and appropriate educational interventions, whereas legal definitions do not.

Low Vision

Various definitions and descriptions of low vision or persons with low vision have been included in the literature. The following examples are offered, but the reader should keep in mind that there is not one universally accepted definition of low vision, and no legal definition has been established

in the United States or, to the authors' knowledge, in any other country. Moreover, many of these attempts to define low vision are based on clinical measures, which, similar to the definition of legal blindness, do not give a full picture of how much vision an individual has or how he or she functions visually.

> A vision loss that is severe enough to interfere with the ability to perform everyday tasks or activities and that cannot be corrected to normal by conventional eyeglasses or contact lenses. (Jose, 1992, p. 209)

> Having a significant visual impairment but also having some usable vision; moderate low vision is acuity of 20/70 to 20/160 in the better eye with the best possible correction; severe vision loss is 20/200 to 20/400 or a visual field of 20 degrees or less. (Levack, 1991, p. 237)

> Bilateral subnormal visual acuity or abnormal visual field resulting from a disorder in the visual system. The defect may be in the globe (cornea, iris, lens, vitreous, or retina), the optic pathways, or the visual cortex. It may be hereditary, congenital, or acquired. Inborn or acquired disease may affect visual acuity or visual field and a variety of other ocular functions: color perception, contrast sensitivity, dark adaptation, ocular motility and fusion, and visual perception or awareness. . . . By definition, the visual acuity cannot be corrected to normal performance levels with conventional spectacle, intraocular, or contact lens refraction. In patients with normal acuity, visual fields must be sufficiently impaired to prevent normal performance. (Faye, 1984, p. 6)

> One who is still severely visually impaired after correction, but who may increase visual functioning through the use of optical aids, nonoptical aids, environmental modifications and/or techniques. (Corn, 1980, p. 3)

> One who has an impairment of visual function, even after treatment and/or standard refractive correction, and has a visual acuity of less than

6/18 [the metric equivalent of 10/60] to light perception or a visual field of less than 10 degrees from the point of fixation, but who uses, or is potentially able to use, vision for the planning and/or execution of a task. (WHO, 1992)

The common thread among all these definitions is the implied discrepancy between what a person with typical vision is able to perform or accomplish and what a person with low vision wishes to perform or accomplish. Although some definitions include clinical measures of acuity or visual field, they seem arbitrary, given that there is no assurance that a person with a specific clinical measure will or will not be able to complete specific tasks that do not require the recognition of letters or symbols at specified distances. The definition of low vision that the authors proposed at the beginning of this chapter is based only on the use of functional vision. This definition is a reflection of the beliefs that persons with low vision function in ways that cannot be predicted by clinical measures and that a change in functional vision can occur without a change in clinical measures.

Visual Function and Efficiency

A functional vision assessment of the individual is the basis of many educational and rehabilitation programs; however, whether the performance of such an assessment is or is not required by a program, it is considered to be "best practice." One may say that *functional vision* is vision that can be used to derive input for planning and performing a task. Visual functions, on the other hand, refer to such visual behaviors as shifting one's gaze or scanning an environment (see Sidebar 1.1).

The extent to which one uses available vision is often referred to as *visual efficiency*. Two individuals may have the same clinical measures, such as a visual acuity of 20/100 and a visual field of 30 degrees, but use their vision differently. One person may make quick visual decisions, use vision for most tasks, and feel comfortable moving from one environment to another. The other may

prefer tactile and auditory approaches to completing tasks and use vision only for facilitating conversations and for locating landmarks and cues during travel. Although neither person may have made a choice regarding his or her visual efficiency, providing children and adults with the opportunity to become visually efficient is at the heart of that for which professionals in low vision services strive. Far more than just clinical measures are important as one learns to use low vision. The development of visual skills, cognitive abilities, experiences, personality, self-esteem, and expectations of self and others are just a few of the factors to consider. The person for whom the use of vision is not preferred, not desirable, or too stressful must be respected for this choice.

Use of Terms

Terms are used for both legal and functional purposes. Although some may argue that those who are blind and those with low vision are both visually impaired, others consider these terms to refer to different populations.

A few examples highlight this state of affairs. The title of one professional journal is the *Journal of Visual Impairment & Blindness*, one professional organization is named the Association for Education and Rehabilitation of the Blind and Visually Impaired (AER), and one school is called the Texas School for the Blind and Visually Impaired. By specifically referring to both concepts—blindness and visual impairment— these names differentiate those with visual impairments from those who are blind.

Other organizations and schools that address the needs of people with and without usable vision may use one term or the other, for example, the American Council of the Blind, the Lions Blind Center of Oakland, the Rockland County Association for the Visually Impaired, and the Visually Impaired Training and Learning Center of Nashville. Many persons with low vision who believe they are not really blind may feel uncomfortable going to an agency for the "blind." The terms used in an organization's name may reflect a variety of considerations. Some organizations

Differences in Terminology among Disciplines

Educators, rehabilitation professionals, and medical professionals have come to use terms, such as *visual function, functional vision,* and *visual efficiency,* in different ways. To educators or rehabilitation professionals, visual functioning and functional vision typically refer to an individual's ability to perform a task; often these terms are used interchangeably. Furthermore, these professionals use *visual functions* to refer to specific visual behaviors, such as fixating on an object and tracking it. To medical professionals, however, visual functions refer to organic features of the eye and visual systems that can be measured clinically, such as visual acuity, field of vision, and contrast sensitivity—measures that educators and rehabilitation professionals frequently refer to as visual *abilities.* Likewise, to medical professionals, the term visual efficiency indicates the absence of limitations on visual functions, whereas to educators and rehabilitation personnel, it relates to how well a person with low vision uses his or her functional vision. In this book, these terms will be used as they generally are in education and rehabilitation settings.

may decide not to have their names reflect both populations they serve because of concerns related to public relations and funding or because they believe that the general public thinks that the term *blind* refers to both people who are blind and people with low vision. Still others may retain the term *blind* in their names for a variety of reasons, such as a belief that it is interchangeable with visual impairment or a wish to maintain their tradition or history.

Although the term *handicapped* has gone out of vogue in many countries, it is still used, for example, in the name of the Nebraska School for the Visually Handicapped. A *handicap* originally referred to a real or perceived disadvantage resulting from a disability. A *disability* meant a condition that prevents an individual from performing a specific task because of an impairment. An *impairment* meant that an organ of the body does not work properly as the result of a disorder. And a *disorder* was thought of as a structural difference that does not necessarily cause an impairment of function, a disability, or a handicap.

As a result, one may hear of persons with *visual disabilities*, a term that encompasses both those who are blind and those with low vision. The term *visual impairments* is also often inter-

changed with visual disabilities, and although an impairment does not necessarily lead to a disability, the field of "blindness and visual impairment" often uses visual impairments interchangeably with visual disabilities.

Examples of the use of the term *disabilities* in the United States include its appearance in the name of the Americans with Disabilities Act of 1990, which was passed in the same year as a new authorization of the Education for All Handicapped Children Act, which became the Individuals with Disabilities Education Act. Since that time, disability has been used in lieu of handicap for many educational purposes.

Other descriptions of persons with low vision have been based on the limitations that low vision is thought to impose. For example, *industrial blindness* has been used when it is believed that a person can no longer earn a living as a result of a visual impairment and *automobile blindness* has been used to signify when a state's motor vehicle bureau determines that it will not issue a driver's license because of a person's visual impairment (Vaughan, Asbury, & Riordan-Eva, 1992). And although, as noted, professionals in the field of low vision do not consider visual acuity measurements to constitute a fractional portion of vision, the AMA provides percentages of "visual loss" based on acuity measures (Vaughan et al., 1992, Appendix I). For example, 20/100 or 6/30 (its metric equivalent) is considered to be a 50 percent vision loss and 20/400 (6/120) is considered to be a 90 percent vision loss. As this text emphasizes, visual acuity is but one of the factors that determines what individuals with low vision are able or choose to do with their vision.

THEORIES AND CLASSIFICATION OF VISUAL FUNCTIONING

Various theories attempt to explain how children and adults with low vision develop or use their available vision. For example, some professionals in the low vision field believe that the sequence of normal visual development in children without visual impairments is a basis for establishing assessment and instructional programs for children with low vision. According to this approach, then, children who have low vision develop visual skills in relatively the same order as do children with normal vision, although perhaps at a different pace. An example of this approach is reflected in the Diagnostic Assessment Procedure, which is part of the Program to Develop Efficiency in Visual Functioning (Barraga & Morris, 1980). This theory does not apply to adults who lose vision, but it explains the milestones in the optical and visual development of children.

Another theory does not discount the typical sequence but proposes that children with low vision bring other internal components to the visual experience that, along with environmental cues, allow for visual function when they are integrated with the child's visual abilities. This theory, by Corn (1983), includes the components of three dimensions—visual abilities, environmental cues, and stored and available individuality—that need to be present for visual function to take place (see Figure 1.1A). The visual abilities dimension includes visual acuity, visual fields, motility, brain functions, and light and color perception (see Figure 1.1B). The environmental cues dimension includes color, contrast, space,

illumination, and time (see Figure 1.1C). And the stored and available individuality dimension includes cognition, sensory development-integration, perception, psychological makeup, and physical makeup (see Figure 1.1D).

According to this model, all the components must be present to some degree for visual function to occur. During development, a child's visual abilities "develop" while other compensations for or hindrances to visual function have an interactive effect. For example, a child with limited visual acuity may need to have the size of an object increased and also need specific physical capabilities to handle an optical device for visual function to emerge or be enhanced. An individual may increase (or decrease) one or more environmental cues or effect change in the stored and available individuality dimension to increase visual function. And adults who have lost vision may adjust their environment and personal variables to function visually. The model is pliable, but there are limitations to its expansion, reflecting the fact that the person with low vision can establish thresholds below or beyond which visual function increases or ceases to be effective.

Hall and Bailey (1989) proposed a third model for increasing visual functioning by differentiating between vision stimulation programs and vision training programs. Vision stimulation programs offer a rich, stimulating environment, and the stimuli provide inherent reinforcement to encourage and facilitate the efficient use of vision. Through direct and planned reinforcement procedures, vision training programs systematically teach a set of specific visual skills that are otherwise learned incidentally. As Figure 1.2A indicates, the specific skills include visual attending behaviors, visual examining behaviors, and visually guided motor behaviors. Undergirding these three sets of behaviors are certain visual capabilities, such as visual discrimination, fixation, and convergence. Hall and Bailey presented three alternatives for teaching specific visual behaviors that are depicted in Figure 1.2B: (1) arranging the environment to foster the use of desired visual behaviors, (2) targeting for system-

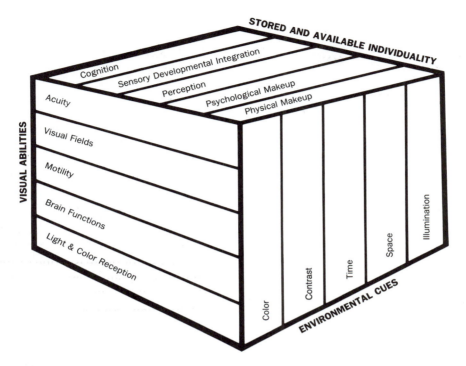

Figure 1.1A. Model of Visual Functioning

Source: Reprinted, by permission of the publisher, from A. L. Corn, "Instruction in the Use of Vision for Children and Adults with Low Vision," 1989, *RE:view, 21,* 26–38. Copyright 1989 by Heldref Publications.

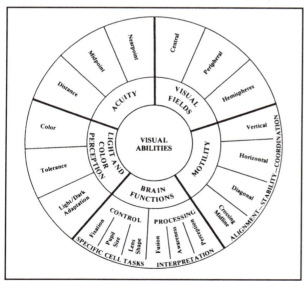

Figure 1.1B. Components of the Visual Abilities Dimension

Source: Reprinted, by permission of the publisher, from A. L. Corn, "Instruction in the Use of Vision for Children and Adults with Low Vision," 1989, *RE:view, 21,* 26–38. Copyright 1989 by Heldref Publications.

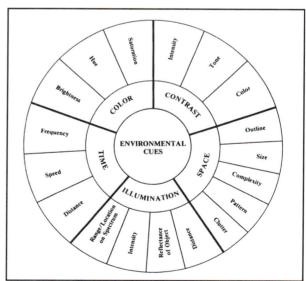

Figure 1.1C. Components of the Environmental Cues Dimension

Source: Reprinted, by permission of the publisher, from A. L. Corn, "Instruction in the Use of Vision for Children and Adults with Low Vision," 1989, *RE:view, 21,* 26–38. Copyright 1989 by Heldref Publications.

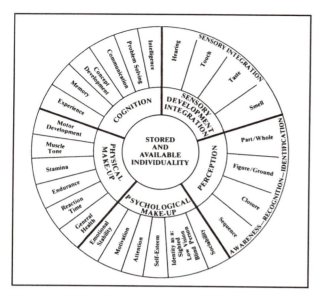

Figure 1.1D. Components of the Stored and Available Individuality Dimension

Source: Reprinted, by permission of the publisher, from A. L. Corn, "Instruction in the Use of Vision for Children and Adults with Low Vision," 1989, *RE:view, 21,* 26–38. Copyright 1989 by Heldref Publications.

atic instruction specific visual attending behaviors that have not developed appropriately, and (3) fostering the use of visual behaviors in specific tasks that are facilitated through the efficient use of vision.

These theories address different aspects of visual development and visual functioning. Together, they lay a foundation from which a professional can understand the visual functioning of an individual with low vision. By no means, however, do any of these theories explain all the processes by which children or adults with low vision experience the visual world. The expectations of others, the need to practice visual skills, and society's concepts of low vision may also have an impact on how and to what extent persons with low vision choose to use their available vision or determine that other methods of functioning are preferable or more efficient.

In addition to theories that attempt to explain functional vision, other methods of classification have been devised. Colenbrander (personal communication, August, 1995) identified ranges of

clinical measures from which one can begin to predict the extent to which persons with low vision will function with vision, with vision and optical devices, or with nonvisual approaches for such tasks as reading and orientation and mobility (O&M) (see Table 1.1). This classification method was based on the *International Classification of Diseases, 9th Revision* (1977) that was recommended by WHO.

DEMOGRAPHICS

Elderly people constitute the largest segment of the population of persons with visual impairments. According to one estimate, 70 percent of the visually impaired population in the United States is over age 60 (Jose, 1992, p. 209). By another measure, 2,907,490 individuals age 65 or over have severe visual impairments (Nelson & Dimitrova, 1993). The proportion of elderly people who are visually impaired ranges from nearly 6 percent of the population age 65 to 74 to over 21 percent of those 85 and older (see Table 1.2). By contrast, only a small proportion of children are visually impaired. The American Printing House for the Blind (APH) maintains an annual registry of school-age children in the United States who are identified as legally blind for the purpose of receiving educational materials from APH. Its 1995 Annual Report listed 54,783 students (American Printing House for the Blind, 1995). Since it has been estimated that about 10 percent of those who are blind have no vision (Kahn & Moorhead, 1973), it can be estimated that some 47,500 of the students in the APH registry have low vision. The actual number of children with low vision in the United States is greater because those who have low vision but who are not legally blind are not included in the APH registry, nor are infants. High-quality educational services for students are vital because their effects will last a lifetime; however, given that the largest percentage of the population with visual impairments is elderly, this group represents the greatest need for specialized services.

Chiang, Bassi, and Javitt (1992) estimated that

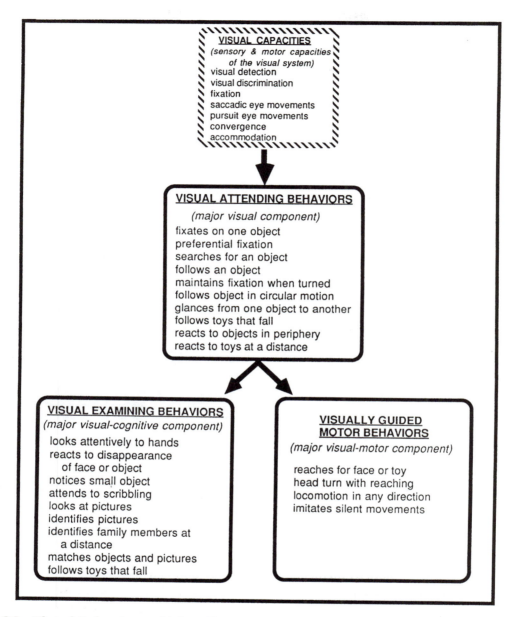

Figure 1.2A. Visual Behaviors of Visually Impaired Children from Birth to Age 2

Source: From A. Hall and I. L. Bailey, "A Model for Training Vision Functioning," 1989, *Journal of Visual Impairment & Blindness, 83,* pp. 390–396. Copyright 1989 by the American Foundation for the Blind.

in 1990, 1.1 million Americans of all age groups were legally blind (both functionally or totally blind and with low vision). If one again uses the estimate that 90 percent of these individuals have usable vision, it would appear that approximately 990,000 Americans who are legally blind have low vision.

Although legal blindness is determined by clinical measures of distance visual acuity and visual field, perceived functional impairment may also be used to estimate the number of persons who have visual impairments. Nelson and Dimitrova (1993) reported on a 1990 survey in the United States in which severe visual impairment

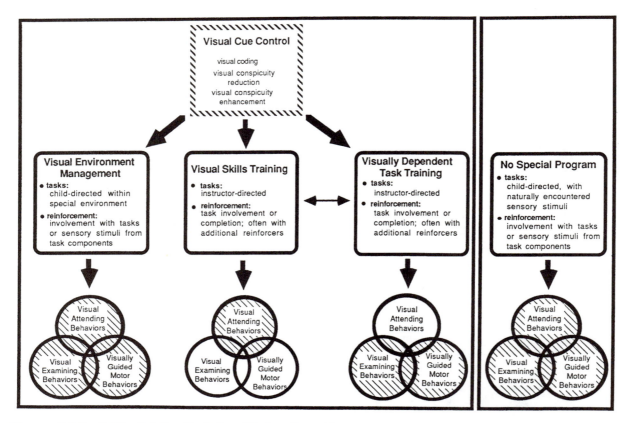

Figure 1.2B. A Model for Training Vision Function

Source: From A. Hall and I. L. Bailey, "A Model for Training Vision Functioning," 1989, *Journal of Visual Impairment & Blindness, 83,* pp. 390–396. Copyright 1989 by the American Foundation for the Blind.

was defined as "the self or proxy-reported inability to see to read ordinary newsprint even when wearing glasses or contact lenses; for children under age six, it is the caregiver's (usually the mother's) report that the child lacks useful vision" (p. 80). (The authors believe that the definition for young children is too restrictive because many children who will not be able to read newsprint in the future have useful vision, and thus the number in this age group may be an underestimate.) Table 1.2 presents the age-specific rates for persons with severe visual impairments reported by Nelson and Dimitrova. Because people who are totally blind are included in these rates, people with low vision will constitute a somewhat lower number than the figures that are given.

According to Barron (1991), 12 million persons in the United States have visual acuities (with conventional eyeglasses or contact lenses) of 20/50 to 20/200. The National Institute on Disability and Rehabilitation Research (NIDRR) (1993, p. 2) stated that "estimates of the numbers of people with visual impairments in the United States range from 6 to 11.4 million. . . . Vision loss has been ranked third behind arthritis and heart disease, among the most chronic common conditions causing a need for assistance in activities of daily living for people who are elderly." NIDRR also stated that 60 percent of those with visual impairments also have additional disabilities.

Demographic data reveal some differences in the presence of visual impairments by gender, racial group, and geographic area. According to data from the U.S. Bureau of the Census (McNeil,

Table 1.1. Colenbrander's Classification of Functional Vision, Based on ICD-9-CM

Functional Ranges	Measured Range of Impairment of Visual Acuity	Estimated Reading Ability[a]	Measured Range of Impairment of Visual Field	Estimated Orientation Ability[a]
Range of normal	20/12–20/25	Normal reading performance	180°–greater than 120°	Normal visual orientation
Near normal	20/30–20/60	Loss of reserves[b]	120°–greater than 60°	Loss of reserves[c] Some scanning
Moderate low vision	20/80–20/100	Near normal with aids	60°–greater than 20°	Near normal with increased scanning
Severe low vision	20/200–20/400	Slow with aids	20°–greater than 10°	Slow, requires constant scanning
Profound low vision	20/500–20/1000	Marginal with aids	10°–greater than 5°	Marginal, requires long travel cane
Near-total vision loss	20/2000 (no light perception)	Inability to read[c]	5° or less	Visual orientation unreliable

Sources: From A. Colenbrander, personal communication, August 1995; and A. Colenbrander, "The Functional Vision Score: A Coordinated Scoring System for Visual Impairments, Disabilities and Handicaps," in A. C. Kooijmans, P. L. Looijestijn, J. A. Welling, and G. J. van der Wildt, eds., *Low Vision Research and New Developments in Rehabilitation.* (Amsterdam: IOS Press, 1994). Copyright © 1994 by IOS Press. Adapted with permission. The classification of visual acuity is based on *International Classification of Diseases, 9th Revision, Clinical Modification (ICD-9-CM)* (Ann Arbor, MI: Commission on Professional and Hospital Activities, 1978).

[a]Influenced by such factors as age at onset of impairment, extent of training, and other individual characteristics.

[b]Refers to excess visual capacity that is available to individuals with unimpaired vision but is typically unused in normal situations.

[c]Refers to visual reading.

1993), in 1991–92, 9,685,000 individuals (5 percent of the general population) were reported to have difficulty seeing words and letters. Of that number, 1,590,000 (0.8 percent) were unable to see words and letters. Overall, women were somewhat more likely to have difficulty seeing words and letters (5.6 percent) than were men (4.3 percent), but the difference was more pronounced in people aged 65 years and older, of which 17.2 percent of the women and 14.1 percent of the men had this difficulty. African Americans were more likely to have this difficulty with vision (7.6 percent) than were Caucasian Americans (4.7 percent). The prevalence among people of Hispanic origin was 5.0 percent.

With regard to people aged 40 years and older in 1990, Prevent Blindness America (1994) found a higher percentage of African Americans who were either blind or visually impaired (defined as having a best-corrected visual acuity of less than 20/40) than of all other groups (Caucasians and others). The incidence of specific conditions among those aged 40 or older was also higher among certain groups. For example, both Mexican Americans and African Americans develop diabetes more frequently than do Caucasian Americans and therefore have a higher rate of diabetic retinopathy; some data suggest that the rate of diabetic retinopathy among those who have diabetes is higher for African Americans and Hispanic Americans. African Americans also have a higher rate of glaucoma than do other groups. However, for unknown reasons, blindness resulting from macular degeneration is extremely rare among African Americans.

There were also geographic differences in the prevalence of blindness and visual impairments in the 40-and-older age group (Prevent Blindness

Table 1.2. Estimated Age-Specific Rates for Persons with Severe Visual Impairments: 1990 (*N* = 4,293,360)

Age	Prevalence[a]	Number
0–17	1.5	95,410
18–44	3.2	349,350
45–54	13.5	340,510
55–64	28.4	600,600
65–74	59.0	1,068,290
75–84	118.4	1,190,520
85 and over	210.6	648,680
Average rate per 1,000		17.3

Source: From K. A. Nelson and E. Dimitrova, "Severe Visual Impairment in the United States and in Each State, 1990," *Journal of Visual Impairment & Blindness* 87 (1993), p. 82. Copyright 1993 by the American Foundation for the Blind.
[a]U.S. rate per 1,000 persons.

America, 1994). For example, Alaska had the lowest rate in 1990 and Washington, DC, had the highest. There appear to be some regional differences as well; for example, in addition to Alaska and Hawaii, the states with the lowest rates are in the West—Nevada, Colorado, New Mexico, Wyoming, and Utah. However, the state averages may mask differences within states or areas, as the high rate found in Washington, DC, compared to the surrounding states demonstrates.

Increases are expected in the number of children and adults with visual impairments. As Crews (1991, p. 52) noted, "Assuming no miracle cure, the number of severely visually impaired older persons will increase from 2 million in 1980, to about 3.2 million in 2000, to 4.6 million in 2020. . . . Elderly people with severe visual impairments make up nearly 80 percent of the population of visually impaired people," a figure that is somewhat higher than Jose's (1992) estimate.

Also, as more infants survive birth at lower gestation rates, more children will experience low vision and multiple disabilities and will need services. According to AFB (personal communica-

tion, Corinne Kirchner, Department of Programs and Policy Research, October 15, 1994), an increase of 6,900 children with legal blindness and severe visual impairments is expected between 1994 and 2000, and a significant number of these children are likely to have multiple disabilities.

Acquired immune deficiency syndrome (AIDS) is another health condition that is associated with visual impairment. Kiester (1990, p. 2) stated that "between 35 and 75 percent of AIDS patients develop visual problems ranging up to total blindness," and the number of individuals with AIDS is increasing.

As the demographic data indicate, professionals will increasingly have to address the needs of persons with low vision. In particular, certain segments of the population will require special attention, including specific age groups, racial populations, and populations with unique additional disabilities, such as those with AIDS.

TEAM FUNCTIONS

A Team Approach

The ultimate goal of most people is to enjoy a high quality of life through mutually satisfying interpersonal relationships and meaningful contributions in a manner that allows them to value themselves and to be valued by others—family members, friends and neighbors, and society as a whole. Generally, early life experiences in the home, school, and community prepare a person to become competent and independent and to develop high self-esteem (Tuttle, 1984). Such a life goal need not be impeded by the presence of a visual impairment. Through ongoing and interactive efforts of a low vision team that are appropriate to the individual's needs, a person with low vision can attain the same life goals that are achieved by others. Although some people will require intensive team efforts and others will need minimal team involvement, it is the coordinated use of a team that is key. No one person has the specialized expertise necessary to address all the needs of the individual experiencing low vision.

SIDEBAR 1.2

Composition of the Low Vision Team

- Individual with low vision and family members (if appropriate)

EYE CARE PROVIDERS
- Optometrists
- Ophthalmologists
- Clinical low vision specialists

EDUCATION/REHABILITATION SPECIALISTS
- Teacher of students with visual impairments

- Rehabilitation teacher
- Rehabilitation counselor
- Orientation and mobility specialist

HUMAN SERVICE/ALLIED HEALTH PERSONNEL
- Speech and language specialist
- Occupational therapist
- Physical therapist
- Transition coordinator

Meeting the specific needs of individuals with low vision requires a team approach that blends the knowledge and skills of a variety of professionals with the needs, desires, and experiences of the individual. Clinical specialists need to interact directly with teachers and rehabilitation professionals and the individual with low vision to translate the outcome of the clinical assessment into meaningful daily functioning. The success of low vision rehabilitation services, including both habilitation and rehabilitation, requires ongoing collaboration among the individual and, when appropriate, family members, clinical low vision specialists and eye care providers, and human service and allied health professionals (see Sidebar 1.2). In this context, *habilitation* is defined as the education and development of children and youths with congenital or early-onset visual disabilities, including the teaching of compensatory and visual efficiency skills as well as daily living skills; *rehabilitation* is defined as the relearning of skills already acquired before the onset of a visual disability, including the relearning of vocational and daily living skills using adaptive equipment and techniques. (The term *vision rehabilitation services* often refers to the full range of clinical and instructional services related to prescribing and learning to use optical and nonoptical devices

while using vision.) Without input from members of any of these groups, addressing the needs of individuals with low vision may result in goals that are fragmented or isolated from real-life functioning (see Sidebar 1.3).

General Responsibilities of Team Members

Individual and Family

As the pivotal member of the team, the individual with low vision communicates personal goals, needs, and desires; interacts with eye care specialists and other professionals to gain needed information and skills; and selects the particular treatment options that will meet his or her needs. For infants and young children, such a process is guided largely by parents and teachers, but when these children reach adolescence and young adulthood, they will assume responsibility for their own decisions. Thus, provided that he or she receives appropriate education and early life experiences, the person with low vision will, in general, move from being a recipient of information to a seeker and synthesizer of information to gain control over his or her visual environment.

Modes of Professional Intervention: The Importance of Teamwork

Low vision rehabilitation requires teamwork from different professionals. The various aspects of vision loss are best expressed in the terms *impairment, disability,* and *handicap* (Colenbrander, 1977), as defined in the World Health Organization's *International Classification of Impairments, Disabilities and Handicaps* (1980). These concepts, which apply to any kind of functional loss (hearing, musculoskeletal, and so on), are best summarized in the accompanying diagram.

The top half of the diagram lists the different aspects of vision loss. The terms *disorder* and *impairment* describe the condition of the organ; disorder refers to anatomical changes (such as cataract or retinal scar), and impairment refers to the functional consequences (such as visual acuity loss or visual field loss). The terms *disability* and *handicap* describe the condition of the person; one can have an impairment of one eye, but not of the other, but one cannot be disabled in one eye. "Dis-ability" refers to a loss or lack of skills and abilities, whereas handicap refers to the ensuing social and economic consequences. These various aspects are

linked, but the links are not rigid. The art of rehabilitation is to influence these links, so that a given disorder results in the least possible handicap. Various professionals need to be involved in this endeavor.

The bottom half of the diagram refers to various interventions. Ophthalmologists provide medical and surgical care to minimize the impairment caused by a certain disorder, but, by and large, they have not been trained to effectively handle the effects of the impairment on the individual's quality of life, mentioned on the right side of the figure. For optometrists and low vision specialists, the medical disorder is a given. They can reduce the disabling effect of the impairment with various optical and nonoptical devices, but most are not prepared to address fully the circumstances and challenges the individual encounters in various social settings, such as the school, the home, and the workplace.

AUGUST COLENBRANDER, M.D.
California Pacific Medical Center,
San Francisco

Aspects of Vision Loss

Visual Disorder	Visual Impairment	Visual Disability	Visual Handicap
←——— the organ ———→		←——— the person ———→	
anatomical changes	functional changes	skills and abilities	social and economic consequences
QUALITY OF THE EYE ↑↑ Medical/surgical intervention	↑↑ Visual aids, adapted equipment		QUALITY OF LIFE ↑↑ Social interventions, training, counseling, education

Modes of Intervention

Eye Care Providers

Eye care providers include ophthalmologists, optometrists, and clinical low vision specialists. An ophthalmologist is a

> physician (doctor of medicine or doctor of osteopathy) who specializes in the medical and surgical care of the eyes and visual system and in the prevention of eye disease and injury . . . [and] can deliver total eye care: primary, secondary, tertiary care services (i.e., vision services, contact lenses, eye examinations, medical eye care, and surgical eye care), diagnose general diseases of the body and treat ocular manifestations of systemic diseases. (American Academy of Ophthalmology, 1992, p. 2)

An optometrist is a health care provider who is licensed

> to examine the eyes and to determine the presence of vision problems . . . [and to] determine visual acuity and prescribe spectacles, contact lenses and eye exercises. . . . (American Academy of Ophthalmology, 1992, p. 2)

In addition, in some states, optometrists also manage and treat eye conditions and diseases (American Optometric Association, 1989).

Either an ophthalmologist or an optometrist serves as a primary eye care provider. A clinical low vision specialist is an ophthalmologist or optometrist who has additional training and expertise with regard to low vision. The clinical low vision specialist

- assesses the clinical visual functioning of persons with low vision
- matches various treatment options to the individual's stated goals for visual functioning
- prescribes various optical and nonoptical devices as appropriate
- provides follow-up services and examinations to ensure that visual skills are successfully integrated into the individual's life.

More information on the roles of these eye care providers and other members of the team is presented in Chapter 8.

Education, Rehabilitation, and Allied Health Professionals

A variety of human service and allied health professionals serve on the low vision team. For children who are visually impaired, the teacher of students with visual impairments is a key member of the team who has primary responsibility for ensuring that a child's educational needs are met and that the child is learning the skills that are the basis for independent life and work after school. This professional has specialized expertise in teaching disability-specific skills to students with low vision, such as the use of low vision devices, and conducting functional vision assessments (see Chapters 7, 8, and 9) and learning media assessments (see Chapter 11). The teacher of students with visual impairments often is the link in the communication chain between the eye care provider and other members of the team.

Rehabilitation specialists work primarily with transition-aged youths and adults with visual impairments. Individuals who are eligible in their states receive rehabilitation services in vocational training, employment, and independent living. Effective transitions between adolescence and adulthood are facilitated by rehabilitation specialists (known as transition specialists) who work with other members of the team to ensure that the individual is adequately prepared for life beyond school (see Chapters 14 and 15). For older persons with low vision, rehabilitation teachers provide daily living instruction as part of a service team that may also include rehabilitation counselors as case managers and physicians, social workers, audiologists, and allied health personnel (see Chapter 16).

O&M specialists provide direct and consultative services to persons of all ages who have low vision. They teach individuals how to use visual cues in conjunction with the other senses to develop basic spatial and movement-related concepts and how to familiarize themselves with the environment and travel safely within it (see Chapter 13).

Other human service professionals are occupational therapists, physical therapists, speech and language therapists, employment specialists, and school nurses. They contribute their expertise in various areas to the vision habilitation or rehabilitation plans of the person with low vision. Although elements of the work of these professionals may appear to relate to areas other than vision-specific needs (such as range-of-motion activities or language therapy), all members of the team seek to integrate the successful use of vision, exclusively or in combination with the other senses, into all activities. In some instances, the use of senses other than vision will allow a person to complete tasks more effectively. Whatever the case, such decisions are best made by considering an individual's needs and desires and the specific tasks to be performed.

Although the appropriate membership of professional teams may appear obvious, and the assembling of effective teams seem a common-sense matter, the gap that exists between the medical and the educational and rehabilitation systems makes the functioning of teams less smooth in reality than in theory. For example, eye care providers do not routinely make referrals to educational and rehabilitation personnel in non-medical facilities. There is a similar gap between allied health care providers, such as occupational therapists, who "take care of most nonvisual rehabilitation, but traditionally learn little about vision," and "the teachers and counselors who are part of the educational system, who have the experience about low vision and about blindness, but traditionally remain at the outskirts of the health care system" (A. Colenbrander, personal communication, August 1995). Given the critical contribution that effective teamwork ultimately can make to the well-being of the person with low vision, the successful delivery of services, and the sense of a job well done experienced by the professional, this issue is one that merits the full attention of the field of visual impairment.

Team Models

Education

The way in which team members interact to meet the vision-specific needs of individuals with low vision varies according to the philosophy of the specific program and local practices. According to Campbell (1987), there are three traditional team models:

♦ *Multidisciplinary teams* include members from a variety of disciplines, each of whom conducts separate assessments and provides isolated services to address an individual's needs.

♦ *Interdisciplinary teams* also include members from various disciplines who conduct individual assessments, but the members share the results of their assessments and jointly plan comprehensive instructional programs.

♦ *Transdisciplinary teams* designate a "primary programmer" who implements the intervention programs in collaboration with various specialists who have designed them on the basis of specialized assessments.

Campbell (1987, p. 108) suggested that the *integrated programming team* is a way of addressing gaps in existing team models: "Parents, educators, and related services personnel team together to determine student goals, provide direct and consultative therapy services, integrate intervention methods, and monitor student progress." Morsink, Thomas, and Correa (1991, p. 5) also found weaknesses in traditional team models and proposed using an *interactive team* in which "there is mutual or reciprocal effort among and between members of the team" to meet the identified goals of individuals.

The philosophy and practices of integrated or interactive teams provide a foundation for an approach that is ideally suited for meeting the needs of persons with low vision. Both clinical professionals and human service professionals are involved in the team, and it is unlikely that any one member will have knowledge in both areas. Therefore, the ongoing collaboration among all members of the low vision team, with a focus on the needs of the individual, is necessary.

The inclusion of the clinical perspective in a team's deliberations and decisions presents a challenge in work with people with low vision. Although primary eye care providers are rarely direct participants in team meetings, their information is fundamental to the development of appropriate educational and rehabilitation plans. Therefore, the teacher or rehabilitation professional in low vision must serve as the link between the eye care provider and other members of the educational team by conveying information from the eye care specialist clearly and articulately to the team and by relaying questions from the team members to the eye care specialist in a timely manner. This communication link is crucial to the overall effectiveness of the team's ability to plan and implement appropriate educational and rehabilitation intervention programs.

Although teams are rarely structured according to the three traditional team models, services for persons with low vision will have the greatest likelihood of success when professionals on a team plan how they wish the team's members to interact. Contacts among various professionals that are informal will result in splintered services and minimal problem-solving strategies. In such cases, persons with low vision who are receiving services may feel that their service providers talk about or to them but not with them and that they do not have the opportunity to work with the team to gain personal empowerment as their needs are being met. It is therefore the important responsibility of schools and rehabilitation agencies to establish working relationships with team members and to provide the structure through which teams become effective.

Rehabilitation

Models formulated for educational teams may also apply to rehabilitation services for adults.

Generally, the rehabilitation counselor at a statewide vocational agency or a social worker at a multiservice private agency will function as a case manager and help to coordinate services for an individual. It is important, however, that the adult with a visual impairment is, to the greatest extent possible, the one to accept assessment information, to select and identify services that will be helpful, and to be responsible for carrying out his or her rehabilitation program. For example, if clients present themselves for services, are told to attend certain classes, and then wait for another person to deem them "rehabilitated," they may not develop a sense of control over their lives or confidence in what they had learned. In contrast, if they are considered to be a guiding member of the rehabilitation team, they can work in concert with professionals who have expertise in promoting the rehabilitation process.

When persons who cannot advocate for themselves have a visual impairment, family members, physicians, or other responsible persons may need to act as advocates for them to ensure that they receive services. At times, it is essential for these advocates to learn about the potential of rehabilitation services to help the person with low vision avoid institutionalization or other changes that would be unnecessary with appropriate rehabilitation.

CURRENT SERVICES

Availability and Use of Services

Educational, rehabilitation, and clinical low vision services have been available to persons with low vision for many years. The following observations can be made about services in these areas:

♦ Teachers of students with visual impairments receive special training to provide educational services to children with low vision.

♦ Governmental and private rehabilitation programs have been established to meet the disability-specific needs of adults with low vision.

- The first low vision clinic was established in 1953, and in 1993, more than 193 low vision centers providing a variety of services (not including private practitioners who provide low vision services) were in existence (AFB, 1993).

- Optical devices and technology are available to solve many of the functional needs of persons with low vision (see Chapters 7 and 8).

- There is an extensive body of literature and research on the specific needs of persons with low vision.

Perhaps the best way to describe the availability and use of services related to low vision is to liken the service delivery system to a patchwork quilt. In some locations in the United States and in various other countries, state-of-the-art services and equipment are available to persons with low vision. Furthermore, professionals from many countries attend international conferences to deliver scientific papers, learn about innovations in services and new equipment, and engage in professional debates. Yet to date, there are no data to indicate the extent to which individuals with low vision are knowledgeable about or able to gain access to services.

In many nonindustrialized countries, low vision services take a backseat to the provision of basic services, such as food and shelter. However, even in countries such as the United States, it is not uncommon to learn of an older adult whose vision has been declining for many years but who first receives O&M services when a spouse, who had been acting as a guide, dies. It is also not unusual to find children with low vision who receive large-type books in school but have never received a clinical low vision evaluation for the use of optical devices to see the chalkboard or to read standard-type textbooks or other printed materials.

Why are low vision services not as readily available in technologically developed countries as might be expected? Several reasons may be postulated:

- Primary eye care providers may not understand the importance of low vision services and do not refer clients to them.

- Individuals with low vision may not be able to afford low vision services because their health insurance plans do not cover them.

- Persons with low vision may choose not to become associated with "blindness" agencies that may offer low vision services.

- There is an insufficient number of professionals and services to meet the needs of persons with low vision.

Standards for Service Providers

In obtaining low vision services, as in obtaining services in other spheres of life, it is advisable for the individual to remember the motto, May the Consumer Beware. Therefore, when individuals with low vision are referred for clinical, educational, or rehabilitation services, they should ask several questions about the professionals who deliver the services. The following sections present information on the training and certification of professionals who provide low vision services that may be helpful in formulating questions.

Clinical Services

Generally, a clinical low vision specialist is an ophthalmologist or optometrist who has had specialized training in providing low vision services. Ophthalmologists go through residencies in low vision services, and optometrists participate in specialized training in low vision, such as diplomate programs, which involve a series of examinations to demonstrate competence in the area of low vision.

A master's degree program in low vision services has been developed by the Pennsylvania College of Optometry. Graduates of this program receive extensive training to work in low vision clinics, but they are not prepared to write prescriptions for conventional or low vision corrections in, or mounted on, eyeglasses or contact lenses. Students who enter this program typically have backgrounds as O&M instructors, rehabilitation teachers, or teachers of students with visual impairments.

Technicians who provide low vision services under the direction of eye care professionals may dispense optical devices, but no professional body certifies them. One may also encounter professionals, such as O&M instructors, with expertise in other areas of low vision services who are hired as low vision specialists but who do not have appropriate training.

When they are referred to a low vision clinic, persons with low vision in all likelihood assume that the individual who is assessing their vision has professional credentials to provide the service. However, since they often cannot read the titles on name tags worn by professionals or the certificates on the walls of offices, it behooves them to ask about the preparation of the people who will perform the assessments.

The National Accreditation Council for Agencies Serving the Blind and Visually Handicapped (NAC) is a private U.S. accrediting body that is recognized by the U.S. Department of Education. NAC sets standards for low vision clinics, as well as for educational and rehabilitation services, and clinics or agencies voluntarily seek accreditation from this body. Persons who are referred for clinical low vision services may want to ask whether the clinics are NAC accredited. Although clinics that are not accredited by NAC do not necessarily provide inadequate services, those that are accredited have met basic standards that committees of professionals have reviewed.

In 1994, the Division on Low Vision of AER approved the establishment of a certificate for low vision therapists, which is in the process of being implemented. "The goal of this program is to bring some uniformity to the field of low vision

in the area of instructional services in [vision] rehabilitation and education" (Jose, 1994, p. 15). The AER certification for low vision therapists is designed for professionals in education, rehabilitation, and health care who provide instruction in visual skills and the use of low vision devices. These professionals must work in an interdisciplinary low vision service in such settings as schools, rehabilitation centers, nursing homes, and day care centers. Consistent with the interdisciplinary nature of low vision services, the low vision therapist works with other professionals, such as eye care specialists and counselors.

Educational Services

In most states, teachers of students with visual impairments are prepared at university undergraduate or graduate programs specifically for the education of students with visual impairments and are sometimes certified to teach children from birth to age 22. Alternative credentialing may include certification by AER, which grants certificates to O&M instructors and to teachers, or through a variety of non-university-based programs approved by certain states.

Parents may inquire about the preparation of the teacher assigned to their child with low vision. In addition to asking about the teacher's certification, they may want to know the extent to which the teacher's training dealt specifically with providing instruction in the use of low vision (see Chapters 9 and 10) and optical devices (see Chapters 7 and 8). They may also wish to know the extent to which the O&M instructor's preparation dealt with O&M for children with low vision.

Rehabilitation Services

Rehabilitation teachers are specialists in the instruction of adults with visual impairments, primarily teaching adaptive communication and daily living skills. Although vocational rehabilitation counselors can specialize in working with persons with visual impairments, there are few such programs at universities, so many agencies prepare their own rehabilitation professionals. Some agencies hire certified rehabilitation professionals and give them training in work with people with visual impairments, whereas others hire individuals, frequently persons who are visually impaired, and then train them as rehabilitation personnel.

AER has adopted guidelines for university-based programs that prepare rehabilitation teachers of persons with visual impairments (Wiener & Luxton, 1994). People with low vision may wish to inquire about the preparation and certification of professionals who provide adults with rehabilitation, O&M, and similar services.

SUMMARY

The imprecise nature of the terms and definitions related to low vision, as well as the lack of agreement among disciplines on a comprehensive definition of low vision, presents a challenge to service providers who are striving to ensure that high-quality appropriate services are available to meet the needs of persons with low vision. Despite the lack of agreement, it is clear that functional definitions allow a direct link to the characteristics of individuals and the provision of services, whereas clinical definitions tend to obscure this link. Given the difficulties of defining the population of persons with low vision, demographic data tend to be muddled. However, with more and more at-risk infants surviving because of medical advances, persons living longer, and medical epidemics, such as AIDS, prevailing, there has been a noticeable increase in the number of persons with low vision.

To meet the needs of people with low vision, cohesive and effective team efforts are generally needed. Given the interactions that are required between clinical personnel and human service providers, a clearly established network of interactions among team members is essential. Also, high-quality services and specially prepared professionals—guided by professionally recognized standards—are needed for coordinated and effective low vision habilitation and rehabilitation plans.

ACTIVITIES

With This Chapter and Other Resources

1. Write a short article that Carol, the journalist in the vignette that opens this chapter, might have written following her interview with people with low vision.

2. You are a new teacher of students with visual impairments who is going to speak with administrators in a school district that has just received a new student with low vision. Write a draft of what you might say to introduce administrators to the professionals who may become involved with the student.

3. You are a rehabilitation counselor who has a new client with low vision—a 53-year-old man who has just learned that, following a farming accident, he is legally blind. Develop a script in which you and he will discuss the term *legal blindness* and you will ascertain his understanding of how the term is applied to him.

4. Write a story to promote understanding of the terms *low vision* and *legal blindness* for the third-grade classmates of a visually impaired child.

In the Community

1. Interview a clinical low vision specialist, a rehabilitation teacher, a teacher of students with visual impairments, and an O&M instructor. Ask them how they participate in the team process of providing low vision services to children or adults with low vision.

2. Ask several members of your family or friends what they perceive to be the definition of legal blindness. Compare their perceptions with what you have learned in this chapter.

With a Person with Low Vision

1. Speak with an adult who has low vision. Ask this person to describe the past and current services he or she has received and is receiv-

ing from professionals who provide services to persons with low vision and the value of the services to his or her overall education or rehabilitation.

2. Speak with two persons with low vision who are legally blind. Ask how the term *legal blindness* has or has not affected their lives.

Also, ask how they describe their vision to others.

From Your Perspective

In what ways can professionals help the general public to understand the distinction between low vision and blindness?

CHAPTER **2**

Psychological and Social Implications of Low Vision

Sharon Zell Sacks

VIGNETTES

Nine-year-old Jenny has had low vision, caused by congenital nystagmus and cataracts, since birth. She wears thick tinted lenses, is able to read her text with a magnifier and can see the chalkboard with a hand-held monocular, rides a bicycle, and enjoys video games. Jenny is an active, social child, and her parents have made every effort to help her to be physically attractive. Lately, however, Jenny has been excluded from team sports and games during recess because she cannot hit a ball as well as her peers. In addition, her friends have noticed that her "eyes move around a lot"; when they mention it to Jenny, she becomes shy and retreats from the group.

One day, while meeting with Mr. Chen, her teacher of students with visual impairments, Jenny burst into tears and explained that she was not as good as her friends in sports anymore and that her eyes looked funny. Mr. Chen discussed alternatives to playing team sports at recess time and then reviewed some reading materials to provide Jenny with some practice in using her new optical device.

Mr. Chen knew that he and Jenny would have to talk again about these concerns, since she needed to discuss her feelings about the appearance of her eyes and the reactions of her friends to her visual limitations. He also planned to speak with the teacher who was on duty at recess, who might be able to suggest

other team sports; for example, Jenny could play volleyball because the volleyball is large.

As Mr. Chen traveled to his next student's school, he thought about how to approach Jenny about her concerns. Just the night before, he had spoken with his own mother about her feelings of isolation because of the onset of macular degeneration. In her early 60s, Mrs. Chen had to give up her driver's license and was feeling that her social life would be limited and that she would no longer be independent. Mr. Chen could not assure his mother that they could find easy solutions to the problems she was facing, and now he had to discuss the same topic with a 9 year old who had her whole life ahead of her.

Carl, aged 28, has corneal dystrophy and approximately 20/600 acuity. When he got a new job, he moved from a large city to a suburb of a mid-sized city. After checking maps to find where the bus lines and grocery stores were located, he purchased a house within walking distance of both. Carl had a slightly rounded back, wore thick eyeglasses, and did not dress fashionably, although he was always neat. He did not need or use a white cane.

After he had been in his new home for about two months, he became well acquainted with one neighbor and learned that several neighbors had assumed he was "slow witted" or possibly emotionally unstable because he had been seen walking in the streets at all hours. No one ever stopped to say hello or offer him a ride; he wondered if he had moved into an unfriendly neighborhood. He also learned that a few neighbors who had been working in their yards had sometimes waved at him while he was walking to or from the bus. However, because he could not see them, he continued on his way without acknowledging them, which further confirmed the neighbors' initial beliefs that there was something "wrong" with him.

Carl decided to hold an open house to meet his neighbors. Because of this party, his neighbors got to know him and accepted Carl into the neighborhood. It turned out that one of the neighbors was employed in the same office building as Carl, and soon he was exchanging rides with Carl for gas money.

INTRODUCTION

Often teachers and rehabilitation professionals who provide services to persons with visual impairments have a solid understanding of ophthalmological terminology, low vision assessments, and training strategies, but they know less about translating clinical knowledge and practice into an understanding of the impact of a visual impairment on a person's lifestyle. Providers of direct services are trained to recommend specific techniques or strategies to enable a child or adult to attain greater independence in the classroom or in the community. However, they do not always address personal issues, such as feelings of isolation or the need to cope with the daily presence and implications of a visual impairment. Many service providers may not address these issues because they feel that there are no clear-cut techniques or strategies for doing so or they are uncertain about the best way to raise these issues.

For many people, the onset of a visual impairment or living with a visual impairment is a mere inconvenience, but for others, it is a lifelong challenge. Thus, teachers or rehabilitation professionals need to be sensitive to the psychosocial needs of adults or children with low vision and should develop practical strategies to help them lead productive, satisfying lives.

This chapter stresses two points. First, it is essential for professionals, family members, and others who work closely with children and adults with low vision to be sensitive to and familiar with what it means to live with this visual condition and its impact on societal perceptions, family support, and levels of independence. Second, it is crucial for those who provide ongoing services and support to develop and implement intervention strategies that promote a positive self-identity, increased understanding and knowledge of low vision, and the social inclusion of people with low vision in the sighted environment. This chapter presents numerous illustrations and examples of how to integrate strategies relating to these goals into traditional service delivery models.

ATTITUDES THAT AFFECT ADJUSTMENT

One's sense of identity, which is influenced by the perceptions and attitudes of others, is central to the development of a positive self-concept. People often make judgments about the abilities and limitations of a person with low vision on the basis of myths or folklore, representations in the mass media, and personal experiences with particular individuals. In general, many people's perception of vision is either black or white—you are either blind or sighted; there is no middle ground. Perhaps this is why children and adults with low vision and their families have great difficulty understanding their position in society. As Faye (1970, p. 415) noted:

> The terms "sighted" and "blind" represent groups possessing well established stereotypes and culturally expected rules of behavior. The position and role of the [partially sighted person] is much less clear owing to the tremendous range of variability in partially sighted types. Generally society views [partially sighted persons] as sighted and expects [them] to function as such.

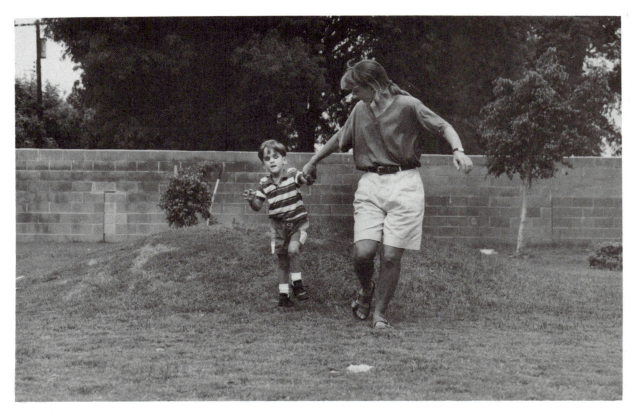

It is important for teachers and rehabilitation professionals to help children and adults develop a positive self-image and greater independence in the classroom and community.

As other chapters in this book indicate, classifications of visual impairment do not always take into account a person's visual abilities. For example, one person who has glaucoma and a measurable visual acuity of 20/400 may read printed material, travel without a cane, and view himself as sighted. Another person with a similar etiology and visual acuity may use braille or print, depending on the situation, and may or may not use a cane for travel, yet consider herself blind. Certainly, societal perceptions and values play a role in how individuals and their families view low vision. For instance, sometimes when an infant is diagnosed with a severe visual impairment, the attending ophthalmologist or pediatrician may recommend to the family that the child should eventually be placed in a school for blind children or may suggest learning strategies, such as instruction in reading braille, based solely on visual acuity levels. In many cases, people with low vi-

sion live with these initial perceptions and believe that they are blind because blindness is something they can understand.

Studies that have compared the adjustment of persons who are blind and persons with low vision have found that those with low vision perceive themselves more negatively than do people who are blind or fully sighted. Freeman, Goetz, Richards, and Groenweld (1991) noted that many of their subjects with low vision refused services from an "agency for the blind" that would have been beneficial because they did not want to be perceived as being blind. Kekelis and Sacks (1992) and MacCuspie (1992) described several children with low vision who had particular difficulty communicating their feelings about their identity to others. As a result, these children placed themselves at risk of social isolation or felt unjustly faulted because their actions were misunderstood, as in the following two examples:

Six-year-old John was playing a board game with his friends in his first-grade class. When it was John's turn to spin the spinner and move his piece according to the number of spaces shown, he accidentally picked up the wrong piece and moved ahead of the others. The other children yelled at John, calling him a "cheater and a dummy." John hung his head and walked away from the group. When the teacher intervened, she abruptly stated to the others in the group, "You know John can't see; let him try again" (Kekelis & Sacks, 1992, p. 70).

While commuting to his job as a paralegal, Steven sat next to a woman on the bus. Because of his macular degeneration, he often appears to be looking in a different direction from where he is actually seeking visual information. Steven was keeping his eyes on street signs, so he could get off at the right stop, when the woman accused him of staring at her. Because the woman was actually in his blind spot and he could not see her, Steven felt wrongly accused, but did not think he should attempt to explain his visual functioning at that time.

The Neither Fish-nor-Fowl Phenomenon

When children and adults with low vision receive mixed messages about their capabilities or others' expectations of them, they may feel confused about their identity, self-worth, or group status. Persons with low vision often say that they are neither blind nor sighted but somewhere in between. Placing oneself in this "gray area" allows for much confusion and misinterpretation of one's abilities and skills by others. For example, because Virginia may hold a book close to her face while wearing eyeglasses and reading, others who do not know her may conclude that she is retarded or weird or may just be nearsighted. Even people who know the individual with low vision may be confused. In the author's experience, friends and colleagues are often surprised to learn that her visual impairment is severe and that she requires assistance to read items or street

signs because they consider her a sighted person. At other times, people assume that she needs help or support with reading or travel when she does not. Instead of asking her, they immediately provide unneeded assistance, which requires her to explain her situation. If people with low vision have difficulty explaining their needs and abilities, cannot advocate for themselves, or feel uncomfortable letting others know about their low vision, then they may become vulnerable to others' negative perceptions of them.

Factors that affect self-perception and group identity are highly contingent on the age at onset of low vision (congenital versus acquired), knowledge of low vision by others who are important to the individual, public awareness, and support from trained personnel. However, even when people with low vision are knowledgeable about their visual impairment, they are still subject to more ridicule and misconceptions about their functioning abilities than are their functionally blind counterparts. The case of Mercedes is an example:

Mercedes, aged 67, has had age-related maculopathy for 10 years. In the past six months, she has noted great changes in her visual functioning. Once a great master of quilting, she found it difficult to continue this avocation. When introduced to a head-mounted magnification device during a low vision evaluation, Mercedes resumed her quilting activities with great enthusiasm. When she again began to teach quilting, however, she found that few of the students asked her for advice, demonstrations, and ongoing support. Soon she learned that the students were reluctant to seek her advice because they believed that she was really blind and was struggling to use her magnification device; thus, each time she used the device, they felt uneasy and physically distanced themselves from her.

Reactions of the Community

Although stereotypes about blindness still exist, when fully sighted people have the opportunity to meet persons who are blind or to see them depicted positively, their preconceived ideas about the capabilities and competence of blind people may change. For example, various films have portrayed blind individuals as active, capable, and competent, rather than as helpless and needy. In contrast, people with low vision have not been the main characters of films and have not even been portrayed in them.

Furthermore, persons with normal vision have difficulty comprehending what it is like to have low vision. Although they may be able to imagine what it is like to be blind when they are in a dark room or they close their eyes (even though these perceptions are unrealistic), they are often confused with respect to low vision. They may have erroneous beliefs about how much and how far a person with low vision can see, about the causes of low vision (often mistakenly assumed to be such factors as reading in dim light or in a moving vehicle, reading small print, or sitting too close to a television set), and about the age at which persons can acquire low vision (commonly assumed to be "old age," which is viewed as an inevitable cause of low vision; it is also commonly assumed that only elderly people can acquire low vision). In addition, they may not believe that persons who appear to have normal vision because they do not use a cane or adaptive devices really do have low vision. For example, one father believed that his 14-year-old daughter was malingering because she could not recognize her aunt's face across a room but could find earrings and other small items on the top of her dresser. Similarly, the neighbors of Carl, in the vignette that opened this chapter, did not know that someone Carl's age could have low vision and could not conceive that he would have to walk on the street in their suburban neighborhood because he was unable to drive.

Even when people with low vision are "well adjusted," they may feel angry or withdraw when they are in situations in which they have to explain their visual status or their actions, as reflected in the following comment:

Once I was in a restaurant reading a menu. Of course, I had to hold the menu close to my face to read it. When the waiter came over to take my order, he looked at me and said, "Looks like you have a bad eye. Don't you wear glasses?" I felt my body tense up, and I said, "Actually I have two bad eyes, and glasses don't help."

Reactions of Family Members

It is not always easy for those who are closest to a person with low vision to understand or comprehend what it is like to live or to function as a person with low vision. Many families view blindness as a punishment, a curse, or "God's will" or share the same erroneous beliefs about low vision as do other sighted people in the community. How families react to and interact with their members with low vision is highly dependent on their perceptions and cultural values. Even when family members are fearful of or devastated by the initial diagnosis of blindness, they can more clearly understand what to expect and how to proceed with daily activities than when the diagnosis is low vision—a condition to which they may react with frustration or impatience because they are not always sure what the person can see or accomplish. In a study of the impact of not being able to drive on the lifestyles of adults who are functionally blind and those with low vision, Corn and Sacks (1994) found that the subjects in the low vision group believed that people who were close to them had less understanding of the emotional or logistical impact of not being able to drive than did those who were in the functionally blind group.

It is not unusual for conflicts to arise between immediate family members (parents, spouses, and children) and extended family members (grandparents, in-laws, and aunts or uncles) with respect to expectations for the person with low vision. Again, preconceived ideas may influence how a relative misinterprets a person's level of visual competence or actions. For example, when the author was a child, her low vision was an issue between her mother and her grandparents. Her grandparents viewed her as sighted and became annoyed and angry when she did not always initiate interactions with them. They could not understand that they had to cue her to get her visual attention. However, they thought that her mother was investing too much time in helping her read assignments and was pushing her unrealistically.

Cultural beliefs also play a significant role in how family members relate to the person who is blind or who has low vision. In some cultures, for example, blindness may be looked on as an embarrassment or disappointment. Yet among other groups, family members may believe that it is their responsibility to care for the person, rather than to foster independence and self-reliance. Research does not indicate whether children and adults with low vision differ on the basis of their gender or cultural or racial group in the extent to which they encounter confusion or rejection from family members.

However, persons who have albinism and who are from minority ethnic or racial backgrounds may frequently encounter reactions that reflect popular mythology in which they have often been portrayed as evil or as having turned white from extreme fear. Furthermore, the development of their sense of identity may be hampered not only by their visual impairment and its associated effects but by their minority status. They may have difficulty relating to any group: They can see, but they cannot see; their features are typical of their cultural group, but their skin appears white. Thus, some people with albinism feel socially isolated because of their "double" marginal status.

Reactions of Classmates, Co-Workers, and Employers

Classmates, co-workers, and employers may have difficulty recognizing or understanding the unique visual needs of persons with low vision. At first, they may be curious about how a child sees or why an adult who already wears thick eyeglasses still needs a magnifier to read or to use a computer. Children generally ask direct questions, such as "Why do you use those big books?" or "Why do you get so close to everything?" or ridicule the child and make cruel comments like "You're ugly; you have four eyes" or "I don't want you on our team; you can't hit the ball."

Co-workers or employers may react more subtly, but their curiosity and discomfort with differences in functioning may still be apparent. Thus, the person with low vision must first decide whether to disclose his or her visual condition during an employment interview and have a plan to assure the employer and co-workers that he or she can do the job with reasonable accommodations and will fit into the social milieu of the workplace.

INITIAL REACTIONS TO LOW VISION

The onset of severe low vision, whether it is manifested at birth or later in life, is a traumatic event and, for many, is fraught with fear, anger, disbelief, denial, depression, and uncertainty. A diagnosis of severe congenital or adventitious low vision is not always indicative of impending blindness but may reflect various degrees of functional vision.

Even before children or adults are diagnosed with low vision, they or their parents and others who are close to them may recognize differences in visual functioning and internally acknowledge that something is wrong. Ophthalmologists and other physicians are not always able to pinpoint the etiology of a condition, such as nystagmus or inconsistent visual responses, especially in children, and may assure a child's parents that the condition is temporary. As a result, many parents feel confused and frustrated about the status of their children's visual functioning and search for physicians who will provide them with a specific diagnosis or cure. This "doctor shopping" may indicate to the children that their low vision is causing their parents much anxiety, and they may link a positive or negative medical prognosis to feelings about their self-worth.

Adults who suspect that they are losing their vision often deny that they have a severe visual impairment and may delay seeking medical attention. Once they receive a definitive diagnosis from an ophthalmologist, they may worry about their future ability to earn a living, drive a car, or be attractive to those who are significant to them.

They may also hide their diagnosis, even to the point of convincing themselves that they do not have a severe visual impairment.

Once the diagnosis is made, the child or adult with acquired low vision and his or her family members may feel a great sense of sadness and mourning in regard to the loss of vision. Sometimes family members search for information to help them understand the complex nature of the visual impairment. Many ophthalmologists provide cursory information: a label, a brief description of etiology, and possibly some literature to reinforce their verbal explanation. As one mother put it:

> Shortly after our daughter was born, an ophthalmologist was called in as a consultant because she was born prematurely. He told us that Karen had retinopathy of prematurity and that she would have limited vision. He left, and I felt lost. I didn't know where to turn, so I went to the library to learn more about this disease.

In some instances, however, an ophthalmologist is ready to explain the medical implications of a visual diagnosis in great detail, but the individual or family members may not be ready to comprehend fully the long-term implications of the diagnosis.

At the time of diagnosis, it is critical for physicians, nurses, and other medical support personnel to provide resources to the person and his or her family to ensure that they establish and maintain a support network. It is particularly important that such support structures are readily available for families of infants and preschool children with visual impairments and for elderly people. For school-age children, the teacher of students with visual impairments assumes a critical role as a liaison between families and eye care providers and as a facilitator to help children and their families understand the nature and long-term implications of the visual impairment. However, it is not always easy for adults with low vision to find established support networks. Many adults find it difficult or choose not to apply to agencies or services for individuals with low vision, even if such agencies or services are available in their communities.

Although family members may have a clear understanding of the visual impairment, it may be difficult for them to communicate to close relatives and friends the nature and scope of low vision, especially for someone whose visual functioning varies from day to day or from one activity to the next. For example, an adolescent who has a severe field loss may be able to watch a play from a backseat in a theater or read street signs from a moving vehicle but may bump into familiar objects at home or when traveling. In addition, conditions such as glaucoma or Stargardt's disease (a form of macular degeneration in children), may not be obvious to others. Confusion and misunderstanding may therefore occur. Furthermore, parents may feel uncomfortable talking about their child's visual impairment and may find it difficult to explain it succinctly and in a relaxed manner. Thus, children or young adults with low vision often learn about their visual impairment from a teacher of students with visual impairments or an eye care specialist. As one girl stated:

> I realized that I was visually impaired when I was in kindergarten. I wore glasses and knew I couldn't see very well. The kids in my class teased me and made fun of my glasses. I knew I was different. My mom told me that I had retrolental fibroplasia. She couldn't give me any more information except that it was the result of my prematurity.

When parents believe that they caused their child's visual impairment, their underlying feelings of guilt or embarrassment may be manifest in denial, anger, or self-abrogation. Even when parents and other family members understand, have adjusted to, and feel comfortable with the child's low vision, any change in visual status, obstacles that the child may encounter as a result of the visual condition, or transitions from one milestone to the next, such as from childhood to adolescence, often revive their guilt or anger.

When parents of children with visual impairments learn that their child's visual impairment was inherited, it is critical for them to seek genetic counseling to determine whether the gene is recessive, dominant, or sex linked. Determining the genotype will help them understand their chances of having another child with the same visual impairment and give them information to share with their child when he or she enters early adulthood.

Initial reactions to an inherited condition vary from family to family. Families in which the parents or other children have low vision often may have less difficulty dealing with the diagnosis. However, for families in which the child is the first person with low vision or in which the visual impairment is detected later in childhood or during adolescence, the process of adjusting tends to be much more difficult.

When an adult with low vision learns that the condition is genetic, he or she must disclose the information to other family members and potential mates. Genetic counseling and testing can determine if family members exhibit signs of a similar impairment or if they are carriers who have passed on the genes to a new generation. Those who are considering parenthood then must decide whether and how they wish to proceed.

FEAR OF LOSING VISION

The idea of eventually becoming "blind" is the greatest fear of many persons with congenital low vision. Because they may view themselves as sighted, any loss in visual functioning may lead to a range of feelings, including anger, disbelief, and confusion, particularly when their visual status has been relatively stable throughout childhood and adolescence and becomes progressively worse during adulthood. Often, individuals who lose vision are unaware that this progression is typically associated with their condition, such as retinopathy of prematurity, aniridia (absence of the iris), and congenital glaucoma (see Chapter 6 for detailed descriptions of the etiologies of various eye conditions).

Once a person finds that his or her visual impairment is no longer stable, he or she may have to deal continually with changes in lifestyle and visual status. Individuals who have had stable vision and then begin to lose visual functioning may feel that they have lost control over their ability to see and will ultimately lose their independence. Furthermore, because the visual impairment may be in flux, visits to eye care specialists may be more frequent and emotionally painful to them.

Having to decide whether to have surgery to maintain relatively effective visual functioning can increase a person's anxiety and frustration. Although an ophthalmologist may present a clear case for surgery and feel confident about the outcome, the individual still has to decide whether to go through with it and weigh the risks that may be involved. For example, a "simple" cataract extraction for an adult with retinopathy of prematurity may cause further retinal detachments; although retinal detachments usually can be repaired, they may compromise the person's level of visual functioning to a greater degree than it was before the surgery.

Individuals with acquired visual impairment often face similar concerns, but their visual condition may slowly deteriorate over an extended period. In cases in which they may be dependent on medical treatment or medication to maintain their level of visual performance, their relationship with their ophthalmologists is pivotal to them. A number of anxiety-producing and potentially sensitive situations may result from this vulnerability. For example, since the goal of ophthalmololgy is to "cure" or to "save" eyesight, an ophthalmologist may believe that medication or another form of treatment is the only alternative for a patient, whereas the patient may not see the merit in taking medication regularly or undergoing painful treatments if there is no improvement in his or her visual status. If the ophthalmologist is not supportive of the person and does not continually reinforce the need for ongoing treatment to preserve visual function, both parties may feel angry and frustrated with each other. In such circumstances, the teacher of students with visual impairments or the rehabilitation professional can act as an objective intermediary to

- ◆ help the individual understand the nature and progression of the visual impairment or, together with the parents, explain the condition to the child
- ◆ include the clinical low vision specialist as a member of the low vision team

◆ accompany the person to an ophthalmology appointment to help the person ask appropriate questions or clarify issues

◆ help the person understand the long-term effects of medication or surgical treatment for maintaining his or her visual performance

◆ give the ophthalmologist information on clinical low vision evaluations and devices.

ISSUES RELATED TO PERSONAL IDENTITY

Many children with low vision perceive themselves as sighted but with limited visual abilities, and their teachers and parents often promote the idea that they are just children who have poor vision. Yet many of their visual behaviors, such as experiencing the rapid eye movements that characterize nystagmus, viewing materials close up, not making eye contact, and wearing thick eyeglasses, cause them to be labeled as different. As a result, many find it difficult to identify with any peer group or to feel comfortable about themselves.

Also, many children who grow up with low vision do not have opportunities to meet adult role models with low vision or to interact with peers who have similar visual conditions. As a result, they may feel isolated or ashamed and lack the confidence to discuss their low vision with others. During the working years, adults with acquired low vision may also find themselves isolated from others who are having similar visual experiences. For fear of losing jobs or changing their social status, they may withhold information about their decreasing vision. Thus, they, too, may resist or have difficulty developing identities as persons with low vision.

When children or adults are legally blind and are referred to as such, they may exhibit a range of emotions. They may be defensive, explaining that they really can see; they may express anger, feeling that they are being categorized with people who are totally blind; or they may experience relief, feeling that they have been given a way to explain their visual functioning to others. Although some people with low vision consider themselves fortunate in comparison to those who are totally blind in that they have retained vision or have been born with sight, others do not compare their visual status to persons who are blind; rather, they relate to those who are sighted, considering that they, too, are sighted individuals.

Passing

Children or adults with low vision who wish to be considered part of the "sighted" society may attempt to cover up their visual status or to pass as fully sighted. In other words, they may act as though they are fully sighted and can accomplish tasks without visual modifications. Many adolescents with low vision may choose to pass when interacting with persons of the opposite sex in order to be accepted as dates or as part of a peer group, as in the following example:

> When I asked Linda out for a date, I didn't tell her that I couldn't see very well. I made plans with my friends, so we could double date and I wouldn't have to tell her why I didn't drive. I wanted her to get to know me before I told her. On our first date we went out to dinner. When the waiter handed me the menu, I held it just like sighted people do. I didn't put on my glasses or use my magnifying glass; I pretended that I could read the menu. I had a pretty good idea of what was on the menu, so I just selected something familiar.

One may argue that passing is emotionally unhealthy and counterproductive to establishing a strong identity as a person with low vision. However, if it is directed in a positive manner, passing can sometimes be a useful strategy. The person with low vision must choose when and under what circumstances he or she should attempt to pass or to avoid doing so. For example, telling a potential employer about a visual impairment needs to be handled delicately. Sometimes passing may assist the person to obtain a job interview, but once the person has a foot in the door, he or she must decide if continuing to pass is appropriate or if disclosure is more effective, as in the next example:

> Monequeka enjoyed community theater. She could both sing and act. But when she auditioned for a show, she was sure to memorize the reading. As she explained, "As soon as they know I can't see very well, they question whether I'll fall off the stage. I'd rather get the part and let the director see me move around before I let him know how poor my vision really is."

Disclosing a Visual Impairment

One of the more difficult decisions for a person with low vision is how to disclose his or her visual impairment to others. Telling people about one's low vision is a real art. The person must determine how much and what type of information needs to be provided and when the visual impairment should be disclosed. Each aspect of disclosure is highly dependent on with whom the person may be interacting and for what purpose. For example, if a child with low vision was being teased by her classmates in elementary school because she could not catch a ball, she could inform them about her visual needs by using the following statements:

> I can't always see the ball because my eyes don't work like your eyes. When I look in bright sunlight, I can't always see you or the ball.

> I'm not blind; I just can't see like you. I just might need a little help.

> I was born with this eye thing. It makes me not see so good, but I can see the ball if it's a bright color.

When children with low vision are talking with a close friend or teachers about their visual impairments, they may choose to use more descriptive information, such as the following:

> My eyes move around a lot because I'm looking for the best way to use my vision. I was born

early, and my eyes were damaged, but I can see you and do all the stuff you can do.

> I have trouble seeing the chalkboard, and glasses don't help. So when you are assigning seats, could I have a front-row seat?

The circumstances may be different when a person with low vision is interacting with individuals in the community. In such situations, he or she needs to be succinct about his or her visual needs while asking for assistance or support, as in these examples:

> I can't see the menu from a distance. Could you read it to me?

> I can't see very well, and I forgot my glasses. Could you help me complete my deposit slip?

> I have a vision problem, and I can't see the street signs. Could you let me know when we get to the Civic Center stop?

On the job, the person with low vision has to educate the employer and co-workers about his or her visual impairment and possible needs while demonstrating poise, competence, and independence, as in the following statements:

> I can do all the computer work using my optical devices, but it would be helpful if I had a larger monitor because it would make the print a bit larger.

> I am willing to purchase a car so I can travel on the job, but I will need some assistance in paying for a driver.

When interacting with professionals in the field of blindness and visual impairment, one cannot always assume that they have comprehensive knowledge of each person's visual status or the effects of low vision on a person's life. In the past, professionals were prepared to work primarily with people who were functionally blind; today, many general eye care specialists may have knowledge of medical conditions but lack specific information about low vision. Thus, the person with low vision may find it necessary to use disclosure strategies even with these specialists.

As one person noted, "Every time I go to a new ophthalmologist, I need to tell the ophthalmic assistant (and sometimes the ophthalmologist) which tests to use to obtain an accurate distance visual acuity."

Once the person informs others, particularly family members and friends, about his or her visual impairment, it may be necessary to provide them with information to help them understand the nature of his or her visual functioning and to clarify misguided perceptions. For example, fully sighted people often initially perceive the individual as "a little" blind or make such comments as "You'd never know she was legally blind; she does so well." Also, it is important for the child or adult with low vision to feel comfortable answering questions or to give examples of how he or she functions using vision. The key is to help others understand that one is neither blind nor normally sighted, but a person who functions with limited visual abilities.

To begin to identify with their visual status, persons with low vision need to discuss their visual impairments with others in a relaxed and safe environment and to be sensitive about the need to protect their privacy. Through practice, persons with low vision may become less sensitive about telling others about their visual impairment and may view their visual status as an integral part of their self-concept. For future communication with another person, it is crucial to know how to place one's low vision in perspective, sometimes with humor and sometimes with statements that diminish the importance of the impairment, as in examples such as these: "You won't have to worry about how you look when I see you; I can't see your eye makeup, anyway." "Once in a while I'll need to be rescued. I made a mistake and went into the wrong washroom today; I guess I'll have to look more carefully the next time."

Whereas some individuals become adept at educating and putting fully sighted people at ease, others feel frustrated about always having to explain or answer questions. As one parent said to her adult daughter with low vision, "When Ella [a family friend of many years] heard you're legal-ly blind, she wanted to know if you were losing your vision. I thought I had answered all the questions I needed to answer when you were little. When does it stop?"

Understanding One's Visual Impairment

Before a child or adult with low vision can use passing or disclosure strategies, it is necessary for him or her to have a clear understanding of his or her visual impairment—its nature, cause, and implications for functioning—adaptations and materials to assist in functional and academic activities, and long-term outcomes. The teacher of students with visual impairments can use a variety of activities (such as those presented in Sidebar 2.1) to enhance a person's level of understanding.

The teacher or rehabilitation professional will see the benefits in devoting instructional time to helping students learn more about their visual impairments on a contining basis. Roessing (1980) designed a curriculum to help professionals assist students from preschool to high school in developing understanding and functioning more effectively as people with low vision by establishing self-advocacy skills, as well as by becoming more knowledgeable consumers with low vision. Sidebar 2.2 presents an example from this curriculum.

Being Sensitive to One's Appearance

Another issue for persons with low vision is how they perceive their physical appearance. Many adults with congenital low vision have commented that they do not think their eyes and general physical appearance are attractive, even when they have no unusual physical characteristics. The authors' experiences suggest that when children are given opportunities to look at their eyes (sometimes with magnification), to meet others with similar visual impairments, and to

SIDEBAR 2.1

Activities to Enhance an Understanding of Visual Impairment in Children and Youths

Have students learn the different parts of the eye through the following:

- Let students examine their own eyes in the mirror (placing a magnifier directly on the mirror may be helpful). Ask them to pay attention to the color and shape of the eyes and to any differences they observe.

- Let students compare and contrast their eyes with others.

- Use a pull-apart model to help students learn the location of different parts of the eye.

- Develop matching games or board games to help students become familiar with the parts of the eye.

Provide opportunities for students to discuss and to learn about their own visual impairments:

- Once students become familiar with the parts of the eye, have them name and identify the source or of their visual impairments. (Use models or drawings.)

- Develop role-play scenarios in which students need to give information about their visual impairments to other children or to regular classroom teachers.

- Provide opportunities for the individual to meet other children or adults with a similar visual impairment.

- Let students share information about their visual functioning.

- Develop a board game in which students who are sighted and students who are visually impaired can learn more about vision and low vision.

- Have students create a story depicting the main character as someone with low vision.

- Have students create television or radio commercials for adaptive equipment used by persons with specific visual impairments.

- Have students keep a journal as persons with low vision, recording positive or successful accomplishments or adaptations used throughout the school year.

have positive experiences related to their visual needs, they develop a more positive sense of their own attractiveness.

It is also important for parents and teachers to recognize that how one looks or appears to others often makes an initial statement about one's social competence. For example, wearing contact lenses may help one feel more attractive than wearing eyeglasses with thick lenses. In addition, contact lenses tend to slow down the rapid eye movements of people with nystagmus and make the eyes of persons with aniridia (absence of the iris) or coloboma (a keyhole-shaped pupil) appear normal, and tinted contact lenses (or eyeglasses) reduce squinting and discomfort from glare for individuals who are photophobic (sensitive to light). (See Chapters 5 and 6 and the glossary for more information.) Furthermore, eye makeup sometimes enhances the appearance of women's eyes by making them appear larger or less sunken.

Ophthalmologists often encourage parents to consider cosmetic surgery for their children with low vision, especially when there is significant

---

Roessing's Low Vision Curriculum: An Example

SIDEBAR 2.2

OVERALL OBJECTIVE

The student shall demonstrate knowledge of how to be an intelligent consumer of eye care services.

OBJECTIVES FOR PRESCHOOLERS

When asked about the sequence of the physical eye examination, the child can relate:

1. the purpose of the eye exam ("to find out how I see")
2. the size and description of the examining chair
3. how and why the examiner occludes an eye
4. the purpose and general description of an eye chart
5. a description of a penlight and how it works.

OBJECTIVES FOR ELEMENTARY SCHOOL STUDENTS

The student can identify the essential sequence of a basic eye exam. He or she also can

1. identify an ophthalmoscope, trial lenses, and other basic equipment
2. define eye dilation
3. understand the purpose of eye charts for near and distance testing
4. describe, in general, the sequence of field testing
5. understand color testing equipment.

OBJECTIVES FOR SECONDARY SCHOOL STUDENTS

The student can formulate questions for the eye care specialist to obtain information about his or her visual functioning. He or she also can

1. state how frequently eye examinations should be conducted and why they may be required more often than annually
2. define testing procedures that are likely to be used
3. prepare a list of questions or concerns to discuss
4. know testing procedures he or she may wish to request for additional information on his or her visual functioning
5. keep personal notes or a journal to record if his or her vision generally fluctuates or if there is any decrease in his or her visual abilities since the last eye examination
6. know that the patient is a co-equal partner in the delivery of eye care services
7. understand the difference between optometry and ophthalmology and the function of opticians
8. define the purpose and scope of the low vision examination.

Source: Adapted from L. J. Roessing, *Minimum Competencies for Visually Impaired Students,* unpublished manuscript. (Fremont, CA: Fremont Unified School District, 1980).

---

eye-muscle imbalance or disfigurement, and adults with such eye disorders may also consider this option. The potential benefits of the surgery should be weighed against the long-term outcome, and surgery for cosmetic purposes, even without potential medical benefits, should not be discounted if it could yield social and emotional benefits. In considering cosmetic surgery, one may find the answers to the following questions helpful:

◆ Will the surgery improve the physical appearance of the eyes?

◆ Can the surgery affect visual status and functioning?

♦ Can the surgery cause other visual anomalies?

♦ Will the surgery be painful and cause discomfort?

USE OF OPTICAL DEVICES

The use of optical devices can enhance the self-concept and self-esteem of persons with low vision in many ways. Among the benefits of using these devices are

♦ a sense of independence when one can gain access to regular print in the environment without being dependent on others

♦ a sense of responsibility for acquiring one's own visual information

♦ increased awareness of the visual environment

♦ a sense of competence because one has some control over the visual environment

♦ greater pleasure from visual aesthetics.

Despite the benefits of optical devices, individuals with low vision sometimes resist using them because they do not always experience the benefits. First, they may be disappointed that a device has not "fixed" their visual impairment. Second, many persons with low vision, especially elderly people, find it difficult to learn to use the devices or think the devices are awkward or cumbersome. Hall, Sacks, Dornbush, Raasch, and Kekelis (1987) found that those who initially did not have a specific purpose for using an optical device tended to use it less frequently than did those who did. Also, the mechanics of using a device prevented many subjects, particularly elderly ones, from persevering until the device became more functional for them.

Children and young adults with low vision may choose not to use an optical device because they think it draws attention to them, making them appear less competent or attractive. Therefore, in prescribing such devices, professionals need to consider not only their functional benefits but their cosmetic appearance and social implications.

On the one hand, parents and professionals may be so anxious for children or adults to use optical devices that they disregard any potential cosmetic and social effects. On the other hand, family members and friends may discourage the use of these devices because they may believe that using them labels people with low vision as "impaired," "blind," or otherwise different. They, too, should be encouraged to recognize the range of functional, social, and emotional benefits of using optical devices, including gaining access to a range of print sizes; being able to view the world at a greater distance; being able to obtain or retain a job; engaging in various recreational activities, such as bird-watching and playing card or board games; and, in some cases, being able to obtain a driver's license.

Professionals can help people with low vision feel more comfortable using optical devices by doing the following:

♦ including games for preschoolers that incorporate the use of optical devices (such as pretending to be a sea captain, astronomer, or photographer)

♦ encouraging the use of optical devices in a safe, comfortable environment for the person to develop skills before they are used in a classroom, in employment, or in the community

♦ providing the person with opportunities to demonstrate and share knowledge about the devices with classmates, friends, and family members who are fully sighted

♦ encouraging the use of optical devices for functional activities (such as using a magnifier to read a menu and a telescope to see a play)

♦ discussing ways that optical devices can be made more attractive (such as by choosing fashionable frames for microscopic lenses and using pocket magnifiers and behind-the-lens telescopes)

◆ demonstrating how adults can use optical devices to resume independent activities (for example, using a closed-circuit television to write checks and a magnifier to read prices in a grocery store and personal items, such as mail, bank statements, and prescriptions, as well as to see jewelry and apply makeup).

THE DILEMMA OF DRIVING

One of the more difficult obstacles that many adolescents and young adults with low vision face is not being able to drive a car. Obtaining a driver's license is not only a rite of passage from adolescence to adulthood in the United States but symbolizes that one has gained independence and has control over one's life. Although some adolescents with low vision may never achieve this milestone, they may long to do so. Therefore, it is essential for parents and teachers of students with visual impairments both to encourage adolescents and young adults to discuss their feelings of frustration and loss and to find constructive alternatives for meeting their transportation needs, so their feelings of self-worth are not diminished. The following suggestions may be helpful in developing strategies to ease the psychological impact of being a nondriver:

◆ If a student wishes, arrange for him or her to participate in classroom instruction in driver's education.

◆ Provide limited experiences with behind-the-wheel driving. Allow a student to drive in an empty parking lot on private property.

◆ Develop alternative ways for the student to travel independently, such as hiring a driver, joining a car pool, using a mass transit or paratransit system, and reciprocating for rides from others.

◆ Arrange for the student to meet adult role models with visual impairments and to discuss being an adult nondriver.

Many adults who lose vision later in life must relinquish their driver's licenses and depend on options other than driving for meeting their transportation needs. Such a transition may occur over an extended period and may require skilled counseling to help them adjust to their changing circumstances. It is often difficult for adults who have never depended on others to give up such control; as a result, they may place themselves in dangerous situations to maintain their sense of autonomy or may choose to remain isolated.

Corn and Sacks (1994) found that women with visual impairments were more isolated and attended fewer social events than did their male counterparts because they were unwilling to travel via mass transportation in unfamiliar areas. The lack of spontaneity in one's life, the circumstances of having to wait for late rides, and the inability to go where mass transportation does not go were themes repeated continually throughout the research. The findings of this exploratory study substantiated the significant impact of nondriving on persons with low vision, both adolescents and adults. The following quote by a respondent in the study exemplifies the frustration and pain someone may regularly endure:

> Boy, am I in a miserable mood today! . . . Does anyone get annoyed that they can't drive? I am very tired of DEPENDING on other people all the time to take me from place to place and know that I'll NEVER be able to drive!

SUMMARY

This chapter has explored the psychosocial needs of children and adults with low vision. Although the needs of persons with low vision are different from those of persons who are functionally blind, many fully sighted people think they are the same, and their perceptions are biased by misguided information, myths about low vision, social mores, and cultural values. Many people are pivotal in helping the person with low vision to establish a healthy identity and a strong self-concept. Therefore, collaboration is essential between the teacher of students with visual impairments or the rehabilitation professional, the family, and eye care professionals with respect to decisions regarding genetic counseling, risky surgical procedures, cosmetic surgery, and the use of optical devices.

Professionals need to develop a curriculum or other program to enhance the psychosocial adjustment of children and adults with low vision and implement it throughout children's educational and adults' rehabilitation programs. The content of such a curriculum might include such subjects as understanding and explaining one's visual impairment to others, developing effective ways to disclose information about one's visual impairment in various environments, learning to maximize one's physical appearance, finding alternatives to driving, and establishing a sense of control and self-identity as a person with low vision.

Although the intent of this chapter is to establish a level of awareness among professionals and family members that persons with low vision have unique social and emotional needs, another purpose is to spur the field to integrate more socially based content into educational, rehabilitation, and clinical direct services for children and adults. It is to be hoped that professionals from all disciplines will become more sensitive to the psychosocial issues of low vision and more willing to implement innovative and creative strategies and curricula on a consistent basis to nurture the positive identities of persons with visual impairments.

ACTIVITIES

With This Chapter and Other Resources

1. Use role-playing to illustrate the discussion between Jenny and Mr. Chen (see the vignette that opens this chapter) regarding her feelings of isolation.

2. Imagine yourself as a professional interviewing a client for intake at a low vision clinic or rehabilitation agency. Develop a method or project to help the person with low vision describe his or her visual needs.

3. Create a two-column chart to compare how fully sighted people perceive persons who are functionally blind and persons with low vision with regard to travel, employment, family relationships, and independent living activities.

4. As a follow-up to two of the situations portrayed in the opening vignettes, describe how you would interact with the persons with low vision and the strategies you would use to help them.

5. Discuss what Carl in the opening vignette might have done to increase his neighbors' understanding of his low vision. Consider whether any of your recommendations would have drawn too much attention to his visual status.

In the Community

1. Form two-person teams in which one person assumes the role of a person with low vision and the other observes the person's actions and the public's interactions with and reactions to the person. Using a variety of vision simulators provided by your instructor that exemplify a range of visual impairments (the less obtrusive, the better), the person who is portraying the individual with low vision should attempt to read a menu or a newspaper in public without the assistance of an optical device and then with a device. After the activity, each team should discuss the following questions in class:

   a. How did the person feel when using the simulator?

   b. Did the person wearing the simulator experience any frustration or physical limitations?

   c. How did fully sighted people react to the person who was using the simulator? What verbal and nonverbal cues did they give to their reactions?

2. As a team, trade tasks, perform the activity again, and discuss the outcomes with one another and with the rest of the class, comparing each other's experiences.

3. Interview a teacher of students with visual impairments or a rehabilitation professional. Find out what activities he or she uses to promote the psychosocial adjustment of students or adults.

4. Interview several people with normal vision to see what they believe people with low vision see, what the causes of low vision are, and how low vision affects people's lives.

5. Interview acquaintances from different cultures and determine if there are cultural differences in their beliefs about low vision.

With a Person with Low Vision

1. Interview an adult with low vision and ask him or her the following questions:
   a. When did you realize that you had a visual impairment? How did the ophthalmologist inform you or your parents about your diagnosis?
   b. How do you explain your visual impairment to family members and friends and to strangers?
   c. Can you recall any instances in which you tried to hide your visual impairment (i.e., engaged in passing)? Was passing a benefit or a problem for you at a later time?
   d. What is your greatest visual limitation? What adaptations do you use to reduce the significance of this limitation in your life?
   e. Do you drive? If so, what have some of your experiences been? If not, how does not driving affect your lifestyle, and what alternatives have you established?

2. Meet with a group of children who have low vision. Together, create a story that illustrates the reactions of others to their low vision and includes examples of statements they could use to help others understand their visual experiences.

From Your Perspective

What would you consider to be indicators of an individual's positive self-esteem as a person with low vision?

CHAPTER 3

Integration of Visual Skills for Independent Living

Gaylen Kapperman and Patricia J. Koenig

VIGNETTE

John, Bjorn, and Peggy are three persons with low vision who were all faced with the same task of grocery shopping on a sunny Saturday morning. John, an energetic youngster with retinitis pigmentosa, who has tunnel vision only, bebopped down the sidewalk with his friends in typical teenage fashion, except that in the group only he carried a white cane. Bjorn, a middle-aged father of three, took the train to a station near his usual weekday commuters' stop. Because of his aniridia, which was accompanied by extreme light sensitivity and poor visual acuity, Bjorn chose particularly strong sunglasses to wear on this bright morning. Peggy, a frail elderly woman with macular degeneration, who had peripheral vision, was picked up at her high-rise apartment complex by the city's paratransit van for people with disabilities; because of her arthritis, she was thankful for the driver's assistance in getting on and off the van.

At the store, Peggy methodically worked her way up and down the aisles, using a well-organized list that she had written with a black felt-tipped pen. Bjorn needed only a few items, so after he changed from his sunglasses to a pair with a tint more effective in dealing with the store's fluorescent lights, he went directly to where he knew the items would be found on the basis of his familiarity with the store. Once Bjorn found the items, he used his pocket magnifier to read the labels and prices. John and his friends were picking up supplies for a Boy Scout outing on Sunday. Knowing that his friends would be busy with their own purchases, John had called ahead to be sure that assistance from a clerk was available, so his first order of business was to head to the Customer Service Desk, where a store clerk met him. John and the clerk worked together from John's grocery list to get the items he needed.

At the checkout counter, John used his vision to select bills, since his acuity was sharp enough to see the denominations, although his visual field was too narrow to allow him to navigate crowded aisles in a grocery store. Bjorn continued to use his low vision devices, as he had done throughout the store, to confirm his change. Peggy wrote out a bold-line check, using a felt-tip pen clipped to the side of her purse. Thus, John, Bjorn, and Peggy made different choices and used different strategies that worked best for them.

INTRODUCTION

As the vignette that opened this chapter illustrated, people with low vision have different needs and learn to maximize their use of vision in different ways, depending on their visual conditions, ages, and other factors, such as the circumstances in which they use vision. Although many persons with low vision perform a variety of daily tasks safely and efficiently with their unaided vision, in some situations, they need to use special devices or techniques for maximizing their functional vision. When this is the case, they can choose from various options, which are discussed in this chapter.

This chapter explores considerations related to the integration of visual skills into daily life by people with low vision. A number of factors, ranging from the manipulation of elements in the environment, such as lighting and contrast, to the individual characteristics of the person's visual impairment, have an impact on the performance of visual tasks. Professionals in the field of low vision can do much to teach and encourage individuals to integrate adaptations and devices into their daily lives. A summary of ways in which service providers can help persons with low vision maximize their visual efficiency and integrate visual skills into their daily lives is presented in Sidebar 3.1. These suggestions are also explored in this chapter. Assessment procedures and guidelines to assist in the process of selecting appropriate devices and techniques to match individual needs are presented in Chapters 9, 10, 11, 15, and 16.

ENVIRONMENTAL MANIPULATIONS

Modifying the environment in which someone lives or works can have a dramatic influence on how efficiently he or she can use vision. Choices related to environmental manipulation are usually based on one or more of the following factors: lighting, contrast, color, distance, and size.

Lighting

Many persons with low vision can determine the optimal lighting for their individual levels of vision. For example, one person may find that a 200-watt lightbulb provides just the right amount of light for reading, another person may find that 200 watts are far too glare producing, and still another may find that the level of lighting is not crucial for his or her visual functioning.

For some visually impaired persons, low vision devices work best with lighting hitting the work surface from over a shoulder; others prefer a low vision device with a built-in light source. Thus, persons with low vision need to experiment to find the best lighting for comfortable viewing and the best way to adjust to lighting conditions they have no control over which. For example, in a dimly lit restaurant, one may use a penlight to read a menu more easily, another person may wear absorptive lenses to cut the glare from directed lighting, and still another may ask for a seat near a window to use the available daylight.

At home, people with low vision may find ways to provide more, less, or different lighting for comfort in performing tasks. For instance, the use of additional lamps can increase the overall levels of light in rooms, as can the installation of skylights (where such modifications are possible). To allow more light to enter dark shower areas, changing from opaque shower curtains or shower-stall doors to clear ones may be helpful.

Contrast

The use of contrast can be beneficial to many persons with low vision. For instance, in the kitchen, a person with low vision may choose to have a cutting board with a dark side and a light side—the dark side to be used for cutting light-colored foods like onions and the light side for cutting dark-colored foods, such as green peppers. In the den or recreation room, a person with low vision may place a dark-colored table on a light-colored floor surface, or vice versa. In the dining room, many persons with low vision place white plates on a dark tablecloth or serve light-colored food on dark dishes; they may also avoid patterned tablecloths and may prefer glasses that are colored or have an opaque design. Sets of stairs may be easier to see with a strip of contrasting tape at the edge of each step. Similarly, needlework, such as knitting, is much easier to complete when contrasting colors of yarn and needles are used. Contrast adaptations are usually not difficult to make, but most persons do not automatically think of them until some adaptations have been identified. Thus, it helps persons with low vision to ask themselves frequently,

SIDEBAR 3.1

Integrating Visual Skills into Daily Life: A Summary of Strategies

1. Teach the individual to manipulate the environment by adapting

   - lighting
   - contrast
   - distance
   - size.

2. Help the individual incorporate the use of low vision devices into everyday activities by

   - selecting low vision devices that are portable and therefore easily available when needed
   - working with the person to overcome psychological obstacles to the use of low vision devices
   - exploring ways for the person to use low vision devices throughout the day for many different tasks in many different settings.

3. Maximize the advantages offered by computers by

   - making the least adaptation to a procedure that will enable

the individual to function efficiently

   - striking a balance among low vision devices, environmental variables, hardware, and software.

4. Encourage the use of all the senses by

   - exploring the use of nonvisual approaches to tasks when appropriate
   - providing instruction in the use and integration of all the senses.

5. Be sensitive to the impact of factors that affect the choices made by a person with low vision by

   - understanding the nature of the person's visual impairment
   - allowing for the effects of fluctuating vision
   - making adjustments for levels of stamina and fatigue
   - respecting the person's characteristics of self-advocacy and self-perception.

"What could I do to improve the contrast in this situation?"

Color

Some persons with low vision who have color deficiencies do not find techniques for manipulating colors to be useful, but others find the use of color extremely helpful. Furthermore, certain colors may be more visible, and hence more useful, under particular lighting conditions. Colors and color combinations that persons who are fully sighted often think are highly visible (such as red on black electronic displays) may not be perceived as such by persons with low vision. Because there are so many variables involved in visual perception, persons with low vision must experiment to discover the best uses of color to maximize their visual functioning.

A common use of color is to organize or code similar items with different colors. For instance, adults with low vision often use color coding systems for filing paperwork (blue folders for information pertaining to income, yellow labels for expenditures, and so forth). Similarly, school-age

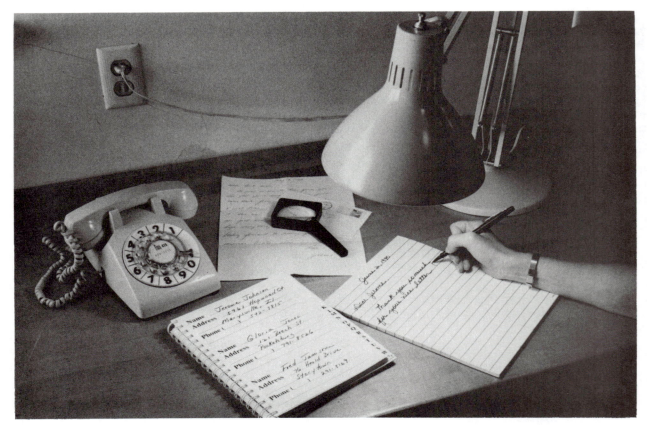

Adjusting the level of lighting according to individual needs is one effective technique to help maximize vision for the performance of specific tasks.

children with low vision may color-code books and materials on mathematics in green; on science, in red; and on reading, in white.

Another common use of color to enhance visibility is to place colored acetate sheets over materials to heighten the contrast. For example, yellow acetate sheets improve the contrast of sheets printed in purple and blueprints when used as an overlay.

Natural colors in the environment can also provide important cues to persons with low vision. For example, in a grocery store, a person may need only to look for many shelves of red-and-white cans to know that soup is in a particular aisle. And while traveling, a person may identify landmarks on a route by color, so he or she knows, for instance, to turn left just after the

yellow house and right between the white and brown fences.

Distance

Virtually everything that can be said about the use of distance by many people with low vision can be summed up in the phrase, "get closer." Persons with low vision who have peripheral field restrictions will find the opposite to be true; they may choose to increase distance to increase the amount of information in their fields of view.

Some examples of distance manipulation include selecting a pew near the front of a church or synagogue, buying front-section tickets at a theater, and sitting closer to the television set at home. When it is not possible to move physically closer, one can use a telescopic optical device to make objects appear closer. For instance, the person who feels self-conscious about walking up to a front porch to see a house number can sometimes read it from the sidewalk using a monocular. For safety reasons, no one should go beyond a certain distance to get close enough to a potentially moving bus or subway train to read a route number, but a telescopic device can make it appear closer and, therefore, larger.

In adjusting or manipulating the factor of distance, persons with low vision need to think about the trade-off between the benefits and the disadvantages. For instance, a front-section seat at the opera may help a person to see better, but it may be much more expensive than a seat in the balcony; thus, the individual must decide whether he or she just wants to hear the music or whether it would be more enjoyable also to see the costumes and scenery. With experience and knowledge of how distance manipulation can assist in optimizing their vision, persons with low vision can make better decisions about how to use distance in their daily lives.

Size

The use of optical devices is generally recommended for enlarging materials for people with low vision, although some individuals with low vision choose to use large-print materials. However, commercially available large-print books, magazines, devotional materials, and bingo cards are only a few types of print materials that people need to read. Some commonly used size adaptations that persons with low vision can make are large-print lists of telephone numbers and addresses written with felt-tipped pens on bold-line paper and blown-up maps, timetables, and charts, enlarged with a photocopier.

In light of the demographic shift toward an older population in the United States, more and more enlarged reading materials and other products are being made. For example, large-print telephone dials or buttons are readily available, as are large-print crossword puzzles and jumbo-type playing cards.

VISUAL AND NONVISUAL TECHNIQUES

Use of Optical Devices

Persons with low vision who use optical devices must integrate that use into their lifestyles. That is, they have to transfer what they have learned about using an optical device in a clinical setting to using it in real-life situations for real-life tasks, such as looking up a phone number in a telephone directory.

Many professionals in the field of low vision know clients who were excited about using optical devices in the clinician's office but whose devices are now functioning only as dust catchers or paperweights. Similarly, many teachers of students with visual impairments have observed children who excel in academic work using a closed-circuit television (CCTV) in the classroom but who do not routinely and comfortably use a CCTV to read leisure materials or to read the instructions on a cake mix box at home. Such individuals have not integrated optical devices into their daily lives, and, as a result, they are not using their vision to maximum efficiency.

To help people with low vision integrate the use of optical devices into their daily lives, professionals can do the following:

- help clients select optical devices that they can carry or otherwise have near them when they need them
- help clients overcome psychological obstacles to the use of optical devices in public
- help clients find ways to use optical devices throughout the day for many different tasks in many different settings.

First, to integrate optical devices into their everyday activities, people with low vision must carry the devices with them (in a large purse, satchel, briefcase, knapsack, or fanny-pack), so they can use the devices when they need them. For example, the best magnifier will do no good to read the dials on a washer and dryer at a laundromat if it is

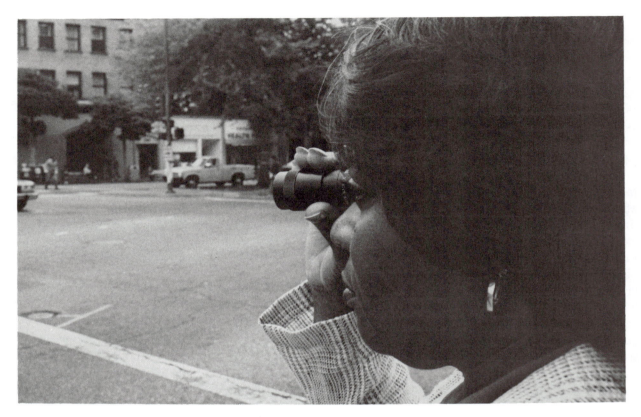

Convenience and portability are two of the qualities that encourage individuals with low vision to integrate an optical device into their daily lives.

in one's desk drawer at home. Thus, optical devices must be selected not only for their optical qualities but for their convenience and portability. Second, it may be necessary to choose one style of optical device over another or to purchase two different optical devices. For instance, a plug-in lighted stand magnifier may be helpful for balancing a checkbook while sitting at the kitchen table, but a similar battery-operated device may work better for reviewing papers at a lawyer's office, where an outlet may not be handy. Third, it may be useful to keep two or more identical devices in different places. For example, many children with low vision have one CCTV at school and another at home, and adults may keep one magnifier in the den, basement, or another area, where they pursue their hobbies; a second in the bedroom for nighttime reading; and a third at work for reading reports and memoranda.

Although it is a big step in the right direction, just carrying an optical device with one does not guarantee that it will be used. Some persons choose not to use their devices outside their homes and schools because they think the devices make them look unattractive and they feel self-conscious, or they do not want to be perceived as being "disabled." Some people feel more comfortable using devices as they progress in their adjustment, and others eventually come to believe that the benefits of the optical devices outweigh any disadvantages. Some even find a way to soften the impact of using particular devices; for example, one teenager found it much easier to pull out a telescope to read the overhead menu in a fast-food restaurant after she decorated it with glitter and stickers and replaced the black strap with a neon-colored thong.

Teenagers may have great difficulty adjusting to the use of optical devices. Because of peer pressure, sensitivity, and other concerns about their appearance and their desire to conform to the group in their lives, many teenagers with low vision prefer to use the most unobtrusive devices possible. Sometimes they may prefer to practice using a device outside the classroom, so their classmates do not observe them learning to use it, and to choose other options for gaining visual information in class, such as asking the teacher to read aloud the notes from the chalkboard as they are written. Teenagers may also be more amenable to using computers to enhance their vision (see the following section) because their peers are also using them for other purposes.

Positive role models can be helpful, especially for discussing sensitive issues with teenagers, such as the use of optical devices in social situations. Although adjustment to the use of optical devices is likely to come with practice and maturity, it is important for teenagers to develop a positive self-image, so they can have successful school experiences and are prepared for the challenges of adulthood.

In general, persons with low vision need to think of ways to use their optical devices beyond those for which they were primarily prescribed or purchased. For example, the optical device that works well for seeing graphics in the workplace may also be used to view photographs in a family album. Similarly, the same device that is used to read labels on cans and jars of food may also work for pill bottles or paint cans, and the telescope used to spot traffic signals may also be used to see birds at a backyard feeder. Persons who have integrated optical devices into their lives can be excellent role models, and they can share the myriad ways these devices are used daily with those who are just beginning to use them.

Use of Computers

Computers are another option in the array of choices that are available for enhancing vision. People with low vision can use special software and hardware to produce large-print images on computer screens and optical devices in conjunction with adaptive technology to enhance their vision further.

A computer has many advantages for a person with low vision. First, the effective distance between the screen and the eye of the user can be adjusted by enlarging the size of the letters through software or hardware modifications and by moving closer to the monitor—a considerable advantage over a typewriter. Second, a computer facilitates written communication, given that many persons with low vision find writing by hand laborious and time consuming, and their handwriting may be difficult to decipher. Third, a computer can be equipped with a speech synthesizer, thereby enabling the person with low vision to process the information on the screen auditorally as well as visually—a special advantage for a person who finds reading the screen to be slow and cumbersome.

Nonvisual Approaches

Sometimes the best method of handling a task is one that does not rely on vision. Although most persons with low vision prefer to think of themselves as sighted, rather than as blind, there are times and circumstances when it is safer, preferable, or more efficient not to use vision alone. For example, in a hotel where the doors to all the rooms look alike, a rubber band slipped over the doorknob will give a person with low vision tactile confirmation that he or she has located the correct room. Similarly, placing a dab of Hi Marks plastic marking paste or using some other tactile cue on the 350-degree mark on an oven control will avoid the need to juggle an optical device in the kitchen. Moreover, listening to an audiotaped book for leisure reading is sometimes faster and less fatiguing after one has used vision for work or school. The use of both nonvisual and visual techniques and of all the senses simply gives the person with low vision a wider range of choices.

FACTORS THAT AFFECT CHOICES

Many factors may influence a person's choices of ways in which to maximize his or her vision with the options just described. These factors include individual characteristics, preferences, needs, and other circumstances.

Type of Visual Impairment

As pointed out in this chapter's opening vignette, the characteristics of a person's visual impairment generally are the primary factors in determining the approaches used to enhance visual functioning. For example, two persons in the vignette, John, who has a restricted central visual field, and Peggy, who has intact peripheral visual fields but reduced visual acuity, will make different choices. If they both go to the movies, John may choose to sit at the back or to use a reverse telescope to increase his field of view, whereas Peggy may prefer to sit up front or to use a telescope in the conventional manner to magnify the images on the screen. John may decide to use a handheld device because he feels less self-conscious about bringing it to his eye, whereas Peggy may prefer a spectacle-mounted telescope because of her arthritis.

Fluctuating Vision

Some visually impaired people have good days and bad days and may even have good and bad times of the day in regard to their vision. The kinds of fluctuation in vision they experience will affect the choices they make. For example, a person who has better vision in the morning and poorer vision in the evening may choose to do most visually demanding tasks in the morning and relax with books on audiotape in the evening. A person whose vision is better in daylight and poorer at night may decide to keep a folding cane in a briefcase during the day and use it only after dusk. A person who is steadily losing vision may opt to learn many nonvisual techniques and begin to integrate them into his or her daily life even with usable vision. Individuals with fluctuating vision can manage their daily routines on the basis of these fluctuations and may learn to deal with certain tasks in several different ways, so they have the ability to handle whatever situations may arise.

Some people may also have to explain their fluctuating vision to others who observe it. For instance, members of her family may not understand why a woman reads her mail visually in the morning but asks to have the directions on the frozen-dinner package read aloud to her in the evening. Classroom teachers may find it difficult to understand why a child with low vision cannot read the chalkboard during an arithmetic lesson just before lunch but can do so well during a social studies lesson at the end of the school day.

Fluctuations in vision can be frustrating to both the person with low vision and others. Using a variety of approaches to gain access to visual information allows people with low vision to engage in activities throughout the day while compensating for changes in vision.

Stamina

Many persons with low vision find that stress and fatigue have a great effect on their vision; generally, the higher the level of stress or the greater the fatigue, the poorer their vision. Thus, although they can begin a task using vision alone or vision plus an optical device, they may need to use a nonvisual technique at a later point, especially if the task takes a long time. Persons with low vision therefore need to develop skills and make adaptations that take into account their levels of functional vision or energy under various circumstances. For example, a student who must read a great deal but who fatigues quickly when reading visually with an optical device may need to augment his or her visual skills with skills in using audiotaped material or in reading and writing in braille or may need to pursue other options.

Typically, people with low vision must look beyond the primary situations in which they use certain techniques or devices and seek to discover which choices will be most helpful in a variety of situations. The professional should keep in mind that visual fatigue affects people in different ways and that persons with low vision experience patterns of fatigue similar to those found among persons with normal vision.

Self-Advocacy and Self-Perception

An individual's willingness to advocate for himself or herself and the level of self-consciousness the person feels can greatly affect the decisions he or she makes related to vision. For example, one person who is struggling to read size tags while shopping for clothing may find it easy to ask for assistance from strangers, whereas another person may prefer to shop only when accompanied by a friend or family member. Although it would be ideal if all people who are visually impaired could have a strong sense of empowerment and self-advocacy, it is more realistic to recognize that, like everyone else, most people with visual impairments make lifestyle choices that are commensurate with their personality traits, level of comfort, and culture. Thus, persons with low vision need to be equipped with skills for completing tasks in a variety of ways, both visually and nonvisually.

SUMMARY

Persons with low vision have many ways to maximize their vision. Environmental manipulation is one approach that includes making changes in regard to lighting, contrast, color, distance, and size. The use of optical devices is another approach. Optical devices are maximally integrated into one's life when they are portable, appropriate, and used throughout the day and for many tasks in many settings. Those who feel uncomfortable or conspicuous using optical devices in public can overcome these obstacles by working with professionals to increase their level of comfort with the devices. The use of computers is still another approach; computers can be integrated into different lifestyles when they provide efficient access to the screen through such options as enlarged image and voice output.

At times, the best method for handling a task is one that does not require vision. Like those who are functionally blind, persons with low vision can benefit from learning to use nonvisual approaches and may sometimes combine these approaches with their usable vision.

Approaches to solving the challenges of low vision are not always clearly evident. Because there is not always a single best solution for performing a visual task, one chooses from among several available options. The type of visual impairment, fluctuations in vision, the level of visual stamina, and the person's self-advocacy skills are among the factors that affect these choices. The professional who takes these factors into account in presenting the many choices that are available will be able to assist the child or adult with low vision to integrate the best visual practices and adaptations effectively into his or her daily life.

ACTIVITIES

With This Chapter and Other Resources

1. Write a memo to John's (see vignette that opens this chapter) classroom teacher explaining why you want to take the time to teach braille reading and writing to a student with low vision who has poor visual stamina.

2. For each of these activities, list as many adaptations, visual and nonvisual, as you can that would be helpful for Peggy (see the opening vignette):
   a. pouring liquids
   b. visiting a local museum
   c. shopping for clothing
   d. setting a microwave oven
   e. playing a piano
   f. reading a newspaper
   g. paying bills.

3. Discuss why some persons with low vision would choose to use nonvisual approaches to complete tasks when they have vision to do so.

4. Identify several activities in your daily life that involve the use of distance vision. If you had low visual acuity, what options would you have for performing them?

In the Community

1. If you were going to adapt your home to maximize the visual functioning of a hypothetical family member with low visual acuity and problems with glare, what specific environmental adaptations would you recommend in each room?

2. Visit a department store and a grocery store. Compare the accommodations they provide for customers with low vision.

With a Person with Low Vision

1. Interview a person with low vision who uses a handheld magnifier. Ask the individual to describe tasks in his or her daily life that are facilitated through the use of this optical device.

2. Ask an individual with low vision who uses computer technology to facilitate his or her job tasks to describe the ways in which it makes the completion of tasks more efficient.

From Your Perspective

In what ways can society help persons with low vision to feel comfortable using optical devices, large-print materials, or other low vision approaches in public?

CHAPTER 4

The Literacy of Individuals with Low Vision

Alan J. Koenig

VIGNETTES

Cecillia, aged 25, is in her third year as a computer programmer for a high-tech company on the West Coast. She was diagnosed with Stargardt's disease in early adolescence and was taught to use optical devices and a closed-circuit television for reading and writing. Also, after several assessments of Cecillia's reading speed and a number of thoughtful discussions with her and her parents about the value of learning to read braille, the teacher of students with visual impairments decided to begin braille reading instruction. When Cecillia graduated from high school, she still used print as a primary reading medium, but used braille, live readers, electronic texts, synthesized speech, and audiotaped materials as well throughout her college years.

In her current job, that combination of literacy tools has proved to be indispensable. For most of the workday, Cecillia uses her spectacle-mounted magnifiers and synthesized speech to read the computer screen. When she needs to scrutinize a computer program to find the bugs, she relies on the braille display that sits under her keyboard. Cecillia's school experiences not only gave her a solid foundation of academic literacy skills, but allowed her to develop essential functional literacy skills by building a range of options to gain access independently to print information. Now Cecillia has taken over that responsibility and will continue to expand her range of

literacy tools to make her work more efficient and her life more enjoyable.

Sam, a fourth-grade student in a regular school program, has a condition that affects the optic nerve, has distance visual acuity of 20/180, and is able to read newspaper-size print at 2 inches. When he was in kindergarten and first grade, he preferred to read from the regular-print books that were in a size he could readily see. Even though the principal ordered "large" large-print books, Sam did not like them because they looked "yucky," since the pictures were not in color.

In second grade, the teacher of students with visual impairments taught Sam to use a prescribed handheld magnifier to read his favorite comic books. Although Sam needed the magnifier to read works in smaller sizes of print, especially the dictionary, he did not need it to read his textbooks. In third grade, Sam learned to use computer software that enlarged print on the screen, allowing him to sit at a comfortable distance as he learned word processing.

In fourth grade, Sam uses the magnifier most of the time to read his regular-print books. The teacher of students with visual impairments is working with him daily to increase his reading rate—now at 110 words per minute—and the amount of time he can read without becoming fatigued. When he feels visually fatigued, Sam uses live readers or listens to audiotapes for a while or takes a short break. Sam's orientation and mobility instructor taught him to use a monocular, so he can see the action at the high school football games his father coaches and read assignments on the chalkboard. Sam's school experiences are building a solid foundation of academic literacy skills and are providing him with specific strategies for gaining access to print materials.

Maria is a curious toddler, always exploring the ins and outs of her home and yard. As a result of her premature birth, she has low visual acuity and restricted visual fields. Her parents and special teachers know that it is important to use strategies to ensure that she interacts continually with her environment, so she will gain a wide variety of experiences. Maria and her parents have spent much time exploring the corner grocery store, the petting zoo, the post office, the community park, and other places. At home, her parents read aloud to her daily from books that have both print and braille on the pages. When the mail arrives, Maria and her mother or father read it together and sometimes even write a letter to someone special, like Aunt Elena. Because the special teachers are unsure whether Maria will learn to read in print, braille, or both, they are exposing her to both through opportunities to scribble with crayons and with the braillewriter, both of which occupy a special place on Maria's small desk. In the community, Maria's parents take time to get close to signs, so she can look at them and feel their shapes. With such planned experiences, Maria is gaining valuable early literacy experiences that will be indispensable for her success later in school.

INTRODUCTION

The topic of literacy is given considerable attention today, and such attention is justly deserved. Few would argue with Geisler's (1994, p.3) statement that in the United States learning reading and writing skills is "usually regarded as a birthright." One of the essential survival skills is the ability to communicate meaningfully through the written word—to gain information from reading and to convey information through writing. To be gainfully employed in the vast majority of jobs and to function independently in life, individuals, regardless of their visual abilities, need to be literate. The value of literacy is held in such high regard in this society that a primary focus of elementary school education is to establish literacy skills. Furthermore, using literacy skills to gain new knowledge and to expand one's experiences is emphasized throughout formal schooling and beyond. In the workplace, literacy skills are required for competitive employment and advancement in almost all occupations.

The written word constantly surrounds us as we go about our daily lives. Literate persons efficiently pick and choose among the multitude of signs, messages, books, magazines, and other forms of abstract symbology to accomplish whatever tasks they are required or wish to perform. Thus, literacy includes not only the selective gleaning of information but the use of it to complete a given task.

If a shopper wishes to locate a certain store at a mall, it is much more efficient for him to use literacy skills to read and interpret the mall directory than to walk up and down the aisles in pursuit of the store. If a homemaker wishes to read for enjoyment or to keep a daily journal, she must have the necessary literacy skills to do so. If a job hunter wishes to gain employment as a medical researcher, she needs technical reading and writing skills to read reports of previous research, plan and conduct new studies, and report the findings. If a grandfather wishes to read a story to his granddaughter, he must use the reading skills he gained as a child or adult to convey the essence and spirit of the book. In short, people use literacy skills to support and guide the activities that are required to function independently in society, as well as to enjoy those that give them personal gratification.

But in a society that places such a high value on the attainment of literacy, problems and issues abound. As Kozol (1985, p. 4) succinctly stated, "Twenty-five million American adults cannot read the poison warnings on a can of pesticide, a letter from their child's teacher, or the front page of a daily paper." And "parents who cannot read often raise children who cannot read" (Bush, 1990, p. 143). Each time the National Assessment of Educational Progress releases new statistics on the reading and writing achievement of American youths, the general public is assaulted with more bad news on the low level of literacy of young people. In the 1992 writing assessment of students in the 4th, 8th, and 12th grades, researchers found that "fewer than 20 percent of students can write at an 'elaborated'— or well-developed and detailed—level to complete a short assignment" ("New NAEP Report," 1994, p. 36).

A multitude of issues also surround the teaching of literacy skills. Proponents of whole language are urging that basal readers—the cornerstone of reading instruction for much of the century—be tossed out the window. Some suggest that teachers, not basal readers, are at the root of the problem. Given the perception that the educational system is failing, national television and radio advertisements—aimed primarily at parents—tout the advantages of programs to teach phonics to children who are having difficulty learning to read. Similar issues confront local and state literacy councils and adult education programs regarding what and how to teach adults who are illiterate. Since so many people have a stake in promoting literacy or benefiting from it, it is not surprising that many are involved in trying to shape literacy practices.

Educators and rehabilitation specialists who work with persons with visual impairments are also dealing with weighty issues concerning the phenomenon of literacy. This chapter reviews some of the issues and concerns that confront these professionals and provides some insights into their impact on instructional practices. Although a child's congenital visual impairment does not prevent the attainment of literacy, and, similarly, an adult's adventitious visual impairment does not prevent the reattainment of literacy, low vision may present unique challenges that must be addressed to ensure full literacy. Given the essential relationship of literacy to employment, independent living, and success in many aspects of life, this chapter presents a framework for understanding the unique aspects of literacy for persons with low vision, along with implications for ensuring the meaningful growth and application of literacy skills.

CONCERNS AND ISSUES FOR CHILDREN AND YOUTHS

Perhaps it is an overstatement to say that a renaissance is now taking place in the way professionals in the field are thinking about, defining, and teaching literacy to individuals with low vision—or perhaps not. The term *renaissance* is defined as "a movement or period of vigorous . . . intellectual activity" and as a "rebirth, revival" (*Merriam Webster's Collegiate Dictionary*, 1993, p. 990). At present, professionals in the education and rehabilitation of persons with visual impairments are engaged in a vigorous reexamination and restructuring of practices related to literacy, especially for those with low vision. Most would agree that this renaissance is much needed and long overdue. And it is interesting to note that the catalyst for this period of renewal has been the subject of braille.

Organizations of consumers—most notably the American Council of the Blind and the National Federation of the Blind—have done much to focus the field of blindness and visual impairment on issues of literacy. These groups staunchly uphold the value and benefits of braille as a means of achieving literacy for people who are blind. They have often been joined by other groups, such as the American Foundation for the Blind, in efforts to ensure that braille is regarded as an appropriate and important option for blind and visually impaired readers. These groups have been instrumental in promoting "braille legislation" throughout the United States. These bills, which have been passed in many states, generally provide assurances that students will receive appropriate assessment for the need for braille and, when appropriate, proper instruction in braille literary skills.

Students with low vision are at the center of the debate over teaching braille reading and writing. All agree that braille must be taught to students who are functionally blind, but the decision is not so easily made with students who have low vision. By definition, individuals with low vision often can use their vision to accomplish a variety of tasks, including reading and writing (see Chapter 1). Consumer groups, however, question the efficiency of a reliance on print reading and writing for many people with low vision, especially those who are legally blind. Issues related to definitions are one area addressed here; other issues that are discussed are the emphasis on the use of vision, the lack of assessment procedures, and various options for gaining access to print.

Issues of Definition

Some consumers and professionals believe that the definition of legal blindness is an appropriate mechanism for identifying people who would benefit from braille reading and writing programs. In fact, some state laws use this definition as a criterion for ensuring that braille instruction is considered for a given student. However, as was indicated in Chapter 1, the definition of legal blindness is an arbitrary measure of visual acuity that has little relation to how an individual uses the sensory channels for learning. Therefore, basing decisions about the introduction of braille reading and writing programs on an arbitrary cutoff point, rather than on the identified needs of individuals, suggests that the value of braille in a person's life may likewise be arbitrary—that the person might or might not benefit from braille reading skills.

Persons with low vision are put squarely in the middle of the controversy about the definition of legal blindness simply by how well they resolve letters on a distance eye chart. Since the majority of them (approximately 90 percent—see Chapter 1) have vision that is useful for learning, most will benefit from learning to read and write in print. Also, legal definitions take into account only distance visual functioning, which is not the type of vision that is used for most literacy tasks. Although no data exist on the proportion of people who are legally blind and who are efficient print readers, a number of people who are legally

blind do attain normal reading speeds and are able to sustain reading for sufficient periods to complete desired tasks.

Legislation on braille that uses the definition of legal blindness generally includes a provision stating that braille instruction is not required if direct evidence can be provided to support such a decision. This type of provision is beneficial in that it allows decisions to be made for individual students, thereby reducing the arbitrariness of using legal blindness as the criterion for offering instruction in braille reading and writing. However, such a provision circumvents the process of assessment and instructional planning. A best-practices approach holds that the findings of an assessment lead to the identification of a student's needs and that these needs are the foundation of a student's Individualized Education Program (IEP). When a need—braille reading and writing instruction—is presumed or determined beforehand, the findings of an assessment must then support what may not be needed, rather than what may be needed.

In contrast to legal definitions, functional definitions of visual impairment provide information about an individual's sensory functioning, generally focusing on whether the person approaches tasks visually or tactilely. On the one hand, individuals who primarily use vision as an approach to learning are likely to use print as a literacy medium, since reading print is a visual skill. On the other hand, those who mainly use touch as their primary avenue of learning are likely to use braille as a literacy medium, since reading braille is a tactile skill.

Although functional definitions provide some information on an individual's sensory functioning and approach to learning tasks, they are insufficient to match a person with an appropriate literacy medium. Some individuals may approach tasks visually at a distance, but prefer tactile methods at near point. Others may clearly be visual learners but have a progressive or unstable eye condition that requires attention to learning nonvisual approaches. Still others may be auditory learners, but few professionals would advocate relying solely on audiotaped books or live readers as the primary literacy medium.

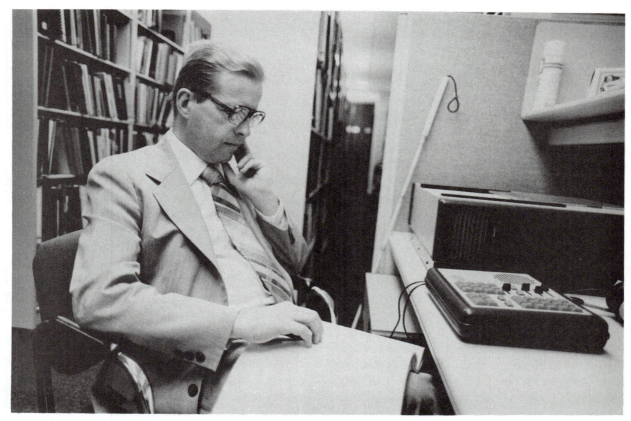

A range of options is available for persons with low vision to gain access to print material; selection of appropriate media is based on individual preferences, abilities, and needs.

The conclusion is that neither legal nor functional definitions of blindness and visual impairent alone are adequate for selecting appropriate literacy media. Rather, decisions on literacy media must be made on the basis of objective information gained through a systematic and ongoing process guided by the principles of diagnostic teaching (see Chapter 11).

Emphasis on the Use of Vision

Educational practices seem prone to the swinging of the pendulum. During the first half of the 20th century, students who were legally blind were routinely taught braille reading and writing. This was an absolute and therefore arbitrary practice, especially in residential schools, that represented an extreme swing of the pendulum in one direction. During the 1960s, the pendulum began to swing rapidly in the other direction with the advent of research on the effectiveness of instructional programs to increase visual efficiency. This emphasis became so ingrained in the 1970s and 1980s that teachers adopted the philosophy of using vision "at all costs," sometimes even when the use of touch or another sense would have been more efficient. (See Chapter 17 for a further discussion of this history.)

The focus on the use of vision led to the belief that reading print was the practice of choice if students had any vision with which to do so. Although some students attained only minimal reading rates with print, print reading was often still considered to be the preferred practice. At the same time, during this period, braille was generally considered to be the medium of "last resort." This perception undoubtedly prevented some students with low vision who could have benefited from braille reading and writing from receiving appropriate instruction in its use.

With the advent of legislation on braille and the renewed focus on issues of literacy for persons with visual impairments, in the 1990s the pendulum is swinging once more. This time, it is to be hoped that it will stop in a moderate and central position. More emphasis is now being placed on using a combination of media to attain full literacy. Braille is included in a repertoire of literacy tools for an individual with low vision more often than in the past. The process of making informed decisions on the contribution of braille to the total repertoire, though, will become increasingly important to the attainment of literacy by persons with low vision.

Lack of Assessment Procedures

Before 1990, there were few, if any, assessment processes and strategies for selecting appropriate literacy media for students with visual impairments. Teachers usually made decisions unilaterally, without much input from other members of the educational team, and on the basis of "professional judgment," which was greatly influenced by the prevailing educational practice of the time that emphasized visual efficiency. When decisions were made on the basis of "conventional practices" and without solid objective data to support them, some students with low vision were not given literacy instruction in an appropriate medium or combination of media. Furthermore, even though many people with low vision were using print as a primary literacy medium, little attention was paid to objective measures of reading rates and stamina.

One of the more positive, although largely indirect, outcomes of the legislation on braille was the initiation of research on appropriate, objective assessment strategies for selecting literacy media for students with visual impairments, since most such legislation mandates the use of some kind of assessment to identify students who will or will not benefit from braille reading and writing instruction. This requirement ensures that all decisions are guided by objective data and informed team decisions. Much work has been

accomplished in this area in the past few years, and much more work is being done today. Chapter 11, which is devoted to the selection of appropriate learning and literacy media, is evidence of the body of knowledge that has been generated in only a short time.

Print Media and Literacy

Large print is a valuable way for some people with low vision to gain access to print information, but it cannot be the only option. Reliance only on large print restricts one's access to information and requires the use of a photocopy enlarger or another means of enlarging materials that are not commercially available.

Whereas some people believe that braille and 18-point type (standard large type) are the only options for readers with low vision, others believe that it should first be determined whether students will benefit from using optical devices. If the only option permitted for students with low vision is braille or large print, then assessment remains incomplete because the size of type and the approach to print access appropriate for the individual may still be issues. However, if those who can read 18-point type are assessed for the use of optical devices, then a meaningful comparison with braille reading and writing can be made. Some individuals who cannot sustain the reading of large print unaided can be efficient readers with optical devices.

Part of functional literacy is the ability to gain access to print independently when information is not in one's preferred medium. Hence, in developing functional literacy in persons with low vision, teachers and rehabilitation professionals should focus on providing a range of options for doing so. Optical devices are an instant, effective, and inexpensive way to gain such access, both at near point and at a distance. The use of nonvisual media, including audiotaped materials, synthetic speech produced on computers, and live readers, should also be learned. Both teachers of students with visual impairments and rehabilitation specialists should take responsibility for expanding children's and adult's options for gaining access to print and should never restrict options because of personal biases or poor-quality, fragmented services.

ISSUES FOR ADULTS

When adults develop low vision, the two major losses they usually experience are the ability to read and the ability to drive a car. Reading is necessary for earning one's livelihood and for caring for oneself and others and is a source of recreation. Therefore, it is imperative that adults with acquired low vision are taught strategies for continuing to read as soon as possible. Whether an individual is interested in learning to play bridge, keeping a job as a bookkeeper, or trying new recipes in cookbooks, life without reestablishing literacy skills can result in feelings of isolation, reduced social interactions, lowered self-esteem, and possible unemployment. (For more information on the rehabilitation needs of working-age and older adults, see Chapters 14, 15, and 16.)

Although the majority of people who are evaluated at low vision clinics for the prescription of low vision devices are adults or elderly people with adventitious visual impairments, many individuals are not referred for clinical low vision evaluations for several reasons. First, ophthalmologists and optometrists are often reluctant to refer their patients to low vision clinics when they are unfamiliar with the benefits that can be derived from such evaluations. Second, many localities do not have low vision clinics, so adults have to travel long distances to obtain specialized clinical services or do not know about them. Finally, eye care providers do not always feel an obligation to refer patients to other professionals for the purpose of regaining literacy skills. Therefore, it is crucial for professionals to give adults information about clinical low vision services.

In prescribing low vision devices for adults with acquired low vision, professionals must match the ready availability and use of the devices with the real-life function and value they provide. Rehabilitation specialists must objectively examine reading rates that are necessary for specific jobs or daily living skills and reading rates that their clients can attain using low vision

devices. If there is a mismatch between need and function or if a person is not taught how to use a device, he or she is not likely to persist, and the device will end up in a drawer.

When an adult receives a prescription for an optical device, he or she may not be given options for the mounting system to be used, which may limit the device's usefulness. For example, a 75-year-old person may be presented with a magnifier embedded in a pair of eyeglasses but be unable to hold reading materials at the close working distance required by the lens for an extended period; a CCTV may thus be a better option for this person, but the eye care provider may not have considered it because of the expense, even though this particular client could have easily afforded it. In addition, for those who cannot or choose not to use optical devices but need more information than is available in large-print publications, computers are an option. However, many adults with acquired low vision are not assessed for and do not receive instruction in computer-generated magnification or spoken output.

A complex issue facing rehabilitation specialists is the teaching of literacy skills to adults who are illiterate and acquire a visual impairment. In such cases, the focus of intervention is not simply on providing an alternate medium, because the person does not have skills to be reestablished. Rather, in such cases, rehabilitation specialists must pair general information on teaching illiterate adults to read with a knowledge of specialized methods for teaching compensatory skills to adults with acquired low vision. This may be a challenge for service providers because they have been prepared to teach compensatory skills, but not necessarily beginning reading skills, to adults.

FACETS AND LEVELS OF LITERACY

A multitude of factors affect the literacy of persons with visual impairments and cannot be presented in a single definition. Koenig's (1992) framework for understanding the unique aspects of literacy for this population includes the following four facets:

◆ There is widespread agreement that reading and writing are the fundamental processes of literacy. Although a variety of related skills—such as computer skills, numeracy (mathematics) skills, and problem-solving skills—are often included as part of literacy, these skills are generally specific applications of reading and writing.

◆ Successful and meaningful communication between a sender (writer) and a receiver (reader) is at the heart of literacy. For communication to be meaningful, the participants must share a common background of experiences and must address each other's receptive literacy demands. For example, an individual may generate a document in braille using an accessible computer and then generate a print copy for a person who reads print. When a person is communicating with himself or herself (such as when writing a list or a diary entry), the person uses his or her preferred literacy medium.

◆ Literacy is demonstrated by the successful and meaningful application of reading and writing to accomplish desired and required literacy tasks in all environments. Thus, it is goal directed and serves specific purposes and functions in a person's life. (See Table 4.1, which presents a number of literacy tasks that are performed in various environments, categorized according to the intended audience.) People demonstrate literacy when they accomplish tasks that they need for daily functioning and those they wish to do for personal gratification. When necessary, a person with low vision must gain access to print independently, such as by using low vision devices.

◆ Literacy is demonstrated at various levels throughout one's life. Koenig (1992) proposed three levels of literacy—emergent, academic (or basic), and functional—gleaned from general literacy theory. Table 4.2 presents the defining characteristics of and a sample of behaviors associated with

each level. The following sections discuss these levels, with special consideration for fostering growth in or reestablishing literacy for individuals with low vision.

Emergent Literacy

Emergent Literacy for Young Children

Emergent literacy is a young child's earliest attempts to bring meaning to reading and writing tasks. Young children show that they are constructing meaning when they listen to someone read and perhaps pick out familiar or repeated words or retell a story later by referring to the pictures. When they draw pictures to convey meaning or scribble and then relate the message conveyed, they are also demonstrating emergent literacy.

As the term *emergent* suggests, these early literacy skills tend to develop naturally in young children with normal vision without much or any planned involvement by adults. Since observation and interactions with mature, literate models are the major stimulators and reinforcers of emergent literacy, children with low vision need direct and planned opportunities to gain these experiences that children with normal vision gain incidentally.

The essential foundation for reading and writing is a range of enriched experiences. When an author writes a story, it is a variety of experiences that makes the writing meaningful to the reader. Thus, to understand what an author has written, the reader must share a similar frame of reference.

Children with normal vision experience many things vicariously—without direct participation—through various means, such as observation of others participating in an activity, looking at pictures in books, and watching television and movies. For example, most people, including children, understand space travel to some extent by watching television news programs of space missions or movies about astronauts. Although such vicarious experiences are not the same as real experiences, it is possible to

Table 4.1. Literacy Tasks Requiring Communication with Self and Communication with Others in Four Environments

Audience	Environment			
	Home	School	Community	Work
Communicating with self[a]	Labeling personal items	Jotting down assignments	Writing shopping lists	Jotting down notes to oneself
	Maintaining an address and telephone book	Taking notes in class	Writing directions to a specific location	Making lists of "things to do"
Communicating with others[b]	Writing personal letters to friends	Reading textbooks and workbooks	Completing deposit slips at banks	Reading memos from supervisors
	Paying bills	Reading periodicals	Reading signs	Writing reports
	Reading mail	Writing term papers	Reading menus	Reading gauges and dials
	Reading for pleasure	Completing assignments	Signing documents	Filling out forms
	Reading newspapers	Taking tests	Writing checks at stores	Reading job manuals
	Reading books to others	Filling out registration forms	Reading labels on items at stores	Writing work-related correspondence

Source: From A. J. Koenig, "A Framework for Understanding the Literacy of Individuals with Visual Impairments." *Journal of Visual Impairment & Blindness,* 86 (1992), pp. 277–284. Copyright 1992 by the American Foundation for the Blind. Excerpted with permission.

[a]The individual is both the writer and the intended reader.

[b]The individual is either the writer or the intended reader, but not both.

gain a basic understanding of events and activities through them.

Children with low vision, in contrast, differ widely in their use of observation and visual media for gaining experiences. Depending on a child's use of vision, experiences gained through passive observation may represent complete information, fragmented information, or inaccurate information. A best-practices approach to educating students with low vision upholds the principles of a multisensory and active experiential approach to learning and gaining basic life experiences. When a student actively participates in learning activities and makes use of all sources of sensory information, he or she will gain meaningful experiences to undergird reading and writing tasks. The use of vision can be meaningfully integrated into all experiences, such as locating a newspaper delivered to one's front door or picking out one's favorite cereal from among boxes on shelves in a supermarket.

Emergent literacy is the earliest phase in literacy learning in which young children are actively engaged in experimenting with reading and writing and in gaining meaning from these activities. Young children with normal vision are continually exposed to literacy events, including the following:

◆ encountering signs that mean something to them (such as the "golden arches" of McDonald's)

◆ hearing parents read a newspaper and comment on its contents

◆ hearing parents read letters from grandparents and friends

◆ seeing people write shopping lists or notes

◆ having parents read aloud to them.

Table 4.2. Levels of Literacy for Individuals with Visual Impairments

Level	Defining Characteristics	Sample Behaviors
Emergent literacy	Development of awareness of the purposes and functions of reading and writing in the preferred medium during the preschool years Meaningful attempts at early reading and writing tasks	Listening to someone read Associating signs in the environment with certain activities or events Scribbling and "reading" a message Recognizing one's name and some letters in print or braille
Academic (basic) literacy	Mastery of reading and writing skills at the eighth-grade level in the preferred medium	Demonstrating reading skills at the eighth-grade level on objective tests, with commensurate skills in writing, in the preferred medium
Functional literacy	Demonstration of literacy tasks required for independent functioning at home, in school, in the community, and at work Use of strategies to gain independent access to print Development of additional communication skills as the demands of tasks and needs change and as new options become available	Asking a store clerk to state the value of bills Using telecommunications and other technology to read a newspaper in an accessible medium Using accessible word processing to prepare reports in print Requesting assistance from a sighted reader to complete a job application Learning to use a new technological device by reading the owners' manual and using the company's technical-assistance hot line

Source: From A. J. Koenig, "A Framework for Understanding the Literacy of Individuals with Visual Impairments," *Journal of Visual Impairment & Blindness,* 86 (1992), pp. 277–284. Copyright 1992 by the American Foundation for the Blind. Excerpted with permission.

As young children observe these literacy events, they naturally try to imitate them. Scribbling and then telling someone what it means is an initial experience in writing, and describing the pictures in a storybook ("reading") is an early experience in reading. The key element in both activities is the meaning that is constructed (through scribbling) and gained (through "reading"). Such meaningful behaviors are part of emergent literacy.

Young children with low vision may not have the same ready access to naturally occurring literacy activities. Therefore, the teacher of students with visual impairments and parents must provide direct exposure to such literacy events. Strategies for doing so are presented in Chapter 12.

Aspects of Reestablishing Literacy for Adults

Adults who are adventitiously visually impaired have already gained extensive life experiences, so there is no need for them or rehabilitation teachers who work with them to focus on experiences or early exposure to literacy events. Rather, in reestablishing literacy skills, attention needs to be paid to relearning visual skills and learning to use low vision devices. If instruction in braille reading is given, tactile readiness activities are necessary. In any case, it is important to keep in mind that the foundation of literacy essentially has already been established.

Illiterate adults with adventitious low vision

pose different concerns. Although they have had life experiences with which to bring meaning to literacy events, the link between written words and meaning has yet to be established. Because these individuals usually make use of some associations with signs and symbols in the environment (such as the knowledge that a red sign at an intersection means "stop"), instruction should focus on linking other written symbols and words with meaningful tasks in their lives. The extent to which an illiterate adult will progress through the emergent literacy phase is probably an academic concern, since the practical aspect of instruction is to move as expeditiously as possible to meaningful literacy events with which the person can perform daily and employment-related tasks.

Academic Literacy

Academic Literacy in Schools

Academic (or basic) literacy is characterized by the mastery of reading and writing skills that one typically learns in school. There is a growing recognition that the types of literacy skills that are acquired in school, such as reading and responding to connected pieces of text and writing stories or term papers, are unique to educational settings. More practical applications of literacy that are used in the workplace or the community, such as writing short memos to co-workers, completing forms, writing checks, and reading signs, tend to be learned through observation and practice, rather than through systematic instruction. Therefore, these two broad types of literacy (academic and practical) are increasingly being differentiated according to the function they serve in people's lives, as well as the process used to gain them.

Academic literacy is important for a number of reasons. First, it is a key indicator of success in school and often is considered more important by society than other skills. Also, some occupations, such as teaching and journalism, require the use of this type of literacy. Second, one can continue to develop and expand literacy skills—

and learning in general—using the basic reading and writing skills that one gains in school (Venezky, 1990). Third, this basic level of literacy allows one to learn or develop more practical uses of literacy if such instruction is not provided directly in school; for example, a person may use academic literacy skills to read the directions on a credit-card application or a menu in a restaurant. Fourth, academic literacy provides the skills needed for many literacy tasks in which an individual may engage for personal enjoyment and gratification, such as writing in a diary, reading for pleasure, and reading aloud to young children.

For children with visual impairments, academic literacy is taught and assessed in the literacy medium that is typically used daily in the classroom. Thus, students with low vision who primarily use large print will be taught academic literacy in this medium. Many students, however, acquire and apply skills in the use of optical and nonoptical devices to gain access to information in regular print during the elementary school years. Although gaining access to information that is not in one's primary literacy medium is a specific characteristic of functional literacy, students with low vision often combine aspects of academic literacy and functional literacy earlier than do students who are functionally blind.

Koenig (1992) proposed an eighth-grade reading level in the primary literacy medium as a standard for judging an acceptable level of academic literacy. This criterion was based on a review of standards proposed by others, as well as an analysis of the readability of various documents, such as newspapers, owners' manuals, and pamphlets and brochures for consumers. It is noteworthy, however, that no commonly accepted standard for judging academic literacy has been adopted by professionals either in the field of general literacy or in the field of visual impairment. In judging academic literacy for children with low vision, a grade-level criterion is not enough. Students must also be able to read at a sufficient rate and level of stamina and with relative comfort to make print reading a viable means of gaining information. Strategies for addressing these unique aspects of assessing reading are presented in Chapter 11.

To develop solid and meaningful academic literacy skills, students with low vision must be continuously involved with teachers of students with visual impairments, either through direct instruction or through consultation, depending on their individual needs. Teachers should not assume that students with low vision will automatically progress like their classmates with normal vision because both groups use some form of print media. Such an assumption fails to take into account the unique aspects of learning to read with low vision and the specific strategies that teachers need to use to ensure that students with low vision develop academic literacy skills. Nevertheless, teachers should not assume that having low vision will limit children's attainment of normal literacy skills. Strategies for teaching basic, academic literacy skills are presented in Chapter 12.

Aspects of Academic Literacy for Adults

For adults with adventitious low vision who have been referred for clinical low vision evaluations, several aspects of reestablishing literacy may present problems. First, they may have already determined that they cannot read any longer and may refuse any optical devices presented to them because using these devices does not represent reading as they recall the process. Second, the close working distance needed to read with spectacle-mounted optical devices is contrary to the method that represented a comfortable experience for them in the past. Third, older adults may accept or reject optical devices on the basis of what reading represents in their lives. For example, if a son or daughter comes each week to take care of paying bills, the older person may be concerned that these visits will not be as frequent if he or she can handle the bills and hence may not want to practice reading with a prescribed optical device.

Furthermore, the techniques for reestablishing literacy with certain age-related impairments may be difficult for some individuals to learn.

Those who have lost the use of their central vision will need to learn to use peripheral vision to read. Those who have slow reading rates, even with instruction and practice, will need to determine whether reading in print is efficient or whether other means, such as braille reading, are more comfortable for them. They may find that academic-style reading is not important but will use optical devices, nonoptical devices, and various techniques for functional literacy tasks. (See Chapters 3 and 7 for more information on these devices and techniques.)

Functional Literacy

Characteristics

Functional literacy "focuses on the specific literacy tasks that are of practical significance in one's daily life and one's success in performing them in appropriate environments" (Koenig, 1992, p. 281). The list of literacy tasks presented in Table 4.1 gives examples of the ways in which literacy is used at home, at school, in the community, and in the workplace. In a sense, functional literacy is the most straightforward type of literacy to understand, assess, and teach because its ultimate criterion is functional utility. If a particular literacy task is of sufficient importance to increase independence or employability, then it becomes part of the functional-literacy curriculum. In general, the literacy tasks performed in the workplace are specific to certain occupations.

Functional literacy should not be misconstrued as a rudimentary level of literacy; rather, it involves practical ways to use reading and writing skills in daily life. Academic literacy includes a knowledge of words and comprehension skills, but does not necessarily ensure that an individual will use these skills to complete practical tasks that require reading and writing. For example, a child may read, understand, and respond meaningfully to a book, such as *Charlotte's Web*, but may not automatically transfer this process to reading directions on a box of frozen food. Thus, one responsibility of a teacher of students with visual impairments or a rehabilitation specialist is to provide direct instruction in the practical uses of literacy and not assume that individuals with low vision will automatically generalize their academic literacy skills to other situations.

There are two interrelated characteristics of functional literacy: the successful performance of literacy tasks that are required in daily life and the use of skills or tools to gain independent access to print information (Koenig, 1992). For persons with low vision, the successful accomplishment of a task is largely dependent on gaining access to the information needed to complete it. Therefore, a variety of literacy tools (including optical and nonoptical devices, live readers, synthetic speech, technological approaches, and large-print or braille materials) should be available to them, so they may assess the demands of a given task and then choose the tool that will allow them to complete it most efficiently.

Self-Advocacy and Critical Literacy

Part of functional literacy is judging the demands of a given literacy task and then skillfully selecting from among a range of options the one that will be most helpful in readily and efficiently completing the task. Sometimes, the option may involve requesting assistance from another person. For example, an individual (with or without low vision) may need to ask a waiter to point to the signature line to sign a credit-card receipt in a dimly lit restaurant. Or a person with low vision may need to ask a receptionist to read the "fine print" to fill out a complex form at a physician's office. Or a high school student may need to ask a teacher who uses transparencies to structure lectures in a chemistry class to provide a desk copy of the transparencies so he or she can study them. All these situations require the individual to advocate for himself or herself to complete the tasks at hand as efficiently as possible. Without such advocacy skills, a person may either not be able to complete certain tasks or may perform them with less accuracy. Therefore, functional literacy is inseparably intertwined with self-advocacy skills.

In addition, a higher level of cognition and problem solving needs to accompany the completion of these functional tasks. Calfee (1994, p. 27) referred to this level as critical literacy, which "includes the capacity for action, but also incorporates a broader sense of understanding and insight." For example, when a person pulls a lever in a voting booth after reading and choosing from a list of candidates (functional literacy), his or her choice is based on a broader understanding of the issues involved in deciding which candidate to vote for (critical literacy).

This distinction between functional and critical literacy is important for teachers and rehabilitation specialists to keep in mind as they teach literacy skills to persons with low vision. For instance, whereas teaching an individual to sign a credit-card receipt is a functional literacy task, developing the understanding that a bill to be paid will ultimately come in the mail and that not paying the entire amount will result in additional charges involves critical literacy. The degree of understanding and insight to be developed depends on the individual's level of cognitive functioning. However, addressing this realm of instruction to the extent possible for each person is important for developing meaningful literacy skills and should not be overlooked by professionals in visual impairment.

Although adults with adventitious low vision may be aware of the additional pieces of information that are needed to make decisions involving critical literacy, students with low vision may not have acquired such knowledge. For example, young adults with low vision may know that credit-card bills have information about the amount owed on the front of the statement. They may not know that some statements include rates for finance charges in light-colored ink on the backs of the statements; yet this information can be critical for determining how much of the bill an individual will pay.

SUMMARY

The attainment and improvement of literacy is a basic right of all people throughout life. To help individuals with low vision attain literacy, professionals in the field of visual impairment need to maintain an ongoing involvement in their literacy programs, providing direct instruction or consultation as needed. The following principles will guide professionals in fostering the development of literacy in both children and adults with low vision:

- Ensure that young children have a wealth of basic life experiences and direct access to early literacy events.

- Ensure that students develop academic literacy skills that allow for reading with efficiency, stamina, comfort, and enjoyment during the school years.

- Teach persons with low vision multiple strategies for gaining independent and ready access to information.

- Ensure that persons with low vision develop functional literacy skills for completing daily tasks that are important for independent living and work.

- Address the unique needs of adults with adventitious visual impairment in reestablishing literacy by teaching them new approaches to reading with low vision.

- Address the needs of illiterate adults with acquired visual impairments by providing opportunities for literacy to be important and meaningful in their lives.

ACTIVITIES

With This Chapter and Other Resources

1. Write a brief description to illustrate how Cecillia (see the vignette that opens the chapter) might have described her literacy skills and tools to her employer.

2. List all the ways in which you use academic, functional, and critical literacy skills during a typical day. Determine the types of adaptations you would need to make if you were a person with low vision.

3. Adults with acquired low vision encounter certain issues in reestablishing literacy skills. Describe how you might address some of these issues during the first and second instructional sessions with an adult who has just received a prescribed optical device.

4. Children with low vision may encounter regular classroom teachers and others who believe they cannot attain academic literacy with their visual impairments. Discuss how one could alter this perception of the literacy potential of children with low vision.

5. Gather three to five definitions of literacy used by conventional literacy theorists. Discuss the implications of these definitions for persons with low vision and whether they would have to be modified to be equally applicable to this population.

In the Community

1. Ask a rehabilitation teacher and a clinical low vision specialist about the special problems that adults face in reestablishing literacy.

2 Spend time with a middle school student with normal vision. List the functional literacy tasks that the student completes after school.

With a Person with Low Vision

1. Interview an adult who has reestablished literacy and discuss the process and emotional impact of doing so.

2. Speak with a teenager who has low vision to learn how he or she accomplishes functional literacy tasks and determine whether additional strategies are needed.

From Your Perspective

In what ways might the focus on braille-related legislation and instructional practices continue to have a positive impact on the literacy of persons with low vision?

PART TWO

Clinical Perspectives

Anatomy and Physiology of the Eye

Marjorie E. Ward

VIGNETTE

At age 8, Timmy really could not understand the long-term implications of having an eye removed, or enucleated. Because one of his eyes hurt and watered most of the time, and he could not see through it, he said he was ready to let it go. Even so, he woke up every night the week before the operation frightened by dreams of armored horsemen racing toward him with sharp, gleaming spears aimed at his face. He confided in his teacher of students with visual impairments, rather than his parents, because he could tell they were upset, and he did not want to add to their worries.

Timmy had many questions about the upcoming operation. How would he wake up? What would he be like? Could he see with just one eye? What about riding his bike and watching television? At the same time, Timmy's parents were wrestling with whether to proceed with the surgery that had been recommended. According to the ophthalmologist, Timmy's congenital glaucoma and cataract in his abnormally small right eyeball, coupled with chronic irritation, led to a situation that warranted immediate action. Timmy's teacher had talked with Timmy's parents several times by telephone and over coffee at their home one morning, and they had given her permis-

The author wishes to extend thanks to Charlie Agnon, M.D., ophthalmologist in private practice in Marysville, Ohio, for technical review of this chapter.

sion to speak with Timmy about the medical aspects of the surgery.

Today, the teacher heard Timmy running down the hall to the library where they met each week. She took a big breath and prepared for another heart-to-heart talk with this bright, perceptive, high-spirited little boy.

Now, Timmy was ready to ask the hard questions. Just what was the doctor going to do and how? What part of his eye was going to be cut, and what would the eye look like when the doctor was finished with surgery? Timmy knew about optic nerves, but he did not know if that part was going to be removed. The teacher's knowledge of anatomy, physiology, low vision, and visual efficiency would certainly be useful, albeit not sufficient, in the next hour.

INTRODUCTION

Much of the discussion in this chapter focuses on the details of the structures and functions of the human eye and how these structures transmit information to the human brain. Although such a discussion is important for understanding low vision, the major focus must remain on the person, the whole and unique human being, who, among many other characteristics, has low vision. Keeping that perspective should help the reader appreciate the many physical, personal, and en-

Table 5.1. Structures of the Eye and Their Functions

Structures	Location/Description	Functions
Around the Globe		
Orbit	Each side of the nose	Provides housing and protection
Orbital septum	The thick front margin of the orbit	Provides protection for the eyeball and contents of the eye socket
Eyebrow	On the thick skin that covers the orbital septum	Provides protection
Eyelid	Above and below the opening of the orbit	Provides protection and control of light
Eyelashes	At the margins of the eyelids	Provide protection
Conjunctiva	The mucous membrane lining the lids and covering the sclera	Provides protection, acts as source of tear elements
In the Lacrimal System		
Lacrimal gland	Anterior temporal orbit	Produces tears
Lacrimal puncta	The openings in the inner upper and lower margins of the eyelids	Collect excess tears
Canaliculi	At the inner corner of the eyelids	Provide passages for excess tears to drain from the puncta to the sac
Lacrimal sac	A lake or pool at the end of each canaliculus	Collects tears that drain into the nasolacrimal duct
Nasolacrimal duct	The tube leading from the lacrimal sac into the nasal cavity	Carries excess tears to the nasal cavity
In the Globe		
Sclera	The tough, white outer layer of the eyeball	Provides protection and form
Cornea	The avascular, clear, front portion of the outer layer	Lets light rays enter the eyes and converges the light rays
Iris	The colored circular disk behind the cornea and in front of the lens	Controls the amount of light entering the eyes
Ciliary Body	The portion of the uveal tract between the choroid and iris	
Ciliary process	Anterior zone of the ciliary body	Secretes the aqueous into the posterior chamber
Ciliary muscle	Area of the ciliary body adjacent to the sclera	Alters the power of the lens
Choroid	The layer between the sclera and the retina	Supplies blood to the retina
Retina	The inner sensory nerve layer next to the choroid that lines the posterior two-thirds of the eyeball	Reacts to light and transmits impulses to the brain
Lens	The transparent biconvex structure behind the pupil	Helps bring light rays to focus on the retina
Optic Nerve	The cranial nerve extending from the optic disk to the optic chiasm	Carries electrical impulses from the retina to the optic chiasm in the brain

(continued on next page)

Table 5.1. *Continued*

Structures	Location/Description	Functions
Vitreous Cavity	The space between the retina and the optic nerve posteriorly and between the lens and the ciliary body anteriorly	Holds the vitreous that helps maintain the shape of the eye
Anterior Chamber	The space between the cornea anteriorly and the pupil and lens posteriorly	Contains the aqueous that drains through the Canal of Schlemm
Posterior Chamber	The space between the back of the iris and the front of the lens and ciliary body	Receives the aqueous from the ciliary body and articulates with the anterior chamber through the pupil

vironmental factors that can influence the manner in which that person receives, interprets, and responds to visual information.

This chapter is organized around four major topics: structures surrounding the globe (eyeball), structures of the globe, the transmission of visual information from the eyes along the visual pathways to the brain, and the process of seeing in relation to vision. At the end of the chapter, the reader should have enough understanding of what vision is in the clinical sense to understand the functional implications of visual impairment (see Table 5.1 for a summary of the structures of the eye and their functions). The material presented in this chapter is based on the following sources: Barraga (1986); Goldberg (1991); Meredith (1975); Newell (1992); Rainwater (1971); Vaughan, Asbury, & Riordan-Eva (1995).

STRUCTURES AROUND THE GLOBE

The eyeballs, which are called globes, although they are not really globe shaped, are situated in bony cavities called the *orbits* (see Figure 5.1). Each orbit opens at the front, so light can enter the eye, and can be closed off by the *eyelids.* With each blink, the eyelids distribute *tears* from the *lacrimal system* across the cornea. The tears also bathe the *conjunctiva,* which covers the white part of the front of each eyeball and lines the inner surface of the eyelids. (In addition to the

following sections, which discuss these and other structures of the eye, Sidebar 5.1 presents some helpful terminology related to orientation of the structures of the eye.)

The Orbits

The two pear-shaped orbits lie on each side of the nose and provide safe housing for the eyeballs. The medial walls of the orbits are parallel to each other, with the nose protruding between them. The lateral wall of each orbit forms an angle, with its medial wall posteriorly at the apex. The angle spreads open to almost 45 degrees. Considered together, these two angles allow the eyes to cover a horizontal field of approximately 160 to 180 degrees and a vertical field of about 120 degrees (see Sidebar 5.2 for additional information on the visual fields).

Each orbit is made of seven bones that resemble triangular plates that fit together with their bases pointing toward the front, resulting in the pear shape. In adults, the orbit is approximately 1.6 inches (40 mm) deep. A major function of the orbit is to provide a safe place for the eyeball. The orbit contains

- ◆ the eyeball, approximately one inch in diameter, which rests in the anterior portion and takes up only about one-fifth of the space
- ◆ the optic nerve, which emerges from the posterior portion of the eyeball

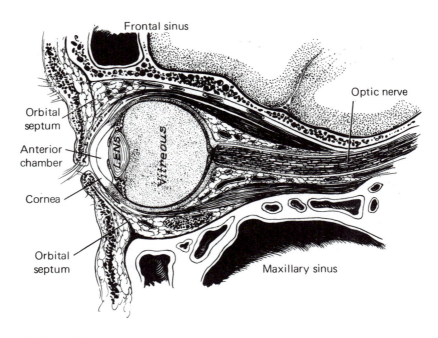

Frontal sinus

Optic nerve

Orbital
septum

Anterior
chamber

LENS

Vitreous

Cornea

Orbital
septum

Maxillary sinus

Figure 5.1. The Orbit and Its Contents

Source: Reprinted, by permission of the publisher, from D. G. Vaughan and T. Asbury, *General Ophthalmology,* 9th ed. (Los Altos, CA: Lange Medical Publications, 1980), p. 208.

- ◆ the six extrinsic muscles that are attached to both the orbit and the globe and move the eye
- ◆ other nerves, including those that innervate the extrinsic muscles
- ◆ blood vessels that nourish the various structures of the eye
- ◆ the lacrimal gland, which produces tears that bathe the front portion of the eye and the posterior side of the eyelids
- ◆ connective tissue that holds the various structures together
- ◆ fat that cushions the contents of the orbit from blows and jarring movement.

The apex of the orbit is the site of the opening for the optic nerve from the back of the eyeball and for blood vessels and nerves to pass through from outside the orbit. Five of the six extrinsic muscles that move the eyeball originate near the apex of the orbit; the sixth originates on the temporal side of the orbit close to the front margin.

The margin of the front opening, the *orbital septum,* is thick, particularly on the top, to provide additional protection for the front of the eyeball. The *eyebrows,* thickened skin from which the eyebrow hairs grow, cover the orbital septum of each eye socket and add another layer of protection.

Eyelids and Eyelashes

The eyelids, the thinnest skin of the body, protect the eye from foreign bodies, including dust, dirt, potentially hazardous liquids, and wind. The lids also help to limit the amount of light that enters the eye. Because the skin of the lids is so thin, however, light rays from the sun can burn it and can even penetrate it to cause damage to the *cornea,* the structure that forms the front part of the eyeball. Burns from intense heat, ultraviolet radiation, and chemicals can also damage the eyelids, as well as the tissues they cover.

By their blinking action, the eyelids also help to distribute tears, the oily film that lubricates the

SIDEBAR 5.1

Terms for Orientation to Structures of the Eye

Anterior	In front of, toward the front of the face	Medial	Toward the nose, nasal
Apex	Top, point of a cone	Nasal	Toward the nose, medial
Lateral	To the side of	Posterior	In back of, toward the back of the head
Margin	Edge, rim	Temporal	Toward the temple, lateral, toward the side of the head

cornea and the transparent conjunctiva. The margin of each eyelid is marked by the gray line, the line that divides the anterior from the posterior portion. The eyelashes are anterior to this line. Modified oil and sweat glands are located anterior to the line as well and open into the follicles of the lashes.

Posterior to the gray line are the tiny openings of the *meibomian glands*—modified sebaceous (oil) glands that secrete an oily layer, one of three layers that make up the tear film. This thin top layer of the tears slows down the evaporation of tear fluid and makes a seal when the eyes are shut, so the eyes do not dry out. The middle thick aqueous layer of tears, which is almost 98 percent water, is mixed with water-soluble salts and proteins that protect the eye from microorganisms and bacteria that could cause infections. The thin inner mucous layer of the tears serves to keep the corneal epithelium wet, so that the aqueous tear layer can spread easily over the surface.

Conjunctiva

The conjunctiva is a thin, translucent mucous membrane that helps protect the eyeball. Starting from the lid margin, it covers the posterior eyelid and then curves around and covers the *sclera*, the white part of the eyeball, and ends at the *limbus*, the point at which the sclera and the cornea meet. The conjunctiva contains many small accessory glands that also contribute to the film of mucous and tears that keeps the front part of the eye moist, smooth, and clean. It serves as a trans-

SIDEBAR 5.2

Visual Fields

The field of vision refers to the area one can see without shifting one's gaze. Because of the location of the eyeballs in the orbits and the position of the orbits in the head, the normal field of vision is approximately 160–180 degrees on the horizontal and 120 degrees on the vertical. The nasal fields of vision from each eye overlap when the eyes look straight ahead, but not the temporal. Field defects are denoted as nasal, temporal, superior, and inferior, terms that refer to space, not to the retinal site. For example, if a person has right superior field loss in the right eye, some of the retinal cells in the inferior nasal retina of the right eye are not functioning adequately or their message is not relayed accurately to the appropriate occipital lobe of the brain. In other words, one way to check retinal function and integrity of the optic pathways is to check visual fields and infer retinal function and integrity from what a person reports in each quadrant of the field.

parent barrier between the contents of the orbit (except the cornea) and everything in front it.

Lacrimal Apparatus

The lacrimal system (see Figure 5.2) consists of structures that produce the tears and structures that drain excess tears into the nasal passage. The lacrimal gland, which is located in the anterior temporal portion of the top of each orbital cavity, produces watery tears when the eye is irritated or when emotions trigger a teary response. Tears travel through ducts that empty onto the conjunctiva. The accessory glands of the conjunctiva, mentioned earlier, and the meibomian glands of the inner portion of the eyelids also contribute to the production of tears.

Tears wash over the surface of the eye and lids, moving toward the drainage system in the inner corner of the eyelid with each blink. The drainage system is made up of the openings called *puncta* at the inner margin of the upper and lower eyelids, the upper and lower *canaliculi* that lead to the *lacrimal sac*, and the *nasolacrimal duct* that extends down from the lacrimal sac

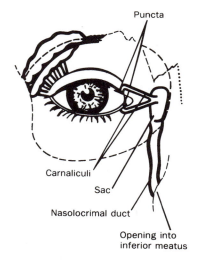

Puncta

Carnaliculi

Sac

Nasolocrimal duct

Opening into
inferior meatus

Figure 5.2. The Lacrimal System
Source: Reprinted, by permission of the publisher, from F. W. Newell & J. T. Ernest, *Ophthalmology: Principles and Concepts* (St. Louis, Mo: C. V. Mosby Co., 1974), p. 43.

and empties into the nose. The system typically floods when one cries, and tears overflow the margins of the eyelids and flow into the nose. In addition to revealing certain emotions and moistening the outer surface of the front of the eyeball, the cornea, and the lids, tears fill in the uneven surfaces on the transparent cornea, nourish the cornea, and wash out or attack microorganisms and bacteria that try to enter the eye.

STRUCTURES OF THE GLOBE

The globe consists of an outer protective layer, a middle vascular layer, and an inner sensory layer called the retina. The *optic nerve* emerges from the back of the globe and carries electrical impulses from the retina to the occipital lobe of the brain (see Figure 5.3).

Protective Outer Layer

The outer protective layer of the eye is made up of the white, fibrous, somewhat elastic, opaque sclera and the smaller, transparent cornea, through which light enters the eye. The sclera and cornea meet at the corneoscleral limbus, which is where the conjunctiva ends. The sclera helps to maintain the shape of the healthy eye; the external muscles attach to the sclera and work together to turn the eyes in the various directions of gaze.

The cornea is a five-layer, avascular, transparent tissue through which light rays first enter the eye on their way to the inner sensory retinal layer. The five layers are the epithelium, Bowman's membrane, the stroma, Descemet's membrane, and the endothelium. The outer layer, the epithelium, is bathed in tears and must be kept moist to maintain its transparency, nutritional status, and proper water balance.

The corneal stroma, the middle layer, makes up about 90 percent of the corneal thickness. It is separated from the epithelium by Bowman's membrane, and from the inner layer, the endothelium, by Descemet's membrane. Corneal

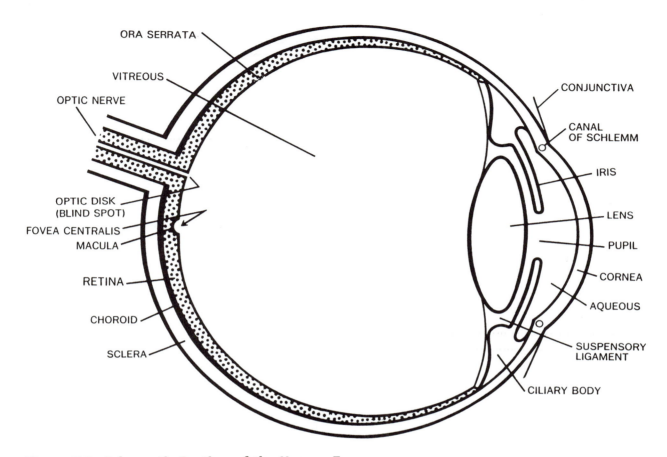

Figure 5.3. Schematic Section of the Human Eye

Source: Reprinted, by permission of the publisher, Prevent Blindness America, Schaumburg, IL.

abrasions that penetrate only the outer epithelium can be extremely painful, but they can heal quickly with little risk if they are cared for promptly. But if the stroma is penetrated, then both the stroma and endothelium become vulnerable to serious infection that can lead to corneal scarring and the loss of transparency. Scarring can interfere with functional vision to the degree that scars block or scatter light rays as they hit the surface of the cornea.

The cornea is transparent because of its uniform cellular structure, its avascularity, and its state of relative dehydration. Because the cornea is the "window" for the eye, any injury or disease that threatens the integrity of its layers puts the entire process of seeing clearly in jeopardy.

The cornea has the most refractive power (ability to bend light, that is, to change the direction in which light travels) of the eye. Light rays that enter the eye through the cornea are bent so they can converge at a point of focus on the retina, which is described later. If the eyeball is too long or too short on the horizontal axis or if the curvature of the cornea is irregular or insufficient, then the points of convergence of light will be in front of or behind the retina, or perhaps both, but on different axes. The eye is said to be *hyperopic* if the rays converge behind the retina, *myopic* if the rays converge in front of the retina, and *astigmatic* if the rays converge on more than one plane. These conditions are termed *refractive errors*. Figure 5.4 presents a diagram showing these condi-

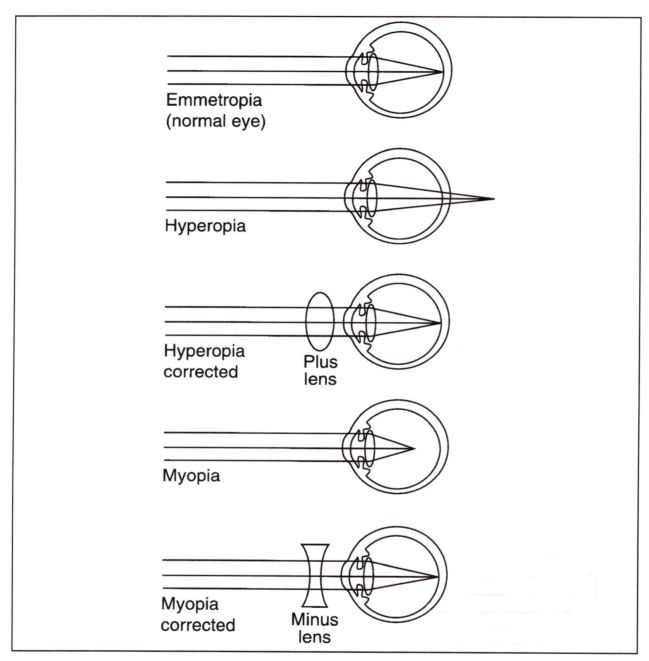

Figure 5.4. Refractive Errors and Lenses Used for Correction

tions and the way in which various lenses are used to correct them. A convex, or plus, lens that bends inward (converges) light rays is used to correct for hyperopia. A concave, or minus, lens that spreads out (diverges) light rays is used to correct for myopia. A cylindrical lens that has variable bending power on different meridians is used to correct for astigmatism. (For additional information on the movement of light and the different types of lenses, see Chapter 7.)

Vascular Middle Layer

The middle layer of the globe that lies underneath the sclera and behind the cornea is the *uveal tract*, made up of the iris, the ciliary body, and the choroid. The word *uvea* comes from the Latin word meaning grape, the color of the choroid. The uvea is a vascular layer that provides nutrition for the retina.

The *iris* (see Figure 5.5) is a circular muscular disk with a hole in the middle, called the *pupil*, that is located behind the cornea and in front of the lens. The iris acts as a diaphragm to control the size of the pupil, through which light rays must pass as they travel to the back of the eye. The color of the iris depends on how much melanin (pigmentation) is deposited within its posterior layers. The two muscles in the iris act to dilate and constrict the iris, thus enabling it to respond to and control the amount of light that enters the back of the eye. The dilator muscle contracts the iris to enlarge the pupil, while the sphincter muscle, located at the margin of the pupil, draws the margins together to decrease the size of the pupil. The size does not depend exclusively on the amount of light arriving at the iris, however; the dilator muscle, innervated by nerves from the sympathetic nervous system, reacts to enlarge the pupil in response to fear, as well as to light. The response of the pupils to light can therefore reveal much about the status and integrity of the central nervous system.

The *ciliary body* consists of the *ciliary process* and the *ciliary muscle*. The ciliary process secretes the *aqueous*, a plasmalike liquid that fills the chambers of the eye in front of and behind the iris. The ciliary muscle controls the amount of tension on the zonule fibers (suspensory ligaments) that attach to the lens capsule, which allows the shape of the lens to vary and hence the lens to accommodate for clear focus at different distances within the field of vision.

The *choroid* is sandwiched between the sclera and the *retina* (the eye's inner sensory layer) and extends from the optic nerve around to the ciliary body in the anterior portion of the globe. The choroid is a rich vascular layer that provides nourishment for the pigment epithelium layer of the retina.

Sensory Inner Layer

The inner sensory nerve layer of the eye, called the retina, lines the posterior two-thirds of the eyeball. It extends anteriorly to end in a scalloped or serrated edge called the ora serrata, continuing with the pars plana of the ciliary body. The retina receives information from the environment and transmits information to the brain. The retina has many layers of differential cells that articulate with each other to transmit information effectively on to the brain. The outer layer of cells that lies next to the choroid and is nourished by it is called the retinal pigment epithelium. The other layers together are often referred to as the sensory retina. In retinal detachment, the retina or layers of the retina split or become separated from the choroid.

Different types of cells make up the sensory retina. The photoreceptor cells, which lie next to the retinal pigment epithelium, activate modulator cells in the inner nuclear layer. The modulator

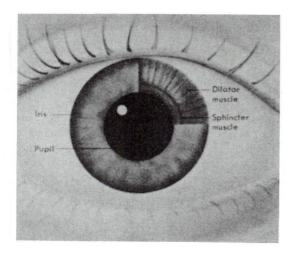

Figure 5.5. The Iris
Source: Reprinted, by permission of the publisher, from "Eye," *World Book Encyclopedia,* Vol. 6 (Chicago: World Book Publishing, 1995), p. 469.

Light and Dark Adaptation

SIDEBAR 5.3

Light adaptation is the ability of the eyes to adapt to different levels of illumination. When the eyes are adapted to dark, the rhodopsin in the rods is more concentrated, and the rod cells are sensitive to extremely low levels of light. At night, people use "night" vision or rods to detect the movement of shapes in dim light. But if lights are turned on, the eyes need some time to adapt to the higher level of illumination, and the pigments of the cone cells go into action. The eyes adapt much more quickly from dark to light than from light to dark because of the speed with which the pigments can be restored and re-formed. Going from dark to light means moving to levels of illumination that activate the cones, but going from light to dark requires time (10–30 minutes or more) for the rods to restore the rhodopsin that the light has bleached out and thus to adjust or adapt to the comparative darkness.

cells, in a sense, serve as condensers to enhance or inhibit the transfer of impulses and relay impulses at their synapses with the transmitter ganglion cells, the cells of the innermost layer of the sensory retina that is closest to the vitreous. The axons of the ganglion cells extend horizontally toward the back of the eye where they exit and become the optic nerve for each eye.

At first glance, the layers of the sensory retina may seem to be in reverse because the photoreceptor cells that are activated by light rays entering the eye lie next to the retinal pigment epithelium, farthest from the layer of the retina that the light rays encounter first. Thus, light rays must penetrate all the layers of the sensory retina before they can reach the photoreceptor cells (see Sidebar 5.3 for information on light and dark adaptation). But further examination reveals the logic of the arrangement.

The photoreceptor cells are of two types: the *rods,* approximately 110–130 million, that contain the pigment rhodopsin and are sensitive to the presence of light and motion, and the *cones,* approximately 6 million, that contain three different photopigments and give us the sense of color and fine detail. The *macula* is the area of the retina, about 0.16 inches (4 mm) in diameter, that is located on the temporal side of the *optic disk* where the nerve fibers from the inner layer of the retina exit the eyeball. The macula contains mostly cones, and the *fovea centralis*, the central portion of the macula, contains only cones. The tightly packed cones of the fovea give us the finest resolution of detail and color. Rods are distributed throughout the peripheral areas of the sensory retina, the area outside the macula.

The significance of the distribution of rods and cones is great. Peripheral vision (side vision) relies on rod cells to alert us to light, even dim light, and motion. When our gaze turns toward whatever catches our attention in the peripheral field of vision, the eye is repositioned, so the light rays reach the macula, where the cones are concentrated to give us detail and color information. The rods can function in low levels of illumination, whereas the cones require higher levels to function. This differential lighting requirement helps explain why we cannot sense colors or detail in dim light but can still detect motion. In that sense, the scotopic (rod) and photopic (cone) systems are independent. This fact becomes important if the rod cells lose function, as in the early stages of retinitis pigmentosa, or if the cones begin to degenerate, as in macular degeneration.

The process of seeing begins when light rays hit the rods and cones that make up the outer layer of the sensory retina. These rods and cones activate the modulator cells, which then communicate with the ganglion cells at their syn-

Where Is Your Blind Spot?

There are no photoreceptor cells at the optic disk, where the retinal ganglion cells collect, become the optic nerve, and leave the back of the globe. Therefore, this spot is a blind spot when visual field testing is done. To demonstrate this physiological blind spot, try this exercise:

+   ○

Cover or close your left eye. Look straight at the + with your right eye. Slowly move this book back and forth until the ○ disappears as you still stare at the +. At the point at which the ○ disappears, light rays from that point are hitting your physiological blind spot, where there are no rods or cones.

apses. The axons of the ganglion cells extend horizontally to the back of the eye and the optic disk, where they leave and become the optic nerve.

The outer segment of each rod and cone, the portion closest to the retinal pigment epithelium, is made up of as many as 1,000 flat disks surrounded by the light-sensitive pigments that mature and must be replaced by new ones. This is where the relationship of the photoreceptor cells to the retinal pigment epithelium becomes critical. The retinal pigment epithelium acts as a waste-management system by engulfing the mature disks and digesting them. If this system breaks down, debris builds up at this site and problems with retinal function can develop.

There are no cones or rods at the optic disk, where the axons from the ganglion cells of the inner layer of the sensory retina exit as the optic nerve. The result is a physiological blind spot in the field of vision where light rays entering the eye land on the disk. We are usually not aware of this spot because what we do not see with one eye we see with the other eye (see Sidebar 5.4).

Other Structures Inside the Eyeball

The lens and the three chambers of the inside of the eye have specific functions that allow light to reach the retina and that keep in balance the internal fluids of the eye. The *lens*, a biconvex-shaped transparent structure within each eye, is the only refractive or light-bending medium in the eye that can change its refractive power. As the ciliary muscle contracts and relaxes, changes occur in the tension of the zonule fibers that hold the lens in place behind the iris. These changes allow the lens to become more or less spherical, thus increasing or decreasing in power to bend light rays. This change in the shape of the lens enables the lens to direct light rays to converge to a point of focus on the retina and is part of the process called *accommodation.*

Accommodation actually includes three distinct changes in the eye. When a person looks from a distant object to a near object,

◆ the lens changes its shape to become more spherical, resulting in more power to bend light rays

◆ the eyes turn toward each other, so the images of an object fall on the maculas of each eye (resulting in binocular vision, or the ability to use both eyes together to form one image)

◆ the pupils become smaller as the iris sphincter muscle contracts.

When the person looks from a near object to a more distant target,

◆ the lens becomes less spherical and thus has less power to bend light rays

◆ the eyes diverge to maintain binocular vision to allow the images of the visual target to land on the corresponding portion of the macula of each eye

◆ the pupils dilate.

The lens capsule holds the lens fibers. These fibers continue to form throughout life and gradually become more and more tightly packed into the center of the lens as the lens matures. By middle age, the lens has usually lost most of the elasticity of its youth, thus decreasing its ability to accommodate. The lens fibers continue to form, however, and to be pushed into the nucleus of the lens.

Chambers of the Eye

There are three chambers in the eye: the anterior chamber, the posterior chamber, and the vitreous cavity. The *anterior chamber* and *posterior chamber* lie in front of the ciliary body and lens. The anterior boundary of the anterior chamber is the endothelium of the cornea, and the posterior boundary of the posterior chamber is the lens and ciliary body. The two chambers are separated by the iris and pupil. The aqueous secreted by the ciliary process flows from the posterior chamber through the pupil forward into the anterior chamber, where it filters through the *trabecular meshwork* into the *Canal of Schlemm*, located in the anterior angle of the eye. The aqueous nourishes the cornea and lens and helps to maintain the shape of and pressure inside the eye. If the flow of the aqueous is impeded, the intraocular pressure can rise, a condition referred to as glaucoma (see Chapter 6 for additional information about glaucoma).

Behind the lens lies the *vitreous cavity* containing the *vitreous*, a clear physiological gel (over 98 percent water) that accounts for two-thirds of the weight and volume of the globe and helps maintain its shape. Light rays emerge from the lens to pass through the vitreous and then enter the layers of the retina. Because light rays entering the eye from the superior (upper) visual field strike the inferior (lower) portion of the retina

and rays from the inferior field land on the superior retina, the image produced on the retina is upside down. The interpretation of what we see as right side up occurs in the brain, as will be discussed later.

Extrinsic Muscles of the Eye

The six *extrinsic muscles* of each eye work in coordination to turn and rotate each eyeball up, down, to the side, and toward the nose. The four rectus muscles arise from the apex of the orbit and attach to the sclera in front of the equator (the midpoint from the back of the eyeball to the front of the eyeball). The two oblique muscles are inserted into the sclera behind the equator (see Figure 5.6).

Each muscle has a primary action or function in turning the globe of the eye in various directions; this action is determined by the muscle's point of insertion in the sclera, its point of origin in the orbit, and the direction in which the eye is pointing when a new direction of gaze is needed. The muscles of each eye must work together to achieve the desired direction, in some cases con-

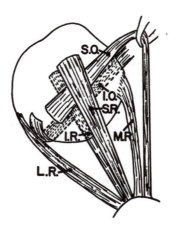

Figure 5.6. Extrinsic Muscles of the Eye
Viewed from above in this diagram, the six extrinsic muscles of the eye are the inferior oblique (I.O.), the inferior rectus (I.R.), the lateral rectus (L.R.), the medial rectus (M.R.), the superior oblique (S.O.), and the superior rectus (S.R.).

Source: Reprinted, by permission of the publisher, from S. Goldberg, *Ophthalmology Made Ridiculously Simple* (Miami: Medmaster, 1991), p. 6.

Table 5.2. Functions of the Extrinsic Eye Muscles

Eye Muscle	Nerve	Primary Function	Condition Caused by Deficit
Medial rectus	Oculomotor (CN III)	Moves eye nasally	Eye is turned downward and outward because of unopposed action of the lateral rectus and the superior oblique muscles
Lateral rectus	Abducens (CN VI)	Moves eye temporally	Eye cannot look temporally
Superior rectus	Oculomotor (CN III)	Moves eye up	Weakness of upward gaze
Inferior rectus	Oculomotor (CN III)	Moves eye down	Weakness of downward gaze
Superior oblique	Trochlear (CN IV)	1. Moves eye down when eye is already looking nasally 2. Rotates eye when eye is already looking temporally 3. Moves eye downward and outward when eye is in straight-ahead position	Vertical double vision Head tilt (compensation for imbalance of rotation)
Inferior oblique	Oculomotor (CN III)	1. Moves eye upward when eye is already looking nasally 2. Rotates eye when eye is already looking temporally 3. Moves eye upward and outward when eye is in straight-ahead position	Vertical double vision Head tilt

Source: Reprinted, by permission of the publisher, from S. Goldberg, *Ophthalmology Made Ridiculously Simple* (Miami: Medmaster, 1991), p. 6.

Note: CN = cranial nerve.

tracting and in others relaxing. For example, the lateral rectus muscle (closest to the temple) contracts and the medial rectus muscle (closest to the nose) relaxes when the right eye turns to the right; the medial rectus contracts and the lateral rectus muscle is inhibited when the right eye turns to the left (see Table 5.2 for the primary actions of the extrinsic muscles).

To coordinate the movements of the two eyes so they can look at the same target at the same time, the muscles of one eye are yoked with those of the other eye that share the same primary action. For example, the right lateral rectus muscle and the left medial rectus muscle are yoked to move both eyes to the right. To accomplish this move smoothly, the right medial rectus muscle and the left lateral rectus muscle must relax. If one considers the many times a minute the direction of gaze typically changes, the importance

and achievement of coordinated and smooth motion are indeed striking.

The rectus and oblique muscles are innervated by cranial nerves (CNs) that come from the brain. CN III, the oculomotor nerve, innervates the superior, inferior, and medial rectus muscles and the inferior oblique muscles. CN IV, the trochlear nerve, innervates the superior oblique muscle. CN VI, the abducens, takes care of the lateral rectus muscle. The optic nerve is CN II.

The correct alignment of the eyes is essential for binocular vision, which gives us depth perception and some appreciation of distance and perspective. For good, clear vision with a sense of depth, the retinal areas stimulated in both eyes should correspond. The brain actually receives two sets of messages, one from each eye and the associated optic radiations. These two sets are processed to make one image of what comes from the two eyes. If the alignment of the eyes is not straight, if tumors push any structure away from its correct position, or if the pairs of muscles in each eye and the yoked muscles of the two eyes are not innervated equally, then the sets of messages transmitted to the occipital lobes of the brain may be sufficiently disparate that diplopia (double vision) results. In children the weaker of the two images is suppressed, or attention alternates between the two. However, suppression does not occur as easily in adults, and diplopia sometimes becomes bothersome.

TRANSMISSION OF VISUAL INFORMATION TO THE BRAIN

When all the structures and functions of the eyes work well, light entering the eyes is transformed into impulses that result in sight. However, it is the brain, not the eyes, which interprets the information being received that results in vision. The transmission begins with light rays, a form of electromagnetic energy, passing through the cornea and onto the retina. The light rays cause chemical changes in the rod and cone cells of the retina, as described earlier. These changes result in electrical impulses being carried along the optic pathways to the occipital lobe at the back of the brain, and connections are then made to link visual images with other brain functions. In the brain, meaning is finally given to what was seen. The scenario that follows illustrates this process (see also Figure 5.7).

The setting is the front porch at sunset. Lou is facing east, not west where the sun is just dipping below the horizon, watching the colors soften in the early evening eastern sky. As the sunlight fades into mauves, purples, blues, and blue-blacks, Lou notices movement to his right. He quickly turns and identifies a white cat staring at him from his neighbor's newly sodded side yard. All this took place "in the twinkling of an eye." What happened?

Lou's eyes were directed to the horizon, so he could observe the gradual changes in light in the sky. His pupils were dilated because of the dimming evening light. Since he was looking east with the sunset's brilliant light behind him, light rays reflected from the white cat located in his right visual field entered Lou's cornea, passed through the aqueous in the anterior chamber, the pupil, the posterior chamber, and the lens, from which they emerged a bit more converged. The light rays continued through the vitreous and the layers of the retina until they came to a point of focus in a nasal portion of Lou's right retina and a lateral portion of his left retina.

The photoreceptor disks of the rods of the peripheral retina of each eye, sensitive to light and motion, reacted by exciting the modulator cells of the retina, which, in turn, excited the ganglion cells that lie next to the vitreous. The axons of these cells extend to the optic disk and form the optic nerve (CN II). Lou's excited ganglion cell axons sent their impulses along the optic nerve through the orbit, out the apex of the orbit, and toward the optic chiasm. The *optic chiasm* is the junction where the fibers coming from the nasal portion of the retina of each eye split off from their optic nerves and cross over to the opposite side to join with fibers coming from the temporal portion of each retina from the opposite side.

What happened next requires additional explanation. Posterior to the optic chiasm, right nasal fibers continued with left temporal fibers and left nasal fibers traveled with right temporal fibers to form the right and left optic tracts that lead respectively to the right and left lateral geniculate bodies. Most of the fibers continued from each lateral geniculate body as optic radiations that end in the occipital lobes of the brain. Some of the fibers, those that carry information related to the pupillary light reflex, bypass the lateral geniculate body and head for the midbrain. (Their departure at this point explains why the pupillary reaction to light is reflexive; it is not mediated by the occipital cortex, but is handled at a lower level in the sympathetic system of the autonomic nervous system.) Lou's optic radiations carried their impulses into the occipital lobes, where they were processed.

"Processing" involves some of the 10 billion

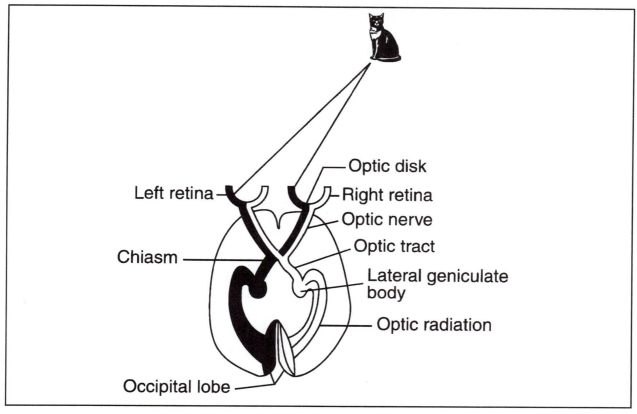

Figure 5.7. Optic Pathways to the Brain

Source: Adapted, by permission of the publisher, from S. Goldberg, *Clinical Neuroanatomy Made Ridiculously Simple* (Miami: Medmaster, 1991), p. 38.

cells of the brain in ways that are not completely understood at present. An information-processing model can be used to understand what may be happening in the brain; what is happening cannot be known by direct observation. What may have happened to the information received by the brain can only be inferred from motor and speech behavior.

In the scene just presented, Lou quickly turned his head to the right. What, perhaps, can be inferred from that movement? The reflected rays from the cat reached the fovea centralis of his maculas, where the discs of the cones received them and produced a chemical change that sent an electrical impulse to the modulator cells. In turn, these cells activated transmitter cells whose axons carried the electrical impulses along the optic pathways back to the occipital lobes of the brain.

In a fraction of the time it has taken to read about what happened, Lou identified the cat and called to it. The cat bounded across the driveway and into Lou's lap, where it purred quietly as Lou turned his gaze again toward the darkening eastern sky. At any point in the transmission, an interruption or degradation in the impulse could have occurred that could have affected the integrity of the signal that arrived at Lou's brain if, in fact, a signal did arrive.

Even if the organs of sight, with all their elaborate and intricate structures, are healthy and functioning, the information they transmit and relay may not reach the brain or may be distorted along the route. And even if the optic pathways are clear and complete, an injury, disease, or deformity in any of the structures of the eye itself or any problem with transparency in the cornea, aqueous, lens, or vitreous could lead to degrada-

Components of the Human Nervous System

Component	Function

Central nervous system
    Brain
    Spinal cord
	Receives, processes, stores, retrieves, and integrates information; assembles, evaluates, selects, and sends out responses via the peripheral system; monitors and coordinates all systems.

Peripheral nervous system
    Cranial nerves (12 pairs)
    Spinal nerves (31 pairs)
	Transmits information from the spinal cord to the body and from the body to the spinal cord.

Autonomic nervous system
    Sympathetic nerves
    Parasympathetic nerves
	Regulates internal structures like the heart, the stomach, the pupils of the eyes, the intestines, the bronchi, and the sweat glands; also regulates the internal environment (blood pressure, respiration rate, temperature) of the body.

tion of the signal or resulting image. Also, a malfunction in any layer or part of a layer of the retina could affect or stop the transmission. Such conditions are discussed in Chapter 6.

An extensive explanation of the brain and nervous systems is beyond the scope of this text. Nevertheless, educational and rehabilitation professionals should be aware of the complex nature of information processing and know something about the divisions of the human nervous system (see Sidebar 5.5 for an outline of the central nervous system, the peripheral nervous system, and the autonomic nervous system).

RELATIONSHIP OF SIGHT AND VISION

This chapter opened with the observation that the information presented about the eye's anatomy (structure) and physiology (function) had to be considered from the perspective of an emphasis on the whole and unique person—body, mind, and spirit. A discussion about the relationship of sight and vision now requires a return to that perspective. Each individual's repertoire of experiences, motivation to perform particular vi-

sual tasks, intellectual skills, persistence, and physical state can affect how visual information of any quality is interpreted and how it may influence vision.

Several years ago, a 70-year-old retired machinist who had lost his vision late in life reminded a group of younger people, gathered around a campfire after a day of tandem cycling, that his dictionary contained 18 definitions of the word "see" and that only 3 of them referred to eyesight. Understanding how light enters the eye and what electrical and chemical changes occur in the various structures and along the optic pathways does explain in one sense how a person sees, but it cannot fully reveal how the person makes sense of what he or she sees. For people with good vision, as well as for people with impaired vision, making sense of what is seen, what is appreciated, and what is perceived can take a lifetime.

SUMMARY

Light rays reflected from objects in the environment are ultimately given meaning at the end of an intricate and complex process involving electromagnetic, mechanical, chemical, and electrical energy. The actual transformation of electromagnetic energy into meaning in the mind begins as light rays enter the eye through the cornea and pass through the aqueous, pupil, lens, and vitreous and land on the retina. As a result of both voluntary (deliberately directing one's visual gaze) and involuntary (accommodation) action, the light rays are focused at a particular place on each retina. The photoreceptor cells in the retina send the information they receive to the optic pathways in the form of electrical impulses that arrive at the occipital lobe of the brain. In the brain, the impulses are given meaning and are interpreted, subject to the particular individual's physical, physiological, and psychological state; repertoire of experiences; and level of attention. Professionals who understand the structures of the eye and how they function are well prepared to help children and adults with low vision better analyze their visual abilities and learn how to use them effectively.

ACTIVITIES

With This Chapter and Other Resources

1. When Timmy (see the vignette that opens this chapter) returns to school after his surgery, he will undoubtedly be asked many questions about what happened to his eye. Using information about the eye and visual system in this chapter and additional information you may obtain from an ocularist (a person who makes prosthetic eyes), write a lesson plan to help Timmy prepare to answer the questions his classmates will ask.

2. A 60-year-old woman has just had cataract surgery but was not a good candidate for replacing her natural lens with an artificial intraocular lens implant (artificial lens). Explain to her why she must now have two pairs of eyeglasses, one for distance vision and one for near vision.

3. Develop a chart or poster to provide information to a support group of adults with retinal problems. Show how the macula, the fovea centralis, and the peripheral retina function.

4. Imagine teaching third graders a lesson on how their eyes work. One student asks why her nose runs when she cries. Explain to the class why we have tears, where tears come from, and where they flow.

In the Community

1. Review several children's books that discuss the eye and visual system. Find books you consider to be especially good at explaining the eye and visual system and those you consider to be unclear or misleading.

2. Request that at least three low vision clinics share with you printed, videotaped, audiotaped, or other materials or models they use to explain the eye and visual system to persons of different ages. How do these various materials compare with regard to the quantity and quality of information and the ease of comprehension?

With a Person with Low Vision

1. With permission from an adult with low vision or from parents of a visually impaired middle or high school student and the student, attend a clinical low vision evaluation. Observe how the clinical low vision specialist and other clinic personnel explain the visual impairment to the person. Do you think that after the explanation the student or adult understands the parts of the eye that are affected and what caused the visual impairment?

2. Interview a person with a congenital form of low vision. Ask at what age and how he or she came to understand what happened to his or her vision. Ask the person to explain what parts of the eye were affected, their function or functions, and how the impairment occurred.

From Your Perspective

Why do you think that many children and adults with low vision have little knowledge of the eye and the visual system? What role can teachers and rehabilitation specialists play in providing this knowledge?

CHAPTER 6

Causes and Functional Implications of Visual Impairment

Virginia E. Bishop

VIGNETTE

Tonight was the first meeting of the discussion group. Laura hoped that all four of her clients would be comfortable talking with each other about their adjustment to low vision. Each had asked for a support group, and Laura was willing to facilitate it. She knew from experience in rehabilitation counseling that each client thought that his or her own problems were unique—that no one else had the same kind of frustrations and feelings of discouragement. Laura had purposely chosen these four people, two of whom were young and two older. Mike, aged 17, and Sandy, aged 22, had been living with their visual impairments all their lives; Mike had achromatopsia, and Sandy had a partially detached retina because of retinopathy of prematurity. June and Tom were both retired and in their early 60s, looking forward to enjoying life for a change. June's diagnosis was macular degeneration, and Tom had central cataracts and could no longer drive a car.

Within the first few minutes of the discussion, Tom mentioned that he was going to have a cataract operation and asked how the ophthalmologist could take his eyeball out and put it back in again. Mike began to laugh. After Laura explained that the eyeball was not removed during cataract surgery, Tom asked Mike, "What happened to *your* eyes?" At that point, Mike had to admit that he knew the name of his condition but not why he had it or why he functioned as he did visually.

This confusion and lack of information about visual impairments was probably a good starting point for Laura. With her knowledge of the functional implications of medical conditions, she was able to provide accurate information and further the four group members' adjustment to their low vision.

INTRODUCTION

Most texts about the causes of visual impairment (both blindness and low vision) first categorize conditions and diseases and then describe the functional implications of the resulting impairments. This chapter strives in large part to take the reverse approach: It categorizes visual impairments primarily by function and describes most of the conditions and diseases included in this discussion as they fit into functional catego-

The author wishes to extend thanks to Stephen Rogers, M.D., ophthalmologist in private practice and Senior Attending Ophthalmologist at The New York Eye and Ear Infirmary in New York City, New York, for technical review of this chapter.

ries. Readers should note that a great many conditions or diseases have similar functional implications, but knowing the actual diagnoses of clients can assist the professional who deals with visual impairments in long-term planning. Because of the complexity of the information that is necessary to comprehend the functional aspects of a condition, some sections of this chapter briefly review information covered in Chapter 5 to highlight what needs to be understood to move from a knowledge of anatomical structures to an understanding of impairments and functional implications (for more comprehensive information, see Beck & Smith, 1988; Gittinger & Asdourian, 1988; Isenberg, 1989; Newell, 1992; Pavan-Langston, 1985; Vaughan, Asbury, & Riordan-Eva, 1992). Many of the terms used in this chapter, however, are defined more fully in Chapter 5. Readers may therefore wish to read these chapters in conjunction with one another.

Low vision can be caused by an anomaly, disease, or injury. However, functional vision involves much more than just vision. An individual's attitudes and experiences as well as organic and psychological factors can contribute to the ways in which a person uses his or her sight. Thus, as indicated in Chapter 1, two people with identical clinical measures may function in different ways. One person with 10/200 visual acuity may be able to move about easily using vision in a familiar area but may miss the social clues of facial expressions or body language. Another person with the same visual acuity may use auditory signals to move freely in a familiar environment and be able to interpret the body language of persons in close proximity for social interactions. Both individuals have the same level of visual acuity but bring different experiences, awareness levels, and skills to bear on the way in which they function. If specific diagnoses are examined, the implications can add a further dimension to program planning.

A final caveat to be noted is that in general it is not possible to compare disabilities based on type of impairment involved. Whom would be said to be more "disabled"—someone with central field loss or someone with peripheral field

loss? The answer is that it depends on what the individual needs or wants to do. The first person would have difficulty with near vision tasks, the second person with mobility. Which is more important? For reasons such as these, it bears repeating that assessments should be based on what the individual needs or wants to accomplish (L. Hyvärinen, personal communication, April 28, 1996).

As described in Chapter 5, for the visual system to function "normally," a number of structures and processes must be present and operative:

◆ The eyes and associated structures must be normal in structure and function.

◆ The neurological pathways from the retina and optic nerve to the visual cortex must be intact.

◆ The brain must be capable of interpreting the information received.

There is no single clear-cut way to classify visual impairments that result in low vision. They can be categorized in a number of ways, including according to anatomy, starting with the eyelid and working back to the visual cortex; according to function, reflecting how an impairment affects the individual's use of vision; or according to cause, depending on whether an impairment results from a disease, congenital defect, or trauma. Although the primary set of categories used in this chapter relate to the functional effects of visual impairments, anatomy and cause are considered as well. Broadly speaking, these categories are low central visual acuity, restricted visual fields, combined loss, and perceptual difficulties. This classification is not precise, however, because there is a great deal of overlap among the categories used and the effects of some diseases or conditions may vary depending on how they progress. Thus, although various conditions may have been discussed under the heading of either low central visual acuity or reduced visual field, it has been indicated when they may have a combined effect as well. In addition, a variety of important issues are not easily discussed within this

Table 6.1. Common Causes of Visual Impairment

| | United States | |
Worldwide	Children	Adults[a]
Trachoma (results in corneal scarring)	Cortical visual impairment	Open-angle glaucoma
Onchocerciasis ("river blindness")	Congenital malformations	Unoperated cataracts
Xerophthalmia (Vitamin A deficiency)	Retinopathy of prematurity	Retinal disorders (diabetic retinopathy; vascular diseases; and degenerative disorders, such as age-related macular degeneration)
Glaucoma	Optic atrophy	
Cataracts (untreated)	Cataracts	
Retinal detachment	Retinal defects	
Diabetic retinopathy	Ocular infections	
Leprosy (corneal scarring)	Albinism	
Herpes simplex keratitis (corneal lesions)	Optic nerve hypoplasia	
	Anophthalmos-microphthalmia	
	Trauma-abuse	
	Retinoblastoma	
	Nystagmus	
	Leber's congenital amaurosis	
	Refractive errors	

Sources: Virginia Bishop, "Preschool Visually Impaired Children: A Demographic Study," *Journal of Visual Impairment & Blindness* 95 (1991), pp. 69–74. Data related to causes worldwide and to adults in the United States are derived from National Society to Prevent Blindness, *Vision Problems in the United States* (Fact Sheet) (Schaumburg, IL: Author, 1993); F. Newell, *Ophthalmology: Principles and Concepts,* 7th ed. (St. Louis: Mosby Year Book, 1992); and D. G. Vaughan and T. Asbury, *General Ophthalmology,* 9th ed. (Los Altos, CA: Lange Medical Publications, 1980).

[a]About one-half of the eye problems in adults occur in those over age 65.

classification scheme, so a number of other conditions and factors, such as monocularity, trauma, tumors, genetics, and progressive visual impairment will be outlined in the chapter's final sections.

In reviewing the visual conditions outlined in this chapter, readers should also note that a great number of diseases and physical syndromes are accompanied by visual effects (see Cassin, Solomon, & Rubin, 1990; Gittinger & Asdourian, 1988; Isenberg, 1989; Newell, 1992; Pavan-Langston, 1985; Roy, 1985; Stein, Slatt, & Stein, 1992; Vaughan, Asbury, & Riordan-Eva, 1992) and that the large majority of medications prescribed may have ocular side effects (see Fraunfelder, 1989; Newell, 1992; *Physicians' Desk Reference,* 1995). These factors further complicate a com-

plex subject, and professionals who work with individuals who are visually impaired need to be aware of their significant influence. Table 6.1 lists common causes of visual impairment and reflects the wide range of possible types of vision loss; the Appendix at the back of this book lists the visual effects of various syndromes and diseases.

CONDITIONS RESULTING IN LOW CENTRAL VISUAL ACUITY

Some persons with adventitious low central visual acuity may describe their condition as "blurry" vision, because they have something with which to compare it, but to those whose low visual acuity has been present since birth, such vision may seem "normal" and "clear." Children, especially, do not know that others see differently from them, and their overall functioning may give the only clues that they have a visual impairment.

Individuals who have low visual acuity do not see details the same way in which those with unimpaired visual acuity do. Instead, they may miss information that is contained within larger areas of an outline. For example, although they may see the crown of a tree, they may not see individual leaves until they are close to the tree; similarly print may appear as gray lines, but individual letters may not be seen as distinct symbols. By getting closer to an object or by spreading the image of the object on the retina, as is produced by magnification, the person with low acuity can benefit from greater distances between edges, lines, and contours within the visual field.

Low acuity is the most common type of visual impairment, and it is accounted for by the largest group of diseases and conditions. It can be related to the following:

- ocular muscle disorders—eyes that are not in proper alignment (strabismus and amblyopia)

- shape of the eye—in extreme cases, eyeballs that are too long (myopia), too short (hyperopia), or too small (microphthalmia)

- corneal disorders and diseases—corneas that are abnormally shaped (keratoconus) or are not clear (keratopathy, corneal dystrophies, corneal scarring)

- absent or dysfunctional irises—irises that are missing (aniridia) or underdeveloped (coloboma)

- conditions of the lenses—lenses that have become dislocated or clouded (cataracts)

- vitreous opacities—conditions in which the vitreous is not clear because of hemorrhage or the presence of foreign matter (diabetic retinopathy)

- retinal disorders—retinas that are not formed properly (achromatopsia, albi-

nism) or are damaged (retinal edema, diabetic retinopathy, retinopathy of prematurity).

Ocular Muscle Disorders

Strabismus and Amblyopia

Strabismus is a term used to describe defects of the eye-muscle system. As explained in the previous chapter, six external ocular muscles are responsible for the alignment and movement of the eyes. When there is a defect in the length, placement, or ability to function of any of the extraocular muscles, the eyes are not aligned correctly and the images that are transmitted to the brain may be too dissimilar to be fused. The brain may then suppress one of the two images, and, over time, this suppression leads to a permanent reduction in acuity in the suppressed eye. *Amblyopia* is a reduction in visual acuity because of nonuse of that eye or marked differences in the refractive errors of the two eyes (see the following section for a discussion of refractive disorders). Since strabismus affects the vision in one eye only, it does not necessarily result in low vision as this term is usually defined (see the section on monocularity later in this chapter). However, it is included in this discussion because strabismus may accompany other eye conditions that do cause low vision.

People with strabismus have either "tropias" or "phorias" (see Figure 6.1). *Tropias* are marked deviations in the alignment of the eyes that cannot be controlled; thus, if a person wishes to look at a specific object and one eye is "turned," he or she will not be able to look binocularly at the object. *Esotropia* is the turning of one or both eyes toward the nose; *exotropia* is the turning of one or both eyes toward the temporal side of the face. *Hypertropia* is the deviation of an eye upward, and *hypotropia* is the deviation of an eye downward. Deviations may occur with either eye alternately or may occur always with the same eye. Hypertropia is the least common and is often compensated for by head tilting on the part of the individual.

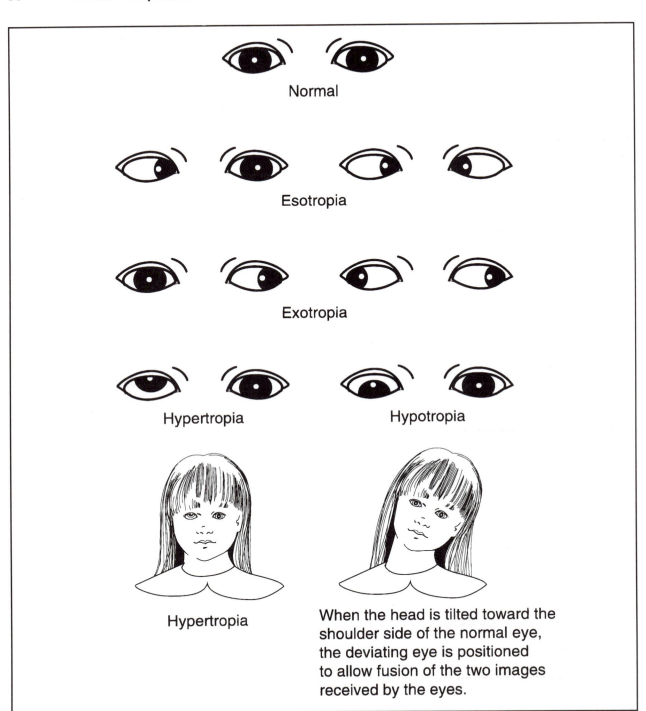

Figure 6.1. Types of Strabismus

Phorias are tendencies for the eyes to deviate and are controlled by the brain's efforts to achieve binocular vision. Because of voluntary control, if an eye is turned and the person wishes to look at an object, he or she will be able to bring both eyes into alignment. The same pattern of terminology used for tropias is applied to phorias. For example, the tendency for an eye to turn outward is referred to as an exophoria.

Strabismus is commonly an inherited condition, although it may also be caused by paresis (partial paralysis) or may be secondary to other visual defects (see the section on genetically determined conditions later in this chapter). Since the muscles of the eyes are responsible for coordinated movements and binocular vision, strabismus should be identified and treated as early as possible, since the younger the child, the better the prognosis for good vision. Vision screening in elementary schools is usually done too late to help children with strabismus; therefore, preschool vision screening is highly desirable. Parents and pediatricians can also recognize strabismus that persists after age 6 months, when eye-muscle control should have been attained, and parents should follow up with a professional eye examination.

The goals of correcting strabismus are good acuity in both eyes, good cosmetic appearance, and binocular vision. Occlusion, by patching the better eye or using medication to blur the vision in the good eye, forces the deviating eye to improve acuity; this treatment should be initiated as early as possible. It is most effective before age 1, becomes more difficult by age 5, and is often ineffective beyond that age.

Early diagnosis and occlusion are the best first steps in preventing amblyopia. When no further improvement of acuity can be accomplished by patching, surgical realignment of the eye muscles is indicated. Occlusion does not straighten the eyes, it only improves the person's acuity. Surgery repositions eye muscles through recession (repositioning a muscle to make it "longer") or resection (in effect, "shortening" a muscle). Strabismus surgery is rarely precise, and sometimes more than one operation may be needed.

Orthoptics, also referred to as eye exercises, are sometimes prescribed before or after strabismus surgery to help improve image fusion.

Nystagmus

Nystagmus is an involuntary, rhythmical, repeated movement of one or both eyes in a horizontal, vertical, or circular direction (or any combination of these directions). Low visual acuity is caused by the inability to maintain steady fixation of the gaze. However, most individuals with nystagmus perceive objects as being stationary. The cause of nystagmus is unknown, and there is no known treatment. However, certain types of jerky nystagmus show spontaneous improvement in the first decade of life and may be amenable to muscle surgery, essentially a repositioning of the muscles to take advantage of the point of least nystagmus or position of relative rest, called the *null point.*

There are basically two types of nystagmus. *Pendular nystagmus* is marked by up-and-down movements of equal speed, amplitude, and duration. *Jerky nystagmus* is characterized by slower movement in one direction, not necessarily up and down, followed by a faster return to the original position; usually, the smaller the amplitude, the faster the rate. Rhythmic head movements often accompany congenital nystagmus. Adults with acquired nystagmus may experience dizziness or vertigo if oscillopsia (the illusion that objects are moving) occurs. Head tilting may decrease nystagmus and is usually involuntary in the direction of the fast component in jerky nystagmus or in a position that minimizes pendular nystagmus. Some individuals voluntarily tilt their heads to position their eyes in the null point to enhance their visual functioning.

Nystagmus rarely appears as an individual's sole visual condition. Congenital pendular nystagmus often accompanies congenital visual impairments, such as albinism, aniridia, cataract, corneal opacity, chorioretinitis, and optic atrophy. Nystagmus may also accompany many neurological disorders and may be a reaction to certain drugs, including barbiturates. The absence of nystagmus may help in discriminating among certain visual conditions; for example, children with cortical visual impairments do not experience nystagmus.

Children with nystagmus may lose their place in reading and may use a typoscope (a card with a rectangular hole) to view one word or line at a time or an underliner or overliner (a card or strip of paper to "underline" or "overline" the line of print being read). As children with nystagmus mature, they seem to need these support devices less often. As is the case with other children and adults with low acuity, magnification for near and distance viewing is helpful.

Disorders Relating to the Shape of the Eye

Refractive Disorders

Refractive disorders cause visual acuity loss only if they remain uncorrected. They are most commonly caused by eyeballs that are longer than average (myopia) or shorter than average (hyperopia) or have an excess cylindrical curvature (astigmatism). These three defects are generally correctable with eyeglasses or contact lenses, and only in extreme or progressive cases would they be considered to constitute low vision.

An unimpaired eye, in which light rays focus on the retina, is called an *emmetropic* eye. In a farsighted, or *hyperopic*, eye, the eyeball is short, and the light rays focus behind the retina (theoretically). In a nearsighted, or *myopic*, eye, the eyeball is long, and the light rays come to a focus before they reach the retina. Myopia and hyperopia are treated by the use of spherical concave and convex lenses, respectively (see Chapter 7 for a discussion of the lenses used to correct these refractive errors).

Astigmatism is a cylindrical curvature of the cornea in one or more of its axes. The lens may also contribute to astigmatism in older people. Astigmatism may be simple, when it is not combined with hyperopia or myopia, or compound, when it is combined with either hyperopia or myopia. Astigmatism may also be "mixed," when myopia is combined with hyperopic astigmatism or when hyperopia is combined with myopic astigmatism. Astigmatic corrections are cylindrical lenses that can be added to any prescription for myopia or hyperopia (see Chapter 7 for an explanation of cylindrical lenses).

Other refractive variations are possible. *Anisometropia* refers to different refractive errors in each eye, and *aniseikonia* denotes a difference in the size or shape of the ocular image of the eyes.

Refractive errors tend to be inherited. The size of the eyeball, shape of the cornea, shape of the lens, and depth of the anterior chamber are all variables that increase the possible ocular combinations of refractive errors.

The symptoms of uncorrected myopia include squinting and frowning. Uncorrected hyperopia may cause a lack of interest in reading; rubbing of the eyes; and even headaches, dizziness, or nausea. Uncorrected astigmatism may cause visual fatigue, headaches, frowning, and squinting. In the absence of disease and other ocular abnormalities, eyeglasses or contact lenses are the primary treatment for refractive errors. Refractive surgery to reshape the cornea may also be used to correct myopia; however, this procedure is still somewhat controversial.

Progressive Myopia

Progressive (or pathological) *myopia* begins with simple myopia. However, in this condition, visual acuity progressively decreases over time and does not stabilize when the eye is fully grown; thinning of the retina occurs in the vicinity of the optic nerve. Vascular leakage can result in increased pigmentation, especially in the macular area, and can result in both nonfunctional retinal areas (blind spots or scotomas) and possible retinal detachment. Although progressive myopia usually causes reduced central visual acuity, it may also be associated with reduced peripheral vision.

Microphthalmia

Microphthalmia is the abnormal smallness of one or both eyes. It is congenital, almost always hereditary, and is usually recessive. Other ocular abnormalities may occur with microphthalmia, including cataract, glaucoma, aniridia, and coloboma, as well as systemic and anatomic abnormalities. Visual impairment results from high hyperopia, that is, hyperopia of a large degree. Treatment includes lens corrections for refractive errors and, often, tinted lenses. Lighting should be tailored to meet the individual's needs and to control glare. Some of the associated syndromes that accompany microphthalmia include cri-du-chat, De Grouchy's syndrome, Edward's syndrome, Patau's syndrome, and the rubella syndrome.

Corneal Disorders and Diseases

The cornea provides about 70 percent of the total refractive power of the eye. To provide best refraction, it must be transparent and spherical in shape. Improper curvature results in astigmatism. In regular astigmatism, there is a cylindrical component, causing the cornea to be sphero-cylindrical (or toric) in shape. In general, this condition is easily correctable with a corresponding cylindrical component in eyeglasses.

Keratoconus

Keratoconus is an extreme type of corneal curvature defect that results in lowered visual acuity and in which the cornea becomes increasingly cone shaped. The central cornea thins and may rupture in advanced stages. Keratoconus is a rare, bilateral, degenerative disease that is inherited as an autosomal recessive trait (for more information, see the discussion of genetics later in this chapter). It affects all races and may appear during the teenage years, progressing slowly up to the age of 60.

Keratoconus is associated with a number of other conditions and diseases, including Down's syndrome, atopic dermatitis, retinitis pigmen-

tosa, aniridia, and Marfan's syndrome. Contact lenses can improve visual acuity in the earliest stages, but a corneal transplant may be indicated when the corrected visual acuity can no longer be improved with contacts. Corneal transplant surgery in keratoconus is successful in more than 85 percent of cases.

Keratitis

Keratitis is a term that is used to define a wide variety of corneal infections, irritations, and inflammations. Because each condition is unique, a correct medical diagnosis and treatment are essential. Corneal ulcers are commonly caused by bacterial or fungal infections that often follow superficial corneal abrasions. Thus, hand washing during periods of illness and after toileting is an essential preventive measure. Among the common infectious agents are staphylococcus, streptococcus, herpes (both simplex and zoster), adenovirus, rubeola, rubella, mumps, trachoma, infectious mononucleosis, and pneumococcus. Keratitis may also result from a vitamin A deficiency. Corneal ulcers may also follow trauma; may be associated with other eye infections, such as conjunctivitis; may be related to other corneal disorders, including degenerative conditions; or may arise from a variety of systemic disorders, especially those of autoimmune origin. The symptoms of corneal infection include extreme pain and photophobia (sensitivity to light).

Immediate medical treatment is essential in cases of keratitis, and even a short delay can affect the ultimate visual result. The causative factors must be identified through laboratory analyses of scrapings or cultures, since medical treatment varies according to the cause. If keratitis is not treated in a timely fashion, tissue can be destroyed and scar tissue can form, interfering with transmission of light through the cornea. Keratitis is usually accompanied by severe pain; however, if the cornea has become desensitized, as in trauma, surgery, or nerve damage, ulcers can develop without accompanying pain.

Corneal Dystrophies

Conditions that cause degeneration of the corneal tissue are classified as corneal dystrophies, and they are often associated with other systemic diseases or syndromes. They are bilateral, not related to inflammation, and affect various layers of corneal tissue. They are often genetically determined and may result in low acuity. The treatment and prognosis vary with each condition or associated syndrome.

Corneal Scarring

Scarring of the cornea may result from infections or penetrating wounds. The five layers of the cornea provide an excellent culture medium for a variety of organisms. The surface epithelium heals rapidly, but the inner layers produce opaque scar tissue in the healing process. Once scarring occurs, that area interferes with light transmission and reduces acuity. In some cases, corneal transplants can restore vision, but not all types of corneal opacities are amenable to grafts.

Disorders Relating to Absent or Dysfunctional Irises

Abnormalities related to the iris of the eye may not directly cause visual acuity loss, but often accompany other ocular changes and conditions that do.

Aniridia

The iris is a circular diaphragm, including radial muscles and a sphincter muscle, pigment, and blood vessels. These are responsible for controlling the amount of light entering the eye. If the iris is absent or not fully developed, the result is called aniridia, a rare, genetically determined condition. Glaucoma is often an associated condition, and cataracts often accompany aniridia as well. There is lowered acuity usually in the 20/200 range. Other associated problems may include photophobia, nystagmus, displaced lens, and un-derdeveloped retina. Visual fields are normal unless glaucoma develops. Treatment includes the control of glare through the use of pinhole contact lenses, tinted lenses or sunglasses, corrections for any refractive errors, and lower levels of illumination. Optical devices may be helpful (see Chapter 7).

Dysfunctional Iris

Some medications will prevent the normal functioning of the iris (constriction in high illumination and dilation in low illumination). Cyclopegic (atropine-like) eyedrops used to treat iritis will leave the pupil widely dilated and may cause light sensitivity. Seizure medications, sedatives, and tranquilizers may also cause dilated pupils. Pilocarpine, an eye drop sometimes used in treating glaucoma, will cause tight constriction of the pupil, causing reduced acuity in low illumination or if cataract is present.

Coloboma of the Iris and Choroid

If the iris does not form completely during the prenatal period, it may not close completely. This condition, called coloboma of the iris, gives the pupil a keyhole appearance. Such a defect results in increased light sensitivity. Coloboma may involve large areas of the choroid and affect the underlying retina, causing marked acuity loss in those areas.

Iritis

Iritis is an example of a type of uveal tract inflammation (or uveitis) that affects the anterior portions of the uveal tract. The onset is usually sudden and is accompanied by pain, light sensitivity, and blurred vision; medical attention is essential for this condition. Another type of uveitis (as in choroiditis and chorioretinitis) involves the posterior portions of the uveal tract and also requires immediate medical attention. Both types of uveitis are common in young and middle-aged persons and are often associated with other diseases (such as arthritis, diabetes, syphilis, toxoplasmosis, and tuberculosis).

Lens-Related Conditions

Dislocated Lens

Because the lens is the second most important refracting element of the eye, any abnormality of the lens will result in impaired visual functioning. If a lens is dislocated, as in Marfan's syndrome (a complex condition involving a number of physical abnormalities, in which lens displacement is a component), it may function minimally or not at all. In such cases, the eye care specialist must provide corrections for both near and distance vision; bifocals or a combination of contact lenses for distance and eyeglasses for reading are common solutions.

Presbyopia

In *presbyopia,* the lens becomes less flexible and less able than previously to accommodate for near point viewing. As a natural part of the aging process, presbyopia usually begins at around age 40 and is often described as "when arms aren't long enough" (that is, many people attempt to move objects beyond arm's reach to see them clearly). Presbyopia necessitates the use of bifocals or eyeglasses for reading to compensate for the reduced flexibility of the lens. (Since it is easily correctable it is not necessarily a low vision problem.)

Cataracts

Cataracts are formed when the lens of the eye becomes opaque. This phenomenon is believed to be caused by chemical changes in the lens protein; primary symptoms are reduced visual acuity and, sometimes, sensitivity to glare. Advanced cataracts may cause overall reduction of the peripheral visual field. Etiologies for cataracts include hereditary causes, congenital anomaly, infection, severe malnutrition, systemic disease

(such as diabetes), trauma (such as a blunt injury or puncture wound), and advancing age.

Age-related cataracts develop gradually and are commonplace because they are a normal part of the aging process. Their characteristics (size, location, and density of the opacity) determine the course of treatment. Most eye specialists do not recommend surgical removal until a cataract interferes with a person's lifestyle. Although eyeglasses or contact lenses are used, intraocular lens (IOL) implants are commonly inserted at the time of cataract extraction. The complications of cataract surgery, though rare, may include glaucoma and retinal detachment.

Congenital cataracts can be caused by prenatal disease, toxicity, or heredity. They also accompany a great many syndromes and other ocular conditions, such as retinopathy of prematurity, congenital glaucoma, retinoblastoma, microphthalmia, and aniridia. Photophobia, nystagmus, or strabismus may also be present. The treatment for congenital cataracts involves their removal as early as possible (even as early as two weeks of age) to prevent deprivation amblyopia, a condition caused by lack of stimulation of the retina by light necessary for this part of the eye to develop properly.

When the natural lens has been removed, the eye is *aphakic,* and an artificial lens must be substituted to perform the major refractive function (although not the accommodative function) that the natural lens would have performed. In infants and young children, these artificial lenses may be in the form of eyeglasses or contact lenses. Occasionally, children receive an IOL implant, but long-term data on the use of IOL implants with children and the effectiveness of these implants are limited.

The management of early cataracts varies. Reduced lighting and lighting from behind the individual can reduce the glare caused by the scattering of light rays inside the eye. A child with a central cataract that has not been removed may exhibit some unusual head positions, because he or she is essentially "looking around" the cataract. In some cases, using magnification is helpful, as are controlling light and wearing visors

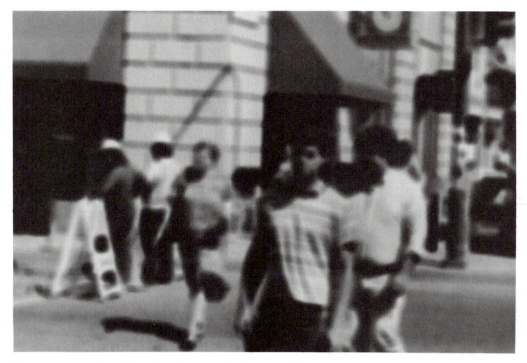

Cataracts result when the lenses of the eyes become cloudy, causing diminished visual acuity characterized by blurred vision.

or hats that have large brims that limit the direction from which light enters the eye.

Disorders Related to Vitreous Opacities

Since the vitreous must be clear for light to pass through it, any significant clouding of the vitreous will result in reduced acuity. However, this condition would be considered a low vision problem only if severe. Trauma and inflammations can produce inflammatory cells and debris in the vitreous. In such cases, functional vision may be variable and is often worse in the morning when debris has settled over the macular area. The most serious problems are caused by bleeding, especially hemorrhage from a vessel in proliferative diabetic retinopathy. *Vitrectomy*, a surgical procedure, is sometimes used to remove hemorrhagic material and replace the vitreous with saline.

Retinal Disorders

The retina contains two types of photoreceptors—rods and cones—that are responsible for different kinds of vision. Rods are involved in peripheral vision; cones in central vision. The cones of the eye are concentrated in the macula; they are responsible for both fine acuity and color perception and require good illumination to function best. A few cones are scattered throughout the retina, although the area of greatest concentration is in the macula. The rods are present only outside the fovea and are responsible for peripheral vision and for the perception of shape and movement; they function best under conditions of reduced illumination. Since most tests of visual acuity describe central vision, they relate primarily to the functioning of the cones. Thus, any discussion of reduced acuity usually refers to problems located in the macula, an area in the central posterior retina, approximately 4 mm in diameter.

Until now, this chapter has mainly discussed conditions or diseases that influence central visual acuity. Diseases of the retina, however, may affect peripheral visual fields, color vision, and contrast sensitivity, as well as central visual acuity. Only a few retinal disorders result in reduced central visual acuity alone. Among them are achromatopsia, albinism, macular edema, and the later stages of diabetes, as described in the discussion that follows.

Color Deficiencies

In many forms of color deficiencies, acuity is normal and only color perception is impaired. However, there are extreme forms of the condition that do affect visual acuity. Within the general population, color deficiency that is congenital (red-green) is usually caused by a sex-linked genetic defect, affecting 8 percent of men and 0.5 percent of women, whereas acquired types (yellow-blue) of color deficiency affect males and females about equally (Vaughan et al., 1992). Color deficiency may also be caused by exposure to toxic substances.

Color deficiencies affect specific types of cone receptor cells. When they are acquired as a result of retinal disease that affects the macula, they result in lower visual acuity. People who are monochromatic (1 in 1 million) have only one of the three kinds of color receptors and may be insensitive to red-green, red-blue, or green-blue colors. Individuals with color deficiencies are classified as protans (who are mildly red-blind), deutans (who experience mild confusion in identifying shades of red, green, and yellow), and tritans (who sometimes confuse blue-greens or orange-pinks).

Achromatopsia

Achromatopsia, also called rod monochromatism, is an extreme form of color deficiency, in which there is a complete lack of cone function (total color blindness). Persons with this condition are extremely light sensitive and have nystagmus and low visual acuity, but their peripheral visual fields are usually normal. The use of sunglasses, tinted lenses, and lowered illumination is the primary management technique for achromatopsia. Since rod function is generally intact, magnification may help the individual perform functional tasks by spreading the image over a larger area of the retina. Often, the effects of photophobia and nystagmus diminish with age.

Albinism

Albinism is a hereditary deficiency of pigmentation that may involve the entire body or only a part of the body. It is believed to be caused by an enzyme deficiency involving the metabolism of melanin during prenatal development.

In oculocutaneous albinism there is a generalized lack of pigmentation in the skin and hair and in retinal and iris tissue. In ocular albinism the skin and hair may vary from pale to normal, and impairments involve the retina, especially the macula; the iris may range in color from blue to brown.

Albinism is usually inherited as an autosomal recessive or sex-linked trait, but there are some rare cases of autosomal dominant inheritance. In the sex-linked type, ocular albinism is visible ophthalmologically only in the female genetic carrier.

Albinism is a nonprogressive condition. Some common visual effects are macular hypoplasia (underdevelopment), nystagmus, photophobia, strabismus, and lowered acuity (20/100 to 20/400, depending on the amount of pigment); color vision is normal. Treatment includes optical correction of any refractive errors, along with the use of absorptive lenses, optical devices, and lowered illumination. Preferential classroom seating may be indicated for youngsters to compensate for photophobia. Individuals with oculocutaneous albinism must be especially careful to protect their skin from strong sunlight.

Retinal Edema

Retinal edema is a swelling of the retina, often in the macular area. It can be the result of a number of vascular retinopathies, is often a complication of diabetic retinopathy, and may be the largest single cause of visual impairment among adults with diabetes (Faye, 1976; Pavan-Langston, 1985). Because the swelling in this condition is caused by capillary leakage, fluid shifts can affect both the edema and acuity, sometimes significantly, as reflected in the inability to read as many as two to three more lines on an eye chart. Variations in the blood sugar levels of individuals with diabetes can also cause changes in refraction and can thereby affect acuity levels, usually in the macular area, as a result of fluid leakage from capillary aneurysms.

Diabetic Retinopathy

Diabetes may affect both central visual acuity and peripheral visual fields. It is a metabolic disease, usually categorized as Type I (formerly called juvenile diabetes) and Type II (formerly called adult-onset diabetes). It can affect retinal blood vessels, causing intraretinal hemorrhaging and the abnormal growth of new vessels into the vitreous, called *proliferative diabetic retinopathy.* In this condition, the vitreous begins to pull away from the retina, and the vessels hemorrhage into the vitreous. The resulting bleeding blocks the transmission of light through the normally transparent vitreous, and functional visual interference is experienced. This can range from floaters (debris in the vitreous that appears to the viewer as existing outside the eye) to blindness. Symptoms of ocular involvement include sensitivity to glare, diplopia, lack of accommodation, fluctuating visual acuity, diminished color vision, and constricted visual fields. Retinal detachment may follow. *Nonproliferative diabetic retinopathy* (also called "background retinopathy") is characterized by microaneurysms (outpouchings on thin-walled capillaries) and "cotton wool" patches (white retinal spots resulting from damage to nerve fibers in the retina). These changes may be accompanied by a swollen macula with reduced visual acuity.

Ocular complications may occur 10 to 15 years after the onset of diabetes. It is believed that if the disease is well controlled in its early years, the onset of retinopathy may be delayed and its severity reduced. High blood pressure can be a contributing factor to diabetes and its effects on the eye, and its treatment and control are vital.

Secondary complications of diabetes may include glaucoma, cataracts, and retinal detachments. Other associated systemic conditions include cardiovascular involvement, neuropathy (loss of tactile sensitivity), and skin and kidney problems.

The control of diabetes is essential and may be accomplished through diet, exercise, and medical therapy. (Insulin is usually required in Type I diabetes, and oral medications are generally effective in Type II diabetes.) Laser photocoagulation may be of enormous value in preserving vision in some types of diabetic retinopathy. This complex procedure involves the use of a laser to cauterize leaking blood vessels. A vitrectomy may help those who have sustained vision loss owing to bleeding. Retinal detachments may be treated with scleral buckling procedures, in which a strap is placed around the eyeball to force the retina into contact with the choroid, as well as with photocoagulation and vitrectomy. Optical and nonoptical devices and increased illumination may be helpful when visual function is preserved.

Retinopathy of Prematurity

Retinopathy of prematurity (ROP) (formerly called retrolental fibroplasia) was first reported in the 1940s and thought to be caused by excess oxygen administered to premature infants in incubators. The term "retrolental fibroplasia" literally refers to fibrous retinal tissue pulled up behind the lens. The effects of ROP on visual functioning start in the periphery of the visual field and become global; therefore the condition produces a combined vision loss.

During the 1950s, as many as 20,000 infants developed ROP (Isenberg, 1989). Changes in the administration of oxygen sharply reduced the number of cases but did not eliminate the disease. As neonatal methodology improved and

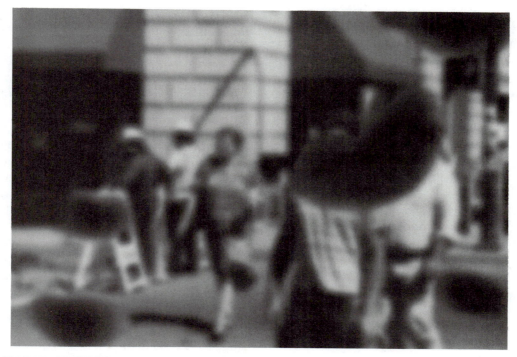

Damage to the blood vessels of the retina causes patches or blind areas that affect the vision of individuals with diabetic retinopathy.

a greater number of preterm infants survived, the incidence of ROP began to rise again in the late 1970s, and ROP continues to be a problem for neonatologists who are saving more and younger infants. Although there are many theories about the cause of ROP, the actual cause is likely to center around factors associated with prematurity and low birth weight. However, occasionally full-term infants who were not exposed to oxygen have been observed to have ROP.

Ocular involvement in ROP follows a pattern of initially constricted ocular blood vessels, followed by vascular dilation and fibrovascular proliferation into the vitreous. In some cases, there is partial or complete regression of the condition, with little ocular damage. Children with ROP have a wide range of visual functioning, from normal vision to total blindness. Children with the regressed types of ROP are at risk of developing refractive errors, amblyopia, strabismus, nystagmus, glaucoma, cataracts, corneal changes, and retinal-vitreous abnormalities. Between 35 per-

cent and 70 percent of the children whose ROP results in blindness or severe low vision experience mental retardation, cerebral palsy, hearing impairment, or epilepsy (Isenberg, 1989). Occasionally, the condition affects only one eye.

Myopia and strabismus are common among children with ROP who retain useful vision, although there is a possibility of retinal detachment later in life. Glaucoma, uveitis, cataract, or phthisis bulbi (a shrunken blind eye) may also occur later.

Treatment consists of early monitoring of the retinal status of premature infants. However, if an infant has respiratory or other problems that require the use of oxygen for his or her survival, it may be impossible to control the progression of adverse ocular conditions. It is important that other complicating eye conditions be monitored and treated simultaneously. Cryotherapy, or freezing areas of the retina to prevent the proliferation of the blood vessels, is among the new treatment approaches being used.

CONDITIONS RESULTING IN RESTRICTED VISUAL FIELDS

The term *visual field* refers to a portion of space in which objects are simultaneously seen by the steadily fixating eye. Reductions in visual field are related to problems in the retina or the visual pathways. Although the term *field impairment* is often used to refer to the peripheral field, it can also refer to central field disorders. When central fields are affected, the macular area of the retina is involved; examples of such impairments include macular disease, cone dystrophies, central scotomas, and optic nerve disease or disorder. When peripheral fields are affected, the retinal area outside the macula is involved; examples of such impairments include retinitis pigmentosa, chorioretinitis, glaucoma, optic nerve conditions, retinal detachments, peripheral scotomas, colobomas, and degenerative myopia. If the optic nerve is dysfunctional, as in the case of optic atrophy, or damage from intracranial pressure or demyelinating disease (in which the nerves' myelin sheath deteriorates, as in multiple sclerosis), the site of the defect can also cause central or peripheral field defects. Although impairments in peripheral vision are less common than impairments in central acuity, they can be more disabling.

Some conditions, such as macular degeneration and achromatopsia, have functional implications that fall within two categories. They are generally characterized by reduced visual acuity but are also among the conditions typical of central field loss; the peripheral fields basically remain intact.

Central Field Impairments

Macular Degeneration

Macular degeneration is a term applied to a group of generally untreatable diseases that affect the macular area of the retina and may have some

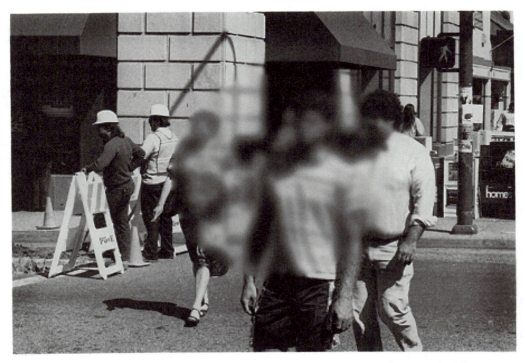

Macular degeneration typically results in gradual loss of central vision.

hereditary component. Some types are familial, bilateral, and progressive, such as Best's vitelliform degeneration (hereafter called Best's disease), fundus flavi-maculatus, and achromatopsia, and some involve the central nervous system. In "wet" macular degeneration, a relatively rare disorder, new blood vessels grow beneath the macula; if detected early, the condition can be treated with laser therapy. In "dry" macular degeneration, a more common condition, a greater number of cone cells atrophy; there is no medical or surgical treatment.

When macular degeneration affects the central choroid, there is a gradual loss of central vision in midlife (such as in central areolar choroidal sclerosis). Other types of macular degeneration affect the pigment epithelium (such as Stargardt-Behr's disease) and may begin at different ages and progress at different rates. Secondary macular degeneration may be a side effect of other causes or conditions (such as trauma or inflammatory disease).

Macular degeneration in childhood can be a result of dominant or recessive genetic inheritance. Best's disease is an autosomal dominant disorder, whereas Stargardt-Behr's disease is autosomal recessive (see the discussion of genetic determinants later in this chapter). Children with these conditions have normal findings on an electroretinogram (ERG), a test of rod and cone function based on the electrical potential between the cornea and retina. Best's disease may result in only minor reductions in visual acuity, despite macular lesions. Stargardt-Behr's disease is characterized by rapid visual acuity loss with few observable ophthalmoscopic indicators until the disease has reached an advanced stage.

Age-related macular degeneration, also called age-related maculopathy, is the most common cause of legal blindness in the United States in persons over age 60; its prevalence increases significantly after age 65 (Gittinger & Asdourian, 1988; Newell, 1992). It is associated with other vascular diseases (such as arteriosclerosis and stroke). Central vision is gradually lost and acuity may decrease to 20/200 or less, but peripheral vision is usually retained.

Cone Dystrophies

Degenerative conditions that affect the cones of the eye are referred to *as cone dystrophies.* They affect both visual acuity and color perception. The ERG can identify the decreased cone function, or photopic vision, since it will differ sharply from rod function, or scotopic vision.

Central Scotomas

Central scotomas are areas of diminished or absent vision that result in a "blind spot" in the center of the visual field. Scotomas may be caused by macular disease, chorioretinal scarring, or damage to the optic nerve.

Central scotomas affect visual acuity and color vision. Individuals who have a central scotoma often comment that they do not see the faces of people unless they shift their gaze so as not to look directly at them. By using this kind of *eccentric viewing*, they are using a more peripheral area and retinal tissue that can accept visual information, even if it is not presented with as much detail as would have been available with macular vision.

Management techniques for central field losses may combine eccentric viewing with the use of magnification, either through bringing objects closer to the eye or using magnification devices. These techniques spread the visual image over a larger area of the retina, thereby allowing the individual to reduce the significance of the scotoma by using a healthy portion of the retina around the scotoma. When peripheral vision is used, detail acuity is lost or reduced; the resolution of images can never be as good as when central vision is used but may be enough to improve the individual's visual functioning. Motivation, past experience, level of ability for performing a task, and the context in which the task is performed may be combined with the increased information received by the brain, resulting in an overall improvement in visual functioning.

Peripheral Field Impairments

Peripheral field impairments are usually caused by a deterioration of retinal tissue outside the macular area, and they have a multitude of etiologies. Some, for example, chorioretinitis, produce scar tissue, while others cause scotomas because of optic nerve damage (as from glaucoma or brain tumors) or congenital malformations (as in colobomas). In degenerative myopia, the changes usually occur in the posterior pole of the eye, including the optic disk, choroid, retina, sclera, and vitreous. There may be secondary effects, such as retinal detachment, cataracts, and glaucoma, that cause field losses. *Retinal detachments* may produce peripheral field losses wherever the retina separates from the choroid. *Hemianopsias* are corresponding peripheral field losses from lesions in the visual pathway anywhere behind the optic chiasm in the brain. *Retinitis pigmentosa* is a group of retinal degenerative diseases that primarily affects the rods of the eye and frequently causes peripheral field loss. If only the periphery is affected and the central fields are maintained, central visual acuity may remain intact; this is often referred to as macular sparing.

Chorioretinitis

Chorioretinitis is a type of posterior uveitis (inflammation of the choroid and overlying retina). It usually follows an infection by a microorganism. The onset may be in utero and can be caused by toxoplasmosis (one of the most common causes). If chorioretinitis is acquired in later life, the onset can be gradual. Fresh lesions seen through an ophthalmoscope appear as yellowish-white patches, often with a hazy vitreous. As healing occurs, the vitreous clears, and pigmentation appears at the edges of the lesions.

In the healed stage, there may be considerable pigmentation and scarring. Scotomas occur corresponding to these lesions. Chorioretinitis can last for months or years, sometimes with remissions, and can cause permanent damage with marked vision loss. It is treated medically, usually with anti-infective agents and systemic corticosteroids. Functional vision depends on the extent and location of the healed lesions. (Peripheral scotomas usually do not affect visual functioning if they are few and are scattered throughout the visual field.)

Glaucoma

Glaucoma is a condition in which intraocular pressure becomes sufficiently high to damage the nerves of the retina and the optic nerve. Causes include the following:

- oversecretion of the aqueous by the ciliary body, exceeding the rate of drainage through the trabecular (filtering) meshwork and Canal of Schlemm (at the junction of the cornea and iris)

- an anatomical aberration that results in a narrow angle between iris and cornea, preventing efficient drainage of the aqueous

- scar tissue from an inflammatory process or surgery that obstructs the drainage of the aqueous (see Chapter 5).

There are three basic types of glaucoma:

- *primary glaucoma,* including open-angle (or chronic simple) glaucoma, the most common type, and closed-angle (or narrow-angle) glaucoma

- *congenital glaucoma,* including buphthalmos and juvenile types associated with congenital anomalies such as aniridia and *Marfan's syndrome*

- *secondary glaucoma,* caused by trauma, uveitis, or surgical procedures, or secondary to prolonged corticosteroid use.

Glaucoma may be present in association with a number of systemic diseases or syndromes, and heredity seems to predispose some individuals to this condition. The treatment of glaucoma varies with the cause and the type. In open-angle glaucoma, the impediment to the free outflow of the aqueous is caused by microscopic changes in the trabecular meshwork. Medication is used to

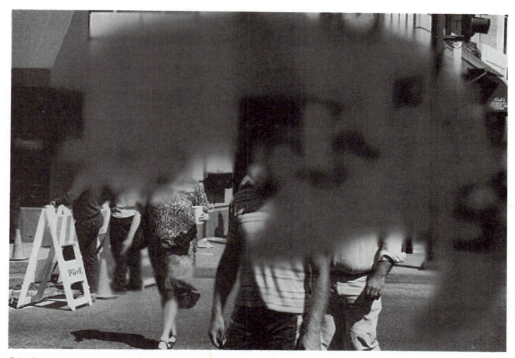

If left untreated, glaucoma may result in the reduction of the visual field and eventual blindness.

lower intraocular pressure, either by decreasing the rate of production of the aqueous fluid or facilitating its outflow. If this treatment is not effective in controlling intraocular pressure, surgery may be necessary. In narrow-angle glaucoma, the peripheral iris is touching the cornea, blocking access to the filtering trabecular meshwork. Surgery is indicated. A peripheral iridectomy (an opening made at the periphery of the iris) relieves the drainage problem permanently. Congenital glaucoma is also treated surgically by cutting away abnormal tissue impeding the drainage of the aqueous. The treatment of secondary glaucoma is usually medical, rather than surgical, and varies with the cause and type.

Early identification and ongoing control are essential if visual function is to be maintained. If glaucoma is untreated, the effects can cause damage to the optic nerve, resulting in reduction of the visual field. Complete blindness can be the result. When treated early, the condition most often can be successfully managed medically. Because the onset of chronic open-angle glau-

coma is so gradual, all adults should be checked regularly for elevated pressure.

Retinal Detachment

In the mature eye, the retina is firmly attached at the optic nerve head and at the ora serrata, the ring marking the retina's most peripheral limit. Elsewhere, the vitreous and general structure of the eye hold the retina in place. If, through disease, trauma, or a puncture wound, the retina is torn, the vitreous can leak behind it and cause it to detach.

If the peripheral retina pulls away, it can usually be reattached with little loss of visual function. If the detachment includes the macula and the retina is pulled away from the choroid, severe visual impairment, even blindness, can result.

Among the predisposing conditions for retinal detachment are high myopia, aphakia, vitreous abnormalities, diabetic retinopathy, retinal degeneration, and trauma. The most common symptom of retinal tear or detachment is the perception of flashing lights.

Immediate medical attention is necessary for retinal detachments because areas that are out of contact with the choroid for a long period may not regain their function. Treatment consists of bonding the retina to the choroid through diathermy (the application of high-frequency current that sears the choroid and retina), cryothermy (freeze bonding), or photocoagulation (laser bonding), all three of which induce scar tissue. It is important to remember that wherever a detached retina is reattached and scar tissue is induced, there will be a scotoma. Scleral buckling to force the retina into contact with the choroid may assist with the bonding procedure. The prognosis depends on the cause of the retinal detachment and the extent and duration of the detachment. Persons with detached retinas in one or both eyes should be careful about engaging in contact sports, diving, and strenuous activity.

Retinitis Pigmentosa

Retinitis pigmentosa (RP) is a group of diseases that result in the degeneration of the retina. The cause is unknown, but it is suspected to be an enzyme in the retina. Most types of RP are hereditary, but the pattern of inheritance varies. Genetic counseling is therefore advisable. In RP, the rods are destroyed, beginning in the midperiphery and gradually advancing inward toward the macula. In many common types, "tunnel vision" (severely restricted peripheral vision) results. In other types, central acuity is diminished. Many individuals who have RP also experience myopia, and many develop cataracts but are unlikely to develop glaucoma or retinal detachment. Night blindness, or difficulty seeing in dim light, is the first symptom and usually occurs sometime during adolescence; deterioration of peripheral vision follows. As the disease progresses and the cones of the eye are affected, central vision may be lost.

There are several types of RP, including congenital RP, or Leber's congenital amaurosis, which is apparent at birth or in infancy and causes a steady, progressive loss of sight; recessive, dominant, and sex-linked RP; and Usher's syndrome, in which vision loss is accompanied by hearing loss (Sardegna & Paul, 1991). No treatment is known for RP. However, a variety of optical devices (magnifiers, handheld telescopes, closed-circuit televisions, and infrared devices for night use) and higher levels of illumination may be helpful in managing it.

Combined Central and Peripheral Field Impairments

Coloboma

Ocular colobomas are defects of embryonic origin in which tissue of the eyelid, iris, retina, or choroid fails to form completely. If the coloboma is near the retinal periphery, functional vision is rarely affected. If it is a large chorioretinal coloboma that includes part of or the entire macula, considerable visual dysfunction may result.

A coloboma of the iris, discussed earlier in this chapter, may cause both photophobia and reduced visual acuity but may also be an indicator of other colobomas that are visible only through an ophthalmoscope. A coloboma of the optic nerve affects both visual function and pupillary reactions; the extent of functional difficulties depends on the location, type, and severity of the coloboma.

Optic Nerve Disorders and Diseases

Conditions of the optic nerve are complicated and difficult to diagnose because the only portion of the optic nerve that can be seen ophthalmologically is the optic disk, the exit point of the nerve from the retina. If there is swelling of the optic disk, suspected causes typically include optic neuritis, orbital tumor, or occlusion of the central retinal vein. If edema is bilateral, other possibilities include malignant hypertension or increased intracranial pressure. There are a number of conditions in which the disks appear normal. These include compressive lesions, tobacco-alcohol-induced amblyopia, vitamin B12 deficiency, and the effects of toxic materials. A third condition, "cupping," in which the optic disk ap-

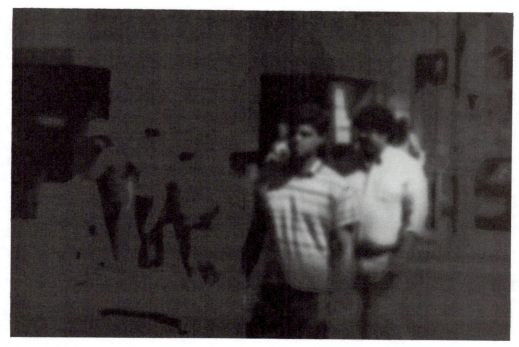

Night blindness and tunnel vision are common characteristics of retinitis pigmentosa.

pears indented, is typical of advanced glaucoma. Optic nerve disease and macular disease may be differentiated by comparing a number of factors, including visual acuity, color vision, visual fields, pupillary response, and sensitivity to light-brightness (Beck & Smith, 1988).

Optic Atrophy

Optic atrophy is a disorder of the optic nerve in which it is difficult for visual stimuli to be transmitted to the brain. There is no treatment, since degeneration of optic nerve fibers is irreversible. Optic atrophy may be congenital or acquired, the congenital type usually hereditary in nature and taking one of two forms. The milder form involves gradual onset of deterioration in childhood but little progression thereafter; the more severe form is present at birth or within two years and is accompanied by nystagmus. In general, optic neuropathy occurs rapidly, commonly in men aged 20 to 30; some vision may be retained.

The acquired type of optic atrophy may be due to a number of causes: vascular disturbances; degenerative retinal disease; pressure on the optic nerve; metabolic disease; trauma; glaucoma; or toxicity relating to alcohol, tobacco, or other poisons. The loss of vision is the only symptom. Treatment varies according to the cause, and prognoses for improvement are generally poor, except in some cases of optic atrophy caused by pressure on the optic nerve, when treatment is given soon after the diagnosis.

Optic Nerve Hypoplasia and Septo-optic Dysplasia

Optic nerve hypoplasia and septo-optic dysplasia are congenital malformations. In optic nerve hypoplasia, the optic nerve fails to develop because of a prenatal neurological insult; some experts believe that the development of the optic nerve actually regresses. Ophthalmologically, the nerve head appears unusually small and is surrounded by a lighter-colored "halo." The anomaly appears to be related to maternal chronic alcohol or drug abuse or to maternal diabetes. The level of visual acuity varies from mild to severe impairment. Occasionally, visual acuity may be normal with only a peripheral field impairment. When optic nerve hypoplasia is severe and bilateral, nystagmus is also usually present; in this case, there is a higher likelihood of other anomalies, such as microphthalmia or colobomas.

In the most extreme cases of this condition, referred to as *septo-optic dysplasia*, there may also be brain abnormalities, including the maldevelopment of the optic chiasm, the absence of the septum pellucidum (the connection between the hemispheres of the brain), pituitary dysfunction, and impairments in the corpus callosum. Those who lack the septum pellucidum may have spatial orientation problems. Low Apgar scores (an index of the physical condition of newborns) are common, and endocrine deficiencies appear after the first year or so of life. Most children with this condition also have some type of neurological difficulties.

Hemianopsia

Hemianopsia ("half vision") results when a specific portion of the optic pathway malfunctions, usually because of pressure from a tumor (see Figure 6.2 for examples of field losses related to the locations of lesions, which are localized, abnormal changes in tissue formation caused by injury or disease). The type, site, and amount of pressure determine the degree of field loss. There are many combinations and variations of field losses, depending on the site and direction from which the pressure is coming (especially at the optic chiasm). Field losses can be corresponding (homonymous, or the same in both eyes) or opposite, involve half fields or quadrants quadrantanopsia, or affect upper or lower fields. They can also affect macular vision or can leave it unaffected.

A retinal lesion, or one that exerts pressure on the optic nerve before it reaches the chiasm, will affect only one eye (see examples 1 and 2 on Figure 6.2), whereas lesions at the chiasm or beyond are more likely to affect both eyes in some way

(see example 3). (The fourth example in the figure depicts a lesion affecting only one eye because of the site of the lesion.) Chiasmal lesions may affect both central and peripheral fields, and the losses are usually bitemporal (referring to opposite sides, as in example 3). Lesions of the optic tract or beyond cause ipsilateral impairments (affecting the same side of both eyes, as in examples 5–7); pupillary reactions are also affected unless the lesion is beyond the optic tract. The closer to the occipital area the lesions are, the more likely it is that the field losses are to be identical in both eyes and that macular function will be spared.

Strokes

Strokes, or intracranial bleeding or infarctions, are another cause of visual field loss. In the case of a stroke, the location of bleeding in the brain will determine the extent and nature of the field loss involved. In general, certain types of visual field losses influence visual functioning more than others do. For example, when there are small scotomas in one or both eyes, functional vision is generally less affected than in other circumstances, as long as the macular area remains intact. When only half the visual fields remain in both eyes, the sites of the lesions determine visual functioning, depending on whether they are corresponding or opposite and which sides are affected. The presence or absence of a pupillary reaction may affect the amount of light that is comfortable to the individual or needed for visual tasks. The report of an ophthalmologist or neurologist should be consulted for a full interpretation of potential visual functioning.

In general, the location of visual field impairments has decided implications for visual functioning and mobility. Mobility, as well as the performance of daily living activities and tasks involving the use of near vision, can be affected by the nature and extent of central and peripheral field losses. Right field losses interfere most with reading in languages that are read from left to right. Inferior (lower) field deficits may interfere with the intermediate walking field, whereas superior (upper) field deficits may obscure over-

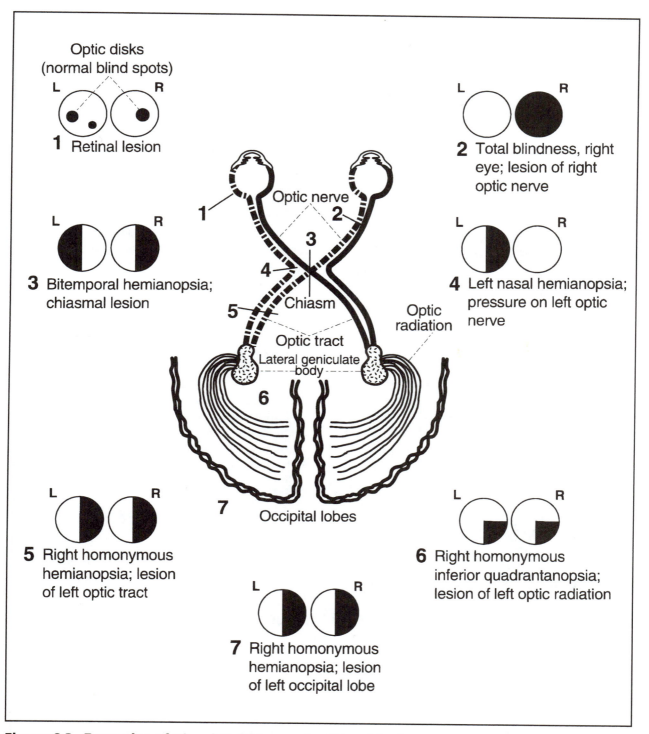

Figure 6.2. Examples of Visual Field Losses by Site of Lesion

Sources: Adapted and reprinted, by permission, from D. G. Vaughan and T. Asbury, *General Ophthalmology,* 9th ed. (Los Altos, CA: Lange Medical Publications, 1980), p. 214; H. Stein, B. Slatt, and R. Stein, *Ophthalmic Terminology* (St. Louis: C. V. Mosby, 1992), p. 225; and J. G. Chusid, *Correlative Neuroanatomy and Functional Neurology,* 17th ed. (Norwalk, CT: Appleton & Lange, 1979).

head obstacles. A perimacular field loss, or "ring" around the macula, may interfere with the use of magnification. RP, sickle-cell retinopathy, and, sometimes, diabetes may produce a marked restriction of the peripheral fields. This type of field loss, when severe, produces tunnel vision and affects both mobility and reading. When a person has visual field loss, a clinical low vision evaluation is essential to determine which, if any, optical devices will be helpful to that individual.

CONDITIONS CAUSED BY EXTERNAL AND OTHER FACTORS

Monocularity

When a person has the use of only one eye, he or she is said to be "monocular." Causes of the loss of vision in the dysfunctional eye usually include injury or enucleation (surgical removal of an eye), amblyopia, and optic nerve lesion. If the visual acuity in the better eye is normal, the only functional vision loss is the lack of depth perception, which is most critical at distances of less than 20 feet. There is also a reduced awareness of about 30 degrees of temporal field on the "blind side," but this reduction can be compensated for by turning the head in that direction. This temporal field loss may cause some problems in activities such as driving and playing tennis, but the individual usually learns to turn his or her head more often for compensation. Thus, if the remaining eye has intact central and peripheral vision, monocularity would not be considered a low vision issue.

Depth perception is a function of binocular vision and occurs primarily when the eyes converge slightly. Each eye sends a slightly different image to the brain; the two images are then fused and interpreted as having three dimensions because of the slight overlap in them. When one image is absent (as when one eye is dysfunctional), the single image received by the brain presents only two dimensions. It is clear and detailed if there is good central visual acuity, but there is no sense of distance or depth.

Individuals who are monocular see in two dimensions, as do binocular individuals at greater than 20 feet. Their near-distance judgments must be based on experience; knowledge of the environment; and other spatial information, such as comparative heights and overlapping objects. Thus, monocular persons must be constantly alert to their surroundings and the judgments needed to operate safely within their environments. In a child, monocularity can cause difficulties in leisure activities, such as errors in judging the speed of an approaching ball and estimating distances to throw a ball, and the child may, as a result, sometimes appear clumsy and uncoordinated; such situations are usually resolved with time and practice, but they can resurface unexpectedly in unfamiliar environments.

For a person who has amblyopia or whose vision in one eye has been suppressed because the eyes are not aligned, it may be important to note that vision has not necessarily been completely lost in the suppressed eye. Although central acuity is generally reduced in that eye, useful peripheral vision may be available. This vision can enhance spatial orientation, since objects and movement may be discernible with both eyes, and the person may "see" with a normal visual field.

Trauma

The eye is surrounded by ocular muscles and fat and is set in a bony orbit. Only a small area of the front of the eye—the cornea and part of the sclera—is visible. This area is protected by the eyelids, which close spontaneously before a threat. Despite these unique, protective structures, humans manage to damage their eyes with projectiles, chemicals, and a variety of other foreign bodies.

Injuries to the eye may include abrasions and lacerations, puncture wounds, blunt trauma, and burns (which can be caused by chemical and thermal causes and by radiant energy). Surface abrasions caused by foreign bodies usually affect only the surface of the cornea or conjunctiva. Medical attention is required in such cases, because damage from an abrasion may be serious and may require the use of an antibiotic and, possibly, patching. Foreign bodies that penetrate deeper than the surface of the cornea or sclera must be evaluated and treated by an ophthalmologist. Lacerations can affect the eyelids, cornea, and sclera. Immediate medical attention is essential.

Puncture Wounds

Puncture wounds can be caused by a wide range of materials, including wood, slivers of metal or glass, arrows, BBs, or pieces of plastic. Wood or plant materials often introduce infection and cause an intraocular inflammatory reaction within only a few hours. Both iron and copper are particularly chemically reactive with eye tissues and, like other metallic foreign bodies generally, must be removed. Most plastics, glass, stainless steel, and aluminum have minimal chemical reactions with ocular fluids but may carry bacteria that increase the risk of infection. Intraocular foreign bodies are removed surgically unless the surgery would cause more damage than the injury. *Sympathetic ophthalmia* (also called sympathetic uveitis) is a delayed hypersensitivity reaction to a penetrating ocular wound. Although rare, it can occur days or years after an injury, but most cases (80 percent) develop within three months (Newell, 1992). In this condition, the injured eye develops uveitis, and the uninjured eye reacts similarly, or "in sympathy." The inflammation can be suppressed medically, but treatment may take years. In general, sympathetic ophthalmia does not occur if the injured eye is removed within seven days of the injury, but enucleation is usually considered only when the injured eye is not visually useful.

Blunt Trauma

Blunt trauma can cause minimal to extensive damage within the eye. Externally, the bony orbit may be fractured; internally, subconjunctival hemorrhages can occur, the cornea can be abraded, the iris or retina can be torn, the lens can be dislocated or form a cataract, and the anterior chamber can become filled with blood and cause intraocular pressure to rise. An ophthalmologist should always be consulted when there has been a blow to the eye area, since damage can exceed what can be seen externally.

Burns

Burns nearly always damage vision, since they usually involve the cornea. Chemical burns should be irrigated immediately and require immediate medical attention. If there is scarring, vision will be reduced; glaucoma may develop if the Canal of Schlemm has been involved. Thermal burns are usually restricted to the eyelids but also require immediate medical attention.

Radiant energy (light) burns are of the ultraviolet (UV) and infrared (IR) types. Ultraviolet light is absorbed by the cornea and lens of the eye, and radiation is cumulative. Mountain climbers, sunbathers, people who are exposed to snowfields, and welders are all at risk of ultraviolet keratitis. Looking directly at the sun allows infrared rays to reach the fovea, where photoreceptors are destroyed and vision may be damaged. Infrared light can also cause cataracts.

People who have no natural lens because of a cataract removal are also at special risk of experiencing damage from UV light because the absence of the light-absorbing lens allows retinal cones to be exposed to whatever light rays reach them. Some types of cones can be destroyed by UV-A rays in the shorter wavelengths, so extreme caution should be exercised when using blacklight (UV light) with children who are aphakic, or have no lens.

Electromagnetic Radiation

Electromagnetic radiation can cause cataracts just beneath the back part of the lens capsule. Such radiation-induced cataracts have been observed in radar technicians, radio operators, air traffic controllers, and airplane pilots. Animal studies have suggested that the retina may be capable of perceiving magnetic fields, thus providing a link between electromagnetic radiation and the central nervous system (Olcese, Reuss, & Volbrath, 1985; Reuss & Olcese, 1986). Although there is insufficient evidence to warn individuals against exposure to electromagnetic fields, this issue should be monitored carefully by practitioners in the field of visual impairments.

Disorders Caused by Tumors of the Eye

Several areas of the eye can be affected by both benign and malignant tumors. Externally, tumors may affect the eyelids and conjunctiva (and only rarely the cornea), and most are benign. They are usually identified early, since they are externally visible. When tumors are present, biopsies should be done to identify whether they are malignant. Early treatment is essential to prevent damage to the eyes.

Intraocular tumors usually involve some part of the uveal tract. The choroid is a frequent location for tumors because of its many blood vessels. Symptoms include unexplained intraocular inflammation, loss of visual field, and retinal detachment. (Since intraocular tumors have been found in the eyes of persons who are blind, regular eye care is important even for persons with no useful vision.) Visual field studies and ophthalmoscopic examination can sometimes differentiate between a benign and a malignant melanoma. Radiotherapy or enucleation are treatment options.

Persons who have cancer in other parts of their bodies are also susceptible to metastatic disease in the choroid. Women who have breast or lung cancer and men with cancer of the lungs, kidneys, testicles, or prostate should be especially alert to this possibility.

Retinoblastoma is a tumor of the eye that is fatal if left untreated. It can be unilateral or bilateral and is usually evident in children aged 1 to 3. When it occurs with no family history, it is thought to be due to a mutated or damaged gene. The gene can become dominant, however, and may then be transmitted as an autosomal dominant characteristic. A considerable amount of genetic research is currently in progress; chromosome 13, the location of the retinoblastoma gene, is being examined for its possible relationship to other types of cancer.

If untreated, such tumors can spread to the brain through the optic nerve and can be fatal. CAT (computerized axial tomography) scans and ultrasound are useful diagnostic procedures. Treatment depends on the status of the tumor and whether it is bilateral or unilateral.

In eyes that have potentially useful vision, radiation therapy, chemotherapy, photocoagulation, and cryotherapy have all been used with varying degrees of success. When there is no hope of useful vision, enucleation is the treatment of choice. Individuals with bilateral retinoblastomas are at a high risk of developing cancer in other parts of the body and should be monitored throughout their lifetime.

Conditions Related to the Eyelids and Lacrimal System

The exterior parts of the ocular system have little effect on functional vision unless they are malformed or infected. However, because persons with low vision may also experience additional conditions related to the eyelids and lacrimal systems, common conditions are discussed here.

The primary impairment of the eyelids that can affect functional vision is *ptosis,* a drooping of the upper eyelid. When it is minor and does not interfere with vision, nothing is done. When it occludes the pupil, even with the eyes wide open, surgical correction may be indicated.

In older persons, the lower lid may turn inward, with the lashes abrading the cornea (*entropion*), or the lid may turn outward exposing the inner surface of the eyelid (*ectropion*). Surgery to return the lid to a normal position is indicated in both instances.

The inner surface of the eyelid, the conjunctiva, is susceptible to *conjunctivitis*, which can be allergic, bacterial, chemical, fungal, or viral in nature or associated with systemic diseases, such as gout or thyroid disease. Because the person usually feels pain or irritation, treatment is generally sought early. Other conditions are related to the lid margins and oil glands, which can become infected, causing a sty, blepharitis (inflammation of the eyelids), or chalazion (inflammation of a meibomian gland).

The lacrimal system can interfere with visual function if the quantity of tear fluid is affected. If there is an excess of tears, the fault is usually a blockage or partial blockage in the eye's drainage system. Excessive tearing can also be a symptom of other ocular problems (conjunctivitis, keratitis, iritis, or a foreign body in the eye). Any associated problem must be addressed before management of excess tearing is attempted. The opposite situation, "dry eyes," often affects older persons and may be a side effect of some medications. Artificial tears in drop form is the treatment of choice.

GENETICALLY DETERMINED CONDITIONS

The visual system is involved in a number of genetically determined disorders or conditions. Some modes of inheritance can be precisely documented; others are inconsistent or unpredictable.

Every human being carries 23 pairs of chromosomes in each cell. Twenty-two of these pairs are somewhat similar and are called autosomal chromosomes; the twenty-third pair contains the sex chromosomes. One of the pair of sex chromosomes is always an X chromosome; the other may be either an X or a Y. Females carry two X chromosomes, and males carry the XY combination. Each chromosome, including the sex chromosomes, contains genes that determine body characteristics. (A gene is a specific locus on a chromosome that carries the genetic information for a particular characteristic, such as eye color.) Genes are arranged in pairs that are similar (homozygous) or dissimilar (heterozygous). If the pairs are dissimilar, one gene will be dominant and the other will be recessive; both desirable and undesirable characteristics can be either dominant or recessive.

Genes can affect hereditary patterns in a number of ways, but both normal and abnormal characteristics are inherited in the same way, through totally random combinations at conception. Genetic disorders are usually one of three kinds: chromosomal, multifactorial, or monogenetic. In chromosomal disorders, one or more chromosomes may be missing, as in cri-du-chat, De Grouchy's syndrome, and Turner's syndrome, or an extra chromosome may be present, as in Down's syndrome.

In multifactorial disorders, a combination of factors, both genetic and nongenetic, are causative influences. Examples of visual involvements of this type are strabismus and some kinds of refractive disorders, such as myopia, cataracts in aging, and glaucoma. Metabolic disorders, although more difficult to trace genetically, probably have multifactorial components. A large number of syndromes are multifactorial and metabolic.

Monogenic (Mendelian) disorders have the clearest inheritance patterns. They fall into three well-defined categories: *autosomal dominant, autosomal recessive,* and *sex-linked.* In the autosomal dominant type, the defective gene is dominant. The parent who has this gene exhibits the characteristic and has a 50 percent chance of passing it on to children; if both parents carry the defective gene, the chance of passing it on increases to 75 percent. If one parent carries two defective genes, all children born will be affected. Examples of autosomal dominant inheritance include aniridia, some kinds of cataracts, most corneal dystrophies, some forms of RP and juvenile glaucoma, colobomas, neurofibromatosis, and Marfan's syndrome.

In autosomal recessive inheritance, the dominant gene is normal, but the recessive gene is abnormal. A disorder will not be manifested in children unless one parent carries two recessive genes and the other parent carries one recessive gene or unless both parents carry the recessive gene. However, carriers can be produced when only one parent has the recessive gene. Examples of autosomal recessive disorders include oculocutaneous albinism; most types of RP; metabolic diseases, such as diabetes; and enzyme deficiencies, such as Tay-Sach's disease. (There are hundreds of metabolic and enzyme deficiency disorders, and many involve ocular disturbances.)

Sex-linked inheritance patterns involve disorders whose genes are contained in the X chromosome. Therefore, in most ocular disorders transmitted by the X chromosome, the mother is the carrier and the father manifests the disorder. With most sex-linked disorders, only males are affected, mothers can pass on the disorder to half their sons, and the disorders are not transmitted from fathers to sons.

Thus, an affected male may have acquired the gene from his maternal grandfather as passed on through his mother. Examples of ocular disorders attributed to sex-linked transmission are ocular albinism, anophthalmia, some kinds of cataracts, color deficiencies, Leber's disease, macular dystrophy, microphthalmia, nystagmus, one kind of RP, and optic atrophy.

PERCEPTUAL DIFFICULTIES

Visual perception occurs in the brain. Thus, even when images are properly refracted and received by the photoreceptors of the eye, sorted, and transmitted correctly to the brain, perceptual problems may occur because, for some unknown reason, the brain is unable to make sense of the impulses sent by the optical system. Perceptual problems relating to vision can range in severity from simple reversals of letters or words to dyslexia—the inability to interpret written symbols, especially printed text.

Although some children with low vision may have perceptual problems that are directly related to their visual impairment, most do not. No specific disease or disorders of the eye are known to cause visual perceptual problems. Among the areas with which children with low vision may have difficulties are visual discrimination, spatial orientation, and figure-ground discrimination. Children with low vision may resemble those with learning disabilities in academic achieve-

ment, motor development (especially visual-motor abilities), and subtest scores on intelligence tests (Daugherty & Moran, 1982).

The educational team of a child who is visually impaired and exhibiting performance deficits or delays in perceptual development needs to determine whether they are caused by the visual impairment or a related brain-based perceptual problem. Since retinal and optic nerve pathologies are directly related to brain function, this differentiation may be difficult, and an interdisciplinary assessment is essential.

CORTICAL VISION LOSS

Vision loss of cortical origin is referred to as cortical vision loss and results from damage or disease to one or both occipital lobes of the brain. The occipital lobes contain the visual cortex, which may be thought of as the screen or canvas on which the visual fields are projected. Damage to one occipital lobe may produce field loss; damage to both lobes may produce a complete or severe loss of vision, often referred to as cortical blindness. Patients with cortical vision loss may deny and actually be unaware of their vision loss, in contrast to individuals whose visual impairment stems from retinal or optic nerve disease. Cortical vision loss is a complex phenomenon, and there is no uniformity in the terms used to describe the condition, which is also sometimes referred to as cortical visual impairment (CVI). In addition, diagnosis and management of the condition are complicated, particularly in regard to young children, because of the range of visual, neurological, and other factors that may be involved.

The main cause of cortical vision loss in adults is a cerebrovascular accident (CVA), or stroke, usually infarctions involving both occipital lobes. Other causes include intracranial tumors and trauma to the occipital lobes. In infants and children, the causes of cortical visual impairment are numerous. In addition to trauma, these causes include hydrocephaly, progressive cerebral degenerations, metabolic disorders, maldevelopment, and meningitis (Beck & Smith, 1988; Gittinger & Asdourian, 1988; Newell, 1992; Vaughan & Asbury, 1980).

The clinical signs of cortical sensory loss include marked decreased vision and visual field in both eyes with normal pupillary responses. Confirmation of this diagnosis is made with CAT scans or MRI (magnetic resonance imaging) evaluations of the visual cortex.

Children may have partial recovery from some of the causes of cortical vision loss. In the classroom and other settings, children with this condition are seen to have the following characteristics:

- normally coordinated eye movements with no nystagmus

- a short attention span

- absence of stereotypical mannerisms, such as eye poking or head shaking, although light gazing is often exhibited

- normal color perception

- normal optical structure

- variable visual functioning

- other neurological involvements (Jan & Groenveld, 1993).

Specific educational approaches that seem to be successful with children who have cortical visual impairment include:

- the provision of a multisensory learning experience that includes verbal and tactile cueing

- the application of simple and consistent teaching approaches

- the spacing of materials (such as objects and pictures) to reduce clutter and crowding

- the use of color, especially red and yellow, in teaching materials

- the use of real objects in learning experiences (Groenveld, Jan, & Leader, 1990).

PROGRESSIVE VISUAL IMPAIRMENT

Age, maturation, and changes in body chemistry and in personal lifestyle can all affect the status of a visual impairment. Regular and routine eye examinations are usually sufficient to manage changes in visual acuity or visual function in the most common visual disorders and diseases.

However, a number of visual conditions require more frequent monitoring. These include glaucoma, corneal dystrophies, macular degeneration, degenerative myopia, and RP, as well as systemic diseases and disorders that may affect vision, such as diabetes, tumors, and demyelinating diseases like multiple sclerosis. People with medical syndromes that lead to visual impairment should have an ophthalmologist on their educational or rehabilitation teams.

Self-awareness and self-monitoring are appropriate goals in an individual's educational or rehabilitation program. In such conditions as glaucoma and diabetes, it is important for the person to understand the implications of the visual impairment and the interaction between his or her lifestyle and health care and to receive direct instruction in monitoring techniques, the administration of medication, and the importance of regular eye care. In the case of RP, macular degeneration, and some demyelinating diseases, the individual needs to understand both the diagnosis and the prognosis of the visual impairment. He or she should be alert to signs of visual changes and should know which are important enough to require medical attention, for in general, responsibility rests with the individual for monitoring his or her own care.

SUMMARY

Vision is a complex process that requires both an optical system (the eye and all its parts) and a perceptual system (the brain and its connections to the eye through the optic nerve and optic pathways). Disorders or diseases in any part of this visual system can result in visual impairment.

Low visual acuity can be the result of a refractive error; macular disease; an optic nerve impairment; a cerebrovascular accident, stroke; or cortical processing difficulties. Retinal diseases or optic nerve disorders can cause field defects. Some conditions result in both central acuity and field impairment. However, two people with the same diagnosis and similar clinical measurements can differ greatly in their level of functioning.

Despite the array of possible disorders and diseases, there is a certain predictability about most visual impairments. The part of the visual system that is affected by a particular disorder can give clues that help the practitioner to anticipate how the person with low vision may function and can help in educational or rehabilitative planning.

ACTIVITIES

With This Chapter and Other Resources

1. Of the four people in the vignette that opens this chapter, two had incomplete or misleading information about their visual conditions. Prepare an explanation for Tom and Mike of the process of cataract surgery and the condition achromatopsia and indicate the functional implications of both.

2. Select one or more ocular defects or diseases and explain what they are in lay terms. Include the functional implications.

3. Review and extract information from an eye report and describe any functional implica-

tions suggested by the diagnosis, etiology, and prognosis.

In the Community

1. Determine what written or other information is generally available for children or adults about specific eye conditions, such as glaucoma, macular degeneration, and albinism. Contact consumer groups and national organizations, as well as local ophthalmologists, optometrists, and low vision clinics.

2. Prepare a presentation for parents of children who have a variety of visual conditions that describes the functional categories of visual impairments, rather than the disease categories by parts of the eye.

With a Person with Low Vision

1. Teach a young student how to explain to others what is wrong with his or her eyes. Help the student emphasize positive functional aspects when possible.

2. Develop a transcript of an interview with parents of a child with sex-linked retinoschisis who are considering having another child, in which the genetic counselor describes the probability of their having another child with this condition.

From Your Perspective

Why do some persons with low vision pursue every avenue to learn about the medical and functional aspects of their visual impairments, whereas others accept and are content with limited knowledge or explanations?

CHAPTER 7

Optics and Low Vision Devices

George J. Zimmerman

VIGNETTE

Billy, a sixth-grade student diagnosed with optic nerve atrophy, had difficulty reading his textbooks and the chalkboard from his desk. He complained of not being able to keep up with the class during reading assignments and of not being able to see what the teacher was writing when she was not directly in front of him. Billy's itinerant teacher of students with visual impairments helped Billy with some of his near vision reading tasks by improving the lighting at his desk. However, Billy continued to have difficulty with the distance vision task of reading the chalkboard from his seat.

The teacher of students with visual impairments recommended that Billy see a clinical low vision specialist, who prescribed two optical devices for him. The first device, a magnifier, allowed Billy to improve his near vision activities, and he no longer needed special lighting. The second device, a telescope, allowed him to see the chalkboard from anywhere in the classroom, which was extremely important to him because, at his height of 5 feet, 9 inches, he felt self-conscious about walking up to the chalkboard or sitting in the front row. Billy received instruction in using both devices from his teacher of students with visual impairments. With this support and assistance he is now able to read his textbooks and to see what is written on the chalkboard independently.

INTRODUCTION

This chapter focuses on the ability of people with low vision to use magnification devices successfully for near and distance vision tasks. It presents an overview of the principles of optics and optical devices, as well as the effect of these devices on the seeing process of individuals who have low vision. With this information, professionals will be better able to assist persons with low vision to enhance their visual functioning in educational, rehabilitation, recreational, and employment settings.

To understand the impact of any optical device (such as magnifiers, contact lenses, or eyeglasses) on the seeing process, one first needs to know the basic principles of light, optics, and lenses. The process of seeing begins when light passes through a variety of ocular media and eventually converges on the inside back of the eye. This chapter begins by discussing what light is, what happens to it during the converging process, and how that process occurs. It then describes various types of lenses and magnification and the latest technology in low vision optical devices and presents information on nonopti-

The author wishes to acknowledge Christine Roman, Ph.D., for her assistance in the conceptualization and editing of this chapter.

cal devices, electronic magnification systems, and field expansion systems. (The material presented in this chapter makes use of the following references: Jose [1983]; Faye [1976]).

Optical devices or aids use lenses or prisms to correct for an optical defect (for example, myopia) and are employed to magnify, reduce, or otherwise change the shape or location of an image on the retina. They may be held in the hand, rested on a base or stand, or be placed in a pair of eyeglasses. They are made for seeing at near point or, with a combination of lenses to form a telescope, to enlarge images seen from a distance. Sometimes, reversed telescopes, which make objects appear smaller, are used to "expand" the visual field by bringing additional information into the usable field. Optical devices may also include mirrors, prisms, and electronics. A closed-circuit television (CCTV), for example, electronically enlarges print or other material onto a television monitor. In general, optical devices vary greatly in price. Many lower power, less optically complex magnifiers and telescopes are priced below one hundred dollars. The cost of other devices is higher because of the quality or complexity of the lenses used. More complex optical systems and electronic devices may cost thousands of dollars.

Nonoptical devices are devices or aids that may be used to enhance visual functioning, especially by controlling illumination or improving contrast. Nonoptical devices may include such items as sunglasses and baseball caps as well as black felt-tipped pens and may range from the use of colored tape on dials, bold-line paper, and enlarged telephone buttons to additional sources of lighting employed to help an individual begin to use vision functionally or perform a task more comfortably.

The effective use of low vision devices depends on the characteristics of both the individual user and the individual device. Readers may therefore find it helpful to read this chapter in conjunction with Chapter 6, which reviews the implications of a variety of visual impairments, and Chapter 8, which considers clinical aspects of low vision and provides additional information about devices.

BASIC OPTICS

The Composition of Light

Two theories explain the composition of light. The first and oldest theory contends that light energy is composed of invisible particles, or corpuscles, and that these corpuscles emanate from a light source or object, such as fire, the sun, or an electric bulb, which are then reflected off objects and enter the eyes. This theory helps explain how light can be used to create electrical energy, such as is displayed in a light meter in a camera (American Optical Corporation, 1986).

The second theory, which is more commonly believed, contends that light travels in electromagnetic waves (American Optical Corporation, 1986) in a manner similar to the wave motion that is caused in water by tossing a rock into a pond. An electromagnetic wave is composed of radiation that, when vibrated at different speeds, provide sound, light, and heat. This theory is useful for explaining why a spectrum of colors can be seen in a rainbow or how prisms work to separate light. To understand why a rainbow or prism produces colors, one must know something about the measurement of light.

The Measurement of Light

As light moves in waves similar to those created in water by a tossed rock, there are both crests and troughs. The distance from the crest of one wave to the crest of the next, as shown in Figure 7.1, can be measured; this distance is referred to as wavelength or wave vibration. In the case of light, electromagnetic sine waves are measured in this manner, which provides a means for measuring different colors of light. The length of the wave is the distance that light travels forward as it goes through one complete vibration. When measured in a one-second interval, for example, longer wavelengths will vibrate fewer times than will shorter wavelengths, as shown in Figure 7.2. The term used to define these vibrations is *frequency,* which means the number of vibrations in a one-

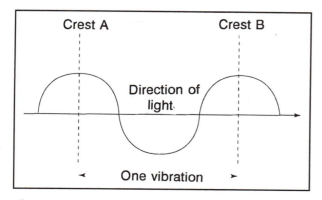

Figure 7.1. Measurement of a Wavelength

Source: Reprinted, by permission of the publisher, from the American Optical Corporation, *The Human Eye* (Southbridge, MA: Author, 1986).

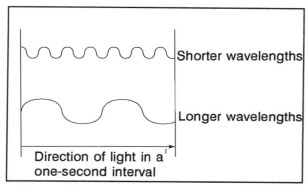

Figure 7.2. Wave Frequency

Source: Reprinted, by permission of the publisher, from the American Optical Corporation, *The Human Eye* (Southbridge, MA: Author, 1986).

second interval. To determine how fast light travels in any medium, the frequency of the vibration is multiplied by the wave length to produce velocity.

White light, a combination of all the colors of the rainbow, is a mixture of the color spectrum of an electromagnetic wave and is the only component of an electromagnetic wave that is visible. When a white light ray is shown through a prism, a piece of triangular glass used to separate light into its various colors, for example, the individual wavelengths are displayed as colors of the rainbow, from red, orange, yellow, green, and blue to

violet. Red is the longest wavelength color, and violet is the shortest. Continuing beyond both ends of the spectrum of visible light are wavelengths that are even longer or shorter. The remaining wavelengths longer than red waves produce infrared radiation and the even longer ones are radio waves. An FM (frequency modulation) stereo uses these wavelengths in the electromagnetic radiation wave band. Wavelengths that are shorter than violet produce ultra-violet, X-rays, and gamma rays.

Light travels at the speed of approximately 186,000 miles per second in a vacuum. Despite the velocity of all white light, there are variations in wave frequencies between the red and violet colors that are so small that the human eye cannot distinguish between them; thus, all visible light appears white and is not broken down into individual color components. Understanding wave-frequency variation is necessary to understand the refraction of visible light passing through various media.

Refraction

If a light ray strikes the surface of an object, such as a flat plate of glass at a 90-degree angle, it will pass through the glass without bending, provided that the two sides of the glass are parallel to each other. This passage is shown in Figure 7.3. The

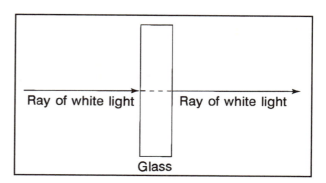

Figure 7.3. Light Passing Through Glass with Parallel Surfaces

Source: Reprinted, by permission of the publisher, from the American Optical Corporation, *The Human Eye* (Southbridge, MA: Author, 1986).

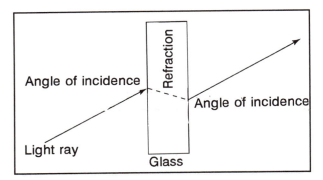

Figure 7.4. Refraction

Source: Reprinted, by permission of the publisher, from the American Optical Corporation, *The Human Eye* (Southbridge, MA: Author, 1986).

Light rays are believed to travel in parallel motion at a distance of 20 feet or beyond from the observer. As the observer gets within 20 feet of a light source (such as a lamp or flashlight), the light rays diverge, rather than travel in parallel motion. Understanding how light rays travel within and beyond 20 feet is important to remember when discussing refraction and concepts such as light, optics, and low vision magnification systems.

Refraction and the Ocular System

The cornea is the first of four transparent layers of the eye through which light passes en route to the retina; the remaining transparent layers, in order, are the aqueous, lens, and vitreous. As light passes through each layer, it is slowed and bent (or converged). Figure 7.5 shows the index of refraction for each of the four transparent media of the eye. These media do not differ significantly in their refractive index ability. Also note that the rays of light begin to converge toward the retina after passing through the various media.

The cornea constitutes approximately 75 percent of the refracting power of the ocular system, and the lens is the second most powerful light-bending structure of the system. The clarity of these internal media may affect the transmission of unobstructed light rays reaching the retina.

light ray (white light) will travel more slowly through the glass than it does through the air but will not bend and will not be perceived as a spectrum of color on exiting the glass.

However, if a light ray strikes a plate of glass with parallel surfaces positioned at an angle other than 90 degrees, it will bend toward an imaginary line perpendicular to the edge of the surface of the glass. The light ray will travel through the glass at a slower velocity. On exiting the glass, it will return to the original line of travel and will be perceived as white light. The angle at which light strikes and exits a surface is referred to as the *angle of incidence*. If the surfaces of the plate of glass are parallel, as in Figure 7.4, a color spectrum is not produced.

Refraction is the bending of visible light rays as they pass through different media. The relative speed of light passing through various media is referred to as the *index of refraction*. The index of refraction is measured by dividing the speed of light in air (186,000 miles per second) by the speed of light passing through the medium (for example, 122,000 miles per second for glass, so the index of refraction is approximately 1.52). For the purposes of this chapter, it is not important to know the index of refraction for various media. It is more important to know that light rays bend when striking and passing through various media at an angle other than 90 degrees.

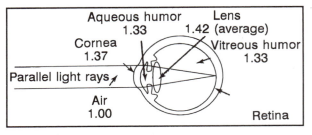

Figure 7.5. Indexes of Refraction of the Ocular Media

Source: Reprinted, by permission of the publisher, from the American Optical Corporation, *The Human Eye* (Southbridge, MA: Author, 1986).

THE OPTICS OF LENSES

Structure of a Lens

Thus far, this discussion has referred to media (such as the cornea of the eye or a flat plate of glass) whose surfaces are parallel. However, it is important to consider what happens to a single ray of light when it passes through media that do not have parallel surfaces. Throughout this section, readers will find it useful to remember that white light is composed of different electromagnetic wave frequencies that are not visible to the human eye. To see the spectrum of color, one must shine light through a plate of glass whose sides are not parallel. Figure 7.6 shows what happens to white light that passes through a plate of glass that does not have parallel surfaces: On striking the surface, the individual color velocities of the ray of white light are slowed, and each is refracted. Each color assumes a different path on exiting the glass. The frequencies are diverging and thus allow the human eye to perceive color.

The same event was described in the discussion of the angle of incidence and parallel surfaces (see Figure 7.4), but because the exiting surface of the glass was parallel to the entering surface, the individual color velocities grouped together and exited the glass on the original angle of incidence. The exiting angle of incidence is dependent on the index of refraction of the media and the angle of the surface of the lens. The greater the angle of the surface and the slower the index of refraction, the greater the refractive power of the media.

By using the information known on angle of incidence and index of refraction and also knowing the angle between the surfaces of glass, one can mathematically calculate the line that light will travel on exiting the glass. This relationship is referred to as *Snell's Law,* and knowledge of it will be useful for understanding lenses and optical devices as discussed later in this chapter.

To begin to understand the principles of how lenses work, one can imagine that four pieces of glass without parallel surfaces and with various

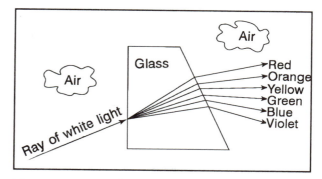

Figure 7.6. Light Passing Through Glass Without Parallel Surfaces

Source: Reprinted, by permission of the publisher, from the American Optical Corporation, *Basic Optical Concepts* (Southbridge, MA: Author, 1986).

degrees of angles are placed on top of each other and that a light is shined through them perpendicularly. Each angle of each piece of glass is greater than the next. The glass can be arranged to make the refracted rays exiting the glass come together and converge on the same point if the lenses are fused together, the imperfections are smoothed out, and all traces of lines separating each glass are removed. This series of steps is the process used when constructing lenses. Figure 7.7 shows what happens to light as it passes through a solid piece of glass (a lens) whose cross section resembles the shape of a cross section of a football.

The single rays of light striking the lens in the exact center or thickest portion are at a 90-degree angle and, therefore, do not bend. The remaining light rays, from the center to the edges of the lens, strike the surface at various angles of incidence. As the rays pass through and exit the lens, they begin to come together or converge at a specific point somewhere beyond the lens.

The discussion of light thus far has focused primarily on light emanating from a single point. Natural and artificial light is all around the environment, and it may be difficult in some instances to determine the exact origin of this light. However, one can assume that a single light source can be pinpointed and shone in close approximation to a lens, as shown in Figure 7.8. The rays of light emanating from the source are not

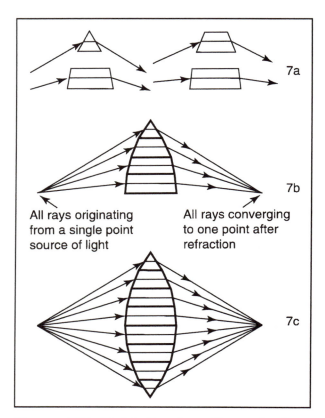

7a

7b

All rays originating from a single point source of light

All rays converging to one point after refraction

7c

Figure 7.7. Light Passing Through Four Pieces of Glass Without Parallel Surfaces and with Various Degrees of Angle

Source: Reprinted, by permission of the publisher, from the American Optical Corporation, *Elements of Optics* (Southbridge, MA: Author, 1959).

parallel to each other. In fact, they are diverging away from the source and each other; thus, if the lens was placed close to the light source, the rays striking the surface of the lens would have various angles of incidence, some greater than others. After passing through the lens, the rays begin to come together or converge to a single point. This point is referred to as the *focal point* or *image point*. Moving the lens closer to the light source, or vice versa, will cause the image point to move farther away from the lens. The closer the light source is to a lens, the more divergent are the rays and the greater the angle of incidence of each ray. Similarly, moving the light source farther away from the lens, and thereby decreasing the angle of incidence of rays striking the lens, will cause the

exiting rays to converge at an image point closer to the lens, as shown in Figure 7.9.

Types of Lenses

A variety of lenses have been developed for use in optical devices, such as microscopes, binoculars, and cameras. This section focuses on the various types of lenses used in devices for persons with low vision that give users the ability to enlarge images and alter the distances from themselves to the objects they are viewing.

Spherical Lenses

Spherical lenses may have two curved sides or one curved side and one flat side. A lens that bulges outward is called a *convex* or *plus* lens. If the lens bulges outward on both sides it is a *biconvex* lens (see *a* in Figure 7.10), whereas if it bulges outward on one side only, it is a *plano-convex* lens (see *b* in Figure 7.10). A convex lens is thicker at the center than at the edges and is used for converging light rays on a specific image point. This type of lens is useful for correcting hyperopia (see Chapter 6) because it converges light rays before the rays enter the eye, thus bringing the light rays to focus on the retina, rather than behind it.

Although light rays that strike the center of the surface of a lens at a 90-degree angle pass through the lens unaffected, rays that strike the same lens away from the exact center and closer to the ends of the lens will be refracted. At the edges of spherical lenses, light may be dispersed, as are colors in a prism (a process called *chromatic aberration*). The greater the aberration, the more fuzzy an image will be when viewed through a lens. In an aspherical lens, such as a magnifier, slight adjustments have been made in the shape of its periphery to reduce apparent chromatic aberrations. Therefore, a person who is reading print materials with a magnifier will experience fewer chromatic aberrations if he or she views the print directly through the center (or thickest portion) of the lens (often called the opti-

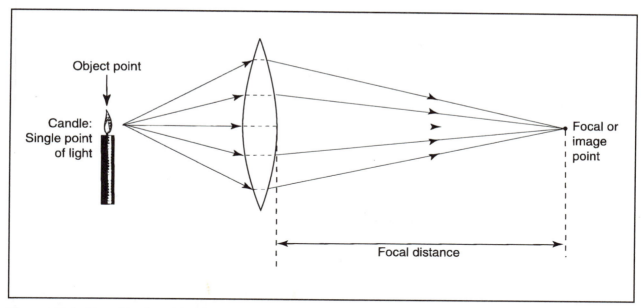

Figure 7.8. Focal Point: Single Source of Light Close to a Lens

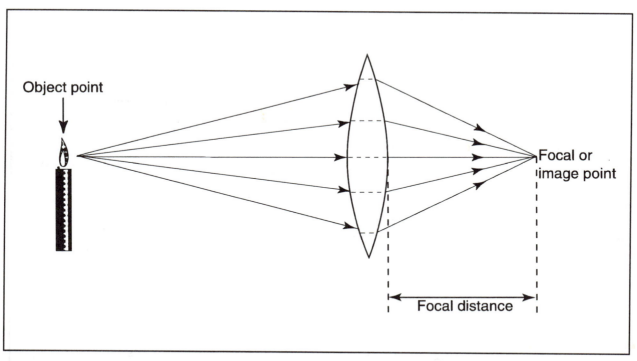

Figure 7.9. Focal Point: Single Source of Light Farther from a Lens

cal center of the lens). If the person views print material toward the periphery of the lens, the print will be distorted, and the person will in all likelihood experience visual fatigue.

The inverse of a convex lens is a *concave,* or *minus,* lens. This type of lens bulges inward and is used to diverge light rays. A concave lens that bulges inward on one side and is flat on the other

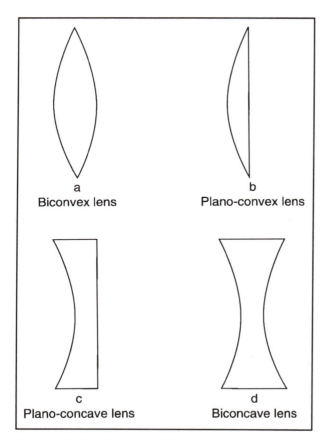

Figure 7.10. Spherical Lenses

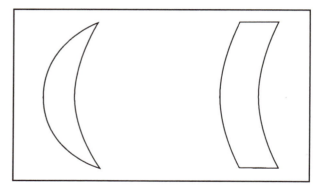

Figure 7.11. Meniscus Lenses

Cylindrical Lenses

A cylindrical lens has curves in one direction but is flat in the other direction, similar to a glass cylinder standing on end that has been cut through the middle from top to bottom (see Figure 7.12). It is useful for correcting astigmatism (see Chapter 6).

Plano Lenses

A lens that is cut flat on both sides is referred to as a plano lens. A plano lens does not bulge inward or outward and is not used for correction in eyeglasses. However, such a lens may be used for cosmetic or safety reasons. When one of two surfaces is constructed without a curve, the term, plano- is used before the term describing the curve of the other lens (as in plano-concave).

is called a *plano-concave* lens (see c in Figure 7.10). A concave lens that bulges inward on both sides is called a *biconcave* lens and is thinner in the middle and thicker at the edges (see d in Figure 7.10). A concave lens is useful for correcting myopia because it diverges light rays before the rays enter the eye and thus brings the light rays to focus on the retina, rather than in front of it. Concave lenses minify rather than magnify.

Meniscus Lenses

Meniscus lenses are spherical lenses with two curves (one a plus curve and one a minus curve) that can be used for either a plus or minus correction in a lens system. The surface with the greater curve will determine whether the lens is a plus or minus lens. These lenses are usually found in standard corrections for people who wear eyeglasses (see Figure 7.11).

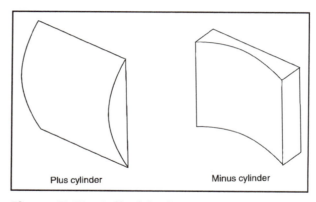

Figure 7.12. Cylindrical Lenses

Combination of Lenses

When constructing eyeglasses or optical devices, eye care specialists may recommend either a single-lens type or a combination of the various lenses just described. Examples of these lenses are biconvex, biconcave, plano-concave, plano-convex, and meniscus lenses.

Prism Lenses

Prism lenses are often prescribed and used with persons who have strabismus or slightly reduced visual acuity who tend to neglect or are unaware of a peripheral field loss. They are also used when optical devices are prescribed with strong plus lenses and the person has the potential to use binocular vision. When prisms are used for strabismus, the purpose of the lens is to redirect the rays of light entering the eye.

Prisms that are used for visual field neglect are more difficult to use when the neglect is in the right peripheral field—a condition that is more common in adults who have had a stroke but that may become apparent in children while they are reading or moving about the environment. Specifically, while reading, a child may tend not to turn his or her head fully to the right and thus will end a line of print before he or she reaches the actual right margin. While moving about, a child may consistently underestimate the distance from objects on either side of his or her body and make contact with those objects. Prism lenses are used to cue the person that additional information (such as the remaining words on a line of print or objects in the periphery) exists, even though it is not immediately apparent.

A Fresnel prism—a common type of prism—can be inserted into a plastic holder that the user can carry in his or her hand. For mobility tasks, a plastic Fresnel prism can be attached to half of each lens in a pair of corrective lenses. Prisms that are prescribed and mounted on a pair of corrective lenses generally require extensive training to be used successfully.

When a person with low vision has the potential to use both eyes together and needs strong plus lenses in a pair of eyeglasses, the lenses must be close to the face. This close working distance may not be sufficient to allow both eyes to converge and thus may place the images of the object on different portions of the retinas of both eyes. A prism is then used to shift the images, allowing for binocular vision.

Measurement of Lenses

As was mentioned earlier, when parallel light rays strike and pass through a spherical lens, the rays exiting the lens come together at the optical axis called the focal or image point. The image point of a lens is determined by measuring the distance from the rear surface of a lens to the point where the rays meet, commonly referred to as the *focal distance (fd)*.

The focal distance and the ability of a lens to bend light rays determine the power of the lens. A stronger, or more sharply curved, spherical lens has a shorter focal distance and converges light rays closer to the lens than does a flatter spherical lens.

The power of a lens is referred to in diopters (D). To calculate the diopter of a lens, divide the focal distance of the lens in centimeters (cm) into 100:

$$D = \frac{100 \text{ cm (40 inches)}}{\text{focal distance of lens (in cm)}}$$

For example, a convex lens with a focal distance of 4 cm has a power of +25D. Similarly, a convex lens with a focal distance of 25 cm has a power of +4D. Lenses with shorter focal distances have more diopters of power than do lenses with longer focal distances.

The same principles apply to concave lenses. The shorter the focal distance, the greater the dioptric power of the lens. However, when this measurement is written for concave lenses, a minus sign is used. For example, a concave lens with a focal distance of 4 cm is written as −25D. These notations for dioptric powers are used in prescriptions for eyeglasses, contact lenses, and optical devices.

TYPES OF MAGNIFICATION

Magnification increases the size of an image that is received by the eye by spreading the image over a larger portion of the retina. For persons with low vision, an image that is too small to be resolved can be enlarged though magnification. The four types of magnification—relative distance, relative size, angular, and projection—all have the same effect of increasing the amount of spread of an image on the retina.

Relative-Distance Magnification

Relative-distance magnification (also called linear or approach magnification) occurs when an object is brought closer to the eyes. As the object is moved closer to the eyes, the amount of information presented on the retina increases. Therefore, the distance is manipulated to gain magnification. For example, the image of a soda bottle can be doubled by moving it from a distance of 4 feet to a distance of 2 feet. Relative-distance magnification is the simplest way to achieve magnification, since it requires only that the individual move closer to the object he or she wishes to view.

Relative-Size Magnification

When the size of an object is increased and this larger object is viewed at a similar distance to the original object, the amount of information presented on the retina is also increased. This type of magnification is called relative-size magnification because the size of the object is manipulated to gain magnification, as with large print. Since it requires modification of the original object, though, it is a more restrictive type of magnification than is relative-distance magnification.

Angular Magnification

The apparent sizes of objects can also be increased through the use of various lenses or lens systems, such as the lenses found in a pair of binoculars. Angular magnification makes an object at a distance appear closer to the eye. Since the object appears closer, the image is spread over a larger portion of the retina, thereby producing a magnification effect. Optical devices are common examples of the use of angular magnification. Because such devices can be used in a wide variety of situations, they provide the user with a great deal of flexibility and independence.

Projection Magnification

When an image is projected, as with an overhead projector or a movie camera, the size of the image is increased. Projection magnification literally increases the size of the image to be viewed through the projection process. For example, a person can double the size of a movie image by moving the projector from a distance of 10 feet from the screen to 20 feet while remaining in the same seat.

Electronic devices, such as computer screens and televisions, also provide projection magnification. For example, a 20-inch television provides twice as large an image as does a 10-inch television. A CCTV, used to project the image of printed and graphic materials to increase their size, is an electronic device used by persons with low vision to gain magnification, generally for reading and writing, and will be discussed later in the chapter.

NEAR VISION OPTICAL DEVICES

The previous discussion of basic optics and the optics of lenses provides a foundation for understanding the application of lens systems in near vision devices, distance vision devices, nonoptical devices, and electronic devices. Table 7.1 presents an overview of the major types of low vision devices. This section describes near vision optical devices that can help students like Jack.

Like most 14-year-old boys, Jack enjoys eating in fast-food restaurants. However, his reasons

Table 7.1. Overview of Low Vision Devices

Type of Low Vision Device	Description	Primary Use	Examples of Devices	Type of Magnification
Near-vision magnification	Any optical device that magnifies the image for viewing tasks within 18 inches. These devices incorporate the use of specific lenses, generally convex or plus lenses.	Used primarily for near tasks within arm's reach, such as reading, writing, sewing, playing board games, and crafts.	Handheld magnifier	Angular
			Stand magnifier	Angular
			Spectacle lenses	Relative distance
			Mirror magnifier	Angular
			Telemicroscope	Angular
Distance-Vision magnification	Any optical system that magnifies the size of an image for viewing tasks from 12 inches to infinity. These devices incorporate the use of both convex and concave lenses.	Used primarily for distance tasks beyond arm's reach, such as spotting street signs, viewing sporting events, or watching television.	Handheld telescope	Angular
			Spectacle-mounted telescope	Angular
			Behind-the-lens telescope	Angular
Nonoptical device	A device that does not involve the use of corrective lenses (convex or concave). Many nonoptical devices do not involve magnification.	Used in near and distance tasks to enhance environmental features, such as illumination and contrast, to sustain visual functioning and to control visual fatigue.	Lighting	None
			Color filter	None
			Large-print material	Relative size
			Reading stands	None
Electronic magnification	A device that magnifies the size of an image through the use of lenses and electronic enhancement. The size of the image is increased as it is projected.	Used primarily for near and distance tasks that require greater magnification and flexibility in adjusting contrast and illumination.	Microcomputer screen	Projection
			Closed-circuit television	Projection
			Low Vision Enhancement System	Projection

for preferring these restaurants may be different from those of other 14 year olds. Jack, who has decreased central visual acuity, primarily uses large-print texts or audiotaped materials in school and finds that he has limited access to nonadapted print in the community. Therefore, he avoids restaurants with printed menus, daily specials, and prices that are subject to change and goes to fast-food restaurants, whose predictable menus he has memorized. Thus, he feels confident that in these restaurants, "one cheeseburger, small fries, and a Coke" will be available.

The use of a magnification device may provide Jack with options to overcome some of the near vision difficulties he encounters when adapted materials are not available. This discussion describes two main categories of near-vision devices—microscopes and magnifiers—both of which could help Jack gain access to print in school and in the community.

Microscopes

Convex (or plus) lenses that are mounted in an eyeglass frame are called microscopes and produce relative-distance magnification. If the object to be viewed is too far away to be seen, the microscope optically brings the object closer. As material to be viewed is moved closer to the eye, the microscope enlarges the image on the retina, so the image appears clearer to the viewer. The closer the material is moved to the eye, the larger the image that falls on the retina. Since light rays entering the eye are more divergent as an object is brought closer to the eye, the eye must adapt by increasing its focusing power to attain a clear image on the retina. Individuals who have a high degree of myopia experience the effect of a microscope when they remove their eyeglasses and use their extra plus-focusing power to bring targets that are near into clear view.

Microscope systems are generally prescribed by the clinical low vision specialist as a monocular lens when a high power is required, such as at the close working distance that is frequently used, and when convergence and binocular focus (the fusion of two images into one) cannot be achieved. Also, the specialist commonly prescribes the lens for use by the dominant eye, or the eye with better acuity. Although prisms can be used to achieve binocularity with high plus lenses, this approach is not effective with prescriptions above +15D.

Individuals who use high plus microscopic devices may find them particularly advantageous for a variety of reasons:

◆ Because microscopes are mounted into eyeglass frames, they allow users to have both hands free for near point activities like reading, writing, or engaging in hobbies, such as needle crafts and even tying flies for fishing.

◆ Because the lens is relatively close to the eye, users have a fuller field of view.

◆ In general, users find peripheral lens aberrations tolerable because they primarily employ the center of the lens for near viewing tasks and are taught to compensate for peripheral aberrations by using lateral head movements or by moving the text to be read or the object to be viewed.

◆ A variety of designs are available, including full-field lenses, bifocal lenses, half-eye lenses, monocular contact lenses, and clip-on loupes. A loupe is attached to the eyeglass frame and flipped up and down when needed by the user for near vision tasks. (Often jewelers will wear loupes to inspect cuts of diamonds.)

However, there are also certain disadvantages to the use of microscopes:

◆ Because the more powerful the microscope, the closer the user is positioned to the target, individuals may experience fatigue in their arms, neck, and shoulders, especially when holding heavy books while reading or maintaining a close working distance for an extended period.

◆ The use of head or arm movements for tracking (that is, for following a line of print) may make the system difficult to coordinate for efficient viewing. (Moving the material to be viewed, instead of the head, may be more efficient.)

◆ Users may feel confused and be unable to see objects beyond arm's reach when they look away from a near point task. This reaction may be a problem for students who

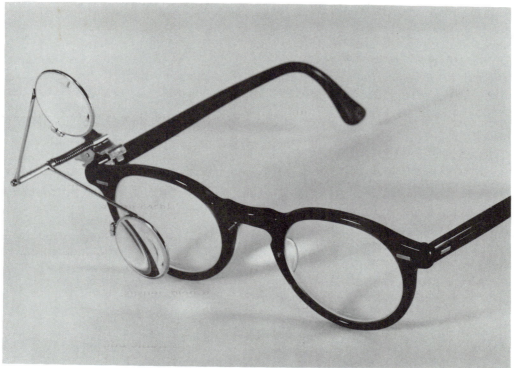

Clip-on loupes can be flipped up and down as needed by the user.

try to copy notes from a chalkboard, especially if they need to remove their eyeglasses each time they try to look at the chalkboard and switch to a telescopic device.

♦ Supplemental lighting may be required to provide enough illumination to see the material viewed.

♦ From an educational and psychosocial perspective, users may find it difficult to adjust to reading speeds that may be slower than expected because of the magnification and limited field of view and may be uncomfortable and conspicuous using extremely close working or viewing distances in public.

♦ Microscopes are relatively expensive. Depending on the type and complexity of

the lenses that are used, microscopes can cost as much as several hundred dollars.

Magnifiers

A magnifier increases the size of the image entering the eye. When this happens, the image may be large enough to stimulate sufficient retinal cells to send impulses to the optic nerve and to the visual receptors in the brain. In other words, if the image is tripled by the magnification lens, the image on the retina, and therefore the number of cells being stimulated, is also tripled.

A variety of magnifiers are generally used for near vision tasks, including handheld, stand, bar, illuminated, and mirror magnifiers. Some examples of the common uses of magnifiers are for reading personal communication, menus, and texts; confirming currency denominations in a wallet or the cost of an item on a price tag; or checking for an address or phone number in a telephone book. Magnifiers are prescribed as part of a thorough clinical low vision examination and from careful assessments of individuals' home, work, educational, and recreational needs.

Handheld Magnifiers

An important consideration in using a handheld magnifier is determining the appropriate focal distance—the distance from the lens of the magnifier to the object or surface being viewed, *not* the distance from the eye to the lens. The focal distance must be held constant and is determined by the dioptric power of the lens. An important principle to remember when working with high plus magnifiers is that the greater the focal distance, the narrower the field of view through the lens.

To establish focal distance in centimeters, practitioners divide the dioptric power of the magnifier into 100:

$$\text{focal distance of lens} = \frac{100 \text{ cm}}{D}$$

Thus, for example, if the magnifier is a +25 diopter lens, the focal distance is 4 cm (or 1.57 inches), and if the magnifier is a +5 diopter lens, the focal distance is 20 cm (or 7.87 inches). (Conversion of centimeters to inches is accomplished by dividing by 2.54, since 2.54 cm equals 1 inch.) It is vital for practitioners to understand and apply this principle when teaching individuals to use handheld magnifiers because the focal distance may be the critical factor in experiencing success with these devices. (However, it should be noted here that manufacturers do not always report the exact dioptric power of a hand or stand magnifier.)

The power of a handheld magnifier is delineated in "X" notation, such as 2X, 4X, or 8X. The strength of the magnifier, or the "X" notation, is determined by dividing the diopters of the lens by 4:

$$\text{"X" notation} = \frac{D}{4}$$

For example, a 40-diopter lens will magnify a target 10 times and is expressed as a 10X lens. The more powerful a lens, the greater the "X" notation number; thus, an 8X magnifier has a stronger magnification than has a 4X magnifier. If it is necessary to find the focal distance for a device for which only the "X" value is reported, the dioptric value must be calculated first by multiplying the "X" value by 4:

$$D = \text{"X" magnification} \times 4$$

See Table 7.2 for a quick reference on determining the appropriate focal distances of various near vision devices.

Another important principle to consider in regard to handheld magnifiers is that the closer the device is to the eye, the larger the field of view and the smaller the amount of obvious distortion of the symbols being viewed. In other words, as the user moves the magnifier closer to the eye while maintaining proper focal distance, a larger and clearer area of the surface being viewed will be present. Conversely, the farther from the eye the user holds the magnifier, the smaller the field of view. When the diameter of the magnifier is held constant, as the dioptric power of the lens increases, the field of view decreases.

The following are other advantages to using handheld magnifiers:

- They are cosmetically and socially acceptable, so users may not feel uncomfortable about employing them in public (such as in restaurants).

- They are lightweight and portable.

- They are relatively inexpensive and are less expensive than are microscopes.

- When appropriate positioning techniques are used, the individual maintains a natu-

Table 7.2. Focal Distance Chart: A Summary

Diopters	Power	Focal Distance (in inches)	Focal Distance (in centimeters)
+ 2	0.5 ×	10.00	50.00
+ 4	1.0 ×	20.00	25.00
+ 5	1.25 ×	8.00	20.00
+ 6	1.5 ×	6.60	16.67
+ 8	2.0 ×	5.00	12.50
+10	2.5 ×	4.00	10.00
+12	3.0 ×	3.30	8.30
+14	3.5 ×	2.90	7.14
+16	4.0 ×	2.50	6.25
+18	4.5 ×	2.20	5.50
+20	5.0 ×	2.00	5.00
+24	6.0 ×	1.70	4.16
+32	8.0 ×	1.20	3.10
+40	10.0 ×	1.00	2.50
+48	12.0 ×	.83	2.08
+56	14.0 ×	.71	1.78
+64	16.0 ×	.62	1.56
+72	18.0 ×	.55	1.38
+80	20.0 ×	.50	1.25

Source: Reprinted, by permission of the publisher, from Bureau of Education for Exceptional Students, *A Resource Manual for the Development and Evaluation of Special Programs for Exceptional Students, Volume V-E: Project IVEY: Increasing Visual Efficiency* (Tallahassee: Florida Department of Education, 1987).

Note: This chart is applicable only to near vision devices.

♦ ral perspective in regard to the surrounding environment.

♦ Prolonged periods of accommodation are not experienced when fixation is shifted from the reading task.

♦ A variety of designs are available (pocket-size, full-page, and ergonomic designs).

♦ If lighting and contrast are factors important to the user, he or she may choose a device that contains a built-in light source.

♦ Magnifiers are more flexible than are other devices for a variety of near vision tasks, since they can be placed anywhere within arm's reach and can be used with other corrective lenses.

However, there are also several disadvantages to using handheld magnifiers:

♦ The focal distance must be held constant.

♦ The field of view is limited, depending on the magnification (the greater the magnification, the smaller the field of view).

♦ Because efficient viewing requires the coordination of the eyes, hands, and head, magnifiers are not advisable for persons with poor eye-hand coordination or poor fine-motor skills.

♦ One or both hands must be used.

♦ Magnifiers with built-in light sources require users to change bulbs or batteries.

Stand Magnifiers

Stand magnifiers, like handheld magnifiers, are convex or plus lenses. The key feature of a stand magnifier is that it sits on a page or surface to be read and is installed in a lightweight platform that secures the distance between the lens and the viewing surface. (Some stand magnifiers are composed entirely of lens material and, therefore, a platform is not required.) The stand magnifier is positioned on the page and over the material to be read and moved across the line of print.

Because the lens is fixed into the stand at a slightly decreased focal length to control for distortions in the periphery of the lens, the actual power indicated on the stand magnifier is generally not the power of magnification realized by the user. Furthermore, some stand magnifiers have an adjustable lens system that can accommodate for the impact of a device user's own refractive errors. Therefore, clinical low vision specialists conduct specialized evaluations when combinations of lens systems are required and may prescribe additional plus, minus, or bifocal lenses so users can achieve optimum magnification.

As was previously mentioned, the clearest advantage of stand magnifiers is the fixed focal distance from the lens to the viewing surface. This fixed focal distance is particularly beneficial for

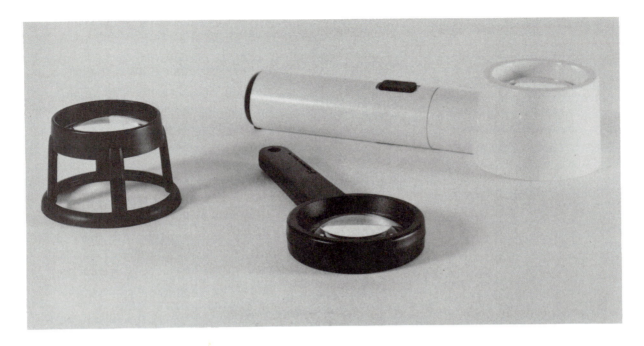

Magnifiers may be used for a variety of near vision tasks, such as reading.

those with poor fine-motor control (such as those with hand tremors) and poor eye-hand coordination who have difficulty positioning materials at specific focal distances or maintaining the focal distance of handheld magnifiers. In addition, magnifiers have the following advantages:

- They are relatively inexpensive.
- They are portable and lightweight.
- They are cosmetically (socially) acceptable.
- They come in a variety of designs (some have a clear plexiglass base to allow for light, and others have legs).
- They are usable with other forms of correction.
- Some models have built-in lighting for added illumination.

Among the drawbacks of using some stand magnifiers is the difficulty of reading or viewing in positions that require the individual to bend forward over the lens and viewing surface to use the optical center of the lens. This position is not only physically fatiguing, but it also causes the user's head and body to block overhead sources of illumination. Newer designs have an angled surface to ameliorate this problem. Other disadvantages are:

- The field of view may be limited, depending on the magnification (the greater the magnification, the smaller the field of view).
- Stand magnifiers are generally bulkier than are handheld magnifiers and cannot be carried in a pocket or handbag.
- One or both hands must be used.
- Stand magnifiers with built-in illumination systems require users to change bulbs or batteries.

Bar Magnifiers

Bar magnifiers are generally considered to be a type of stand magnifier because of the fixed focal distance that is achieved when they are placed directly over a line of print. They are typically not available in high powers of magnification. Because they magnify one line of print at a time, they can be particularly useful for individuals who have difficulty maintaining the smooth, continuous tracking required in reading.

Illuminated Magnifiers

Illuminated magnifiers are especially helpful for people who use high-powered devices, who require supplementary lighting, or who wish to avoid reflections from ceiling lights. The construction of these higher powered magnifiers results in a lens that transmits less light, since the light reaching the viewing surface is decreased, and more light is absorbed by the thickness of the lens itself.

With a high-powered near vision device, the focal distance between the lens and the printed material is generally shorter than with less powerful systems. Because of this decreased focal distance, the user needs appropriate levels of illumination that generally cannot be provided from supplementary sources without causing uncomfortable levels of reflective glare. Thus, illuminated magnifiers are a solution to this problem.

Illuminated magnifiers are available as both handheld and stand devices. The built-in light sources may be incandescent, fluorescent, or halogen; may provide a constant intensity of light or may be adjusted by using a rheostat; and may be battery operated or electrical. However, all illuminated magnifiers supply light that is intended to clarify the symbols being viewed evenly without producing shadows or glare to interfere with the viewing field. Therefore, these magnifiers permit individuals with low vision to be less affected by the lighting conditions of an environment, as in a dimly lit church, restaurant, theater, or store or outdoors in the evening.

Mirror Magnifiers

In most magnifiers, the lens is parallel to the reading surface, which forces the reader to align his or her body parallel to the device. Users report that this posture increases their physical fatigue, which hampers their ability to read for long periods. One way to ameliorate this problem is to place on the page, one line above the line to be magnified, a mirror magnifier with a 45-degree viewing angle. When a magnifier is placed in this position, the need for the user to be in parallel alignment with the viewing surface is eliminated.

DISTANCE VISION OPTICAL DEVICES

Optical devices for distance viewing, known as telescopic devices, include handheld monoculars, clip-on monoculars, spectacle-mounted telescopes, and contact lens systems. People with low vision, like Amanda, can increase their independence by using these devices.

After work, Amanda, aged 26, goes to a health club that is less than one mile from her home. Because she has decreased visual acuity and peripheral field restrictions from retinopathy of prematurity (ROP), she generally uses a cane while traveling outdoors. Amanda's orientation and mobility (O&M) instructor helped her learn to use both visual and auditory cues to cross intersections. However, Amanda continues to have difficulty visually discriminating the "stop" and "go" signals at corners. Although she often relies on sighted pedestrians to tell her when it is safe to cross the street, she is uncomfortable with what she believes is an inefficient and unsafe street-crossing system. The use of a distance viewing device, such as a handheld monocular telescope, will enable Amanda to see the "stop" and "go" signals and to combine these visual cues with the auditory cues she is receiving for safer and more independent crossings.

Telescopes: General Information

The basic purpose of telescopic devices is to enable an individual to bring distance information into closer view so that objects appear larger. Telescopic devices may be used for orientation, for localization, for short-term spotting activities, or for mobility. Although refinements have been made in a variety of telescopes for distance viewing, the Galilean telescope is often the device selected by clinical low vision specialists for individuals with low vision. This telescope is made of two lenses: the objective lens is a plus or convex lens and the ocular lens is a minus or concave lens. In discussions of telescopes, the *objective* is the end nearest to the object being viewed, and the *ocular* is the end nearest to the eye. The two lenses in a telescope are separated at a distance that is equal to the sum of the focal lengths of both lenses. The optics and power of the two lenses and the length of the telescope barrel determine whether objects can be viewed at nearer versus more distant ranges.

Some telescopes, termed *afocal,* are prefocused at optical infinity. Although any focusable device can be set at infinity, afocal devices may be selected for individuals who are beginning to undertake distance training. Objects that are at distances of 20 feet or more will be in focus at this setting.

A reading cap (plus lens) is an adaptation that permits focusing distances of 16 to 18 inches. When placed in front of the objective lens of a telescope, the reading cap creates a system called a *telemicroscope,* which provides additional plus lens power to an existing system, transforming the telescope into a viewing device for intermediate distances. People who need to view small features but must maintain greater distances and must have both hands free (such as someone who plays an instrument in a community orchestra and must be able to read the music on a music stand) may find a reading cap especially useful.

An important characteristic of telescopes is that as the degree of magnification increases, the extent or degree of the visual field decreases. For example, one type of monocular (see the discussion that follows) that has 6X magnification power provides an 11 degree field of view, whereas a monocular with 8X magnification provides only a 8.2 degree field. Thus, the user may have difficulty judging objects that are moving through the restricted field of a telescopic device and may perceive that his or her body is less stable in space. Therefore, instructional techniques should include methods that enable the user to find a secure and comfortable viewing position.

Another general consideration is that light transmitted through the lenses of a telescope is altered and usually decreased. Therefore, some people with low vision may need a device that has an increased surface area of the objective lens and hence increased light transmission, whereas others who are intolerant of brightness may benefit from a telescope that transmits lower levels of light. In addition, some users may require several devices to correspond with various levels of illumination.

In general, the amount of brightness an individual can tolerate is determined by the size of his or her pupil and the amount of light passing through the telescope. To determine the amount of light transmission through a telescope, one must know the magnification and the diameter of the objective lens in millimeters (mm). For example, a 6×30 telescope (the first number indicates the power of the lens, and the second number indicates the amount of light entering the telescope) will transmit a 5 mm bundle of light rays to the eye. If the width of the person's pupil is 5 mm, the person will benefit from a brighter image than would be obtained by using a 6×18 telescope, which would reduce the overall brightness from 5 mm to 3 mm. Thus, the clinical low vision specialist must select a telescope that corresponds to the size of the user's pupil size, as well as consider the amount of magnification and the width of the objective lens.

Handheld Monocular Telescopes

Handheld monocular telescopes, which are perhaps the most extensively prescribed devices, are used for short-term distance viewing tasks, such as reading a street sign or a chalkboard at school, checking a shopping mall directory, reading signs in grocery store aisles, or viewing plays and sporting events. These telescopes are commonly available in 2.5X, 2.8X, 3X, 4X, 6X, 8X, and 10X powers. As the power of a telescope increases, the field of view generally decreases; therefore, it is important to determine whether an individual can compensate for the reduced field of view provided by a particular device.

For people with low vision, handheld monoculars are often the preferred distance viewing devices. Some of the advantages of these devices are as follows:

- They are small and lightweight and can be carried in a pocket or handbag or worn on a cord around the neck.
- They are less expensive than spectacle-mounted devices of comparable power.
- They generally can focus on objects whose distance is from 10 inches to infinity.
- The user can choose the preferred eye or dominant hand and can position and adjust the focusing mechanism with either hand.
- A full range of magnification is available (from 2.5X to 10X or more).
- A plus lens can convert the device into a telemicroscope.
- Reverse telescopes expand the visual fields of persons with poor peripheral vision.

Some of the limitations of using handheld monocular telescopes are the following:

- They require specialized instruction in how to align an object, the lens, and the eye and in how to scan stable and moving objects.
- They are generally used for monocular viewing.
- They inhibit the transmission of light.
- They cannot be used for activities that require two hands because one hand is needed to hold and focus them.
- Higher-power telescopes have a small field of view and require good arm-hand-eye control.
- The user may experience upper-body and visual fatigue if he or she has difficulty

maintaining a stable arm position for brief or extended periods.

- Motion that is viewed is exaggerated as magnification increases.

Clip-on Monocular Telescopes

A clip-on monocular is an adaptation of a handheld telescope. It can be attached to or removed from an eyeglass lens, using a wire clip, at the user's discretion or can be flipped up and out of the viewer's visual field to allow for mobility. A clip-on telescope is generally intended for monocular use and has the advantage of enabling the wearer to have two hands free once the focus has been adjusted for a given task. Other advantages are as follows:

- Clip-on telescopes are relatively inexpensive.
- They are beneficial for prolonged distance viewing and for persons with poor fine-motor coordination.
- They offer lower-power magnification, which increases the field of view.

However, it is important to note the following disadvantages:

- Although a variety of magnification is available (from 2.5X to 6X), magnification powers greater than 3X are generally not available.
- A clip-on monocular adds extra weight to eyeglasses and therefore may not be comfortable.
- Because the lens of the telescope is mounted on the spectacle frame at a greater distance from the eye than a handheld monocular would be, the visual field is reduced.
- Some individuals may find it necessary to occlude the unaided eye during the initial stages of instruction to avoid visual interference from that eye.

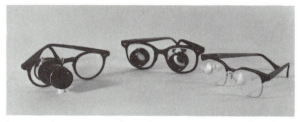

Spectacle-mounted telescopes or telemicroscopes are useful to people who need to view small features at greater distances and must have both hands free to perform tasks.

Spectacle-Mounted Telescopes

Full-Field Telescope Systems

Spectacle-mounted distance systems use telescopes that are permanently fixed to the individual's eyeglass lens and are positioned in front of the pupil. Like clip-on types, spectacle-mounted telescopes permit the user to use both hands for activities and do not require sustained motor control and coordination for their use.

A full-field spectacle-mounted telescope provides magnification over the entire lens in the eyeglass frame and is prescribed for individuals who need a larger field of view primarily for leisure, recreational, or vocational purposes, such as for watching television or repairing a car engine. The permanently attached lenses are available in higher powers of magnification and in some prism lenses; can have either an afocal or an adjustable system; can be manufactured to include more than one type of correction, including corrections for astigmatism; and are available in half-frame lenses for easier adjustment in transferring from near distance to far distance tasks.

No other correction or viewing option can be exercised while a full-field spectacle-mounted telescope is worn; the user sees only the magnified images. In addition, the user will experience significant peripheral distortion that severely limits the possibility of safe movement. For these reasons, as well as the higher cost of these full-field devices relative to handheld or clip-on telescopes, their conspicuous appearance, and the need to use a greater number of head movements

and more frequent scanning to keep an object in view with them, full-field spectacle-mounted telescopes are infrequently prescribed.

Bioptic Telescope Systems

Bioptic telescope systems are miniature telescopes mounted into an individual's regular spectacle lenses, positioned above or below what is the direct line of sight as the individual is facing forward. The placement of the bioptic telescope is determined by the tasks the user intends to perform with it (in some states, certain persons with low vision can receive special licenses to drive while using bioptic telescopic lenses). With most bioptic telescopic systems, users employ specific head movements, either up or down, to view through the telescope as needed and then reverse the movement to use the correction in their other conventional lens.

For people who have the potential for simultaneous binocular vision, binocular telescopes are mounted into both lenses of a user's spectacles for short-term distance viewing. For those who have similar vision in both eyes, binocular telescopes may provide the depth and spatial advantages of binocular vision.

As with all spectacle-mounted distance-viewing telescopes, users of bioptic telescope systems experience reduced fields of view. In addition, some people, especially those whose lenses are prescribed binocularly, report the presence of a "ring scotoma" resulting from the housing of the telescope and the bioptic system of lenses. Other limitations are that these devices are heavier and more cumbersome than other spectacle-mounted devices and require training in their use.

Contact Lens Telescopes

A full-field telescopic system, which produces a visual field of approximately 50 degrees and nearly 2X magnification power, can be created for continuous wearing for some individuals. This arrangement creates a Galilean telescope system by fitting a high-power minus contact lens on the eye that serves as the ocular lens and a high-powered plus lens in spectacle frames that serves as the objective lens. Although this system requires careful attention to alignment and distance and many practitioners have found that their clients have limited success with it, some people may want to try it for its cosmetic advantage and the benefit of being able to wear it full time.

Behind-the-Lens Telescopes

Another type of distance optical device, called a behind-the-lens system, was developed primarily because of the cosmetic issues surrounding the use of bioptic or frame-mounted telescopic systems, which protrude from the lenses into which they are mounted. Behind-the-lens telescopes incorporate a Keplerian or astronomical telescope, which uses two convex lenses and a prism to invert the perceived image, unlike the Galilean telescope, which uses a convex objective lens and a concave ocular lens.

In this system, the telescope is frame mounted behind the lens and directly in front of the cornea, as opposed to the Galilean bioptic system, which is frame mounted but more conspicuous. Because the telescope is placed in the inferior field of the carrier lens, it does not inhibit central visual functioning, and there is less midline distortion of an image. A behind-the-lens system is used like a bifocal; that is, the person moves the eyes down and views through the lens. At present, behind-the-lens systems are available only in 3X and 4X powers and require training in their use.

NONOPTICAL SYSTEMS

Bess is a first-grade student who has been diagnosed with aniridia. Because of her limited visual acuity, she is seated at the front of the classroom, where most instruction takes place. Although the size of the print in the first-grade

texts appears adequate for Bess at this time, her performance relative to both near and distance activities seems erratic. Sometimes Bess avoids activities, does not complete assignments, or puts her head down on her desk. The classroom teacher is puzzled by Bess's inconsistency and wonders if Bess may have a behavioral or emotional problem.

During a meeting of Bess's educational team, the itinerant teacher of students with visual impairments offered several nonoptical solutions to make learning easier for Bess. First, because of photophobia associated with aniridia, the teacher suggested that Bess wear tinted lenses and, at times, even sunglasses in class. Second, since Bess's fluctuating performance could be related to fluctuating lighting conditions, she recommended that Bess be seated with her back to the windows, that a light-absorbing blotter be placed on the surface of her desk to reduce reflective glare, and that worksheets be reproduced with darkened high-contrast characters for Bess.

Each of the interventions suggested by Bess's teacher represents a nonoptical solution to the effects of the little girl's visual impairment. The discussion that follows examines some of the nonoptical systems that can make visual information more accessible for individuals with low vision.

Illumination

Illumination is the amount of light on a surface. The amount of illuminance present is measured in footcandles of power. Reflectance, or luminance, is the amount of light from a task, surface, or similar point of focus, to the eye; reflected light is the light to which the eye responds. Reflectance is measured in foot lamberts. Various surfaces produce or are characterized by different amounts of surface reflectance; ceilings, walls, and floors all produce distinct levels of illumination. A light meter provides measurements of the quantity of light that is present on the surface of a viewing target or its surrounding surfaces.

What is considered a comfortable or sufficient quantity of light for the performance of a task varies from individual to individual. The Illuminating Engineering Society publishes a list of recommended levels of illumination expressed in footcandles for specific environments or tasks. For example, the minimum lighting recommended for writing by hand in pencil is 70 footcandles of luminance. The list may be useful to practitioners when deciding upon secondary levels of illumination for an individual who is performing a task. (For additional information, the society can be contacted at 120 Wall Street, New York, NY 10005-4001; (212) 248-5000; http://www.iesna.org/iesna.) For persons with low vision, the amount of illumination for comfortable viewing may be related to many individual factors, such as the extent and location of a visual impairment, the time of day, and personal preference.

Types of Light

Illumination also relates to the type of light that is present. The source of natural, full-spectrum light is the sun; however, specific combinations of incandescent plus fluorescent light can produce near full-spectrum conditions. For some individuals with low vision, natural light or sunlight may be the optimal viewing environment, whereas other individuals may react with extreme sensitivity in sunlight.

Incandescent light, which is similar to natural light in regard to the continuous light energy that it produces, is usually associated with indoor household lighting. Although it tends to produce the least irritating lighting environment for viewing tasks, it may not permit the high levels of contrast that some people with low vision need.

The third category of light, fluorescent light, is a cooler light source that yields higher levels of illumination, but it produces visual fatigue because of its potential strobelike effect. Although the blue-white type of fluorescent light is usually found in overhead fixtures, "daylight" or "pink" types are preferred for prolonged viewing periods. Since proper lighting conditions are essential for persons with low vision, practitioners must carefully consider not only the amount of light, but the type and position of lighting when evaluating how to modify the environment to maximize an individual's use of vision.

Position of Light

There is no formula for determining the proper position of light for a given person, so when the issue of positioning is considered, an individual should be assessed according to his or her eye condition, the type of task to be performed, the setting, the available light sources, the time of day, and the individual's personal preference. In general, supplemental light sources are positioned so that the light comes over the shoulder opposite to the individual's preferred hand (that is, if the person is right-handed, the light is positioned over the left shoulder) to prevent the person's body from casting shadows in the work area to be viewed. If the person functions monocularly, the light may be positioned so that it comes over the shoulder nearest the functional eye. Those who use supplemental light sources should position the light as close to the task or object to be viewed as is comfortable because the greater the distance from the source of light, the lesser the effect of the lighting.

As people grow older, changes tend to occur in the ocular system, for example, the amount of light transmitted to the retina may be reduced. In such cases, the elderly individual may move closer to the object being viewed or may turn on more lights, both of which are normal adaptations to increase contrast. With increasing levels of illumination, the person not only feels greater comfort, but the size of the viewed image is enhanced.

In many cases, a reading stand can be used to provide increased lighting without shadows and to help the reader place material in a position that is comfortable for viewing. Positioning the stand appropriately can allow the user to sustain a close working distance without experiencing strain in the neck, back, or arm muscles. Furthermore, when a stand with an adjustable shelf is used, the individual can adjust the stand, rather than continually change his or her posture, and thus will have greater access to information toward the end or bottom of a page. Some reading stands have built-in gooseneck lamps that enable the user to choose from a variety of lighting positions. Reading stands are available in table-top, floor, and clip-on models.

Adaptation to Light and Dark

Movement from brightly illuminated settings into dark settings requires 10 to 20 minutes for the light-sensitive cells of the retina, specifically, the rods, to adjust to lower levels of light. Because the cones of the eye adapt more quickly, a person can in general adjust from lower levels of illumination to brighter environments in 2 to 6 minutes. It is, therefore, important for professionals who are providing low vision services to monitor the individual's ability to adjust to various lighting conditions and to consider the use of adaptations, such as red or amber lenses, to facilitate smoother transitions between differently lit environments.

Glare

An important factor that must be considered in a discussion of illumination is glare, of which there are three types: discomfort glare, environmental glare, and disability glare. Discomfort glare is stray light that reduces visual comfort but generally does not interfere with the resolution of an image on the retina. For example, because of this type of glare, a student whose desktop reflects the ceiling lights may experience visual fatigue when working on materials placed on the desktop.

Environmental glare actually interferes with the resolution of visual information. This type of glare can be caused by tiny particles in the air or on a viewing surface or by highly reflective surfaces, such as high-gloss pages in a book. Disability glare is related to aspects of the visual system and can be caused by the clarity of the ocular media, corneal scarring, or cataracts. For instance, corneal scarring will cause light passing through the eye to radiate or scatter throughout the eye, producing a distorted image and, at times, an uncomfortable level of glare.

Modifications can be made in the environment and to materials and to work surfaces to provide light-absorbing, rather than light-reflecting, settings and hence to decrease the interference of glare in an individual's visual activities. A reduction in objects suspended from a ceiling, the placement of a carpet remnant under a work station, the use of a desktop blotter, or the wearing of a cap with a visor are all examples of such adaptations.

Illumination Control

Rheostat switches, which are devices mounted on lamps and other light sources to manipulate lighting levels, can be installed on both overhead and tabletop sources of supplemental light to allow a person with low vision, especially one with photophobia, to adjust lighting for various near and distance viewing tasks. An individual can use rheostats to create appropriate levels of illumination to compensate for changes in light in a room at different times of the day, to perform various tasks and hence to avoid visual fatigue, or to accommodate lighting to different types of materials.

Other devices that are used to control illumination and reflective glare are sunglasses and sunfilters. Sunglasses are generally designed to provide comfort and protection from high levels of light and glare for people with average sensitivity to light. However, those who have such conditions as cataracts, corneal scars, or vitreous hemorrhages may find even average levels of light to be excessive or painful. Conditions that cause light to scatter in the eye and diminish functional vision can create hazards for individuals with low vision. Sunglasses or sunfilters that are carefully chosen to meet the optical requirements of the user can significantly improve a person's vision.

Choosing appropriate sunglasses for an individual entails the consideration of several factors, including the transmission of light, the reduction of glare, the control of ultraviolet and infrared rays, the suitable color for the lenses and the design and shape of the frames, and the compatibility of the sunglasses with prescription lenses. Because each person has a different threshold of sensitivity to both indoor and outdoor light, if possible, sunfilters should be tested in the environments in which they will be used. In addition, cosmetic factors should be discussed with the individual; for example, a young child may respond differently to the use of sunglasses in settings in which his or her peers may be encountered than may a teenager or an adult.

Sunglasses are generally manufactured with lenses having light-transmission rates ranging from 60 percent to 20 percent (indicating an absorption of 40 percent to 80 percent of the light)—levels of transmission that are more appropriate for individuals with normal sensitivity to light. However, much useful vision remains even in the presence of lower transmission levels, such as those below 20 percent, and light-absorptive lenses can be manufactured with light-transmission levels as low as 1 percent. Therefore, when sunglasses are being used, professionals working with people with low vision should be alert to any decrease in visual acuity caused by the presence of lenses that transmit low levels of light.

People with photophobia may require greater amounts of light absorption to function comfortably. Sunglasses that eliminate up to 99 percent of reflective glare are available in various colors that provide further protection to the user who is sensitive to particular spectral wavelengths. For example, red or amber-yellow tinted sunglasses eliminate most blue and green light wave lengths that persons with retinitis pigmentosa (RP) typically find uncomfortable.

Nonoptical Magnification

As was indicated earlier in this chapter, relative-size magnification involves increasing the size of an object. According to the principle governing relative-size magnification, the increased size of the target increases the number of retinal cells being stimulated. (A target that is too small will not stimulate a large enough area of retinal cells

to be visually resolved and perceived by a person with low visual acuity.) When a sufficient area of retinal cells is stimulated by the object to be viewed, the cells send impulses to the optic nerve; the visual information is then perceived and ready to be interpreted by the body's processing centers.

Large-print materials are an example of non-optical relative-size magnification that allow a person with low visual acuity to maintain a more normal distance from the material to be viewed when reading; however, large-print materials are not universally available and may be considered cumbersome because of their typically increased length.

Relative-size magnification may not be useful for a person who has less than 5 degrees of visual field because the image produced would fall outside the viable area of the retina, and the person would receive only partial image input. To view the entire enlarged image, the individual would have to scan the image visually and hence would need complex viewing and processing skills.

Relative-distance magnification involves the reduction of the distance between the eye and the object being viewed, as when a person brings a photo closer to his or her eyes to distinguish the details. In the nonoptical approach, the object is not actually being magnified, but as the object approaches the eye, the image on the retina increases and the brain perceives it as larger.

This approach requires no special adaptation to materials. However, there are several drawbacks that warrant consideration. First, the closer the material is to the eye, the less information is presented in the available field of view, and the individual may need to learn visual scanning techniques. Second, the reduced viewing distance and limited visual field may result in visual fatigue, and some may perceive the need to reduce viewing distance as a socially unacceptable behavior in public. Third, there are some circumstances in which relative-distance magnification is not feasible. For example, in a grocery store, it is not possible to bring labels on high shelves closer to the eyes; in such situations, a hand magnifier may be beneficial.

ELECTRONIC SYSTEMS

Manuel uses braille primarily for assignments that require reading in his fifth-grade class. His best visual acuity is approximately 20/400 in his better eye, and he becomes visually fatigued after reading print for a few minutes. Although he is supplied with large-print adaptations of maps and charts for social studies, because of variations in the size and contrast of the print, Manuel frequently asks to take these assignments home so he can get help from his mother. His teacher of students with visual impairments recently requested that the school acquire a CCTV, so Manuel could have easier access to print in sizes and contrast levels that meet his visual needs and hence could perform tasks independently.

A CCTV is an example of an electronic magnification system. Such systems are the focus of the discussion that follows.

Common Electronic Magnification Systems

Electronic magnification systems are machines that produce enlarged images. Although overhead projectors, slide projectors, and rear-projection systems successfully use the principle of projection (or electronic) magnification, a number of factors make these devices impractical as low vision devices. First, most of these machines are not portable. Second, because they generally require decreased room light to achieve appropriate levels of contrast, they must often be used outside the classroom or work environment. Third, with both slide projectors and rear-projection systems, as an image is magnified, resolution and contrast are decreased. Fourth, some devices, such as overhead projectors, may produce levels of illumination that are too intense for comfortable prolonged viewing. In short, these systems may offer short-term occasional solutions for individuals who require enlarged images, but they are rarely the solution of choice for the person with long-term magnification needs.

The advantages of near-vision electronic magnification systems, such as CCTVs and computer monitors, can be summarized as follows:

- CCTVs and microcomputers allow magnification up to 64X.
- Brightness and contrast can be controlled.
- Postural fatigue is reduced.
- Near vision systems can be used for reading and writing.
- Text shown on the monitor screen can be blocked for reading a single word, a line, or a paragraph.
- Some CCTVs can be linked to a microcomputer.
- Some microcomputers are portable.
- The possible working distance for the user is increased.
- Software with a variety of fonts is available.

However, the limitations of these systems are the following:

- They are expensive.
- Many systems are not portable.
- Training may be required.
- One or both hands are required to operate these systems.
- An external power source is needed.

The discussion that follows explores these advantages and disadvantages in more detail.

CCTVs

A CCTV provides electronic magnification by means of a video camera that, when directed at an object or symbol, projects the image onto a television monitor. Although the CCTV is generally thought of as a near vision device, external cameras are available that permit distance viewing as well. Most CCTVs use systems that are "in line"; that is, the camera, the monitor, and all the electronic parts are arranged in a vertical position above the viewing material. Monitors are available in a variety of sizes, from 12 to 19 inches, and, although most monitors are black and white, amber or green monitors are also available. CCTVs that electronically enlarge color images are also available.

Some individuals prefer larger monitors on which greater amounts of information can be presented at one time. Below the monitor, reading material can be placed on an X/Y table, which permits horizontal and vertical manual (or, in some versions, motorized) movement of the material being viewed. Other features of CCTVs are focus, enlargement, and contrast controls; reversed polarity features (that is, a black-on-white background or white-on-black background can be selected); and window options, so portions of the text projected on the viewing screen can be blocked or blacked out for single-word, single-line, or paragraph viewing. Some CCTVs can be interfaced with computer systems so that the monitor can display information as well as printed material; in addition, handheld models have been introduced.

The benefits that CCTV systems provide to users are enlargement that can be controlled by the viewer; enhanced contrast; clarity of images; increased size of the viewing field; reduction of shadows or smearing of symbols; and the ability to maintain more comfortable, natural reading positions. As the technology improves, CCTVs that are lightweight and more portable, including types making use of hand scanning, are becoming more widely available.

The CCTV is generally suggested as a secondary device for educational or vocational purposes because it is not portable. As with the use of all vision devices, it is important to evaluate the individual's visual skills, motor skills, and motivation to learn to use an electronic magnification device when a CCTV is being considered for use by a particular person. CCTVs are costly, but when they are selected for appropriate users, they can be a highly effective means of enlarging and viewing information.

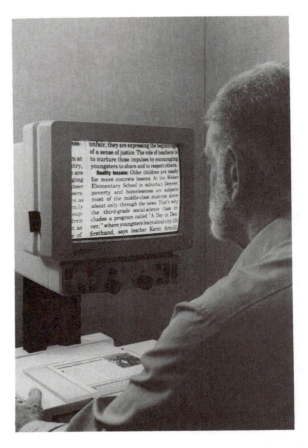

Closed-circuit televisions project an enlarged image of reading materials onto a television-type screen.

Computer Systems

Computers are another effective type of enlarging system for various tasks. Software with variable sizes and types of fonts, enlarged monitors, and screen magnifiers are readily available for computer use. Computers also provide users with choice of colors for print and background shown on the screen, control of the speed and type of scrolling of material to be viewed, and control of the size and location of the viewing window. The vertical position of a computer screen is also advantageous to persons with low vision who cannot see the type on a typewriter, which is positioned a greater distance from the eyes.

In addition, many computer printers can produce printed information in various sizes and styles of type. For example, someone who prefers to work with 18-point type on the computer screen can then print it in 24-point type, such as a lecturer who needs to read material at a greater distance from the page when presenting a talk to an audience.

Other Magnification Systems

The advancement of microchip technology has spurred the refinement not only of microcomputers, but of optical systems that are most apparent in televisions, CCTVs, and videocassette recorders (VCRs). Because microchips have become smaller and faster and are capable of performing multiple tasks at once, researchers and manufacturers have begun to develop new devices that persons with low vision can use. These systems incorporate the latest technology to produce images that are optically correct, and they are capable of modifying images.

The Johns Hopkins Low Vision Enhancement System (LVES) is an example of a device that reflects these advances in technology. This head-borne device is worn on the face like a pair of giant eyeglasses. Three miniature cameras, which are engineered into the frame, function similarly to an on-line camcorder; they display their black-and-white video images back onto a screen in front of the person's eyes. The images produced by the LVES are equivalent to those one would see when sitting in front of a 60-inch television screen at a distance of four feet.

The LVES may be connected to a VCR to allow the user to view movies. It can also be connected to a computer or a compact video disk to allow a person to scroll across a screen. Individuals who will benefit the most from using the LVES are those who have visual acuities ranging from 20/100 to 20/800 in the better eye.

electronically enlarges images seen at a distance

FIELD-EXPANSION SYSTEMS

Field-expansion systems offer a variety of options for individuals with reduced visual fields. There are two categories of systems: field selective and full field.

Selective field-expansion systems allow the user to employ a system selectively for specific visual tasks. A prism, discussed earlier as a means of enhancing reduced peripheral fields, is a good example of such a system that can displace and enhance the field of view that is not readily apparent.

Full-field expansion systems allow the user to view a visual array in its totality. An example of a full-field expansion system is a reverse telescope, which is a Galilean telescope that is viewed through the objective versus the ocular lens (exit pupil) of the telescope. Reversing the telescope allows the user to view an entire setting because the image is not magnified, but minified. A reverse telescope may be used for familiarizing oneself to unfamiliar rooms. To benefit from its use, however, the individual must have good central visual acuity and reduced peripheral fields, as is the case with persons who have RP.

An advantage of using either a field-select or full-field expansion system is that a greater amount of additional environmental information is available to the user; objects that would normally not be viewed because of a field restriction can be enhanced and displaced closer to the field of view. A disadvantage of using either system is that the user's perception of where objects are located in actual space is disrupted. Therefore, a period of training in the use of either system is recommended.

SUMMARY

This chapter discussed a number of principles related to basic optics, lenses, and the visual system and presented numerous descriptions of various optical, nonoptical, and electronic low vision devices. Understanding the task-specific visual difficulties that persons with low vision may face and knowing how to resolve those difficulties through the use of optical and nonoptical devices requires knowledge and expertise in all these areas.

The vignettes in this chapter provided examples of optical and nonoptical devices and addressed the specific visual needs of the individual in relation to the particular task and setting described. The factors listed for the consideration of the use of various devices relate to the quality of services that can be provided to people with low vision. The more familiar that professionals are with these considerations and the characteristics of various optical and nonoptical devices, the more enriched the services they offer clients will be.

ACTIVITIES

Using This Chapter and Other Resources

1. Consider the vignette of Billy that opens this chapter. Billy's teacher has asked you to prepare a lesson plan on basic optics for his class and to include how the principles of Billy's new devices are applied to help people with low vision to see. Billy thinks this lesson is a good way in which he can introduce his devices to his classmates. Write the lesson plan that will be used with Billy's class.

2. Develop a fact sheet about optical and non-optical devices that summarizes the options available to persons with low vision.

3. Compare the features of three telescopes of different powers, including field of view, light-gathering features, size, and magnification.

4. Compare a child's or adult's reading rate as the person uses a handheld illuminated magnifier versus a magnifier used with ambient or supplemental room light.

In the Community

1. Prepare a list of local, regional, and national suppliers of optical, nonoptical, and electronic devices and include methods for obtaining and repairing the devices.

2. Observe a teacher of students with visual impairments or an orientation and mobility instructor teaching the use of an optical device to a child who has low vision. Discuss the goal or goals of the lesson, the method used to teach the use of the device, and whether the child's visual functioning was enhanced when the device was used.

With a Person with Low Vision

1. With a preschool or early elementary school child with low vision, pretend to be a person who uses optical devices in daily life. This type of play may prepare the child for the later use of optical devices. Examples of persons who use optical devices include sea captains, detectives, photographers, and jewelers.

2. Observe an older adult using a recently prescribed optical device. Consider whether the person is using the device efficiently. For a near vision magnifier, consider aspects of use such as whether the person is holding the device at focal length, coordinating movements across a line and to the next line, feeling comfortable when holding the device, and experiencing reasonable reading speed and stamina. For a spectacle-mounted magnifier, consider the individual's eye and head movements, as well as movements involving the lens and the object being viewed. Are there any techniques that may help the person become more efficient?

From Your Perspective

Optical devices have been used by persons with low vision for many years. Why do you think that some school systems and rehabilitation agencies still do not include training in the use of optical devices in their services?

CHAPTER 8

Clinical Low Vision Services

Mark E. Wilkinson

VIGNETTE

Larry is a 35-year-old former golf pro with multiple sclerosis who uses a wheelchair for mobility. In an effort to stay in the field of golf, Larry recently became a partner in a corporation that was building a golf resort. He came to the low vision clinic because of decreased vision owing to his illness.

During the clinical low vision evaluation, Larry said that he wanted to acquire a low vision device that would allow him to be both binocular and more comfortable with sustained near point activities than he was with his current 4X monocular spectacle-mounted telescope. Although Larry had done well in the past with this telescope, he was uncomfortable not being able to use both eyes together, especially for near point activities, and he had a great deal of fatigue when using this device for extended periods. Larry was interested in a binocular system that would allow him to read more comfortably, without having to adopt the closer working distance that reading spectacles require.

Larry's distance acuity was 20/200 with either eye, and his near acuity was 6M print at 12 inches with either eye through his standard spectacle correction. With the 4X spectacle-mounted telescope for the left eye, Larry's distance vision improved to 20/70.

As a result of the clinical low vision evaluation, the clinical low vision specialist prescribed a 4X bin-

ocular reading telescope system that allowed Larry to read 1M continuous-text print at 13 inches without difficulty for extended periods and gave Larry a 5X hand magnifier that he could carry with him. Because Larry needed to do a great deal of reading and writing, a closed-circuit television (CCTV) was also demonstrated and loaned to him for a trial period. Larry eventually acquired a CCTV because he found it to be useful for reading the many contracts and other paperwork he needed to review daily.

INTRODUCTION

The clinical low vision evaluation determines whether an individual with low vision can benefit from optical and nonoptical devices, as well as adaptive techniques, to enhance visual function. Clinical low vision services encompass not only the clinical low evaluation, but also such related services as instruction in the use of prescribed devices, loans of devices for a trial period, and all necessary follow-up. These services help people with low vision gain greater independence in using vision and the ability to accomplish many of their goals and meet their needs. Clinical low vision services also encompass referrals to a variety of individuals and agencies providing services to individuals with visual impairments, including orientation and mobility (O&M) specialists, general rehabilitation services, educational services, technology assistance, and additional medical or surgical care when indicated.

Clinical low vision evaluations should be recommended for all individuals with low vision, regardless of their ages or the severity of their additional disabilities. This service should be ongoing and integrated into the care provided by a team of professionals, as described in Chapter 1.

In general, clinical low vision care may often be overlooked by eye care providers as an integral component in the treatment of persons with low vision. Often individuals with low vision are told that nothing more can be done to enhance or improve their visual functioning, when what is actually meant is that nothing more can be done medically or surgically. Children with congenital low vision often receive their initial ophthalmic care from eye care specialists who may tend to be pessimistic about the children's functional vision because they significantly underestimate the children's future visual capabilities. Frequently, adults with low vision have similar experiences and hence consider that the visual problems that have brought them to an ophthalmologist, such as the inability to read, are a permanent result of a nontreatable visual condition. For reasons such as these, attention by service providers to the need for sound low vision care is vital.

Eye care services for persons with low vision are generally provided in three phases:

1. an initial evaluation by an eye care professional (optometrist or ophthalmologist), who provides a diagnosis and medical treatment or referral for medical treatment or surgical care, when appropriate, for the eye condition

2. an evaluation by a clinical low vision specialist, who provides optical and nonoptical devices to enhance visual function for specific tasks

3. educational or rehabilitation services by professionals who provide instruction and meaningful practice in the use of prescribed devices.

This chapter reviews the components of a clinical low vision evaluation, the techniques and equipment used in these evaluations, factors that go into the choice of the most appropriate optical and nonoptical devices, and the information that should be given to individuals following their evaluations. Readers may find it helpful to read this chapter in conjunction with the previous chapters in Part 2 of this book, which deal with the visual system, the causes of visual impairment, and optics and low vision devices.

BACKGROUND

Purpose of an Evaluation

A clinical low vision evaluation should be recommended for all individuals with low vision as an adjunct to the care they receive from their eye care providers—ophthalmologists or optometrists. Whereas the role of the eye care provider is to maximize a person's visual capabilities through all available medical, surgical, and optical means, the role of the clinical low vision specialist is to maximize a person's functional vision capabilities. The clinical low vision evaluation differs from the evaluation of the eye care specialist in many ways:

- It starts with a comprehensive, goal-oriented case history.

- It uses special charts and materials for the assessment of distance and near visual acuity that are not routinely used in general eye examinations.

- It goes beyond the prescription of standard spectacles to provide optical, nonoptical, and/or nonvisual devices to help individuals meet their specific visual needs for distance, intermediate, and near activities.

- It includes the gathering of information about the individual's functional use of vision by a clinical low vision specialist, even when optical devices may not be beneficial, to provide techniques for maximizing the functional use of vision.

The clinical low vision specialist initiates and maintains ongoing communication with other members of the low vision team. At the conclusion of the low vision evaluation, the team members review the person's capabilities to be sure that he or she can easily and efficiently use the optical devices that have been recommended to accomplish specified goals. The low vision evaluation also results in referrals to other services or resources, when appropriate.

Low vision care must be comprehensive to ensure that people with low vision have the devices and techniques they need to assist them in their educational, vocational, self-help, and recreational activities. It must also be ongoing, since individuals' visual needs may change over time because of changes in their visual system and their goals.

Referral for an Evaluation

Once a person has been diagnosed as having low vision by a primary eye care provider, he or she should be referred for a clinical low vision evaluation, as part of the overall multidisciplinary rehabilitation services, to review what, if any, optical and nonoptical devices and other rehabilitative techniques, such as O&M, would be beneficial. However, many individuals are not referred. The reasons why they are not referred are not always well understood, but some possible explanations are that many eye care specialists:

- ◆ spend more time reviewing the eye disease than the functional effects of the eye condition on the person
- ◆ underestimate the individual's functional visual potential
- ◆ are unfamiliar with the benefits of vision rehabilitation or sources of services for referral
- ◆ may not be acquainted with individuals who have made maximum use of their vision
- ◆ lack training in referral procedures or believe that such referrals are not part of their responsibility.

The following case histories of Louise and Wanda illustrate the importance of not underestimating a child's capabilities early in life.

Louise was 13 years old and had a history of tyrosinase-positive oculocutaneous albinism when she underwent her first clinical low vision evaluation. She had received ongoing eye care since she was 2 weeks old and received her first spectacle correction at 6 months. When she reached school age, she was enrolled in a residential school. When her family moved to a new state, Louise was not enrolled in that state's residential school for the blind. During the low vision evaluation, Louise stated that since she had headaches and eye fatigue when reading regular-size print, she was reading large print. At this visit, Louise, her mother, and her teacher of students with visual impairments were interested to see what could be done to enhance her overall visual functioning and to improve her ability to read regular-size print comfortably.

Louise's best-corrected distance acuity was 20/200 OD (right eye), 20/100+1 OS (left eye), and her near acuity was 1M print at 4 inches OD and 6M print at 4 inches OS. Louise could read .8M continuous text print at 4 inches without difficulty and could identify 1M size words at 16 inches. When Louise's distance spectacle correction was combined with a 4.00-diopter add, her near vision improved to the point where she could read .5M continuous text print without difficulty. Louise demonstrated that she could read 9-point print in *Seventeen* magazine without difficulty, and both she and her mother noted that with this bifocal addition, Louise was able to read smaller print more fluently than in the past.

With the hopes of enhancing Louise's overall visual functioning further, the eye care specialist fit Louise with contact lenses, which improved her binocular distance acuity to 20/63 − 2. With the contact lenses and a pair of +4.00 prismatic half-eye magnifiers, Louise could continue to read .5M continuous text print without difficulty (see Chapter 7 for descriptions of optical devices). With these relatively simple modifications, Louise's overall visual functioning improved significantly, and she was able to function comfortably and efficiently in a regular educational classroom. Furthermore, with the improvement in her distance acuity, Louise now had the visual qualifications to attempt to acquire a restricted driver's license in her state.

At age 4 months, Wanda did not respond visually to her mother's face and had a wandering nystagmoid eye movement. Electrodiagnostic testing was performed; the results were found to be below normal. When Wanda came for her initial low vision consultation at age 13 months, she had been diagnosed as having Leber's congenital amaurosis, and her parents stated that she had become significantly more attentive to faces in the past several months.

During that initial evaluation, Wanda did not respond to formal visual acuity testing, including Teller visual acuity testing. It was noted that she could consistently find a 15-mm size object at a three-foot distance, which corresponded to 20/200 or 3/30 (its metric equivalent) vision. Since a significant amount of myopia was also noted, it was recommended that she wear spectacles. With the addition of spectacles to her life, Wanda's parents immediately noted that she was much more visually attentive and wanted the spectacles as soon as she awoke.

Over the years, Wanda was reevaluated on several occasions. When she was about 3 1/2 years old, her unaided binocular distance acuity was in the 20/200–20/250 range, and her uncorrected near acuity was .8M print at 2 inches. With the appropriate myopic spectacle correction, Wanda's binocular near acuity improved to the 20/120–20/150 range. When Wanda was last evaluated at age 5 1/2, her uncorrected binocular acuity was 20/160, and at near, she could read .63M print at 5 inches. With the appropriate spectacle correction, her binocular distance acuity improved to 20/80.

Wanda's case illustrates several points. First, when large refractive errors are present, specta-cles should be prescribed, even for infants, to provide the individual with the clearest optical image possible. Second, it is difficult to predict how much the visual function of a child with a congenital visual impairment may improve over time and whether a congenital ocular condition will be progressive. For these reasons, it is important to give such children every opportunity to develop their visual potential to its highest level by providing visual stimulation and optical corrections at as young an age as possible. Third, although Wanda had a large myopic refractive error, she did not experience as large an improvement in visual acuity with the spectacles as would a normally sighted individual. Nevertheless, she definitely sees better with the spectacles on, and her overall visual functioning would likely not be as good today if she had not started wearing spectacles at a very young age.

Early identification and low vision care give families and teachers of children with congenital visual impairments, like Louise and Wanda, the opportunity to develop realistic goals and expectations of what can be expected visually, in both the short and long term. Early care may allow children to have more visual control over their environments and early access to visual details.

MEMBERS OF THE LOW VISION TEAM

The low vision team consists of a variety of professionals, including an eye care specialist, teacher of students with visual impairments or low vision educator, O&M instructor, rehabilitation teacher, vocational rehabilitation counselor, occupational therapist, physical therapist, social worker, and gerontologist, depending on the needs of the individual and the location and structure of the services. The clinical low vision specialist, either an optometrist or ophthalmologist who is specifically trained and has experience in low vision care, provides the clinical low vision evaluation. This specialist will have had training in low vision either during his or her optometric or ophthalmological training or in a fellowship program and will have gained experience in low vision care in a mentorship program. It is essential that the specialist has had experience evaluating individuals with low vision of all ages and with a variety of eye conditions.

For a child with low vision, the teacher of students with visual impairments addresses the child's specific educational needs, and the O&M instructor reviews the child's functional abilities for independent travel, both indoors and outdoors. The teacher of students with visual impairments and/or the O&M instructor often perform a functional vision assessment and provide a report to the clinical low vision specialist before the clinical evaluation (for assessment procedures and methods of instruction, see Chapters 9, 11, and 13). A functional vision assessment reviews the child's visual field preference, tracking abilities, ability to shift visual attention, scanning abilities, ability to reach or move toward an object, and visual curiosity. It also examines what objects attract the child's attention the most.

For an adult with low vision, the low vision educator, who is specially trained to provide instruction in the use of optical and nonoptical devices, helps the person adapt to the devices that have been recommended. Low vision educators come from a variety of backgrounds, such as O&M, rehabilitation teaching, and the education of students with visual impairments. At one national agency, all low vision educators are registered nurses who have been specifically trained in techniques for instructing individuals with low vision.

A rehabilitation teacher, an O&M instructor, a vocational rehabilitation counselor and, sometimes, a rehabilitation engineer may also be involved in the clinical low vision evaluation and instruction of adults. The O&M instructor or the rehabilitation teacher conducts the functional vision assessment, and the rehabilitation engineer may evaluate a work station and provide input about the types of optical devices that may help the person perform tasks. The input from these professionals guides the clinical low vision specialist's decisions about such factors as the distances at which visual function needs to take place and which mounting systems of devices—that is, devices that are spectacle mounted and can be permanently attached to a frame, in contrast to clipped on or flipped up—will be beneficial.

SEQUENCE OF A TYPICAL EVALUATION

The typical clinical low vision evaluation is conducted over a period that can range from one to several sessions in one day to a few sessions weeks or months apart. This time frame differs from that of the general eye care examination because the clinician may want to determine how a person's vision may change as a result of health conditions (such as diabetes), may desire to prevent visual fatigue, or may need to monitor visual functioning at different times of the day. Furthermore, the clinical evaluation may be done both indoors and outdoors to assess the person's need for and use of optical devices and light-absorptive lenses. The typical clinical low vision evaluation consists of a sequence of steps, which are summarized in Sidebar 8.1.

Case History

A comprehensive case history covers the following points:

- the person's main visual problem or problems
- any other visual problems
- onset and cause of vision loss
- other disabilities
- family history
- developmental milestones (when appropriate)
- ocular and general medical history
- educational and employment history
- current distance and near visual functioning

SIDEBAR 8.1

The Clinical Low Vision Evaluation: A Typical Sequence

- Comprehensive case history
  - √ Review of functional vision assessment (when available)
  - √ Review of previous spectacles and/or optical devices
- Interpretation/review of medical eye information
- Ophthalmic health evaluation to confirm/ review previous diagnosis
- Distance and near visual acuity measurements
- Objective and subjective refraction
  - √ Retinoscopy
  - √ Keratometry
  - √ Binocular vision evaluation (if appropriate)
- Color vision evaluation
- Contrast sensitivity assessment

- Visual field assessment
- Prescription of low vision devices
  - √ Optical device evaluation for distance, intermediate, and near vision tasks
  - √ Preliminary determination of low vision devices
- Optical device instruction, trial, and follow-up
  - √ Instruction in the use of recommended devices
  - √ Loaning of optical devices
  - √ Follow-up visit to review the efficacy of the loaner devices and to see what if any additional problems have been identified
  - √ Additional visits as necessary
- Recommendation of accessory or nonoptical devices
- Final dispensing of devices.

- previous low vision care
- previous optical devices used (and not used)
- current reading media
- goal and objectives for distance, intermediate, and near point vision enhancement
- concerns about independent travel.

The case history should be taken at intake before the clinical low vision evaluation is conducted, since it helps set the tone of the evaluation and ensures that the individual's specific goals and objectives are identified and visual problems and needs are understood. Without a proper understanding of a person's goals and objectives, it is virtually impossible to proceed with the clinical low vision evaluation. For example, recommending a CCTV to an individual who is not interested

in reading is inappropriate, regardless of how much better he or she could see with the device. However, if the person is an enthusiastic model airplane builder, a CCTV will enlarge the pieces of a model and allow the person to have both hands free and thus may be an appropriate recommendation. The Adult Data Sheet included at the end of this chapter is a sample of a form typically used to record the history of an individual. In the case of children, parents or teachers may be asked to provide information, which can be gathered prior to or at the time of the low vision evaluation. (Sample forms for this purpose also appear at the end of the chapter.) Overall, the information requested allows the low vision clinician to know how to structure the evaluation for the maximum benefit of the individual by providing data that gives a comprehensive picture of the person's abilities and needs. For this reason, the clinical low vision specialist will at this point also frequently read any medical eye reports (discussed later in this chapter) available on the person.

Preliminary Observations

When the individual with low vision enters the examination room, the clinical low vision specialist observes his or her gait, posture, head position, visual curiosity, ability to navigate in unfamiliar settings, and need for assistance. On the basis of this brief observation, the specialist gains preliminary information on how well the person is functioning with his or her current level of vision. By keeping the level of illumination in the examination room the same as in the waiting area, the specialist will ensure that the preliminary observations are based on the individual's usual visual functioning, rather than his or her ability to adapt to different levels of light. It should be noted in addition that dilation of the pupils impairs the focusing ability of people under age 50 and can cause increased light sensitivity and blurred vision at any age. For this reason, a person's pupils should not be dilated during the clinical low vision evaluation. When necessary, they can be dilated at the end of the examination to check or confirm the cause of the vision loss.

Since the visual functioning of individuals with low vision varies considerably, some may need assistance in traveling safely in the office and examination areas. Therefore, the clinical low vision specialist and other staff members should be skilled in using basic O&M procedures, particularly the sighted guide and room-familiarization techniques (see Jacobson, 1993).

Distance Visual Acuity Testing

Distance visual acuity testing is the first procedure performed at the clinical low vision evaluation. It establishes a baseline of how well the individual with low vision is able to see symbols of different sizes. This baseline can be compared to findings at the end of the evaluation to deter-

mine how much the person's distance vision has been enhanced by the recommendations made as a result of the examination.

Measurement Charts

Standard projection charts (such as the Snellen Chart, the traditional eye chart whose top line consists of the letter *E* and which is used in routine eye examinations) that are used by most eye care specialists are ineffective for assessing the distance visual acuity of individuals with low vision because these charts:

- have lower contrast
- do not attempt to determine acuity levels between 20/100 and 20/200, between 20/200 and 20/300, and between 20/300 and 20/400 and thereby do not allow for finer discriminations in acuity levels of persons with low vision
- have only one letter to represent acuities of 20/200, 20/300, and 20/400, respectively, and hence include fewer stimuli for correct responses than are presented for the higher levels of visual acuity
- are presented at the standard distance of 20 feet, which is too far for many individuals with low vision to maintain fixation. *Fixation* refers to the ability of the individual to hold his or her attention on the object being viewed and also defines the direction from which the person needs to look to see the object best.

Because the design of the eye chart used in a low vision examination can influence measurements of visual acuity, it is an important consideration when evaluating an individual with low vision. Bailey and Lovie (1976) found that the number of letters per row and the relative spacing between letters and between rows can cause substantial variation in acuity scores. For this reason, the Bailey-Lovie charts and their derivatives (such as the Lighthouse Distance Visual Acuity Chart) follow the principle of proportional or logarithmic spacing. That is, these charts use almost

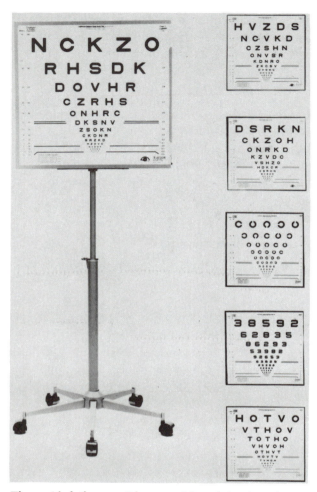

These Lighthouse Distance Visual Acuity Charts are commonly used to assess individuals with low vision.

Usually, the test distance is determined by the type of chart used and the visual acuity and age of the person being tested. Children are often less distracted when a shorter test distance (such as 5 to 10 feet) is used. The Designs for Vision Distance Chart is particularly useful for individuals with very low vision because the largest symbol is a 700-foot number; when this chart is used at a distance of one foot, visual acuity can be measured to the level of 1/700 (20/14,000).

The LEA Symbols (depicting a circle, house, apple, and square) are useful for testing a child's visual acuity because they use readily identifiable pictures that can be verbally identified or matched. These tests are typically used at a distance of 10 feet, although the distance can vary from 1 to 20 feet. The HOTV test, another useful test for children, uses four optotypes (symbols/pictures, letters, or numbers used on acuity testing cards): H, O, T, and V. It is designed for a 10-foot test distance, similar to the Lighthouse Flash Card Test. The Tumbling E test—a Snellen letter test—consists of Es oriented in one of four positions: to the right, to the left, up, or down. The Landolt C test is similar to the Tumbling E, except that it substitutes Cs for Es. It consists of open

equally legible symbols with the same number of symbols in each row and spacing between symbols and rows proportional to the size of the symbol.

Low vision charts provide higher-contrast letters and flexibility in the distance used during testing. Most low vision charts are used at either 2 or 4 meters (such as the Lighthouse Distance Visual Acuity Chart) or at 5 or 10 feet (such as the Designs for Vision Distance Chart for the Partially Sighted and the Lighthouse Flash Card Test for Children).

The distance used for distance visual acuity testing can be varied for a number of reasons.

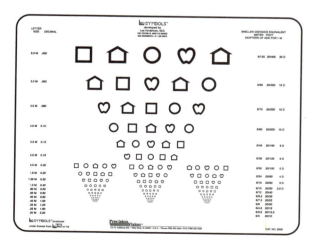

LEA Symbols are helpful when testing children because the familiar pictures they use can be readily identified or matched.

circles with diminishing diameters in which the break in a circle is placed in one of the four principal meridians. For many children, the Landolt C test is more difficult than is the Tumbling E test. Furthermore, with both these tests, visual acuity measurements can be artificially lowered by a child's problems with directionality or laterality.

During the distance visual acuity test, the right eye is tested first, then the left eye, and then both eyes together. With young children, it is often beneficial to retest the right eye for accuracy if visual acuity in the left eye is significantly greater than in the right eye because young children often do not fully understand the visual acuity test at first and thus perform better with the left eye after they have become familiar with the test.

Distance Acuity Notations

During the distance acuity test, the individual stands at a predetermined distance from the chart. This distance is the first (or top) number in the acuity notation. The second (or bottom) number indicates the smallest size symbol that the person accurately identified and represents the number of feet at which a person with 20/20 acuity could identify that size letter. In other words, a person with 20/70 acuity can see at a distance of 20 feet a letter that a person with 20/20 acuity could see at 70 feet. In countries in which metric measurements are used, the nota-

tions are represented the same way; a person with 6/60 (20/200) acuity sees at 6 meters what a person with 6/6 (20/20) acuity sees at 60 meters. The test distance of 20 feet was selected as the standard test distance because 20 feet is considered to be optical infinity. At this distance, no focusing or accommodation occurs, and for this reason, a more accurate assessment of refractive error can be obtained.

In the measurement of visual acuity, the resolving power of the eye, or minimum separable acuity (the ability of the eye to see a gap between two objects or two parts of the same object), is being determined. Early astronomers determined that the normal eye's ability to discern a gap between two stars required a minimum of 1 degree of arc. A 20/20 letter is one that subtends 5 degrees when a line is drawn from the top and bottom of the letter back to the observer who stands 20 feet from the letter. Therefore, a 20/20 letter will subtend 5 degrees of arc at 20 feet (see Figure 8.1). It should be noted that a visual acuity of 20/20 does not indicate "perfect" vision. The majority of individuals with normal sight see better than 20/20, and for optimum visual functioning, many of those with 20/20 vision still need an optical correction for such conditions as latent hyperopia, presbyopia, and astigmatism.

When testing visual acuity, the examiner records the correct number of responses as, for example, 20/100+2 or 20/70−1. The notation

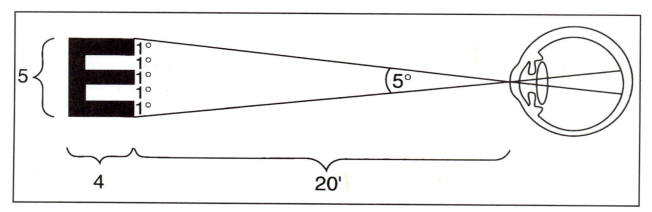

Figure 8.1. Standard Snellen Acuity Measurement
The 20/20 letter is 5 parts high by 4 parts wide. The bars of the E are equal to the open spaces in size. The angle subtended to the eye at 20 feet is 5 degrees.

20/200+2 indicates that the individual being tested correctly identified all the letters, numbers, or symbols on the 20/200 line as well as two letters on the next smaller line, whereas the notation 20/70−1 indicates that the person correctly identified all but one letter on the 20/70 line. The majority of acuity charts used to test individuals with low vision have four to six symbols per line.

If the distance acuity test is conducted at a distance other than 20 feet, the first number is written as the test distance and the second number is written as the size of the smallest line of letters identified, as was noted earlier. If an individual reads all the 80 line at a 10-foot distance, for example, the acuity is written as 10/80. To convert this notation to a 20-foot equivalent, one would multiply both the first number and the second number by the appropriate multiplier to make the first number equal 20. In this example, the first and second numbers would be multiplied by 2 to obtain 20/160. Similarly, a visual acuity of 5/60 would be converted to 20/240 (4 × 5 = 20 and 4 × 60 = 240).

When measuring visual acuity, a low vision clinician should not use "counts fingers," a method in which the examiner records the number of inches at which the individual can differentiate and count upheld fingers, often used with someone who cannot see the 20/400 line on the standard Snellen eye chart. The results of this method are often regarded as a measurement that does little to quantify acuities, particularly when the test distance is not accurately recorded.

If a person cannot see a large test letter or symbol at any distance, a visual acuity of hand motion (HM) should be noted if he or she can appreciate gross object and motion perception without detail discrimination (for common abbreviations used by eye care specialists, see Sidebar 8.2). The distance at which the person can see hand motions should be noted (such as HM at 1 foot).

Individuals are said to have light projection (LProj) when they are able to locate light in a minimum of nine quadrants in each eye: superior temporal, superior central, superior nasal, inferior temporal, inferior central, inferior nasal,

temporal central, nasal central, and central (see Chapter 5 for information on the structure of the eye). From a practical standpoint, many clinicians note that a person has light projection if he or she can identify light in any quadrant. A more accurate way to record the visual acuity of an individual who is able to identify light in only a few quadrants, however, is to record his or her visual acuity as light projection in the specific quadrants in which light can be seen.

When a person cannot locate the direction of light but is aware that light is on or off or present or absent, he or she is considered to have light perception (LP). Total blindness occurs when no external light is seen and is often referred to as no light perception (NLP).

Assessment of Young Children

Numerical visual acuity measurements may not be obtainable until a child is 2 to 3 years old because many children younger than age 2 do not understand how to perform a standard acuity test and do not have the abilities to verbalize the pictures they see or match them. To maintain the attention and interest of younger children, a working distance of 5 to 10 feet is needed. When acuity measurements are obtained for young children with low vision, it is important to remind parents that the children's visual functioning will probably improve with visual maturation—a process that usually occurs until approximately age 7 to 9, as was the case with Wanda described earlier in this chapter.

Observation. Observing a child's visual functioning before visual acuity measurements can be obtained is helpful in assessing current visual functioning. Areas of observation may include:

- ◆ visual attention
- ◆ eye preference
- ◆ visual field preference
- ◆ tracking ability
- ◆ visual attention to central and peripheral targets

Common Abbreviations Used by Eye Care Providers

SIDEBAR 8.2

ACL	anterior chamber lens	NLP	no light perception
ARMD	age-related macular degeneration	OD	right eye
BDR	background diabetic retinopathy	OS	left eye
b.i.d.	two times a day	OU	both eyes
BVO	branch vein occlusion	PCL	posterior chamber lens
Cat.	cataract	P.D.	pupillary distance
c̄c	with correction	PDR	proliferative diabetic retinopathy
CC	chief complaint	PERRLA	pupils equally round and reactive to light and accommodation
CF	counts fingers		
CL	contact lens	PROS	prosthesis
CVA	cerebral vascular accident	PVD	posterior vitreous detachment
CVO	central vein occlusion	q.	each, every
d.	day	q.d.	once a day
Dx	diagnosis	q.h.	every hour
ENUC	enucleated	q.i.d.	four times a day
FC	finger counting	q.2h.	every two hours
FHx	has a family history of . . .	RD	retinal detachment
GL	eyeglasses	RP	retinitis pigmentosa
gtts	eyedrops	Rx	prescription
h.	hour	s̄c	without correction
HA	headache	sig.	label
HM	hand motion	Sx	symptoms
h.s.	at bedtime	t.i.d.	three times a day
Hx	history	tono	tonometry
IOL	intraocular lens	Tx	treatment
IOP	intraocular pressure	ung.	ointment
LP	light perception	UTT	unable to test
LProj	light projection	VA	visual acuity
		VF	visual field

- ability to shift visual attention
- scanning ability
- movement toward lights or targets
- preferential viewing of visually stimulating targets
- optokinetic nystagmus.

The examiner can determine whether the child favors one eye or appears to have equal vision in both eyes by observing the level of visual curiosity and visual skills that the child exhibits. A trained low vision specialist can determine the severity of a visual impairment even in a young child and can use this information to anticipate how well a child is likely to function visually with maturation.

Tests of visual functioning are done at a relatively close working distance (2 feet or closer) because they were designed for young children who cannot respond to distance visual acuity testing even at 5 feet and because young children's visual attention is greater for closer objects. As a child's visual skills mature, testing distance can be increased to allow for better quantification of visual acuity.

Tests of Visual Functions.   When a visually stimulating target, such as a finger puppet or toy, is presented and a child's monocular fixation (that is, viewing of an object with one eye as the other eye is occluded) is found to be central, steady, and maintained through a blink, it is thought that the child's visual acuity is reasonably good. With regard to fixation preference in the presence of an obvious strabismus (exotropia, esotropia, or hypertropia), the eye that is preferred for fixation is likely to have better visual acuity.

In standardized techniques to determine visual acuity through preferential viewing, a child is presented with two targets simultaneously, one consisting of stripes and the other consisting of matched luminance gray, at specific test distances. If the child can see the grating pattern, the examiner will observe the child fixating on it. There are several methods of testing visual acuity using preferential viewing techniques, such as using Teller acuity cards, which consist of alternating light and dark stripes. These cards are a method of testing acuity on children who are unable to respond to standard acuity testing, such as children who are preverbal or nonverbal.

When a child is unable to respond to a standardized test of preferential viewing and it is difficult to assess the fixation pattern, an alternate technique is to present two light boxes, one with a visually stimulating pattern and the other with no pattern (or light only). If the child is able to view the more visually stimulating target preferentially, it indicates that the visual system is capable of a higher level of visual functioning than light perception or projection.

In the past, an optokinetic drum (a cylinder with black stripes spaced a certain distance apart on a white background) was used to assess an infant's visual acuity. The examiner would hold the optokenetic drum vertically in front of the child's eye and slowly spin it. If the child could see the target, optokinetic nystagmus (OKN)—an involuntary rhythmic oscillation of the eyes produced by a repetitive stimulus passing in front of them—would be induced. OKN occurs because the child fixates on a line and follows it with a slow eye movement until it goes out of view; then he or she makes a fast refixation on another line, repeating the behavior again and again. If the child cannot see the vertical stripes, OKN does not occur. However, there are at least two problems in the use of an optokinetic drum:

- If the drum is spun either too quickly or too slowly, it is impossible to detect the nystagmoid movements.
- Since the stripes are so wide, a child with a visual acuity as low as 20/1000 may respond positively when the drum is held at a distance at which the child will attend.

For these reasons, it is difficult to quantify a child's visual acuity with an optokinetic drum. The use of the drum primarily establishes the presence or absence of vision, although its accuracy is still questionable.

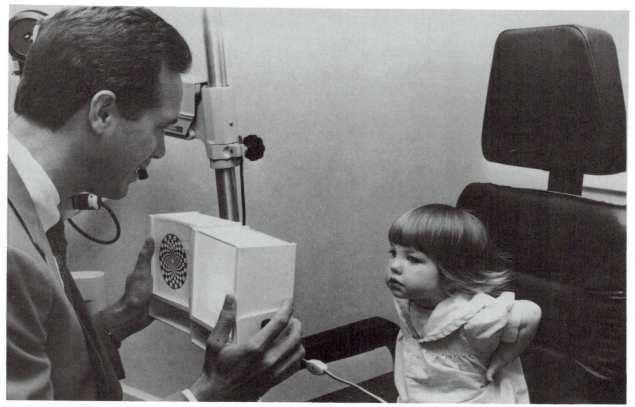

A clinical low vision evaluation is essential for individuals with low vision. Here, a child's preferential viewing is being tested with light boxes.

When children cannot verbally identify or match LEA symbols or the HOTV, the STYCAR Toy test is an option. This test uses a miniature set of toys and eating utensils that the child verbally identifies or matches at a distance of 10 and 20 feet.

When it is difficult to assess the visual acuity of a child who is young or who has multiple disabilities in the traditional manner, an approximation of the child's acuity can be obtained with familiar objects (food or toys) in which the child is interested. Those objects are placed at various distances, and the child is asked to find them. The distance at which the child becomes aware of an object is estimated. When a consistent distance is established after several trials, the size of the object is measured and converted into an equivalent Snellen letter size. Once the working distance at which the child became aware of the

object is determined, an approximate distance acuity can be established that will serve as a reference point for comparison at follow-up low vision evaluations. (Sidebar 8.3 contains information on converting the sizes of objects to visual acuities.) This procedure is illustrated as follows:

◆ A child locates a 2-inch (51-mm) car at a distance of 4 feet. The size of the car is equivalent to approximately a 20/180 Snellen-size letter. Therefore, the visual acuity estimation is 4/180, the first number being the distance from the object and the second number being the size of the letter. The acuity of 4/180 converts to 20/900.

◆ A child locates a Cheerio at a working distance of 2 feet. A Cheerio is a 0.25 inches (6 mm), which is equivalent to a 20/20-size

Size of Objects for Distance Acuity Comparisons

SIDEBAR 8.3

Millimeters	Inches	Distance Equivalent	Metric Conversion
3.0	1/8	20/10	6/3
3.8	5/32	20/12.5	6/3.8
4.8	3/16	20/16	6/4.8
6.0	7/32	20/20	6/6
7.6	9/32	20/25	6/7.5
9.6	3/8	20/32	6/9.5
12.0	15/32	20/40	6/12
15.0	19/32	20/50	6/15
19.0	3/4	20/63	6/19
24.0	31/32	20/80	6/24
30.0	1 3/16	20/100	6/30
38.0	1 15/32	20/125	6/38
48.0	1 29/32	20/160	6/48
60.0	2 3/8	20/200	6/60

letter. Therefore, the visual acuity is 2/20 or 20/200.

- ◆ A child sees a 1 1/2-inch rubber ball at a distance of 5 feet. The size of the ball is equivalent to a 20/125 letter, so the approximate distance acuity is 5/125 or 20/500.

The case study that follows suggests several issues involved in assessing children with low vision.

Gregory was born with a midline facial anomaly that resulted in microphthalmia with an eccentric lens and pupil (see Chapter 6 for a discussion of various eye conditions). At his initial low vision evaluation at age 3, his parents wanted to know whether he had any useful sight.

Gregory was an active, verbal, and observant child. During the evaluation, the clinical low vision specialist observed that he had reasonably good vision in the inferior temporal portion of his right field and a visual acuity measurement of 5/200 in the right eye, but only light perception in the left eye. At near, Gregory could see 3M print at 2 inches.

Gregory's parents were advised that Gregory had useful vision and that his visual functioning was particularly good at near [i.e., at reading distance]. However, further work was needed to develop his visual potential to its highest level to increase his visual functioning.

At age 6, when Gregory was learning to read in braille, he received a follow-up assessment to review his visual functioning. At this evaluation, his unaided distance visual acuity was 10/160, and at near he could see 1.4M print at 4 inches. A spectacle correction enhanced Gregory's distance acuity to 10/100 and allowed him to read 1.5M continuous-text print at near. The clinical low vision specialist recommended that Gregory receive a learning media assessment (see Chapter 11) to determine whether braille reading and writing should be continued and/or whether to have Gregory concentrate on using his vision more efficiently.

Gregory was evaluated next at age 8. At that visit, his uncorrected distance acuity had changed to 10/125 − 1, and with a spectacle correction his distance vision improved to 10/100.

With the use of a bifocal correction, Gregory could now read .7M print at 1 inch and 1M continuous-text print fairly comfortably; without the bifocal correction, he could read 1.5M continuous-text print comfortably. Therefore, it was recommended that he discontinue the use of large-print material and the CCTV that he had been using on and off over the previous year. Bifocal spectacles were ordered to reduce fatigue for sustained near point activities.

When Gregory was last evaluated at age 9, he was reading regular print in school and had no difficulty keeping up with his classmates. At this visit, his distance acuity was 20/125−2 (10/63−1), and at near he could read .8M print continuous-text print at 2 inches. A separate pair of reading spectacles was recommended to allow for a larger field of view when reading than Gregory could get with his bifocal correction.

This case illustrates two points. First, with maturation, the overall visual functioning of children with congenital low vision can improve significantly, particularly with the use of the appropriate spectacle correction. Second, it is important for evaluations to take place regularly. If Gregory had been evaluated yearly, his needs could have been addressed more consistently, and it is likely that he would have not started a braille program or used a CCTV, both of which later proved to be unnecessary.

Special Considerations

If macular disease has been diagnosed or is suspected, when testing distance acuity, the examiner should direct the person's fixation to points either to the right, left, above, or below the letters the person finds difficult to view (for a discussion of macular disease, see Chapter 6). If there is a change in the visibility of the letters when this is done, eccentric viewing strategies should be discussed with the person. Eccentric viewing strategies teach individuals with a loss of central vision to view with an off-center point in which they are not looking directly at the object they are trying to view but instead are looking a few degrees off to the object's side. This technique can allow them to see better than when looking directly at an object. When individuals try to view an object by looking above, below or to the left or right of it, they can find their best eccentric viewing position and then, with practice, learn to use this eccentric point for better visual functioning. Those who were born without central vision learn to use an eccentric fixation point almost automatically because their central vision has always been impaired.

Many people with low vision have negative feelings about how well they can see because they believe they have often performed poorly on acuity tests during regular eye examinations or vision screenings in school. Therefore, it is important to show them that they do have useful vision by starting with significantly larger test letters, so they can recognize several lines of letters, which will encourage them and motivate them to try harder.

Near Visual Acuity Testing

Near visual acuity testing is performed after distance acuity testing to establish a baseline of how well the person with low vision is initially able to see at his or her habitual near working distance. To make an accurate assessment of the initial near visual acuity, the examiner asks the individual to hold a test card at his or her normal reading distance and then compares this finding to the size of print the person wants to be able to read. This comparison gives the low vision specialist an approximation of how much magnification will be needed to enable the person to achieve his or her goal. The finding is also compared to the best near visual acuity findings at the conclusion of the low vision evaluation to determine how much enhancement of near vision was possible.

Measurement Charts

The Lighthouse near acuity cards for adults and children are commonly used to measure near acuity. In addition, the Lighthouse "continuous text cards" for both adults and children are well

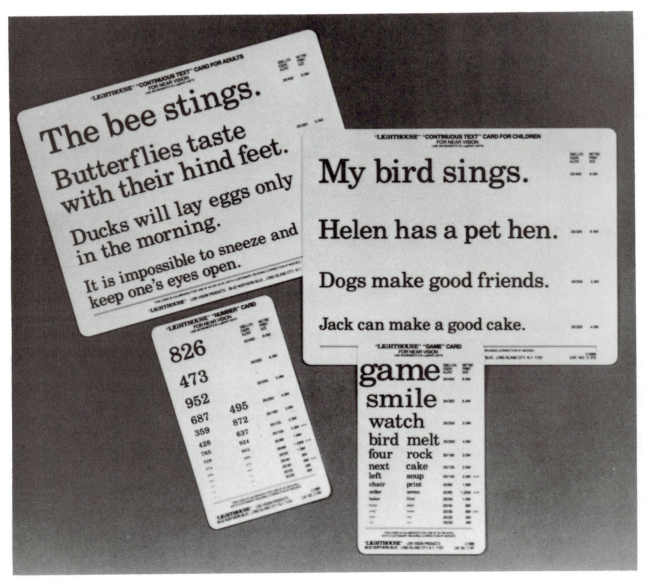

Lighthouse near acuity cards are among the assessment materials used to evaluate near acuity in adults and children with low vision.

designed and are useful for evaluating what a person can read.

A common practice in the past, which some eye care specialists still use, was to express print size as a reduced Snellen equivalent. This was done in an attempt to determine the equivalent distance acuity to read a particular print size at a viewing distance of 16 inches (40 cm). However, because most people with low vision do not view near targets at this working distance, it is both confusing and inaccurate to record visual acuities in this manner. Another system that has been used for some time in ophthalmology, but is becoming less common, is the Jaeger system, which consists of words and phrases in various print sizes. Because this system has not been standard-

SIDEBAR 8.4

M-Size Equivalents for Near Visual Acuity Comparisons

M-Size Equivalent	Point Size	Common Examples	Sample of Point Size
2.00	18	Large print Books for grades 1–3	Sample of 18 point
1.60	14	Books for grades 4–7	Sample of 14 point
1.25	12	Books for grades 8–12	Sample of 12 point
1.00	9	Newsprint	Sample of 9 point
.60	6	Telephone book	Sample of 6 point
.40	4	Small bible	Sample of 4 point

ized, print size is not the same from one test card or chart to another, and test results therefore cannot be regarded as standardized.

Once single-letter or single-word near acuity has been measured and the appropriate working distance has been noted, the individual's ability to read continuous text is assessed. It is expected that a person's ability to see single words or letters will be much better than his or her ability to read continuous text. This information is helpful in determining just how much magnification is needed to meet a particular reading goal.

Near-Acuity Notations

Near visual acuities are recorded as both the smallest print size read and the working distance at which that print size was obtained, such as 1M print at 3 inches. Bailey (1978) reviewed a number of systems for noting near acuity and recommended the use of the M system for clinical low vision specialists because of its compatibility with the traditional Snellen method of denoting visual acuity. M units express the distance in meters at which lower-case letters subtend 5 degrees of arc. (See Sidebar 8.4 for a list of M-size equivalents, point sizes, and examples.)

Special Considerations

Because near-point activities such as reading can be significantly more difficult for people with macular disease (who have central scotomas) than can viewing an object in the distance, these individuals can have near-acuity readings two or more times worse than what would be expected on the basis of their distance acuity measurements. Therefore, it is unreliable to predict how much magnification will be needed to accomplish a specific near point task solely on the basis of a measurement of distance visual acuity. Conversely, children often have significantly better visual acuity at near in comparison to their distance visual acuity. In addition, individuals with hemianopic field loss need special instruction to learn to look all the way to the beginning or end of the line they are reading, depending on whether they have a left or right homonymous hemianopia.

Refraction

Determination of Refraction

Because the refraction, or testing of refractive error, of individuals with low vision can be time consuming and thus exacting, it may sometimes be done incompletely during a general ophthalmologic or optometric evaluation, and hence the refractive errors of many people with low vision are either uncorrected or undercorrected. However, when a refraction is done correctly, significant improvements in distance and near point visual functioning can occur with the use of conventional spectacle lenses, and thus the importance of a careful refractive analysis cannot be overemphasized. Significant refractive errors are often found with disorders such as albinism, aphakia, cataracts, corneal scarring, keratoconus, Marfan's syndrome, degenerative myopia, retinitis pigmentosa (RP), and retinopathy of prematurity (ROP) (for a discussion of these conditions, see Chapter 6).

Refractions can be done both objectively (based solely on the clinician's findings) or subjectively (based on the individual's responses to which lenses appear "better"). Objective evaluations are emphasized for children from birth through age 4 or for individuals who cannot respond subjectively. Refractions are recorded as prescription for lenses that are then prepared by opticians or technicians who are specially trained (see Sidebar 8.5 for examples).

Retinoscopy. The first step in refraction is retinoscopy, an objective evaluation that is performed with a retinoscope, an instrument that projects a streak of light into the person's eye. The light is reflected off the retina and back toward the examiner, who observes the movement of the light coming back through the pupil through the retinoscope's eye piece. The examiner uses handheld lenses or lens bars to determine the presence of myopic, hyperopic, or astigmatic refractive errors.

Retinoscopy under noncycloplegic, or "normal," conditions is the standard method for evaluating the refractive status of persons with low vision. A noncycloplegic examination is done without the use of medications to freeze the accommodative system of the eye by having the individual fixate on a distant target. When accommodation can be controlled, there is no difficulty determining an accurate prescription.

However, if an individual is unable to carry out the steps required during retinoscopy, a cycloplegic refraction can be helpful in determining the starting prescription for someone with low vision. A cycloplegic refraction involves instilling into the eyes special medications that freeze the focusing mechanisms. Refractions of this kind are helpful when there is difficulty controlling fixation or accommodation.

Instruments for Refraction. The mainstay device for routine refractive analysis of individuals with normal vision is the phoroptor, which is routinely placed in front of the individual's face as various lenses are tried to determine the best correction. The phoropter is in general not recommended for use with individuals with low vision because unimpaired peripheral vision is helpful in its use. If the individual's primary visual input is from the peripheral retina, it will be difficult for the person to view through the phoroptor and give accurate information about what is seen. In addition, persons with low vision need to have the head and eyes free to move to the best viewing position during an examination, which allows the clinician to observe the eye movements and head positions necessary for optimum visual functioning.

Trial Frame and Lens Set. For people with low vision, a trial frame and a trial lens set can be used to determine the best correction. Occasionally, the use of lens clips (such as Halberg clips) to place loose lenses over the individual's current prescription is appropriate when the current refractive error is large or when small changes in the refractive error are anticipated.

Keratometer. Keratometry provides objective data that, when combined with retinoscopic findings, increases the examiner's ability to determine a final refractive correction. In this test, a keratometer is used to measure the curvature of the two primary meridians of the cornea, which is helpful in determining whether there is a large amount of astigmatism (for descriptions of eye

SIDEBAR 8.5

Prescriptions for Conventional Spectacles: Examples of Refraction

EXAMPLE 1

O.D. + 2.50 − 1.25 × 155 with 1.25 Prism Diopter − Base in
O.S. + 1.25 sphere with 1.25 Prism Diopters − Base in

In this example, the right eye has a toric (astigmatic correcting) lens and the left lens has a spherical lens. In the case of the right eye, the first number (+2.50) indicates the spherical power that will correct for hyperopia. The second number (−1.25) indicates the cylindrical power that is the correction for astigmatism. The third number (155) indicates the orientation of the 1.25D of astigmatism correction. These numbers indicate that there is 2.50D of correction for hyperopia at 155

degrees and there is 1.25D of hyperopia correction at 65 degrees. The left lens power indicates that the left eye requires a spherical correction (that is, has no astigmatism) of 1.25D for hyperopia.

In addition, a prism power of 1.25 prism diopters has been added to both lenses, base in. This notation means that the thicker portion of the prism, in both lenses, is positioned towards the individual's nose.

EXAMPLE 2

O.D. − 1.25 − 2.25 × 20 Add 2.25
O.S. −2.00 − 1.75 × 105 Add 2.25

In this example, both lenses are toric (astigmatic correcting) lenses that have a bifocal correction incorporated into them. The first number for the right lens (−1.25) shows the spherical power that will correct for myopia. This notation is combined with the second number (−2.25), which is the amount of astigmatism correction needed. The last number (20) shows the orientation of the astigmatism. Therefore, the right eye has 1.25D of correction for myopia at 20 degrees and there is 3.50D of myopia correction at

110 degrees. In regard to the left eye, the first number shows that there is 2.00D of myopia correction, which is combined with 1.75D of astigmatism correction oriented at axis 105. This notation indicates that there is 2.00D of myopia correction at 105 degrees and there is 3.75D of myopia correction at 15 degrees.

In addition, this distance spectacle correction is combined with a 2.25 diopter add, which is the additional strength of the bifocal, added to the distance prescription of each lens, to give the reading power of the lenses.

---

conditions, see Chapter 6). The keratometer also alerts the examiner to distortions of the corneal surface that may make refracting the patient more difficult.

When a standard keratometer is not available, a *keratoscope* can be used. A keratoscope is a device with a series of concentric rings that

can be alternating light and dark, as in the Placido's disk, or illuminated, as in the Kline keratoscope. By observing an individual's cornea through the viewing aperture of these devices, the clinician can observe irregularities in the corneal curvature and the presence and orientation of astigmatism.

Special Considerations

Persons with low vision are often less sensitive to refractive shifts than are those with normal vision. As a general rule, as visual acuity decreases, so does central visual function, which often results in decreased sensitivity to refractive changes of the eye. However, this is not always the case. Many individuals with visual acuities of less than 20/400 are sensitive to even small refractive shifts, and individuals with relatively good acuity often do not see significantly differently with even large refractive shifts. It should also be noted that many individuals with a significant loss of central vision report that their visual acuity with a standard spectacle correction has not improved, even when they have a fairly large refractive error. They do not experience greater visual acuity because central vision, not peripheral vision, improves the most with optical correction.

Color Vision Testing

Color vision testing is conducted for at least three reasons:

- Testing can assist in the detection and diagnosis of pathological changes in the visual system if an acquired anomaly in color vision is noted.
- Color deficiencies can cause functional difficulties with color discrimination tasks.
- People with low vision should be aware that they have difficulty discriminating colors and know which colors they confuse.

Color vision testing requires fairly good central visual acuity, so it cannot be conducted with individuals with significant reduction in central acuity. In addition, since a quantitative color vision assessment requires subjective responses, it is difficult to perform with young children or others who have difficulty understanding the test.

The two primary objective tests of color vision are the use of Ishihara color plates and the Farnsworth D15 test. With the Ishihara color plates, which are used to screen for color deficiencies, the individual is asked to identify numbers and symbols or to follow a winding line within a patterned background. Some younger children can trace the pattern with their fingers, rather than identify the symbols verbally.

The Farnsworth D15 test, a diagnostic test to determine the type of color deficiency, has 15 color chips that the person arranges to appear in order according to chromatic similarity. Because these color chips are small, a jumbo version of the Farnsworth D15 test can be either fabricated or purchased. The Farnsworth D100 test—containing 100 color chips—is not routinely used for people with normal vision and should not be used for people with low vision because these individuals in general do not have the resolving ability (near acuity) to see and discern the changes in hues this test requires.

Color matching is a test that can be used with young children. Although it can be helpful in identifying children with gross color vision problems, it is of limited value because it does not test more refined color discrimination.

Congenital color vision problems cannot be medically or surgically resolved. If reduced color vision is the result of an eye disease or condition that affects the visual system, it may be resolved or improved when that disease or condition is ameliorated (such as with the removal of cataracts). Acquired color vision disorders involving the discrimination of red and green typically represent optic nerve disease, whereas those that involve the discrimination of blue and yellow are the result of retinal or macular disorders.

Contrast Sensitivity Testing

The testing of contrast sensitivity is a subjective measurement of an individual's ability to detect pattern stimuli at low contrast. Spatial frequency refers to the frequency or number of light and dark stripes in a given area. Higher spatial frequencies involve a greater number of alternating stripes in a given area, whereas lower spatial frequencies have a lesser number of alternating stripes. Because Snellen visual acuity letters measure the eyes' ability to discriminate fine detail (high spatial frequencies) with high contrast (black letters on a white background), they cannot be used to determine visual function in day-to-day activities, when people experience much lower contrast and lower spatial frequencies (coarser details) than is found with standard Snellen letters. For this reason, the testing of contrast sensitivity function gives a more accurate representation of the eyes' visual performance, and hence an individual's overall quality of vision, than does only a distance acuity finding.

Contrast sensitivity testing can be performed using electronically generated sine-wave gratings with video monitor displays, the Pelli-Robson charts, the Arden Plate test, or the Vistech Vision Contrast Test System. The Vistech system, developed by Ginsberg (1984), and the Pelli-Robson charts (see Pelli, Robson, & Wilkins, 1988) are most often used in a clinical low vision evaluation. The Vistech system is made up of six rows of 3-inch diameter sine-wave gratings (that is, a pattern of alternating white and dark stripes); the Pelli-Robson charts contain variably contrasted alphabetic letters that can discriminate normal from abnormal contrast function.

Contrast sensitivity testing has proved helpful in understanding why individuals with similar distance visual acuities function so differently for both distance and near point activities. It is also useful for identifying persons who need both increased magnification and contrast for improving visual function and for completing the diagnostic workup of a number of conditions, including glaucoma, optic nerve disease, macular degeneration, albinism, and amblyopia. Furthermore, when an individual complains that things do not look clear, but no observable decrease in visual acuity is found during the eye examination, the examiner can use contrast sensitivity testing to review how the person is seeing in the lower- and midspatial frequencies, not just in the high spatial frequencies of standard eye charts.

Individuals with reduced contrast sensitivity in the lower and midspatial frequencies and who have relatively normal contrast sensitivity in the higher spatial frequencies usually have relatively good distance acuity but severely reduced near acuity because near visual tasks require finer detail vision than do distance tasks. For this reason, they require more magnification than might be expected on the basis of their distance acuity. For example, a person with macular disease may have a best-corrected distance acuity of 20/100 but a best-corrected near acuity for single words of 5M print at 10 inches. On the basis of their distance acuity, one might expect that such persons need 5X magnification (100/20) to see 1M continuous-text print at near, when they probably need 10X or more magnification to do so.

Decreased contrast sensitivity can be improved in certain cases. For example, when cataracts, which can cause decreased contrast sensitivity, are removed, the individual's overall visual functioning can improve significantly, even when retinal problems are present. Also, absorptive lenses can improve an individual's ability to see with more detail, both indoors and outdoors (for more information on absorptive lenses, see the section on these lenses later in this chapter).

Visual Field Testing

Visual field testing can be helpful in understanding which portions of the individual's visual field are functional. The loss of central vision peripheral vision can have profound and yet different effects on the person's ability to function visually, and the normal field of view can be restricted by such features as eyeglasses, droopy eyelids, a large nose, or heavy eyebrows (see Chapters 5 and 6 for more information on visual fields).

Since impairments or reductions to the visual field (rather than to visual acuity) have the greatest effect on visual functioning (Faye, 1984), a visual field assessment is essential for understanding the functional effects of a visual impairment. The Amsler Grid, confrontation fields, tangent screens, and manual and computerized bowl perimeters are methods for assessing central and peripheral visual fields.

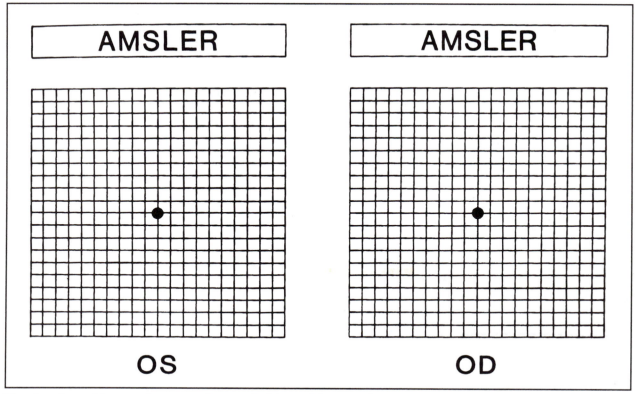

The Amsler grid tests the area of central vision. This reproduction of the grid has been reduced from the actual size.

The *Amsler grid* test is done to analyze the disruption of visual function that occurs when pathological conditions affect the macula, the area of central vision. This test is conducted at an 11- to 13-inch (28–33 cm) working distance, with the observer monocularly viewing the center spot on the grid and pointing to any disturbances.

Confrontation visual fields is a widely used rapid and practical technique to detect gross defects in the central and peripheral fields. In this test, the examiner and client face each other, approximately 2 feet (0.6 m) apart, and the examiner wiggles an index finger in each of the four quadrants of the visual field and asks the person whether he or she can see it. The test can be more sensitive if the examiner increases the working distance to 10 to 13 feet (3m to 4m) and uses a finger-counting field examination, rather than a wiggling finger, to assess the peripheral visual field out of 40 to 60 degrees from fixation (straight ahead). This technique can detect only the most gross defects, and a negative result is often recorded as a normal field when there may be deficits of considerable size and density. Therefore, it should be considered an adjunct to the more precise methods of perimetry represented by tanget screen, manual-bowl, and computerized-bowl perimetry.

Tangent screen perimetry is a flexible technique for examining the visual field within 30 degrees of fixation. The individual is asked to fixate monocularly on the center target of a 2-meter black felt target at a distance of 2 feet (0.6 m). The examiner then moves a wand with a small target at the tip from a point where the person cannot see the target to a point where he or she can just see the target and marks that point on the tangent screen with a pin. This process is repeated at various points around the tangent screen to establish the individual's field of vision.

Manual-bowl and computerized-bowl perimetry are used to test the central and peripheral fields. Bowl perimeters are essentially half a hollow sphere that places the person's eye at the center of the sphere as the person places his or her chin in a chin rest. The individual is asked to fixate on a central target monocularly and to report when he or she sees a light either flash on (static perimetry) or just move into his or her field of view (kinetic perimetry). With manual bowl perimetry, visual field testing is sensitive, and the eye care specialist or experienced technician can quickly adjust and easily record the size, brightness, and color of the test object. Computerized-bowl perimetry has become the accepted standard in clinical practice; it is much more time efficient, precise, and consistent than is manual bowl perimetry and can do threshold testing with statistical analyses of an individual's visual field in comparison to age-matched normal fields.

Interpretation of the Eye Report

Reviewing the medical eye report can be helpful in understanding the functional implications of low vision. In addition, information on the prognosis of an eye disease or condition can be helpful for developing a plan to enhance a person's visual function and to improve overall independence. The special equipment and procedures that are used in a medical eye examination are presented in Sidebar 8.6.

The medical eye report may not contain fully accurate information about how the individual is currently functioning, as well as what may affect his or her visual function in the future. For example, in many cases, parents of young children with low vision may be told their children are blind or will become blind. When incomplete information is provided, it may delay or prevent the timely receipt of appropriate clinical low vision services. Furthermore, since an eye condition can significantly influence a person's ability to respond to visual enhancement with various forms of magnification (Faye, 1984), knowledge of the most likely course of a visual condition over time is important for planning strategies to compensate for low vision and for determining the most appropriate optical device for the individual's needs.

In many cases, particularly with stable congenital conditions, such as albinism, nystagmus, or optic atrophy, it can be expected that a person's visual functioning will not deteriorate or, in the case of young children, that it will improve as they mature. With other conditions, such as congenital glaucoma, RP, or macular degeneration, it can be more difficult to anticipate a person's future visual capabilities. Nevertheless, in the majority of cases, individuals with low vision retain useful vision throughout their lives that can be enhanced by low vision services.

When reviewing a medical eye report, one should be aware whether ocular surgery is being considered. In many cases, a person will see significantly better following cataract surgery. When laser treatment is done for diabetic retinopathy or "wet" macular degeneration, the person's vision can be slightly or significantly decreased. (Individuals with Type I diabetes often have better visual acuity with less daily fluctuation of vision and a better overall quality of vision if their diabetes is tightly controlled.)

The clinician must weigh the immediate need for vision rehabilitation against the likelihood that the person's vision will change significantly in the near future as a result of medical problems or upcoming surgery. If the person's vision is likely to change significantly in the near future, the prescription of more elaborate optical devices should be deferred until the vision has stabilized, and less expensive devices and alternate techniques should be used in the interim.

Prescription of and Instruction in Low Vision Devices

Most individuals with low vision can benefit from optical devices to enhance their visual performance. The optimum combination of optical and nonoptical devices depends on the visual tasks a person wishes to perform, the person's visual capabilities, and his or her attitude toward both optical devices and the visual disability.

Magnification is often the first optical parameter considered for enhancing visual functioning

Additional Equipment and Procedures Used in General Ophthalmic Evaluations

Direct ophthalmoscope	Provides a small-field, high-magnification view of the posterior pole of the retina. Examination can be performed through dilated or undilated pupils.
Binocular indirect ophthalmoscope	Provides a less magnified view of the ocular fundus, allowing for visualization of both the central and peripheral retina. Examination is performed through dilated pupils.
Slit lamp (biomicroscope)	Used to evaluate the anterior structures of the eye, including the cornea, the lens, and the anterior portion of the vitreous.
Gonioscope	Used in conjunction with the biomicroscope for viewing the filtration angle of the anterior chamber. Gonioscopes are prismatic contact lenses, some of which have a central lens that is used to view the posterior pole of the retina.
Electroretinogram (ERG)	Records the mass response of the retina to an intense flash of light. One electrode is placed on the anesthetized cornea with the aid of a contact lens, and a second electrode is placed on the face or forehead; the individual is then subjected to the intense light. The ERG records information from the inner segment of the rods and cones, the bipolar cells, and the retinal pigment epithelium. Its use is an important diagnostic technique when a rod abnormality is suspected, such as in retinitis pigmentosa.
Electrooculogram (EOG)	Records the response to movements of the eye. One electrode is placed near the inner canthus of the eye, and the other is placed near the outer canthus; the individual is instructed to fixate back and forth between two fixation points that are 40 degrees apart. The potential difference between the cornea and the back of the eye is then measured under conditions of dark adaptation and light adaptation. Abnormal EOGs are useful in the differential diagnosis of abnormalities of the retinal pigment epithelium.
Visual evoked response (VER)	Records the electrical response of the visual cortex created when the person views an osculating checkered board or striped stimulus pattern. In this test, an electrode is placed on the scalp near the Inion, and the individual views the osculating pattern. This test records the potential of the visual cortex. (At this time, the VER should be considered experimental because only a few controlled clinical studies have been performed using this technique. Also, its known lack of specificity is a major drawback in clinical assessment.)
Gene testing	Seeks to identify the genes that carry various forms of hereditarily acquired conditions. By looking at specific genes, a more accurate prognosis of a person's future visual capabilities can be made. Although this technique is still relatively new, more and more genes that govern certain visual conditions are being identified by researchers.

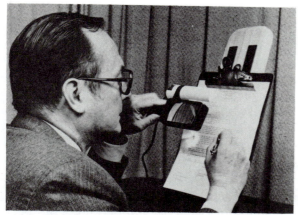

Many people with low vision can benefit from using a combination of optical and nonoptical devices, such as a magnifier with a reading stand, as shown here.

(see Chapter 7 for a discussion of the four types of magnification—relative size, relative distance, angular, and projection). As noted in Chapter 7, magnification allows the size of the retinal image to be increased to the point that enough retinal cells are stimulated to send a detailed image to the brain, thereby allowing the individual with low vision to see the magnified object. The amount of magnification necessary for a given individual is generally not determined until after the distance refractive error is assessed and corrected.

Simply magnifying an object to the appropriate size does not always allow the individual with low vision to view that object comfortably, however. Some individuals will benefit from other alterations of the visual image, including those produced by field expansion systems and prisms. With eye conditions such as cataracts or other problems relating to the ocular media (in addition to many retinal conditions), contrast enhancement will also be required.

Many factors go into making decisions about the most appropriate optical device for an individual with low vision. Individuals are often concerned about ease of use, portability, working distance, cosmetic appearance, and cost of devices. In general, an individual with low vision will receive more than one optical device. Because most people wish to accomplish a variety of tasks at varying working distances, one device will usually not meet all their visual needs.

The prescription of low vision devices is never solely the decision of the clinical low vision specialist. Because low vision care is goal oriented, the prescribed device or devices should be designed to meet the needs of the individual being evaluated. With this in mind, the clinician will present different options that provide the needed level of visual enhancement, tailoring recommendations about an optical device or devices (such as handheld, spectacle mounted, monocular, and binocular) to the specific personal, vocational, and avocational needs of the individual. In doing so, the clinician will keep in mind the process that has caused the individual to have low vision and make sure that the appropriate amount of image alteration (magnification, minification, and/or contrast enhancement) is provided to allow the individual to accomplish tasks. The individual can then choose the combination that best suits his or her needs and goals. (For a discussion of various types of optical and nonoptical devices, see Chapter 7).

The following case history illustrates how various devices can be considered and tried out to meet the particular needs of the individual with low vision.

Mark, aged 39, a plant manager for a large manufacturing company, experienced a loss of vision secondary to histoplasmosis, a fungal infection, at age 31. At his last low vision evaluation seven years ago, he received a handheld monocular telescope and a stand magnifier that he has used successfully since then. During a recent medical eye examination, Mark's ophthalmologist suggested that he should have another low vision evaluation to see if any additional optical devices might be of assistance to him.

Mark's best-corrected visual acuities at this evaluation were 10/80−1 (OD) and 10/125 (OS) through the following spectacle correction: OD −5.75 −.50 × 170, OS −6.00 −.50 × 95. His near acuity was 2.5M print at 5 inches OD and 4M print at 5 inches OS through this myopic spectacle correction. Mark's binocular near acuity improved to .8M print at 5 inches when the spectacles were removed. His 16-diopter stand magnifier improved his near vision to the point where he could read .4M print at 1 inch. Mark did not bring his monocular telescope with him to the low vision clinic.

A number of optical devices were tried at this visit, and Mark was sent home with the following: a pair +12 prismatic half-eye magnifiers in addition to +12 full-frame reading spectacles, both of which improved his near vision to the point where he could read .5M continuous-text print at a 2-inch working distance without difficulty; two different types of 4X microscopic spectacles, which allowed Mark to read .4M continuous-text print with minimal difficulty; a 20-diopter hand magnifier, which also allowed him to read .4M continuous-text print at 4 inches; and a 6X monocular handheld telescope, which improved his distance acuity to 20/32 and allowed him to read .6M continuous-text print at 14 inches. In addition, a CCTV, which Mark took to try at home for several days, allowed him to read newsprint comfortably and easily at a 14-inch working distance using approximately 10X magnification.

After a two-week trial of the various devices that he took home, Mark decided that he really did not need a CCTV because he could read so well with both the spectacle-mounted and handheld optical devices he had tried. Therefore, he chose to acquire the 20-diopter hand magnifier, two 6X monocular telescopes, and a set of 4X microscopic spectacles, which he found useful for the various tasks he needed to accomplish and more comfortable than his previous hand magnifier and monocular telescope. It was recommended that Mark be reevaluated in two years.

Spectacles and Contact Lenses

Spectacles can significantly enhance an individual's ability to see at both near and far distances. For this reason, refractive error must always be assessed and properly corrected.

For individuals with high refractive error, or anisometropia, contact lenses can be of great value in improving overall visual functioning and are often cosmetically more acceptable than thick spectacles. People with nystagmus or distorted corneas will often see significantly better with the use of contact lenses. Individuals with field problems have also found contact lenses particularly useful when they have high refractive errors.

High plus aphakic spectacle lenses can be quite disorienting to some persons because of problems with visual perception and depth perception, in addition to the field restrictions and a "jack-in-the-box" effect created by these lenses. Contact lenses minimize these effects and can significantly improve the overall visual functioning of the aphakic individual. Contact lenses can be colored or painted to reduce photophobia by creating an artificial pupil that will decrease the amount of light entering the eye. In addition, such a contact lens provides a better cosmetic appearance for individuals with conditions, such as aniridia and iris coloboma.

Monocular and Binocular Reading Spectacles

When an individual with low vision requires greater resolution at near than he or she can obtain with the best spectacle correction, the clinical low vision specialist needs to increase the reading power of the prescribed device. This increase in reading power simultaneously reduces the working distance. The closer working distance increases the person's ability to read small print as a result of relative distance magnification.

The Lighthouse Plus Estimation Card is helpful in reviewing an individual's reading acuity at an 8- or 16-inch working distance. With this information, the low vision specialist can estimate how much additional plus power will be needed to read newsprint-size materials (1M continuous text). (Plus lenses are converging/convex lenses that are thicker in the middle; minus lenses are diverging/concave lenses and are thicker on the edges; see Chapter 7 for more information.)

When binocular vision is present, it is possible to maintain binocularity with the use of base-in prisms in the person's reading spectacles to powers of 10 to 12 diopters. In eyeglasses with base-in prisms, the thicker portion, or base, of the prism is placed toward the nose. The base-in prism allows the two eyes to work together more comfortably because the eyes do not have to converge (turn in) as much as they would if the prism, which bends the light, were not present. When individuals need more magnification, they must learn to perform near point visual tasks monocularly. Because many individuals with low vision have significantly better vision in one eye than in the other or can only use one eye at a time, the lack of binocularity tends not to be as much of a problem as the close working distance required.

Because children with low vision have considerable ability to accommodate to varying working distances, they can sustain the prolonged accommodative effort needed for close working distances when doing near point activities for an extended period of time without eyestrain and fatigue. For this reason, a reading correction is often not required by an individual until the second decade of life.

The advantages of monocular and binocular reading spectacles are that they offer the widest field of view while allowing the wearer to keep both hands free. Also, they tend to be relatively inexpensive, as well as inconspicuous. The primary disadvantage of these spectacles is the close working distance they require. Maintaining this distance can result in arm fatigue and increased head movement when reading and so can be uncomfortable for the person to use for sustained near-point tasks.

Hand, Stand, and Mirror Magnifiers

Magnifiers are particularly useful for individuals with reduced central vision, as well as for those with low visual acuity and normal visual fields. Since individuals with central vision loss need to view with an off-center (eccentric) point to have their best vision, they often have a difficult time viewing through high-powered reading spectacles or telemicroscopes because the optics of these devices require viewing through the center of the lens. When these individuals are able to use an optical device at a longer working distance, such as a hand, stand, or mirror magnifier, eccentric viewing is easier to accomplish. Many persons with more advanced forms of macular disease do much better with these devices than they do with spectacle-mounted ones. Because of their portability and flexibility, handheld devices are often very helpful, although they are not useful for certain tasks, such as playing a musical instrument. Stand magnifiers are helpful for individuals with hand tremors because they do not require the individual to maintain a specific working distance.

A source of great confusion about hand and stand magnifiers is the problem of lens size versus magnification power. Many older individuals with low vision want a large, high-powered magnifier. However, the practical optics of strong lenses require smaller lens diameters as power is increased. The smaller lens size and resulting field of view can be frustrating for individuals who need a higher powered magnifier.

Head Loupes

Head-mounted loupes are primarily used for tasks where both hands need to be kept free and a relatively close working distance is not a problem. Loupes are relatively inexpensive. They are simple convex lenses for magnifying that can be used in monocular or binocular forms, mounted in front of the eye, for viewing small objects at a very close distance. The lenses can be moved in and out of the line of sight as necessary, which makes them fairly convenient to use. The maximum power of head loupes is 10.00 D (4-inch working distance) for binocular units, and 60.00 D (1.5 inch working distance) for monocular units.

Distance Telescopes and Telemicroscopes

Telescopes are useful for individuals who need to be able to spot objects in the distance and do not have the ability to get closer. Monocular handheld telescopes are quite helpful for such tasks as O&M and the reading of chalkboards; they tend to be relatively inconspicuous. The ability of some telescopes to adjust to variable viewing distances (10 inches to infinity) makes them flexible for use in a number of tasks.

For some individuals with low vision, the small field of view associated with a handheld or spectacle-mounted telescope can be difficult to use. This difficulty is particularly evident for individuals with central scotomas and can result in their inability to use this type of device.

For driving purposes, bioptic telescopes can be legally used in many states to provide enhanced distance resolution ability for briefly spot checking distant targets. This capability can allow some individuals with low vision, who are carefully screened and who receive appropriate driver's education, to drive a vehicle.

Binoculars are another type of optical device. Because they are used with both eyes, they provide a wider field of view, and they may be easier to manipulate and focus than a monocular handheld telescope. The disadvantages of binoculars are their weight, size, and inability to focus at intermediate and near distances.

Over the years, clinical low vision specialists have attempted to create a telescopic system by using a high minus powered contact lens with a high plus powered spectacle lens to create a Galilean telescope. Because of alignment problems as well as relatively low magnification and narrow field, this approach has rarely met the needs of individual users.

Telemicroscopes, or intermediate and near-vision telescopes, can be quite helpful for individuals who need a longer working distance and hands-free magnification, such as keyboard operators, but who cannot function comfortably at the closer working distances required by other spectacle-mounted systems. Telemicroscopes can be set for any working distance desired but are not focusable. Disadvantages of telemicroscopes are that they are more conspicuous, more expensive, and have a smaller field of view than other reading devices.

A binocular system is the logical approach to take for telemicroscopes when the visual acuity between the two eyes is essentially equal. If visual acuity is not equal, the better eye should be fitted with the telescope. As with all optical devices, the specific needs and visual abilities of the individual should determine whether a monocular or binocular fit is most appropriate.

With a spectacle-mounted system, arm fatigue is not a factor, and the hands are kept free to do various manipulative tasks. However, the weight of the system can limit the length of time an individual can wear a spectacle-mounted telescopic system. Also, spectacle-mounted systems require additional head movements and are often considered less cosmetically appealing than handheld devices.

CCTVs

When an individual requires magnification greater than can be provided by optical devices or when contrast enhancement is needed in addition to magnification for best near point functioning, a CCTV becomes the logical and often only option. The CCTV is the only device that provides both enhancements. CCTVs can also be very helpful if a larger field of view or a longer working distance is required with higher degrees of magnification.

However, the disadvantages of most standard CCTVs at present are their cost and relative lack of portability. The majority of portable CCTVs have some limitations, including the need for greater manual dexterity on the part of the user than with full-size models, the small size of the monitor, decreased contrast, availability only in black and white, limited magnification range, and a smaller objective field of view. Portable CCTVs are beneficial for a select group of individuals using them for specific tasks, such as college students studying in the library.

Another form of projection magnification is enlarged text on computer screens. Such systems typically are provided through educational and rehabilitation programs rather than low vision clinics.

Absorptive Lenses

In the prescription of absorptive lenses, decisions about appropriateness are typically based on reported symptoms of photophobia, which can occur indoors and outdoors. Also, the perception of the effect of the filters by each individual weighs heavily in the decision as to which absorptive lens is best. Often, individuals with conditions such as albinism, aniridia, achromatopsia, and iris colobomas can be highly photophobic, although this is not universally the case. Absorptive lenses may be placed in frames with shields on the tops and sides to prevent ambient light from entering the eyes.

Field Expansion Devices

According to Faye (1984), there are three options available to an individual who wishes to compensate for a large area of missing field:

- Compress the existing image to include more of the available area.
- Provide prisms that relocate images from the blind area into the seeing area.
- Use a mirror to reflect an image from the nonseeing area.

Fresnel lenses are pliable, soft plastic lenses that can be temporarily attached to a regular spectacle lens. They are are recommended as a trial lens in either spherical powers, bifocal segments, or prisms. One of the more common uses of Fresnel prisms is in the treatment of field loss. Fresnel prisms with powers of 10 to 15 diopters are placed with the base in the direction of the field loss. The prisms can be presented over the entire lens or just out from the midline into the area of field loss. When the individual directs his or her eyes into the prism area, a lower contrast image from the missing field will come into view. Because of the decrease in visual acuity as a result of the reduced contrast, most individuals will reject Fresnel prisms as a permanent solution for field enhancement. However, a trial is helpful to see if the individual would benefit from having a prism incorporated into a spectacle correction.

Reverse telescopes have been used to enhance the effective visual field for persons who have concentric peripheral field loss. With this technique, the individual looks through the objective end of the telescope (the end closest to the object being viewed) rather than the ocular end (that part of the telescope normally placed up to the eye).

For many years now, monocular hemianopic mirrors have been used to reflect an image from a nonseeing area into the seeing field of view. This technique is of value to a select group of individuals. In some cases, a −1.50 diopter lens mounted in a hand magnifier carrier held at arms' length can provide a simple yet effective method of expanding an individual's field of view.

Follow-Up

Once initial optical and nonoptical devices have been determined for an individual, instruction in the use of these devices is critical if the person is to learn the skills needed to become efficient in their use. Because elderly persons are sometimes less able to adapt to the use of unfamiliar devices, some older individuals may require additional training to use recommended devices.

Once the person with low vision has received initial instruction in the specific use and care of the devices prescribed, arrangements should be made for him or her to take the devices home for several days or weeks. A teacher of students with visual impairments, an O&M specialist, or a rehabilitation specialist can then provide additional instruction and guided practice in school, living, and working environments. This additional instruction should be ensured by the low vision clinician and be provided by the clinician, by his or her staff, or by referral. A follow-up visit is necessary after the trial period with devices to reassess how effectively the person is using them on a day-to-day basis and to decide if any modification of the trial devices or any additional devices are needed.

Accessory and nonoptical devices are usually demonstrated at the conclusion of the clinical low vision evaluation. These devices also can be reviewed and recommended by other professionals who work with individuals with low vision, such as educators, rehabilitation specialists, O&M specialists, and low vision educators.

Accessories

Accessory and nonoptical devices take many forms. Large-print material, adjustable illumination, and felt-tip pens are helpful for near-point tasks. Technological advances to assist persons with low vision include computer speech synthesis, variable-size type fonts, and image intensifiers. Outdoor glare can be controlled with wide brim hats, visors, photochromic lenses, wraparound and clip-on sun filters, and absorptive lenses.

Other accessory devices include talking clocks, watches, and calculators. Reading stands can be useful for individuals of all ages by allowing the user to maintain a more normal body posture while moving material to be viewed closer and keeping both hands free. There are a variety of reading stands available, some of which have movable shelves, a feature that is often quite helpful.

Lighting

Many elderly persons find that they see worse at home than they do during their clinical low vision evaluations. This discovery may be the result of inadequate task lighting in the home. Rosenbloom and Organ (1986) stated, "Poor lighting in the home is virtually a universal problem" (p. 343).

The quality and quantity of illumination is critical for optimum visual functioning. General advice on how to arrange lighting for prolonged near point tasks is important. Light can be positioned and adjusted to avoid glare problems. For example, some persons have found that a light angled over the shoulder nearest the better seeing eye and adjustments in the positioning of material to be viewed help to reduce glare. An adjustable lamp with an incandescent indoor floodlight bulb of from 60 to 100 watts provides a useful means of controlling task illumination and

enhancing contrast. Also, placing a television a reasonably short distance from the eyes not only enlarges the image, but increases the illumination to see the image.

Report of Clinical Findings

After the clinical low vision evaluation is completed, the clinician should convey essential and important information to the person with low vision, family members (if appropriate), and other professionals of the low vision team. The report should present the findings in a clear and understandable manner, so the educational or rehabilitation specialists can use them to develop an individual educational or rehabilitation plan. It should be stressed here that the clinical low vision specialist should guard against making educational suggestions, such as the most appropriate literacy medium, or any recommendations for the most appropriate academic placement for a specific child. Typical components of a report include history, diagnostic data and treatment, and follow-up, although the components vary among practitioners. (More specific areas are presented in Sidebar 8.7.)

OTHER CONSIDERATIONS

Individuals with Multiple Disabilities

Because individuals with multiple disabilities have additional impairments besides vision, it can be difficult at times to sort out whether any lack of visual attention they display is related primarily to low vision or to other factors, such as head position, medications, difficulties with arm and general motor control, or stimuli or information processing delays. Therefore, it is critical for the clinical low vision specialist to work with the teacher of students with visual impairments, rehabilitation professional, adult care providers, and occupational and physical therapist (if appropriate) to develop an educational or rehabilitation plan to help the person improve his

SIDEBAR 8.7

Components of the Low Vision Report

◆ The eye diagnosis and prognosis, as well as any other physical or mental problems experienced by the person

◆ A brief history of the person's current visual conditions

◆ Specific questions or concerns presented to the low vision clinician by the person, referring doctor, agency, family, or teachers or other service providers

◆ Distance visual acuity

◆ Near visual acuity and working distance

◆ Reading acuity (continuous text)

◆ Distance spectacles or contact lens recommendations

◆ Effect of prescribed lenses on both distance and near vision

◆ Recommendations concerning removal of distance spectacles for reading or other visual tasks

◆ Magnification devices prescribed for near, intermediate, and distance vision tasks

◆ Optimum working distance

◆ Initial findings concerning print size, with recommended devices indicated

◆ Seating and lighting recommendations

◆ Difficulties the person had with the initial devices recommended

◆ Significant visual field defects discovered

◆ Color vision deficiencies

◆ Activity restrictions (if any)

◆ Recommendations for additional testing

◆ Recommendations for the next low vision follow-up evaluation

---

or her visual functioning. (Chapter 10 reviews additional techniques for evaluating the functional visual capabilities of children with multiple disabilities.)

Emotional Aspects of the Evaluation

People with low vision and their families often feel anxious and confused when they visit a low vision clinic. Furthermore, many adults who have recently acquired low vision, as well as parents whose children have recently been diagnosed with low vision, are looking for a "magic cure," such as a new pair of spectacles, to restore sight. Thus, it is important for the clinical low vision specialist to explain the goals of low vision care and to indicate that such services can enhance visual functioning but not restore sight, to describe the sequence of the evaluation, and to

stress that the purpose of the clinical low vision evaluation is to look at someone's functional abilities for both distance and near-point activities and then to work to maximize those abilities with optical and nonoptical devices that the person finds comfortable.

Many children with low vision are afraid and uncertain of what to expect during a clinical low vision evaluation because of their previous experiences with such items as eyedrops and bright lights during medical eye examinations. In addition, parents are often anxious about what having low vision will mean for their children, personally, educationally, and vocationally. Adult patients are frequently concerned about losing their independence, particularly in relation to driving, reading, and maintaining their personal affairs. For teenagers and adults with congenital low vision, a clinical low vision evaluation may be the deciding factor in whether they will be able to drive or be employed in a job requiring vision.

Furthermore, both children and adults may be concerned about the cosmetic effects of optical devices, which they may think will make them conspicuous. For reasons such as these, the low vision specialist and other members of the low vision care team need to be sensitive to the emotions, fears, and anxieties of the individual and his or her family.

Funding Issues

At present, low vision devices vary in price from $1.00 to several thousand dollars. The majority of handheld and stand magnifiers typically cost less than $75, and many reading spectacles can be acquired for less than $100. Monocular telescopes usually cost $100 to $200; spectacle-mounted telescopes and telemicroscopes cost from $300 to $2,000, depending on their style and whether they are monocular or binocular. Electronic magnification devices, such as a CCTVs, range from $1,000 to $3,500.

Low vision care and optical devices are not covered by most insurance policies, including Medicare, but partial reimbursements are frequently provided for visits to ophthalmologists and optometrists. However, rehabilitation agencies in many states fund clinical low vision evaluations and devices for select individuals who are receiving vocational assistance and for students who will attend college; some states' public aid programs fund select low vision care and devices. Funding is also sometimes available from school systems and service organizations, such as the Lions Clubs. Whatever the source of funding, it is crucial that the person with low vision receive appropriate optical and nonoptical devices, which are an integral part of the rehabilitation process.

SUMMARY

Comprehensive low vision rehabilitation requires a transdisciplinary team approach because the clinical low vision specialist alone cannot provide an individual with the multidimensional care that is required. Clinical low vision care emphasizes the functional capabilities and functional potential of each person with low vision and does not just look at the person's static distance or near visual acuity, because it does not accurately reflect a person's visual function or predict how that individual will function in the real world. Furthermore, low vision care must be ongoing to provide any additional assistance that the individual may require as his or her visual needs change over time. By providing comprehensive, thorough, and sensitive care and paying attention to individual needs, the clinical low vision specialist and other members of the low vision team can play a pivotal role in helping people who are visually impaired fulfill their personal and professional goals and potential.

ACTIVITIES

With This Chapter and Other Resources

1. Consider Larry's initial problems when he came to the low vision clinic in the vignette that opens this chapter. Describe the problem solving that he and the low vision clinician needed to do to arrive at the best combination and type of devices. Would other options have been available to Larry?

2. Interpret a report from a clinical low vision evaluation for parents of a child who has low vision. Use the information in this chapter, especially the case examples, if other reports are not readily available.

In the Community

1. Visit a low vision clinic and observe clinical low vision evaluations of both children and adults with different causes of low vision. Write a description of a clinical low vision evaluation.

With a Person with Low Vision

1. Interview a person who has been to a low vision clinic. Ask him or her to compare how

the low vision evaluation differed from a general eye examination by an ophthalmologist or optometrist.

2. Ask the parents of a child with low vision or an adult with low vision about their expectations for the help they would receive during the visit to a low vision clinic. Were their expectations realized? What do they recommend that people should know before they go for a clinical low vision evaluation?

From Your Perspective

In a community without a clinical low vision service, what actions might professionals take to establish access to such evaluations?

Adult Data Sheet

Patient's name _____ Date of call _____

Address _____ Appointment date/time _____

Telephone number _____ Social Security No. _____

Insurance carrier _____ Emergency room contact person _____

Referred by _____ Send reports to _____

_____

Chief Complaint _____

_____

Medical History

General health _____

Medical doctor _____

Allergies _____ Medications _____

Recent surgery _____

Education/Work/Social

Highest grade completed _____ Employed/retired _____

Occupation _____

Living situation _____

Visual History

Eye doctor _____ Last eye exam _____

Diagnosis _____

Have you had eye surgery? ☐ Yes ☐ No If yes, when? _____

What type? _____

Have you had laser treatment? ☐ Yes ☐ No If yes, when? _____ Why? _____

How long has your vision been a problem? _____

Do you take any eye medications? ☐ Yes ☐ No If yes, which? _____

Do you have eye pain or discomfort? ☐ Yes ☐ No If yes, describe: _____

_____

Do you have fluctuations in vision? ☐ Yes ☐ No If yes, describe: _____

_____

Have you had a previous low vision exam? ☐ Yes ☐ No If yes, When? _____ Where? _____

Are you currently using any low vision devices? ☐ Yes ☐ No If yes, which one(s)? _____

_____

(continued on next page)

Appendix A. Sample Intake Form

Adult Data Sheet (*continued*)

What is your preferred eye? ☐ OD ☐ OS ☐ No difference

Do you wear glasses? ☐ Yes ☐ No If yes, are the glasses helpful? ☐ Yes ☐ No

Is sunlight bothersome? ☐ Yes ☐ No

What is your preferred lighting? _____

Do you have problems seeing at night? ☐ Yes ☐ No If yes, describe: _____

_____

Near Assessment

Do you read printed material? ☐ Yes ☐ No If yes, do you read: ☐ Large print ☐ Regular print

What types of things would you like to be able to read better? _____

_____

Intermediate/Distance Assessment

What types of things would you like to be able to see better? _____

_____

Other Difficult Visual Tasks

Do you have difficulty seeing objects on a particular side? ☐ Yes ☐ No If yes, which side? _____

Do you turn your head or look to the side to see better? ☐ Yes ☐ No If yes, which side? _____

Mobility

Do you drive a vehicle? ☐ Yes ☐ No

Do you use public transportation? ☐ Yes ☐ No

Do you walk indoors? ☐ Yes ☐ No   Outdoors? ☐ Yes ☐ No

Do you use a cane? ☐ Yes ☐ No

Leisure Activities

What leisure activities are you presently involved with? _____

_____

What activities do you miss doing? _____

_____

Goals/Objectives

Comments

Interviewed by _____ Date _____

Preexamination Report from Teacher of Visually Impaired Students

Teacher _____ Student _____

Subject area _____

Date report completed _____

Student's physical abilities? _____

_____

Student's ability to walk from one place to another _____

Indoors _____

Outdoors _____

Does the student run? ☐ Yes ☐ No

Student's visual functioning _____

_____

What is used as the student's primary learning medium?

☐ Braille

☐ Regular print   What working distance is used? _____

☐ Large print   What working distance is used? _____

☐ Auditory (tapes, talking books, etc.)

☐ Reader

Has the child used optical devices or magnification of any kind?

☐ Yes ☐ No If yes, what kind? _____

Please list any behavior(s) you have noticed, on a regular basis, that relate to this child's visual ability

_____

_____

Education and extracurricular activities _____

Achievement level _____

Grade or school placement _____

Work experience _____

_____

Vocational plans _____

_____

Hobbies _____

(continued on next page)

Appendix B. Sample Preexamination Report Form

Preexamination Report (*continued*)

Does the student express or show a positive attitude toward the use of his/her vision in daily living? Explain.

_____

_____

Does the student express or show a realistic interest in additional use of vision as a learning modality?

_____

Parental attitude: ☐ Positive ☐ Negative   Explain. _____

_____

What specific information would you like from this evaluation? _____

_____

_____

_____

Has a functional vision assessment been performed by an educational consultant and/or an orientation and mobility specialist?

☐ Yes ☐ No If yes, please attach that report to this form.

Additional Comments _____

_____

_____

_____

_____

Preexamination Report from Parents

Name of child _____ Date of birth _____ Date _____

Your name _____ Relationship to child _____

Address _____ Telephone _____

Medical History

When did your child last receive a physical examination?

Date _____ Physician _____

Address _____

List the medications your child is currently taking and any special medical treatments he or she has

had or is receiving _____

If your child has undergone any surgery, please explain and give date(s). _____

_____

_____

What is your child's current overall physical condition (good, poor, unstable, etc.)? _____

If anyone in your family has similar medical problems, please explain _____

Observations or Other Pertinent Data

Does your child have a hearing loss? ☐ Yes ☐ No

If yes, explain the degree of hearing impairment _____

Does your child have any learning difficulties other than visual? ☐ Yes ☐ No

If yes, explain _____

Does your child have any balance, posture, or movement problems? ☐ Yes ☐ No

If yes, explain _____

Visual History

Indicate the date of your child's last eye examination and the eye doctor who performed the

examination:

Date _____ Ophthalmologist/optometrist _____

Address _____

_____

Most recent visual acuity measurement:

Distance: Right eye _____ Left eye _____

Near: Right eye _____ Left eye _____

What is the cause of your child's visual impairment? _____

_____

(continued on next page)

Appendix C. Sample Preexamination Report Form

Preexamination Report (*continued*)

Explain any treatment, medication, or surgery related to your child's eye condition _____

At what age did your child's visual impairment occur? _____

Which eye seems to be your child's better eye? ☐ Right ☐ Left ☐ No difference

Explain any recent changes in your child's vision _____

_____

Has your child ever had a low vision evaluation? ☐ Yes ☐ No

If yes, when was your child's last low vision evaluation? _____

Visual Functioning

Does your child watch TV? ☐ Yes ☐ No If yes, at what distance does he or she sit from the screen?

Does your child see better or more comfortably on ☐ bright/sunny days? ☐ overcast/cloudy days?

Does your child use sunglasses, visor, or hat? ☐ Yes ☐ No

Is your child bothered by glare? ☐ Yes ☐ No

Does your child read any of the following?

Print?	☐ Yes ☐ No	If yes, at what distance? _____
Newspaper headlines?	☐ Yes ☐ No	If yes, at what distance? _____
Large print?	☐ Yes ☐ No	If yes, at what distance? _____
Books?	☐ Yes ☐ No	If yes, at what distance? _____
Typed print?	☐ Yes ☐ No	If yes, at what distance? _____
Magazines?	☐ Yes ☐ No	If yes, at what distance? _____
Newspaper text?	☐ Yes ☐ No	If yes, at what distance? _____
Telephone book?	☐ Yes ☐ No	If yes, at what distance? _____

Does your child use reading glasses or a magnifying glass?

☐ Yes ☐ No If yes, which one? _____

Does your child use any of the following?

Braille	☐ Yes ☐ No
Talking books	☐ Yes ☐ No
Cassettes	☐ Yes ☐ No
Readers	☐ Yes ☐ No
Tapes	☐ Yes ☐ No

(continued on next page)

Preexamination Report (*continued*)

Mobility

What kind of transportation does your child normally use? (bus, walking, etc.)? _____

Does your child:

Travel alone? ☐ Yes ☐ No

Indoors in familiar places? ☐ Yes ☐ No

Indoors in strange places? ☐ Yes ☐ No

Outdoors in familiar places? ☐ Yes ☐ No

Outdoors in strange places? ☐ Yes ☐ No

Has your child received any mobility training? ☐ Yes ☐ No

Has your child used any devices or aids been used in mobility? ☐ Yes ☐ No

If yes, what has been used? _____

If appropriate, what are your child's future vocational objectives? _____

_____

What information would you like from this evaluation? _____

_____

_____

_____

_____

Additional Comments _____

_____

_____

_____

_____

_____

PART THREE

Functional Perspectives

Functional Vision Assessment and Instruction of Children and Youths in Academic Programs

Jane N. Erin and Beth Paul

VIGNETTE

Even though school has been in session only four days, Tracy feels as if she has been in school for weeks. As a new teacher of students with visual impairments, she is overwhelmed by the number of things that need to be done. With two students who use braille in her caseload, her week has been occupied with book orders and reassurances to classroom teachers who have never taught a student who is blind. She spent most of the previous day in a classroom that included two children with severe and multiple impairments, working with the physical therapist on positioning these students so that they could see the other students and participate in classroom activities.

This morning, Tracy finally found time to stop by the middle school to see Andrew, a seventh grader with low vision. The note from last year's teacher of students with visual impairments said "consult only," and Andrew's records indicated that he was doing well academically. Therefore, Tracy was surprised when Andrew said, "It's been a terrible week. I wish you'd come to see my teachers earlier." When she asked why, Andrew said, "So you could tell them that since I use my monocular, I don't have to sit in the front row; that it's OK for me to take physical education; and all those other things they don't understand." Tracy felt as if she had failed Andrew and her other students with low vision already, but she had assumed that they could get along fine without her for the first few weeks. She wondered whether she could have managed her time differently, but she is not sure how.

As Tracy thought about her first week, she realized that her role in working with students with low vision was not as clear as her role in working with students who are blind. Students who read braille need skills that only she could provide, but what is she expected to do with students who have low vision and who read print? Her university professor had said, "You're not a tutor, and you aren't there to help with homework," but some of the students with low vision have trouble keeping up academically. What skills can she teach that would help them to perform better in the classroom? And how can she decide when a skill is important enough to remove the student from other classes to teach it? Finally, when should she advocate for students like Andrew, and when should they be expected to do so for themselves?

INTRODUCTION

Although Tracy is new to her role, she is struggling with questions that challenge much more experienced professionals. The role of the teacher of students with visual impairments can vary widely with respect to students with low vision. The age and abilities of the students, as well as their need for specific skills, will influence whether the teacher works directly with a particular student or interacts primarily with the educational team or classroom teacher. The teacher's role as an advocate for the student with low vision is critical. Because the student uses vision, others may not realize that experiences, such as social interactions and independent living activities, can require specific instruction and practice during the school day; therefore, the teacher may need to educate other school staff in these matters, as well as to provide direct instruction in non-academic areas. As a member of the team, the teacher is responsible for interpreting clinical diagnoses and assessments to other educational personnel and for acting as a bridge between the provision of information and the transfer of information into practice.

In many instances, the teacher of students with visual impairments will be the first to prepare a functional vision assessment for a child, and this chapter begins with this assumption. However, in some countries, pediatric ophthalmologists, physiotherapists, and others may become involved in the early assessment of functional vision. Hyvärinen, an ophthalmologist with a specialty in low vision, has alerted ophthalmologists, pediatricians, and others to the "developmental emergency" that occurs when a child is born with a visual impairment. She recommends that "the ophthalmologist should be aware of this and make the appropriate referrals as soon as there is well-founded suspicion that the infant's visual development deviates from normal, rather than waiting for a confirmed clinical diagnosis" (1994, p. 219). Hyvärinen discusses this emergency by contrasting the development of normal and visually impaired infants. When, for example, there is a delay in visual maturation, she states that an infant's eyes will remain turned up and out, as during sleep, for a longer period of time. This results in the child not bringing his or her hands to midline, but ap-

proaches can be employed to facilitate this aspect of development. For service providers to be aware of a child's needs for intervention, early assessments need to be performed. During the clinical assessment, Hyvärinen states that there are three core questions that should be asked:

- How much and what kind of vision is available for the development of various functions?

- How well can the infant use his or her vision?

- How much visual information must be compensated for by information from other modalities?

The teacher of students with visual impairments plays a vital role in ensuring that these and other essential questions are asked on an ongoing basis in a child's life.

This chapter first reviews how vision develops in children with normal vision as a foundation for understanding how vision develops in children with low vision. It then discusses the assessment of functional vision, which, when combined with the clinical evaluation, provides a thorough understanding of a student's visual capabilities and visual behaviors. Next, it describes the planning and implementation of instruction for students with low vision, both in skills related to the use of vision and in curricular areas that may require adaptation. Finally, it presents approaches by which the teacher of students with visual impairments ensures that the student has functional visual skills that can be generalized to other settings.

DEVELOPMENT OF VISION

Teachers of students with visual impairments participate in decisions that take into account the students' visual capabilities, so it is important that they understand the changes in vision that occur as children grow. Although the questions they ask may be similar for different children, the answers may vary, depending on the ages of the students. During the first year or two of life, changes in visual capacity are possible because the structures of the brain are still unspecialized; however, older children are unlikely to experience major increases in visual ability. For this reason, goals for younger children may be developmental, whereas those for older ones focus on adaptations that result in the best visual function or use of vision in regular life activities. An understanding of the developmental progression of vision gives teachers the background to plan age-appropriate activities that challenge students' visual abilities. (See Sidebar 9.1 for a sequence of normal visual development.)

Newborns

Newborns immediately begin to gather information about their world through the use of vision. Light and form engage their interest, even though they cannot yet accommodate well to changes in viewing distance or respond to detail.

Although there is disagreement about the visual acuities of newborn infants, some studies (see, for example, Isenberg, 1989) have suggested approximate acuities of 20/400. The eye structures of newborns are fully formed, with two exceptions: The optic nerve takes several months to become fully myelinzed, and the macula fully develops midway through the first year of life.

Newborns have had no experience with the appearance of real objects or people, but some perceptual responses are present at birth. Newborns are innately aware of the fact that an object increases in apparent size as it draws nearer; the existence of this awareness has been determined through "looming," or presenting an enlarging stimulus to elicit a defensive response (Sekuler & Blake, 1990). They notice primary colors within a week of birth (Isenberg, 1989) and have a preference for human faces within a few weeks.

First Year of Life

During the first months of life, infants begin to coordinate eye movements and develop fixation. Although they initially may transfer visual fixation from one eye to the other, by the third month, their eyes work together, and binocular vision has developed well. Eye movements become increasingly smooth during the first six months, at which time most infants are consistently able to track and shift their gaze. A preference for yellow, orange, and red emerges in the second or third month. The field of view, which is central at first, expands during the first year as the retina develops and the infant learns to coordinate head and eye movements.

A critical stage in visual and motor development occurs at around 5 months, when infants begin to reach and grasp. Then they can manipulate objects, and because of their developing accommodative abilities, they are challenged to notice near and distant objects. Physical control of the visual environment provides infants with the opportunity to pair active touch or haptic feedback with visual experiences, so they can now explore their world and examine it deliberately. As babies manipulate objects, they begin to make use of and refine their understanding of the following perceptual phenomena and concepts, which develop at age 3 to 5 months:

- *Size constancy*: Objects retain their size even though they appear smaller at a distance.
- *Shape constancy*: Objects remain the same shape even though their shapes may appear to alter when viewed at different angles.
- *Depth cues*: Nearer objects overlap with those at a distance.
- *Figure-ground relationships*: Single figures can be visually selected from backgrounds, and elements of a scene can exist at different distances from the eye.

By age 6 months, movements are more controlled, and infants can examine objects visually, pursue moving objects smoothly, and shift their gaze among objects. Convergence is now fully developed so that a child can use both eyes together to view objects moved toward him. He can

A Visual Developmental Scale

Age	Visual Characteristics or Skills
Birth	◆ Can see patterns of light and dark, but specific objects are blurry ◆ Has some degree of fixation
1 month	◆ Can focus eyes at 1 1/2 inches ◆ Displays beginning of conjugate following movements (binocular coordination) ◆ Follows slow-moving objects ◆ Follows horizontal movement of objects to the midline
2 months	◆ Displays development of protective blink reflex ◆ Prefers faces to complex patterns ◆ Follows vertical movement of objects
3 months	◆ Displays smoother eye movements ◆ Smiles at visual stimulus ◆ Displays improving visual acuity ◆ Displays improving binocular vision ◆ Notices gross color differences ◆ Seems aware of objects only when manipulating them ◆ Anticipates feeding by visual stimuli
4 months	◆ Displays accommodative flexibility (can now shift focus) ◆ Displays improved hand-eye coordination ◆ Shows interest in small, bright objects ◆ Attempts to move toward objects in visual field ◆ Recognizes familiar faces ◆ Visually explores new environments ◆ Follows objects across the midline ◆ Shows horizontal, vertical, and circular eye movements ◆ Makes unsuccessful attempts at reaching ◆ Mouths and looks at objects in hand
5 months	◆ Develops eye-hand coordination ◆ Grasps objects successfully ◆ Looks intently at objects held close to the eyes ◆ Examines objects with the eyes, rather than uses objects only for light play
6 months	◆ Shifts visual attention from one object to another in a field of various objects ◆ Recognizes faces up to six yards away ◆ Rescues toys dropped within reach ◆ Turns object in hand and explores visually ◆ Has capability of both eyes holding fixation and converging equally

A Visual Developmental Scale (continued)

9–10 months
- Imitates expressions
- Looks around corners
- Spills, to watch liquid spill
- Is visually alert to new things
- Plays games
- Develops object permanence

1 year
- Has distance and near visual acuity near normal
- Displays improved binocular vision
- Displays improved accommodation

1 1/2 years
- Displays vertical orientation: builds 2–3 block towers
- Matches identical objects: 2 spoons, 2 blocks, and so forth
- Points to pictures in a book
- Imitates vertical and horizontal strokes

2 years
- Inspects objects with eyes alone
- Imitates movements
- Seeks missing objects or persons visually
- Has increased color vision
- Has increased visual memory

3 years
- Matches simple forms, does simple form board or puzzle, but still relies on some tactile clues
- Pretends to pick up objects from the page of a book
- Can draw a crude circle

4 years
- Can accurately discriminate sizes
- Has good depth perception
- Displays free hand-eye coordination (does not require conscious effort)
- Discriminates length regardless of orientation

5 years
- Displays mature coordination: picks up and releases objects precisely
- Colors, cuts, and pastes
- Demonstrates knowledge of concept and muscle control of size by assembling nesting blocks with facility, not trial and error
- Can draw a square

6 years
- Handles and attempts to use tools and materials
- Prints capital letters but has common reversals
- Can draw a triangle
- Begins to read

7–9 years
- Prints sentences
- Has speed and smoothness of eye-hand preference
- Includes details in drawing.

Source: Reprinted, with permission of the developer, Mark E. Wilkinson, O.D.

also use both eyes together to receive a three-dimensional image, known as binocularity.

During the remainder of the first year of life, visual changes include the further refinement of visual acuity and more the precise use of vision at near point. The most notable changes during this period are due to the pairing of visual abilities with aspects of memory and thought; thus, infants can search visually for missing objects, imitate other people's facial expressions, and show visual interest in the results of cause and effect in the world around them (Barraga, 1982).

During infancy and early childhood, the availability of visual experiences has a critical impact on children's later use of vision. Because the cells of the brain become specialized in response to the type of stimulation that is provided during early childhood, it is important for children to have experiences that allow them to be actively involved with the visual environment. An absence of these early experiences may inhibit the ability to use vision effectively during later years.

Childhood

As children emerge from infancy and venture into a world that is rich with experiences, vision is the catalyst of accomplishment. Their increasing ability to think about and remember events influences the development of visual memory, as well as their ability to notice details of objects and people. During the second year of life, they are aware of similarities and differences among objects and can match like things. At about a year of age, they can recognize simple pictures, and over the next several years, they show increasing interest in detail and in relationships between elements. Between ages 3 and 5, they refine these skills to include assembling pictures from puzzle pieces, locating a single object in an entire picture, telling stories based on pictures, and categorizing pictures.

Gross motor activities in early childhood also require the use of vision to monitor distance and position in space. The coordination of eye and head movements is required for activities that reach further beyond the individual's immediate body space. Children can now move independently, and they need vision to help them chase friends, catch balls, search for favorite toys, and orient themselves as they somersault, do cartwheels, and wrestle.

Fine motor tasks occupy increasing amounts of time in early childhood. The refinement of the scribbling of a 1 year old into the imitation of specific strokes of an 18 month old and the drawing of rough forms and shapes by a 3 year old requires hand-eye coordination, including the ability to follow the path of a crayon on paper and to make spatial judgments about leaving room for the unwritten lines to follow.

By the time that children enter elementary school, their eyes have grown to full size, and their mature visual functions are intact, although some children experience minor changes in acuity throughout the school years. Many children who have refractive problems first demonstrate functional difficulties during the early elementary school years because of changes in their eyes or the visual demands of school.

After Grade 1, there is also a greater and greater demand on children to use their near vision in the highly detailed task of reading for prolonged periods. The eyes learn to identify a printed symbol instantly and to channel it to the brain, where it is associated with both sound and meaning; as reading ability develops, the eyes become increasingly efficient through small visual movements called saccades, which take place at the rate of four or five per second for efficient readers.

In early childhood, primary visual abilities are established, and experiences shape perceptual development. However, minor changes in visual ability or efficiency can occur throughout the school years because of refractive changes, additional growth or structural changes in the eye, or changes in a visual-perceptual response, based on experiences, such as playing baseball, which leads to the better eye movements when following objects.

To assist school-age children with low vision effectively, teachers of students with visual impairments must be aware of the developmental

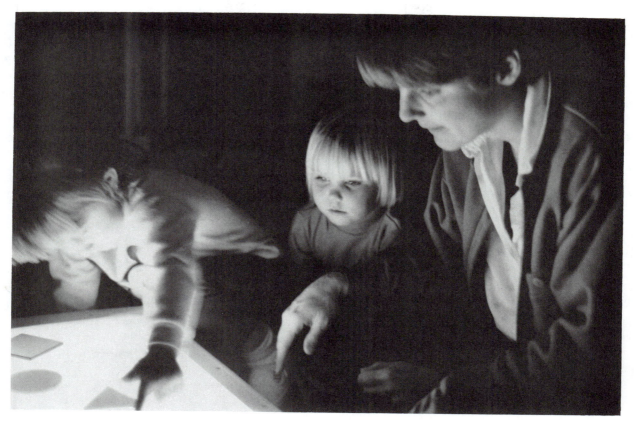

Providing preschool children with visual experiences early will have a critical impact on how they will use their vision when they are older.

visual characteristics demonstrated by children of various ages. The Program to Develop Efficiency in Visual Functioning (Barraga & Morris, 1980) is a detailed source for new professionals in this area. With a thorough grounding in the sequence of visual development, teachers will be better prepared to assess children's vision accurately and to plan an appropriate educational program.

APPROACHES TO THE ASSESSMENT OF FUNCTIONAL VISION

Many people assume that the amount of vision that an individual has can be accurately represented by a visual acuity figure, such as 20/20 or 20/400. They may not be aware that vision can vary in many dimensions and that the results of an evaluation of vision in an eye care specialist's office only partly describe how an individual sees. Experienced teachers of students with visual impairments can often describe two people whose visual acuities are the same, but whose use of vision varies. For example, Pamela, a 6 year old with 20/200 visual acuity, explores visually, runs fearlessly in unfamiliar settings, and learns readily from pictures and observation, whereas her classmate Henry, who has the same visual acuity, moves cautiously and uses his hands to explore before looking. Since each person's use of vision is unique, an assessment of vision as a child uses it in his or her daily routines is essential for gaining a complete picture of the child's educational needs.

Role of the Functional Vision Assessment

Previous chapters have emphasized the importance of a thorough evaluation by a clinical low vision specialist. Although such an assessment provides details that cannot be obtained outside the clinical setting, it is limited because it is generally done in one setting during just a few visits. To develop a complete picture of a student's visual functioning, the teacher of students with visual impairments must also assess the student's functional vision. The assessment should reflect the student's typical use of vision during a series of ordinary activities, as well as the student's potential for developing new visual functions. Ideally, it should be conducted before the clinical low vision evaluation, and the report should be forwarded to the clinical low vision specialist.

In many cases, the clinical evaluation represents a conservative estimate of a child's visual capabilities. Children may feel apprehensive in a clinical or medical setting and hence may not respond as they might otherwise if an unfamiliar procedure is presented. Even the most skilled ophthalmologist may not elicit a child's best response because of time limitations and differences in children's behaviors in an office. When a clinical evaluation indicates that a child has limited vision, it is still important to observe the child functioning in familiar settings, under various lighting conditions, and in situations that involve moving objects.

A professional should not assume that the visual responses reported in the clinical evaluation are representative of a child's typical use of vision. Some parents have been told since their children's birth that their children could see nothing, but evidence of vision has been noticed later; therefore, it is important to approach an assessment open to the possibility that a child has some vision. However, it is also possible that a clinical low vision specialist may report that a child's visual function is better than what is apparent during observations. For example, a child may see a certain size print during the clinical evaluation, but may not be able to read textbooks in that size of print for a long period.

The teacher of students with visual impairment must not communicate the philosophy that it is better to have vision than to be totally blind or that the visual function of all students with some vision can improve significantly. Thus the evaluation should include activities that can be performed by students with and without vision, and students should be praised for their cooperation and involvement, not for their successful use of vision. The investigation of vision does not exclude observations of the use of the other senses, which can provide further information about the usefulness of vision in the accomplishment of tasks.

The purpose of a functional vision assessment is to indicate instructional goals for visual habilitation, including these:

◆ to identify a student's visual competencies and capabilities with and without optical devices
◆ to identify visual skills that need to be learned
◆ to convey information to the student and to other members of the educational team about how the student uses vision
◆ to identify the student's preferred environmental cues
◆ to help the student become familiar with ways of alleviating visual fatigue or discomfort.

Functional vision assessments should be conducted when a new student becomes part of the teacher's caseload, at regular intervals throughout the year, and any time the environment changes. In many states, a functional vision assessment is required at specified intervals to determine a student's eligibility for special education services and equipment. Regardless of whether there is such a requirement, the best practice is to conduct functional vision assessments on an ongoing basis for all students with low vision.

The professional who conducts the functional vision assessment should review the background information on the student's eye condition and medical treatment. Following the clinical low vision evaluation, additional functional assessments may be done to ascertain the benefits of prescribed optical devices, determine if instruction is needed for devices, and view changes in visual function that are the result of the clinical evaluation.

The functional vision assessment should include observations of the student in several environments, including the classroom, gymnasium, hallways, nonacademic classes, extracurricular activities, and social or leisure-time settings. During the assessment, the teacher asks a variety of questions, including these: When lighting, familiarity, contrast, time constraints, and other factors vary, how does the student's visual function change? What tasks present difficulties in the use of vision, and which tasks are easily accomplished?

Some teachers find it useful to videotape or audiotape their functional vision assessments, especially with young children or those who cannot respond to formal assessment procedures. However, it should be noted that taping may increase the time needed to develop the final report because entire sections of the assessment have to be reviewed.

Some professionals conduct standardized developmental assessments as an additional means of gathering information about a student's use of vision. The Diagnostic Assessment Procedure (DAP) (Barraga, 1980), for example, provides a profile of a student's visual responses to a series of developmentally sequenced tasks that tap a variety of visual responses. The DAP is appropriate for children who are developmentally above age 3, and its results can be used to plan a teaching program using the extensive activities described in its companion project, the Design for Instruction. These assessment and instructional programs are also part of the Program to Develop Efficiency in Visual Functioning (Barraga & Morris, 1980), mentioned earlier. Although it can provide a basis for investigating a student's use of vision through successively more complex tasks, it cannot take the place of a complete functional vision assessment, which must reflect a student's typical activities and visual efficiency.

The section that follows describes the information that can be included in the functional vision assessment, which consists of the following elements:

- background information: visual history, medical history, educational history
- observation of the environment
- visual responses and activities: structure of the eyes and reflexes, near vision, distance vision, fields of vision, color vision, motility, other visual responses (such as to lighting and contrast)
- summary
- recommendations.

Although certain visual behaviors, such as ocular motility, may be observed, the functional vision assessment emphasizes how these visual abilities affect a student's visual functioning.

Components of the Functional Vision Assessment

The evaluation should take place over a number of sessions with a student and should involve a representative cross section of the student's typical activities. Initially, the teacher of students with visual impairments (the evaluator) should arrange to observe the student in the classroom and in other settings. Later, he or she can plan activities and conduct formal and informal measurements of acuity.

If the student routinely uses optical devices, prescription eyeglasses, contact lenses, or light absorptive lenses, these should be used as appropriate during activities for the functional vision assessment. If the student does not routinely use an optical device and the evaluator believes that the student may be able to use one in the future, the evaluator may introduce a magnifier or monocular for brief functional activities, such as looking at a insect or spotting a car at a distance. However, the goal should be to observe the student's motivation and functional application, and the report should include a recommendation for a full clinical low vision evaluation for the prescription of appropriate devices.

Gathering Background Information

Before the functional vision assessment, the evaluator should review the results of earlier clinical low vision evaluations and general information about the student's development and other impairments, including etiology and age of onset of the visual impairment and previous eye reports, especially the measured visual acuity from the most recent evaluation and descriptions of devices or eyeglasses currently being used. General information related to the student's developmental and educational history should also be reviewed to identify any additional impairments and current functional levels.

This background information is crucial for planning the directed visual tasks and observations that will take place during the functional vision assessment. For example, if a student has a restricted visual field, the evaluator will plan to observe activities that involve eye scanning in the classroom and playground. If a student has a progressive eye condition, the evaluator will plan to observe situations in which functioning may have changed since the previous assessment.

Observing in Natural Environments

The functional vision assessment should begin with an evaluation of the physical attributes of the classroom, as well as all the other areas in which the student will be observed, including the gymnasium, cafeteria, library, and playground, to understand the conditions under which the assessment will be conducted. Figure 9.1 presents a form on which the environmental features to be considered can be recorded.

The location of the room, time of day, and general weather conditions (such as sunny, overcast, raining, or snowing) should be recorded. A sketch of the classroom space or primary observation site that indicates the location of doors, windows, chalkboards, the student's desk, and other pertinent features, as well as the compass directions of the room, may be helpful. The color and pattern of the floor, as well as the amount of visual clutter, distraction, and reflective glare in the room, should be noted. In addition, furniture and equipment, such as the type of desks (whether top or side opening); the presence of storage places for nonoptical, optical, and electronic devices; access to electric outlets for additional illumination; and the color and condition of the chalkboard, should be described.

The classroom teacher's routines and patterns should also be noted. Does the teacher stay primarily in one place for instruction or circulate throughout the room? Does the teacher use gestures and facial expressions to convey information? Does the teacher tend to move close to students? Does the teacher tend to stand in areas that have high- or low-contrast background or in front of a window?

Before the actual observation, it is helpful to measure approximate distances in the observation area. Small pieces of tape or colored stickers can be placed at specific distances from the student's desk to estimate distances accurately. How far is the classroom teacher from the student? How far is the chalkboard from the student? How far is the window lighting from the student's desk?

Before the observation, it is also helpful to note the daily schedule of activities in the classroom, which provides a framework of the visual requirements during the student's day and can be helpful in identifying priorities for instruction. Figure 9.2, the Low Vision Classroom Observation Form, can be used to note the activities, as well as the degree of independence and consistency, that a student demonstrates throughout his or her daily routines.

Carrying Out Activities

Most activities that are observed during the assessment are chosen because they are typical daily activities that demonstrate the student's use of vision, and most include different aspects of visual function. However, it is important to select

Physical Environment Observation Form

Student _____ Compass Direction _____, _____ feet

Class _____

Date and time _____

Recorder _____

Sketch in ink:
   Windows
   Door or doors
   Chalkboards
   Pertinent desks and tables
   Other critical information
Pencil in the location of
   Lights
   Outlets

_____ feet

Floor covering
Color _____
   _____ Tile
   _____ Carpet
   _____ Other _____

Walls
Color _____
   Visual clutter _____ Yes   _____ No

Ceiling
Color _____
   Visual clutter _____ Yes   _____ No
   Type of lighting _____

Chalkboard
   Color
   _____ Black
   _____ Green
   _____ White
   _____ Other _____
   Condition of board—Contrast:
   _____ Good   _____ Fair   _____ Poor

Copy Machine
   _____ Teacher can use
   _____ Teacher of students with visual impairments
       can use
   Enlarges?   _____ Yes   _____ No
   Enhances contrast? _____ Yes   _____ No

Ecological Suggestions
   Seating from the chalkboard
      Location: _____
   Seating from the videotape machine
   Seating from a demonstration
   Writing for group:
   _____ Thin chalk
   _____ Thin marker
   _____ Standard pen or pencil

Type of Desk
   _____ Open back
   _____ Top open
   _____ No storage
   _____ Chair attached

Videotape Machine
   Frequency of use
   _____ Daily
   _____ 1–2 times a week
   Size of screen _____ inches

Organizational Potential
   _____ Shelves (space available)
   _____ Shelves (no space available)
   _____ Closet
   _____ Location for the safe storage of the device
   _____ Coat storage

Window Covering
   _____ None
   _____ Shades
   _____ Blinds
   _____ Curtains

_____ Feet (with the device)   _____ Feet (without the device)
_____ Feet (with the device)   _____ Feet (without the device)
_____ Feet (with the device)   _____ Feet (without the device)

_____ Thick chalk (railroad)
_____ Bold marker—color _____

Figure 9.1. Features of the Physical Environment: A Checklist

Classroom Observation Form

Student ______________________ Date ______________________

Class ______________________ Recorder ______________________

Time	Subject or Activity	Objective of the Task	Specifics	Yes Unaided	Yes Aided	Identified Needs Inconsistent Unaided	Inconsistent Aided	No Unaided	No Aided
				☐	☐	☐	☐	☐	☐
				☐	☐	☐	☐	☐	☐
				☐	☐	☐	☐	☐	☐
				☐	☐	☐	☐	☐	☐
				☐	☐	☐	☐	☐	☐

Figure 9.2. Low Vision Classroom Observation Form

enough activities to demonstrate a variety of skills. The functional vision assessment should include items that reflect abilities in the following areas: structure of the eyes and reflexes, near vision, distance vision, fields of vision, color vision, motility, and other visual responses (such as to lighting and contrast).

Structure of the Eyes and Reflexes. The functional vision assessment should include some description of the appearance of the eyes and related structures. The evaluator should take care not to use diagnostic terms, unless they have been included in medical reports, because it is not the evaluator's role to make a medical diagnosis. For example, the evaluator may note, "Frank's right eye consistently turns outward when he is reading," but should not say, "Frank has a right exotropia." Other observations may relate to cloudiness of the eye; irregularities in the pupil and iris; deviations in either eye; irregularities of eye color; and any abnormalities of the lid or redness in or discharges from the eyes. If any unexpected characteristics are observed, the student should be referred to his or her primary eye care provider.

The evaluator should also check for a blink reflex and a pupillary response (see Chapter 10). Although these responses are not a clear indicator of the presence or absence of vision, they can provide information about whether both eyes respond similarly to moving stimuli and whether the student may have unusual reactions to light. Because both procedures can be uncomfortable or intrusive, the evaluator should take the time to explain them to the student and may allow the student to try them on him or her, so the student can understand the process and its purpose. The evaluator can use the information obtained as a basis for observing more functional activities. For example, if the student has difficulty with pupillary reflexes, the evaluator will want to observe the student when changing environments, such as when walking from a well-lit hallway to a darkened auditorium.

Near Vision.   Although near vision activities are usually thought of as related to reading, it is important to include those that involve the performance of other tasks, including sewing, stamp collecting, artwork, and electronics. One way of discovering a student's visual requirements in daily tasks is to ask the student to list the ways in which he or she spends leisure time. Observing a student doing an activity like assembling a model car, threading a needle, or chopping vegetables for a salad provides an opportunity to note how far away the student places materials, how he or she angles them, and what types of background and lighting are chosen. For an evaluator who is new to assessment, it may be easiest to take anecdotal notes describing the student's behaviors during the activity, after explaining the purpose of the notes to the student.

The evaluator should also plan to use a variety of materials. Thus, the student should be observed reading not only typical school materials, both silently and aloud, but materials that vary in contrast and format, including magazines, comic books, newspaper display advertisements and classified advertisements, food and clothing labels, and telephone books. A notebook can be assembled that includes samples of these items; in addition, the evaluator can use a selection of age-appropriate books that include various typographic and picture formats.

For example, a classic book for young children, *Goodnight, Moon* (Brown, 1947), includes pictures of a child's bedroom as the light is dimming during the evening. An interesting game associated with this book can be to find various objects in the room as it becomes darker, and this activity provides an opportunity to observe the child's response to decreasing contrast. Printed materials that vary in boldness, density, contrast, and style should be used because the student's preferences among these materials may indicate his or her visual comfort and interests.

The evaluator should measure the student's reading speed under various conditions because many students with low vision use large or standard print for years without any comparison being made of their efficiency in various print styles. Although standard print is more efficient for many students with low vision, as a study by Koenig and Ross (1991) indicated, it is often assumed that because a child has low vision, he or she will benefit from enlarged print. As other chapters have discussed, enlarged print is a less desirable option than standard print or the use of a low vision device. This is because it is more expensive, requires enlargement of each book or material, and is often more cumbersome to transport. If a state does not require an assessment of learning media to be conducted separately from the functional vision assessment, a thorough assessment of the efficiency of reading media should be conducted and reported in the functional vision assessment (for additional information on the learning media assessment, see Chapter 11).

In evaluating near vision, it is also important to observe the student after sustained silent reading. Some students can read efficiently for short periods, but their speed and efficiency decrease after five or ten minutes. The student who fatigues easily when reading silently will need alternative approaches for longer tasks: audiotaped materials, readers, and braille in combination with print. Such alternative approaches will allow the student to manage increasing quantities of materials as he or she advances in school.

A student's handwriting abilities should also be evaluated in the functional vision assessment. Handwriting can be particularly difficult for students with low vision because it requires hand-eye coordination in a sometimes uncomfortable working posture. Some students can write legibly but have difficulty reading their own handwriting; therefore, students should be asked to read material that they have written, especially material that has been written several days before and is no longer familiar. The students' writing speed may be slower than that of their fully sighted peers, and this fact should be noted so that alternatives for note taking can be considered. Tasks

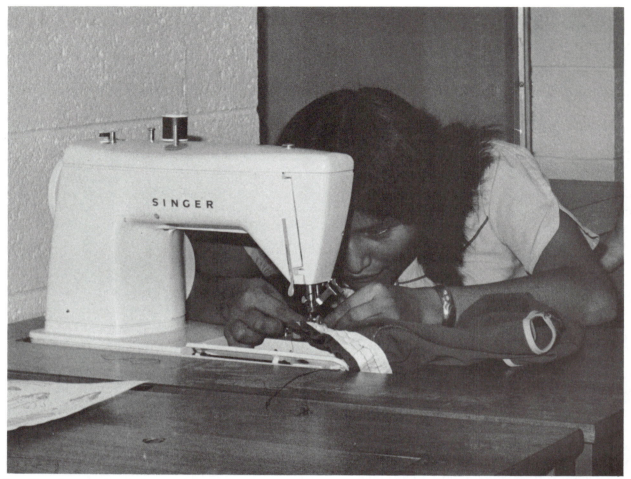

Reading is not the only way to evaluate near visual acuity. Observing a student performing other activities that require near vision will help a teacher evaluate a student's functional vision.

such as writing a letter to a friend, making a grocery list, or entering homework assignments on a daily schedule will reflect a student's handwriting skills. Students should be encouraged to select their own handwriting tools and paper, and the teacher should explore the efficiency of these and other options. Although many students prefer a felt-tipped pen because of its bold line, individual preferences and efficiency vary greatly. Typical near vision activities include the following:

search-and-find puzzles	reading a map
cutting out pictures	putting together puzzles

writing a letter	making a shopping list
looking up a library reference	looking up telephone numbers
completing a job application	reading magazines
labeling tapes	reading a recipe.

The formal assessment of near vision can be made using a standard near point card that includes a variety of sizes of print. These are presented at specific distances or "points" from the eye. This assessment is typically administered at 14 or 16 inches, and the evaluator records the smallest line of print that can be read at that distance. When the student is unable to read a line of print, the evaluator can ask the student to move the card closer until the line becomes visible. Near point cards may use a variety of measurement systems, including points or the American Medical Association system. Although the formal testing of near point visual acuity can provide information about the smallest-size letter a student can see, measured visual acuity should be considered in conjunction with informal methods, since eye charts consist of individual, separate letters that are easier to distinguish than are words or various print styles.

Distance Vision.   As with near vision, activities used to assess distance vision should be varied and should reflect the student's interest and capabilities. Thus, the assessment should include classroom activities, such as reading the chalkboard, as well as activities that take place outside the classroom, such as reading a banner in a hallway, catching a ball in a physical education class, or identifying the bus after school.

A formal distance-screening procedure should be included in the functional vision assessment to act as a comparison with clinical measures provided in the report of the clinical low vision specialist. Many evaluators use Lighthouse Flash Cards or use LEA Symbols, developed by Hyvärinen, because the symbols (apple, house, circle, square) are easy to identify, and the test is portable and easy to administer. In response to the need for assessment materials for children with low vision, Hyvärinen has developed a variety of charts, games, and toys. These "user friendly" materials, when used in a clinical setting, can provide information about an individual's visual acuity, contrast sensitivity, color vision, and visual fields. In regard to formal distance screening, however, any of the formal screening charts described in Chapter 8 are appropriate: the Snellen wall charts, the HOTV, or the Feinbloom charts. The formal vision acuity screening represents only the beginning of the evaluation of a student's use of distance vision.

Functional tasks using distance vision should include familiar and unfamiliar ones under different lighting conditions. In the classroom, the most common activities for the use of distance vision are reading the chalkboard and overhead transparencies. The evaluator's observation should include an assessment of the student's ability to read brief phrases, such as the next day's homework assignment, as well as longer passages, such as classroom notes, located on different parts of the chalkboard, and to copy written material from the chalkboard or overheads. The teacher should also note the student's preferred seating arrangement for these activities, including the approximate viewing distance from the material and lighting. Other typical distance activities in the classroom are reading bulletin boards, recognizing pictures and posters, viewing slides and videotapes, locating classmates and one's desk, seeing the teacher's facial expressions, and retrieving dropped objects from the floor.

Outside the classroom, there are several areas of the school and its grounds in which students commonly use distance vision, and students should be observed in these areas as well. First, outdoor playing fields and indoor gymnasiums are difficult environments for some students with low vision because of variations in lighting and the need to respond to moving objects and people at different distances, such as when playing ball. Second, the cafeteria requires the use of distance vision for proceeding through the line, identifying foods, and recognizing the faces of classmates against a busy and colorful background. Third, hallways necessitate the use of distance vision for recognizing friends, since the inability to recognize others can be misinterpreted as unfriendliness; otherwise, students with low vision may need to greet an approaching student aloud to receive a response and identify the speaker's voice. Fourth, the auditorium requires the use of distance vision for viewing a performance or a speaker during assembly. In this setting, it is important to note how the student responds if he or she cannot see enough detail to enjoy a performance: Does the student ask a classmate to provide essential information,

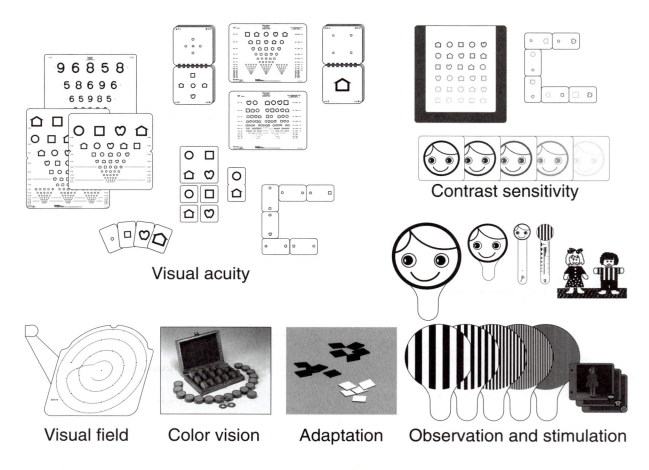

Visual acuity

Contrast sensitivity

Visual field   Color vision   Adaptation   Observation and stimulation

Materials such as these developed by Hyvärinen are used to gather a variety of information during clinical assessments and may be encountered by professionals who are formulating a comprehensive picture of a child's visual abilities.

use a monocular, or select a seat close to the front but away from friends and classmates?

In the community, there are numerous occasions for using distance vision. Some common activities are finding hidden objects, spotting airplanes and oncoming traffic, blowing bubbles, reading street numbers and signs, reading signs in stores, and watching birds.

It should be noted that the assessment of and instruction related to distance vision are not the sole responsibility of the orientation and mobility (O&M) instructor. Rather, the teacher of students with visual impairments also assumes this responsibility, both inside and outside the class-

room, depending on the student's needs and the composition of the educational team.

Fields of Vision. Although an informal assessment of visual fields cannot yield an exact measurement, it can yield a gross estimate, as well as information about how a student compensates for differences in his or her visual fields. Older students can respond to clinical evaluations, such as the tangent screen and the Amsler grid tests, described in Chapter 8. A confrontation test, also described in Chapter 8, can be used to identify areas of the visual field to which the student does not respond as readily. There are a variety of functional activities, however, that can also provide information about a student's visual fields.

A student's scanning of an array of objects or looking for a missing object can demonstrate his or her functional visual field at near point. For example, a compensatory head turn suggests a peripheral field loss to the side of the head turn, since the student has learned to compensate by moving the usable visual field toward the side where information is missing. The performance of activities, such as scanning a map or doing a word-search puzzle, can also suggest where scotomas (areas of absent vision) may be located, because if students are asked to keep their heads perfectly still while doing them, they may miss information in some areas of the tasks.

Students who walk with their heads turned slightly to one side may be compensating for a difference in visual fields. It is particularly revealing to watch students with low vision traveling in crowded hallways at a school where other students are moving past or overtaking them; by asking them to say when they can see another student approaching them from the side, the evaluator can compare that point on either side to determine whether there are differences in the visual fields.

Eye preference, evidenced in typical tasks, can also be evaluated. One quick way of determining eye preference is to ask a student to look through a cardboard tube or monocular; the eye to which the student brings the device is usually the preferred eye. Another way is to observe the student's head tilt and orientation of materials during a task. Some students with low vision use one eye for distance tasks and the other for near-point tasks, so it is important to evaluate their eye preferences in both situations.

Students who use only one eye experience a moderate field loss (about 20 degrees) on the side where vision is not present. This field loss may be most noticeable if they drive a car, during which they will need to check and look carefully when traffic is merging, or when they play fast-moving games that use balls or projectiles. The role of the evaluator with respect to field loss is to help the student define the parameters of the loss and find ways of compensating for it in specific tasks, such as scanning from side to side while walking down a crowded hallway and switching to tactile means when applying makeup to the usable eye.

Color Vision. Because difficulty seeing colors is common among students with low vision (Knowlton, 1989), it is important to assess color vision as part of the functional vision assessment. A variety of activities can be used to supplement clinical evaluations in this area.

Simply asking a student to identify colors by name is not sufficient to determine his or her ability to distinguish among colors and shades. Therefore, some evaluators organize a set of cards that include lighter and darker shades of the same hue and ask the student to arrange them from lighter to darker shades or in families of related hues. They also evaluate a student's ability to identify colors in real situations. In this regard, they observe whether a student can select an item by color or distinguish between associated colors in following directions in a primary workbook or reading graphs and pie charts in a textbook. For older students, visiting a store to match items of clothing may provide an opportunity to note how they perceive and describe colors. For younger students, since many classroom activities depend on the ability to identify color, it is important to notify the classroom teacher, as well as the students, of any differences in color recognition, so tasks that are color dependent can be modified, such as working with a lab partner with normal color vision in chemistry experiments.

Motility. Eye movement, which allows a student to scan a broad array or follow a moving object, can be observed in activities that require horizontal tracking, such as watching a passing car, fish swimming in a tank, a football soaring through the air, or a moving character in a video game. The smoothness of the tracking movement should be noted; some students have a jerky tracking movement, while others track irregularly across their midline. Vertical eye movements can be observed as a student follows a bouncing basketball or the direction of a dropped object. The performance of many tasks that involve combinations of eye movements, such as scanning a bookshelf for a particular book or examining a painting in an art gallery, can demonstrate diagonal and circular patterns, as well as horizontal and vertical movements. The functional vision assessment should evaluate whether both eyes move together during tracking activities and whether the student typically moves both his or her head and eyes while tracking and scanning. Generally, the lower the student's visual acuity, the more the student will move his or her head when visually searching (Jan, 1986).

Other Visual Responses.   Students with low vision may demonstrate variations in other responses to their environment. Lighting is one area in which comfort levels may vary. Some students, particularly those with retinal conditions, prefer brighter lighting, whereas others, particularly those with ocular media opacities, such as cataracts that refract and intensify light, may be more comfortable with moderate lighting. The evaluator should include both indoor and outdoor activities in the evaluation and, if possible, observe the student when he or she is moving into and out of brighter lighting.

Some students, including many who have albinism, experience photophobia and find bright light unpleasant; they prefer light-absorptive lenses or visors when outdoors. Others find flickering or flashing lights unpleasant and thus have difficulty adjusting to lighting conditions when fluorescent lights flicker in classrooms or strobe lights flash during rock concerts.

For students who use computers, the evaluator should observe their preferred lighting effects and color combinations while viewing a computer screen. Some students with low vision prefer screens with colors other than the standard ones, and some use theater gels to adapt the screen material to their preferred color (Allan & Erin, 1993). Although it has not been determined whether these strong preferences are based on actual color or simply differences in contrast produced by color variations, if the student believes

that it improves his or her performance then varying colors may increase motivation.

Some evaluators also observe students' perceptual differences, such as difficulties perceiving figures and forms, identifying visual directionality, discriminating figure-ground, and perceiving depth. Even though it may not be possible to determine whether perceptual differences result from a student's low vision or whether they result from other physical or neurological factors, they should be reported because they are closely associated with visual skills and adaptations.

Developing Recommendations

The functional vision assessment is most effective when it yields clear recommendations for practice. Since effects of instruction in the use of functional vision are more fully realized in activities of the student, family, and other members of the educational team, the recommendations must be specific, easy to understand, and practical. Several types of recommendations can be included in the report: referrals, adaptations, instructional strategies, and service delivery.

Referrals.   The evaluator may note areas of function for which additional information is needed from other specialists. In these cases, he or she may include recommendations for an assessment by a clinical low vision specialist, an occupational or physical therapist, a speech-language therapist, or an O&M instructor. The evaluator should also note the reason for the specific recommendation in the report, for example, "Maria should be evaluated by a clinical low vision specialist to consider her use of optical devices for distance tasks."

Adaptations.   The evaluator may also recommend modifications of environmental characteristics to facilitate the use of vision. These modifications can include variations in lighting, color, contrast, distance, and other characteristics that enhance a student's visual efficiency. When possible, they should be described with respect to the student's responsibility for making the adaptations, for instance, "Steve may be provided with a choice of papers for writing, but he should also have the opportunity to compare his performance using several types of paper so that he can make an informed choice."

Instructional and Compensatory Strategies. Recommendations for instructional and compensatory strategies should include the actual areas that will require intervention. They may include instruction or guidance in the development of specific visual skills, the use of equipment or optical devices, or the practice of compensatory skills. For example, a recommendation may state, "Pedro will locate and identify specific items on maps in his social studies texts by using systematic scanning techniques."

Recommended Services. The report may also include recommendations for the amount and type of services that should be provided by the teacher of students with visual impairments or the O&M instructor (or both). Although decisions about services are ultimately made by the educational team, the evaluator's recommendation is important because it is from the perspective of an experienced professional with regard to how much time will be required to meet a student's specific needs in regard to visual functioning. The teacher may recommend regular consultative visits, so he or she can provide feedback to the student's teachers, or regularly scheduled direct instruction in disability-specific skills, as in the following example: "Lee should receive direct service from a teacher of students with visual impairments for 30 minutes per week for 3 months to teach the use of a prescribed telescope in a variety of applications."

Writing the Report

After the evaluator completes the observations and assessment, he or she presents the results in a report, which is the primary written source of information on the student's vision. The report of the functional vision assessment should be:

- *Specific*—with details about the student's performance on individual tasks in clearly described situations
- *Factual*—with conclusions based on clear, objective observations, rather than opinions or broad generalizations
- *Applicable*—with direct links made to the tasks and activities normally performed by the student.

The report should be detailed but clearly understandable to the student's family and other members of the educational team who may not be knowledgeable about visual impairments or familiar with the terminology used to describe them. Typically, the report is in narrative form, although checklists can be included or attached. A sample functional vision assessment report is included at the end of this chapter (for other suggestions about the format and organization of the report, see Bishop, 1988).

The section of the report that describes the student's vision is usually divided into several subsections for ease of reference. It should be noted here that even though an evaluator may have a preferred format for organizing the report, the sequence of the activities may not necessarily follow that format. In other words, a single activity, such as reading a bulletin board, includes opportunities for observing several aspects of vision, such as near vision, visual field, and scanning. Similarly, while opening a can of soup, a student demonstrates the use of near vision (reading the label), depth perception (inserting the wheel of the opener under the rim of the can), and field preferences (arranging the materials). A student's visual behaviors in each area may be described in different sections of the report even though they have been observed during a single activity.

The report often includes a statement for the educational team indicating, from the evaluator's perspective, based on the functional vision assessment, whether the student is eligible to receive services as a student with a visual impairment. However, the final decision about the student's eligibility is made by the entire educational team.

The report should also include a summary for use as a quick reference by members of the educational team. Although it does not contain program information, the summary supports the student's needs for specialized services and can be included in general educational reports. Finally, the report should include practical and specific recommendations that will assist the team members in providing for the student's educational needs related to the visual impairment.

INSTRUCTIONAL GOALS AND PROCEDURES

The report of the functional vision assessment is the blueprint for instruction of a student with visual impairments. On the basis of this report, instructional goals and procedures must be carefully planned to foster a student's progress. Selecting appropriate materials, sequencing the learning process, and creating a motivating learning environment will ensure that the student uses his or her vision efficiently. The teacher of students with visual impairments acts as a facilitator in this regard, encouraging the student to assume more and more responsibility and thereby to gain more independent control over the visual environment. This section describes the planning and implementation of instruction for students with low vision and presents strategies for instruction in the use of optical devices, as well as describes instructional resources and explores the teacher's role.

Planning and Implementing Instruction

The functional vision assessment is the basis for identifying the goals of a student's instructional program that are related to vision. However, students can have similar goals, yet learn in different ways, so their programs must be individualized. For example, whereas Beth may be highly motivated to use her monocular and may want to become proficient as quickly as possible to copy

notes from the chalkboard during an algebra class, Tyrone may be self-conscious about his monocular and may want to use it only to spot signs when traveling away from the school grounds. Thus, in planning these students' programs, the teacher of students with visual impairments will emphasize one-handed focusing and manipulation of the telescope with notetaking for Beth, but will explore and implement options for Tyrone to gather information from the chalkboard independently, without using a telescope. Hence, the implementation of an instructional program requires consideration of the student's needs, the identification of instructional areas, and the development of a teaching sequence.

Student's Needs

The educational team must approach instruction in the use of vision as a holistic endeavor in which visual skills are taught within real applications. Thus, an instructional program that does not incorporate the recommendations of the report of the functional vision assessment may place the student at risk of developing fragmented or unnecessary skills. For example, if Juan, a fourth-grade student, is taking twice the amount of time as other students to copy and complete long division problems, further instruction in long division may seem to be needed. However, a review of the report may show that Juan needs instruction in scanning pages to help him copy the problems faster, rather than instruction in computation.

Instructional Areas

According to Bailey and Hall (1989), instruction in the use of low vision involves three primary areas: making environmental adaptations, enhancing visual skills, and integrating vision into activities. The educational programs of many students will include goals in all three areas.

Environmental Adaptations. The need for changes in the learning environment to maximize the use of vision should be included in the

Individualized Education Programs (IEPs) for all students. Although the teacher of students with visual impairments can guide progress in these areas, ultimately the goal is for the students themselves to make the necessary adaptations. This goal may require students to learn to recognize environmental difficulties and, in some cases, to learn appropriate skills for being assertive or for requesting assistance from others. The adaptations themselves are identified during the functional vision assessment and include factors related to color, contrast, time, space, and lighting, as identified by Corn (1983) and described in Chapter 1. Students' activities in this area may involve adjusting seating, lighting, and distance, as well as positioning, to use vision efficiently.

For the student who is beginning to respond to visual stimuli and attach meaning to the environment, the teacher controls environmental factors to increase the student's visual attention. For example, Tasha's instruction might begin in a dark room with the presentation of the lit face of a toy clown that is held within 6 inches. The initial object (the clown's face) is large, the distance is very close, and the dark room provides maximum contrast with the highly visible light source—the clown's face. Future instruction would then expand Tasha's visual horizons from the ideal to the real, to the extent that she is capable, in the following areas:

◆ *Distance:* Objects are initially presented at near point and then are moved farther away, to the most natural viewing distance.

◆ *Size:* At first, large objects are presented. In later instructional sessions, the size of the objects is consistently decreased.

◆ *Contrast:* Initially, objects are presented against an uncluttered background and, subsequently, the contrast between the background and the object of regard is slowly normalized. Black-and-white patterns and contrasting primary colors are presented first, and then patterns are reduced to colors with less contrast, pastels, and, finally, shades of the same color.

◆ *Illumination:* In the beginning, a dark room provides maximum contrast with the lighted object or light source, but subsequent attempts allow more and more light into the room. At first, a light source, a reflective object, or ultraviolet light is used; later, these features are eliminated, and natural lighting and the features of an object are substituted.

◆ *Time:* Initially, the student may need more time than would someone with normal vision to interpret what he or she is seeing. In subsequent steps, the duration of the presentation of objects or the speed of movement of objects can be altered, so the student makes more time-efficient visual interpretations and decisions.

In this process of gradual naturalization, the student moves from activities in an artificial, highly controlled environment to those in a natural environment in which he or she can tolerate distraction and multiple features. Such may be the case of a student who increases his or her reading speed for longer and longer periods.

On the one hand, students with few visual skills may be visually efficient if their visual function is considered in relation to their visual capacity. On the other hand, students with many visual skills and better visual acuity may be visually inefficient with regard to their visual capacity. Therefore, the extent of the increase in visual efficiency should not be related to the number or type of visual skills, but to the expansion of the individual's visual capacity and potential. As was discussed earlier, children should receive reinforcement for their efforts, not for their ability to function more closely to the way that children with normal vision function.

Older and more capable students can learn to adapt their own visual environment, but they must first recognize the advantages of the adaptations. To help a student understand the benefits, an adult may have to prepare the environment and allow the student to experience the difference, by saying, for example, "See whether you can find the pen better when I put it on the

Basic Visual Skills

Skill	Definition
Attention (attends to . . .)	General visual orientation to an object of regard
Fixation (fixates on . . .) or localization (localizes . . .)	Sustained visual attention to an object of regard
Tracking (tracks . . .)	Ability to fixate on and follow a moving object, using eye and/or head movements
Shifting of attention (shifts attention between . . .)	Changes in fixation from one object to another
Scanning (scans . . .)	Ability to shift fixation among three or more objects along one line of direction before shifting direction
Reaching for objects (reaches for . . .)	Ability to attend to and extend a body part toward an object of regard

table surface instead of on the printed placemat." Later, however, the student may need only a reminder to make the adaptation himself or herself: "Before you start reading, think about what you can do to make reading comfortable." When a student routinely makes these adaptations after being prompted, the teacher of students with visual impairments should develop a plan to generalize them to the home and classroom. Encouraging students to adapt their environments reinforces their sense of control over factors related to vision.

Visual Skills.   Visual skills instruction includes learning to use visual skills, such as tracking, scanning, and attending to visual stimuli (see Sidebar 9.2 for definitions of the basic visual skills). Although these skills may be taught through highly controlled activities whose main purpose is to stimulate and encourage the use of vision, this type of instructional activity is of limited effectiveness for most students with visual impairments. Very young children, students who are recovering from neurological insult, and stu-

dents who have experienced sensory deprivation (such as after the removal of long-term cataracts) may be candidates for the development of specific visual skills because of the need to activate organic brain function. In most cases, however, responses that are encouraged through visually stimulating activities should be reinforced and integrated into functional activities, as in the following example:

Three-year-old Wendy, who has a visual impairment, had meningitis at age 2. Although she is able to perform cognitively at a 3-year-old level, her visual skills need to be further developed. In addition to encouraging Wendy's use of vision during functional activities, such as at mealtime and while dressing, the teacher of students with visual impairments spends 10 minutes twice a day doing play activities with Wendy under special lighting conditions. The teacher has developed a play routine in which she shakes a fluorescent toy under the light, encourages Wendy to reach for it, and provides reinforcement to Wendy when she grasps the toy. Since

Wendy enjoys this attention, she is using her vision more frequently to search for the toy. The teacher chooses smaller and smaller toys and dims the light to more normal levels so that soon Wendy will be able to perform the activity without the environmental adaptations.

Integration of Vision into Tasks. Most students with low vision have educational goals that focus on the efficient accomplishment of classroom tasks and life skills. Skills are taught within the actual activities in which they are needed, and students learn to become more efficient in performing those tasks. For example, Ray may work on scanning by searching his social studies text for vocabulary words that he is required to define and by scanning the school menu for that day's meal. Initially, his teacher of students with visual impairments highlighted the important words or sections with a yellow marking pen, but as Ray becomes more efficient, this adaptation may be reduced or eliminated.

Instruction in this area emphasizes an ecological approach, first identifying the tasks and activities that a student must accomplish to be successful in a particular current classroom, as well as in other environments. The teacher will then determine whether the student will learn the task using vision, the other senses, or all the senses. For example, if the 10th-grade home economics class is using recipes from a variety of cookbooks, Maria can practice scanning the indexes of the cookbooks for a particular recipe and locating the titles of recipes. The opportunity to practice using vision to locate the information she needs will enable her to participate in the activity. Building speed in accomplishing a task may be the result of practicing a particular visual skill, but the ultimate goal is the efficient performance of the task.

Skills Instruction Sequencing

In all three areas just described, the process involved in teaching the targeted skill should be specifically planned to ensure that the student acquires the skill and becomes more independent. The teaching plan should be geared to mov-ing the student from structured practice to independent, self-initiated action. The following steps should be included in the instructional process: setting goals, modeling, guided practice, and independent practice.

Setting Goals. Goals that relate to a student's use of vision are the basis for the development of the instruction plan. These goals should be developed from the recommendations of the report of the functional vision assessment and, like any others' goals, should be specific and measurable. Ideally, they should provide the student with an understanding of his or her learning objectives and should be simple enough that the student can monitor his or her own progress.

Modeling. It is essential for a student to see others using a skill to understand its importance and to observe the activity. If there are no other students with low vision in the school, the teacher should arrange for the student to meet others with low vision outside the school and to observe them functioning efficiently. The student can also learn techniques, such as the use of a prescribed monocular device for watching a play or spotting license plates of cars, that are used by everyone, with or without low vision. One child for whom modeling enhanced motivation was 6-year-old Henry:

> Henry attended the High Vision Games with his brother, who had low vision. These games involved activities to encourage interest and curiosity about optical devices. Six months later, when Henry was diagnosed with a visual impairment, his response was, "Now I can get a scope of my own!" Modeling by other children who used low vision devices had clearly shaped his attitude and motivation.

Guided Practice. At first, students should receive enough prompting and instruction to gain confidence as they learn a visual skill. Students should experience some success during each teaching session, and steps should be discrete enough that the mastery of individual elements of the task can be identified. Checking to see that a student properly understands the instructional steps involved is important because guided practice reinforces the development of correct skills. The student must then demonstrate successful mastery of the entire sequence of steps before being expected to replicate that practice independently.

For example, the student who is learning to use an optical device will learn discrete elements, such as spotting and focusing, that will later become well integrated into activities. So the student does not have to learn a new visual skill at the same time as he or she is learning new information in the classroom, the teacher of students with visual impairments begins instruction by presenting the use of the optical device outside the class. The teacher will then use guided practice in the classroom, if necessary.

Independent Practice. Only after the student experiences repeated success within the time constraints that are normally required in a particular setting is he or she ready to practice the task independently. Once the student reaches the level of independent practice, it is important for him or her to have frequent opportunities to use and reinforce the skill. In addition, the teacher of students with visual impairments should maintain close contact with the regular classroom teacher and the student's parents to monitor the student's use of the skill in various settings. For example, if the student's goal has been to monitor his or her own lighting, the teacher can check weekly with the classroom teacher and parents to see that he or she is doing so, until this practice becomes routine.

In implementing an activity through this four-part process, it is important that the student's motivation be considered. Although some skills and activities naturally motivate some students, others may need the reinforcement of interesting materials or a reward after achieving them. Whether a reward is the choice of an activity after a difficult task is accomplished, the search for a dinosaur sticker with a monocular, or the opportunity to earn points by maintaining orderly study materials, the student should associate his or her efforts with a pleasant result. Some students have heard only negative or pitying comments about their vision, and it is particularly important for them to feel positive about their visual capabilities.

Providing Instruction with Optical Devices

Basic Approach

The effective use of an optical device begins with a thorough low vision evaluation that considers a student's individual needs and preferences, as described in Chapter 8. Because devices vary in size, portability, ease of use, and strength, it is necessary for them to be prescribed by a qualified low vision specialist who can evaluate specific needs, ideally in cooperation with the student's educational team. For a school-aged child, efficiency in the use of an optical device may play a role in determining his or her academic success and self-confidence.

Since the 1980s, children as young as age 3 have been successfully taught to use distance optical devices (Corn, 1993; Cowan & Shepler, 1990; Paul, 1992). Although some children may seem to adapt to using a telescope after a 10-minute demonstration, most preschoolers benefit from ongoing instruction. Lessons can be fun and can begin as soon as a child has the motor ability to manipulate the device, as well as the desire to see something at a distance.

For young children, Cowan and Shepler (1990) recommended that highly stimulating activities be introduced during short instructional sessions of 15 to 20 minutes and that instruction should begin with a variety of activities, so a child considers a particular optical device to be a versatile and worthwhile tool, not an object that is connected only with schoolwork. Generally, the instructional program includes positioning, localizing, scanning, tracking, and focusing. Some suggestions by Cowan and Shepler (1990) for young children, as well as additional ideas for older students, are provided in Sidebar 9.3A/B.

Activities for Using a Magnifier

With Preschool/Elementary School Students	With Middle School/High School Students
1. Observe interesting objects: rocks, shells, fossils, feathers, money, fingerprints, leaves, flowers, and so on. Try to identify them by referring to a (regular print) guide.	1. Scan computer printouts for specific information.
2. Use a magnifier to identify stamps and find the country of origin in an atlas or on a globe.	2. Read newspaper classified sections, sports pages, and stock reports to search for specific information.
3. Use a game board approach to move forward when cut-out pictures pasted on individual cards are identified.	3. Locate information about food ingredients on grocery store labels.
4. Find hidden pictures (similar to those found in the *Highlights for Children* magazine). Encourage systematic left-to-right scanning by placing a clear piece of acetate over the page with a grid or scanning plan mapped out at first.	4. Read bus and train schedules to plan routes to and from school and work.
5. Read recipes off boxes during a cooking lesson.	5. Make an address book by looking up names and addresses of friends in the telephone book.
6. Life skills reading activities include reading the following: menus, newspapers, album covers, food cans, maps, charts, graphs, television guide, and bus schedule.	6. Make a chart to compare reading speed using a magnifier with different sized print.
7. Read and play board games which require reading fine print, e.g., Monopoly, Clue, Trivial Pursuit.	7. Read instruction manuals for computers or new appliances.
8. Read Lego assembly instruction sheets to Lego toys.	8. Use a magnifier to locate geographic areas mentioned in current news broadcasts in an atlas.
9. Place magnifier on mirror to observe eyes and open a discussion on the child's eye condition.	

SIDEBAR 9.3B

Activities for Using a Monocular

With Preschool/Elementary School Students	With Middle School/High School Students
1. Use a monocular for observing moving targets: birds, animals, children on the playground, kites, traffic, bubbles.	1. Identify license plates and makes and models of automobiles.
2. Find toys "hidden" around the classroom or outside in several different places.	2. Identify musical instruments in a band or orchestra on stage.
3. Find specific aisles and products in the grocery store.	3. Identify signs in stores in a mall and locate signs for a particular type of product.
4. Play a (Velcro) dart game or go bowling. Use the monocular to tally scores.	4. Visit an airport or bus station and read departure/arrival postings.
5. Use an overhead projector to check and develop focusing skills. Allow children to manipulate the focusing knob.	5. As a passenger in an automobile, assist the driver by locating specific street signs and location information when the vehicle stops.
6. Tape pages of a picture book along a wall and use the monocular to view pictures and tell the story.	6. Visit a college class and observe the visual requirements; use the monocular to view overheads and instructor notes.
7. Encourage monocular use at concerts, plays, and sporting events; during story time; and on field trips.	7. Locate a particular player in a spectator sports event.
8. Have children observe your facial expressions from a distance with the monocular and mimic them.	8. Visit a museum or art gallery and practice viewing items and information in glass cases.
9. Teach copying by preparing activities on one-inch ruled chart tables that are portable. Some interesting items to copy include poems, limericks, tongue twisters, instructions to a recipe or a science experiment, sentences pertaining to an amusing topic, and novel or unusual formats (columns, crossword puzzles, fill-in-the-blank).	9. Make a chart that compares speeds of copying material from an overhead or chalkboard, and compare reading speeds weekly over several months.

Source: C. Cowan and R. Shepler, "Teaching Techniques for Teaching Young Children to Use Low Vision Devices," 1990, *Journal of Visual Impairment and Blindness, 84* (9), 419–421.

Low Vision Device Assessment Form

Student _____   Date _____

Class _____   Recorder _____

Type of device _____

Brand _____

Power of magnification _____

_____ Use with glasses   _____ Use without glasses   _____ Either

_____

Kinds of activities for which the device could be used

_____

Length of time for use

_____

Methods for enhancing the student's comfort

_____

Plan for storage of the device in the classroom

_____

Plan for transporting the device between environments

_____

Important factors for the care of the device

_____

Figure 9.3. Assessment Form for Low Vision Devices

Figure 9.3 is a form that can be used to record basic information about a student's use of an optical device. Because elementary classroom teachers are often unfamiliar with these devices, they may appreciate written information about the use, maintenance, and storage of the devices. This form can also be copied and circulated to other members of the educational team to ensure that a device is used consistently.

The student who uses an optical device should have the opportunity to observe others who use low vision devices successfully. The student also should be encouraged to share his or her experiences with others in the classroom.

With the student's approval, the teacher of students with visual impairments can tell the entire class the purpose of optical devices, emphasizing their usefulness in many contexts for all children and adults. This may also be the appropriate time to allow classmates to examine and try out a handheld device with supervision. However, they should be told clearly that the device belongs to the student for whom it was prescribed, and classroom personnel should reinforce the importance of careful storage and handling.

Instruction in the use of optical devices moves the student from familiar to unfamiliar situations, from supported to unsupported use, and from high-contrast to low-contrast environments. With a graduated sequence of instruction and opportunities to observe others using optical devices successfully, even very young students can become competent in their use.

Resources for Instruction in the Use of Vision

A variety of resources on vision enhancement have been developed that may be valuable for teaching basic visual skills, such as attending and scanning, as well as for applying these basic skills. Although it is tempting for new professionals to rely heavily on one or two of these resources for program development, it should be emphasized that the characteristics of individual students vary and that no one resource will provide a framework for learning for all students. Therefore, to be effective in enhancing the use of vision, it is necessary to be familiar with a wide variety of resources and to apply elements that are appropriate for each child. A sampling of materials is listed in Sidebar 9.4.

Professional Roles and Responsibilities

The vignette at the beginning of this chapter introduced Tracy, a new teacher of students with visual impairments, whose confusion about her role with students with low vision is not uncommon. The role of the professional who works with students with visual impairments varies according to the capabilities and needs of each student. The concept of vision stimulation or vision usage as a discrete service that is delivered at pre-scheduled times is often inappropriate. Rather, the teacher often decreases or increases his or her direct involvement with a student over time as the student masters a skill or moves into a school setting that poses new challenges. Flexibility in short- and long-term scheduling is important. Scheduling should be openly discussed with family members during the annual IEP conference, so they clearly understand the teacher will provide the services.

The activities carried out by the teacher of students with visual impairments should be directly related to a student's visual needs. These activities can focus on the more efficient use of vision or on skills, such as listening, that are necessary because of the student's visual needs. It is sometimes tempting for the teacher to serve as a tutor or to assist students with homework because this is the students' and classroom teachers' most immediate concern. However, the role of the specialized teacher is to assist a student to acquire skills related to his or her visual needs. Although such skills can often be taught in the context of regular daily assignments, they should be generalizable to other situations. For example, if Sharon's history teacher has asked the class to answer questions about a map of eighteenth-century Europe, Sharon's teacher of students with visual impairments can use this assignment as an opportunity for Sharon to practice using her hand-held magnifier.

With respect to the student with low vision, the role of the teacher of students with visual impairments may include any of the following:

- providing information on low vision to other members of the educational team
- performing functional vision assessments
- arranging for necessary clinical evaluations and, in some cases, attending the evaluations with the student and his or her parents
- obtaining or helping to obtain appropriate optical and nonoptical devices
- providing information about low vision and low vision devices to classmates with normal vision
- providing initial instruction in visual skills, including the use of low vision devices, to the student in a controlled environment
- facilitating the transfer of visual skills to the child's natural environments as early as feasible
- developing and implementing an individualized curriculum in all areas specific to low vision, such as daily living skills and social skills

SIDEBAR 9.4

Vision Enhancement Materials and Resources

These resources are appropriate for use with students who are becoming aware of visual features of the environment and are learning to associate meaning with visual stimuli.

AWARENESS AND MEANING

Materials

Bright Sights (American Printing House for the Blind, Louisville, KY): This kit includes a variety of reflective and light-stimulating materials that are designed to attract visual attention.

Light Box, Level I (American Printing House for the Blind, Louisville, KY): The light box provides a lighted background with rheostat controls to vary lighting. Level I materials rely on movement, light, and color without symbolic representation to gain visual attention.

Publications

Harrell, L., & Akeson, N. (1987). *Preschool vision stimulation: It's more than a flashlight.* New York: American Foundation for the Blind. This book, intended for parents and professionals, presents ideas for activities to encourage the use of vision in young children.

Langley, M. (1980). *Functional vision screening inventory for the multiply and severly handicapped.* Chicago: Stoelting Co. An assessment and teaching program that is appropriate for students who are functioning at developmental ages 0–2. It includes a screening instrument, a visual assessment, a teaching program, and a list of instructional materials and resources.

Project strive (1987). Houston: Education Service Center, Region IV. This curriculum includes goals and activities that are designed to develop visual responses in students with severe impairments.

Smith, A., & Cote, K. (1982). *Look at me: A resource manual for the development of residual vision in multiply impaired children.* Philadelphia: Pennsylvania College of Optometry Press. This book provides developmental

activities that are designed to increase responses to visual stimuli in students with developmental delays.

SKILL ACQUISITION

Materials

Light Box, Levels II and III. (American Printing House for the Blind, Louisville, KY): These light box activities, which are more advanced than Level I, address the visual needs of students who can comprehend symbolic representation and who have some visual memory.

Publications

Barraga, N. & Morris, J. E. (1980). *Program to Develop Efficiency in Visual Functioning.* Louisville, KY: American Printing House for the Blind. An assessment and instructional program that provides a developmental profile of vision for students aged 3–16, which can be used as a basis for program development. The instructional program includes a variety of teaching activities in eight areas of visual development.

Levack, N. (1991). *Low vision: A resource guide with adaptations for students with visual impairments.* Austin: Texas School for the Blind and Visually Impaired. A guide to programs, services, and educational practices for students with low vision that addresses environmental and instructional adaptations for school-age students of all levels.

Project IVEY. (1987). Tallahassee: State of Florida, Department of Education. This comprehensive program guide is intended for professionals in the field of visual impairment. It includes guidelines for vision assessment and teaching activities.

Smith, A. & O'Donnell, E. (1992). *Beyond arm's reach.* Philadelphia: Pennsylvania College of Optometry Press. This publication presents a comprehensive program for instructing low vision students in the use of distance vision.

- assessing a student's need for learning media and recommending the most appropriate literacy medium or media to the educational team
- arranging access to adult role models who have low vision
- referring the student for additional services, such as those provided by an O&M instructor.

Other members of the educational team, particularly the classroom teacher, need to understand the role of the teacher of students with visual impairments. Meeting with team members at the beginning of the school year and providing them with a brief, clearly written description of this specialized teacher's activities can promote understanding of his or her role.

PROMOTION OF FUNCTIONALITY AND GENERALIZATION

Instruction in Decision-making Procedures

The primary goals for students with low vision are to recognize their options for gaining information and to make the most appropriate choice among those options. This process begins early, when young students are encouraged to consider such questions as: Do you prefer sitting in front of the teacher or to the side? Do you want to sit close to the teacher or use your monocular to see the teacher? The critical element is that the student perceives that he or she has opportunities for making decisions within a given context. Students who have received reinforcement for thinking of themselves as handicapped may recognize the obstacles that vision loss presents to efficient functioning because friends and relatives have emphasized these obstacles. They have heard, "You can't see that" or "Let me help you" so often that they may not realize that there are many ways of accomplishing a task independently, as in the following example.

Rebecca attends story time at the local library with her friend Jason. Since she cannot see the pictures that the storyteller displays, she has several options: She can arrive early and ask to sit close to the storyteller, she can ask whether a second copy of the book is available, she can ask Jason to tell her about each picture, she can use a monocular to view each picture, or she can ask to see the book after the storytelling session. The best solution may be different from week to week. For example, when there are only a few children who know Rebecca well, she may be comfortable sitting near the storyteller. However, when the group is larger, she may prefer to use her monocular.

For a student to make a responsible choice about gaining access to information, he or she must first recognize that options exist. For a preschooler, it may mean choosing between two alternatives: Do you want to hold the book closer or look at the picture under the closed-circuit television? For an older child, it involves brainstorming to think of all the options with regard to a complex task. For example, when looking for a particular store at a mall, the student may choose to use a monocular, to look for nearby landmarks that he or she has memorized, or to follow the lead of a friend. Having identified the options, the student can then make a choice about which solution is most appropriate. To do so, the student needs to be aware of the advantages and disadvantages of each option, including such factors as the need for the equipment, as well as the size and portability, efficiency, social acceptability, and ease of access of the equipment. For students who are just learning this process, it may help to list the advantages and disadvantages of each choice.

Finally, students must learn to use known skills to make decisions in unexpected situations, such as when dealing with a missed school bus, a lost monocular, or a spontaneous invitation to go shopping with friends, when all the desirable options are not available. In such situations, students must learn to consider whatever options are available and to see themselves as the ones who make the ultimate decision, even if the decision is to accept more assistance from others than would normally be required. Ultimately, students who can recognize and apply a decision-making process will be more successful in generalizing skills and using them efficiently.

Developmental Requirements for the Use of Vision

Skills in efficient learning related to low vision also vary as students grow older. For students to be responsible, they will need to generalize skills learned in specific situations as life tasks become more complex.

The learning of academic tasks is one example. A child in kindergarten or first grade may have learned to use a magnifier to enlarge small pictures and closely spaced mathematics problems in a workbook. When map reading is introduced in third or fourth grade, the teacher of students with visual impairments may again work with the student on skills in using a magnifier, this time to search for particular symbols on a map and to read the key. When the student is required to read computer printouts in eighth grade, additional practice may be helpful to apply skills in the use of the magnifier to these tasks. Even though the student has a basic understanding of how to use a magnifier, he or she expands those skills to deal with new tasks.

The generalization of social skills also becomes more complex as students advance in school. Social learning in elementary school may involve mainly the use of conventional social routines—knowing how to introduce oneself, how to stand in line, or to raise one's hand in class—which may require additional learning for students with low vision. By adolescence, however, social experiences involve independent decisions that require students to weigh options. For example, do they want to go to a football game with classmates even though they cannot see the activity on the playing field? If so, is it important to ask someone else to keep them informed of the action on the field, or is the opportunity to talk with friends more important than knowing what is occurring at every point in the game?

Options for leisure activities change as children grow older, and the decisions to be made broaden in number and complexity. In elementary school, recess time often involves fast-moving games with chasing and running. Children with low vision may be at a disadvantage in competitive games such as these and may choose other playground activities in which they can compete more successfully. Later on, they may develop skills in games involving complex thinking and planning. Then, they can choose recreational activities that interest them and can take the initiative in adapting activities for their visual requirements. For example, children who enjoy playing board games may select playing pieces that contrast with the board, and those who like to ice-skate may ask their friends to wear brightly colored clothing so they can locate their friends in a crowd or at a distance.

It is important for students' leisure decisions to be based on their own interests, not on the limitations imposed by their vision. Since the interests of peers direct choices to a great degree beginning in elementary school, the teacher of students with visual impairments should be aware of the preferred activities of a student's peers to help the student find ways to participate in them.

Career development is an area in which the use of functional vision has a different impact at different points in a child's development. During elementary school, low vision may limit a student's ability to gather details about the work roles performed by adults. Direct participation is more important for the student with low vision than for the student with normal vision, who is able to gather information incidentally through the use of sight. However, photographs or videotapes may provide information that is not visually accessible; for example, the activities of a construction worker, which may be dangerous to observe at near point, may be more richly represented through photographs or videotapes.

For older students, career development involves a consideration of the impact of vision on job roles. Only a few jobs, such as an airplane pilot or a truck driver, are not possible for the person with low vision. The great majority of jobs are possible but may require adaptations. Therefore, a variety of work experiences are desirable at the secondary level to enable students to solve specific problems related to their vision and to evaluate their interest in the activities that may be related to a desired job.

For students to lead satisfying adult lives, it is important for them to make responsible decisions related to using vision during typical activities. In addition, they will use skills learned in controlled situations in a greater variety of other settings as they mature. For instance, children who consider the monocular a tool that can enrich their enjoyment of hiking or enable them to read a menu in a fast-food restaurant have more options than do children who believe the monocular is a tool only for reading the chalkboard in school.

SUMMARY

The teacher of students with visual impairments is responsible for translating the implications of a student's low vision into activities that will enable the student to be effective in school, at home, and in the community. Through the use of specific information gathered during the functional vision assessment that can be applied to a student's individual needs, the teacher provides the vehicle to move the student into a world of choices and opportunities to become increasingly independent.

ACTIVITIES

With This Chapter and Other Resources

1. In the vignette that opens this chapter, Andrew was upset that his teacher of students with visual impairments had not visited him to ease his first few days at school with the regular classroom teachers who did not understand his visual needs. Write three objectives for Andrew to become an advocate for himself by explaining his visual needs to his teachers for the next year.

2. Use the form in Figure 9.1 to analyze an environment, such as your home or apartment. Write a concise narrative report of this analysis.

3. Prepare a brief explanation about functional vision assessments and the roles of the teacher of students with visual impairments for an audience that may include optometrists, ophthalmologists, regular classroom teachers, and parents.

4. Choose a visual task that you might teach a student with low vision, such as taking notes from a chalkboard by using a monocular. Following the sequence of instruction found in this chapter, write a plan for a seventh-grade student.

In the Community

1. Observe an experienced teacher of students with visual impairments conducting a functional vision assessment. Discuss with the teacher his or her preparation for conducting the assessment and the recommendations that will be developed.

2. Ask a clinical low vision specialist how he or she uses the functional vision assessments provided by teachers of students with visual impairments when planning for the clinical low vision evaluation of patients.

With a Person with Low Vision

1. Conduct a functional vision assessment of a student with low vision and write a report containing the components described in this chapter.

2. Interpret and discuss the recommendations in a report of a functional vision assessment with a classroom teacher and a parent.

From Your Perspective

In what ways can teachers and eye care professionals promote the use of optical devices in school systems that rely solely on large-type materials?

APPENDIX
SAMPLE FUNCTIONAL VISION ASSESSMENT REPORT

Student: Sandra Aguilar

Date of birth: March 9, 1983

Evaluator: Jack I. Chen, Teacher of Students with Visual Impairments

School: Cross Creek Elementary School

School district: Dry Gulch Independent School District

Date of evaluation: September 15, 1996

Date of report: September 20, 1996

This functional vision assessment was performed to update Sandra Aguilar's educational program. Sandra has been eligible for services as a student with a visual impairment since 1985. Her last functional vision assessment was performed in May 1994.

BACKGROUND INFORMATION

Medical. Sandra was born after 32 weeks' gestation; her mother, Maria Aguilar, who has had diabetes since age 12, experienced medical complications during her pregnancy with Sandra. During her first year, Sandra had chronic respiratory difficulties that required three hospitalizations. She has a moderate hearing loss in her left ear, which presents little functional disadvantage, and is reassessed annually by the school audiologist.

Visual. Sandra was diagnosed with cataracts at age 6 months; surgery was performed in November 1984 by Dr. Iris Lopez at the Valley Medical Center in Valley, Texas. She received eyeglasses following the surgery; in 1988 Dr. Mark Smith prescribed contact lenses for Sandra, which she wears regularly at school. Her current prescription is +14 left eye and +12 right eye, with a mild astigmatic correction in both eyes; her measured acuity is 20/300 in the left eye, 20/150 in the right eye, and 20/200 for both eyes. Sandra has mild peripheral visual field limitations (approximately 15–20 degrees on either side) in both eyes. She continues to be seen annually by Dr. Smith and was last examined in November 1995.

In May 1994, Sandra was evaluated by Dr. Connie Jenkins at the Valley Medical Center Low Vision Clinic. Dr. Jenkins recommended a 4X monocular for use during distance activities, which Sandra uses routinely in the classroom and for activities at home and in the community.

Educational. Sandra, who has received educational services since age 2 because of her visual impairment, attended an early childhood program at Cross Creek Elementary School from 1987 to 1989. During her preschool years, she demonstrated language delays of approximately one year and received speech-language therapy from 1987 to 1990. She entered first grade with her age peers and has received average grades throughout elementary school. She is currently in sixth grade, where she is having difficulty with mathematics and history; she is receiving Ds in both subjects. She also expresses a dislike of physical education and has asked to be placed in adaptive physical education, in which she was enrolled in fourth grade. Sandra says that she enjoys school, except for mathematics and mentioned several good friends in her class. She wants to be a hairdresser or a child care worker when she leaves school.

OBSERVATION OF THE ENVIRONMENT

The functional vision assessment was based on observations of Sandra in her classroom and in physical education on September 9; at lunchtime and in class on September 10; and in a conference room on September 14, where Sandra participated in activities presented by the evaluator.

Sandra's classroom includes about 30 desks and chairs arranged lecture style, facing Ms. Ramirez's (the teacher's) desk, which is in the center. The students' desks have surfaces that are hinged at the back and can be raised at the front to store books and papers. The students were permitted to choose their seats at the beginning of the year, and Sandra chose a seat in the center of the room, about four rows from the front. The classroom lighting is from a bank of windows along the east wall (to Sandra's left as she faces the teacher), as well as from overhead fluorescent lighting. The classroom door is at the right rear of the room; the door and frame are brown wood. The floor is brown tile with a white mottled pattern, and the walls are pale blue.

There are green chalkboards on the front and right walls. General announcements, a daily schedule, and exemplary student work are posted on a brown bulletin board at the front of the right wall, posters are above the chalkboard at the front of the room, and emergency evacuation instructions are posted beneath the light switch to the right of the classroom door. At the back of the room is a shelf of library books and two beanbag chairs on a large carpet square. Two Apple computers in study carrels are against the back wall, to the left as one enters the room.

An overhead projector on a cart is next to the classroom teacher's desk; Ms. Ramirez used it to project lecture material during both the classroom observations, and during that time she placed it in front of her desk and projected material on the pale blue wall above the chalkboard. Most classes are conducted in a lecture format, with students facing the teacher, who lectures from the front of the room.

Physical education and lunch both take place in a large multipurpose room located on the same hallway as the classroom. The room has a green tile floor that is highly polished and reflects glare from the window light on the north side of the room. At one end of the room, lunch tables with attached benches are arranged in rows, with an aisle about six feet wide between the table and the line through which students move to pick up lunch items.

VISUAL RESPONSES AND ACTIVITIES

Structure and reflexes. Sandra's eyes appear aligned. She showed a normal blink response to a ball tossed to her and during a reading task.

Near vision. Sandra reads standard-print texts for her classes, with a reading distance of six to eight inches. This year she requested and received enlarged print for her mathematics text because the print size of individual problems varied greatly.

Sandra read the 9 point (1.0 M) line of the Lighthouse near vision acuity card at about nine inches. When asked to hold the card at a 12 to 14 inch distance, she could read print down to the 14-point line. During the evaluation, she read selections aloud from several textbooks, a comic book, and a popular magazine. She was offered a bookstand but declined, saying that the bookstand "looked weird." She had no difficulty reading printed material that had a predictable format; however, when reading comic books and mathematical problems, she turned the material sideways, tilted her head, and squinted when the print size, style, and format were irregular. She read aloud from her reading book for three pages and then stated that she was tired; she made three errors in reading, all of which involved the misidentification of words for similar ones (for example, "again" for "against"). Other near vision activities included using a calculator, playing jacks, and handwriting.

With regard to the calculator, Sandra could read the numerals on the screen, which were quarter-inch red letters against a gray background. However, she stated that the glare made reading the numerals difficult and tilted the calculator to block out glare from light sources.

Sandra said that the sixth-grade girls often played jacks at recess and that she was not very good at it. When the evaluator asked her to show him how to play, she explained the rules accurately; however, she was unable to shift her gaze from the bouncing ball to the jacks quickly enough to pick them up after the first bounce.

For the handwriting activity, Sandra wrote a one-page letter to a friend and read it back. Her handwriting is larger than is typical for sixth graders, and she prefers a felt-tipped pen on standard notebook paper. She had difficulty distinguishing n's and m's and i's, u's, and w's when reading back her writing.

Distance vision. Distance screening was conducted using the Feinbloom chart, and Sandra's acuity was 20/200 in her left eye, 20/150 in her right eye, and 20/150 for both eyes.

In the classroom, Sandra used her monocular to read material from the chalkboard and overhead projector. The classroom teacher offered her a printed copy of material from the overhead, but she declined. She was able to take notes from the chalkboard within the time expected for the rest of the class, except during mathematics class, when vertical and horizontal problems were presented on the board. When she fell behind, she asked the student beside her to allow her to copy the problems.

During physical education, Sandra participated in calisthenics and a game of volleyball. She positioned herself to avoid the ball during volleyball; on the two occasions it came to her, she returned it successfully once. When her team was facing the window, she stood sideways to avoid looking directly toward the window.

When going through the cafeteria line, Sandra read the posted menu using her monocular and located and selected her own foods visually. She had difficulty locating her friends' table in the cafeteria and asked another student for assistance. When traveling in the halls, Sandra exhibited no difficulty in travel or locating destinations; she appeared to recognize acquaintances by voice and called them by name after they had greeted her aloud.

Visual field. When scanning for a moving object, such as a volleyball or a moving vehicle, Sandra turned her head more than is typical. When traveling, she looked directly ahead but occasionally was startled by someone passing her from either side. During near vision tasks, she scanned maps for specific labels and completed a word-search puzzle; during these tasks, she also moved her head to a greater degree than would be expected.

Other visual responses. Sandra successfully identified colors and shades of objects on request and was able to sequence the shades accurately using the Farnsworth test. She described other students' color combinations of clothing that she preferred and mentioned that a classmate's skirt "didn't match" her blouse because they were different shades of blue.

Sandra stated that she did not like bright lighting, especially in the multipurpose room where it reflected on the floor. When a study lamp was provided during the evaluation activities, she arranged it at a 45-degree angle at her left elbow and asked whether she could use it in the classroom.

When using the computer, she turned the screen slightly to avoid the reflected light from the window. The evaluator suggested that she should try several contrast effects on the computer, and although Sandra liked the red letters on blue background, she eventually returned to the black on white, saying, "This is the best because it's what I'm used to." She also stated that she disliked computer activities that have rapidly moving stimuli, which bother her eyes.

SUMMARY

Sandra manages near vision tasks in the classroom by adapting her viewing distance and angle of vision. She demonstrates the greatest difficulty with materials that combine different sizes of print or include vertical and horizontal materials together. For distance viewing she uses a monocular and extra head movements and requests assistance to meet her needs. She uses her monocular appropriately but slowly and finds it tiring to use it for long periods. She experiences discomfort from irregular lighting, glare, and some types of moving visual stimuli. Her difficulty with mathematics and physical education may be linked to the specific visual demands of these subjects.

RECOMMENDATIONS

The following activities will assist Sandra in learning effectively:

Referrals

1. Sandra should receive an evaluation from the technology outreach consultant at the Texas School for the Blind and Visually Impaired to determine the most effective print size, contrast, and color effects for computer usage.

Adaptations

1. The teacher of students with visual impairments will obtain a study lamp for Sandra's use in the classroom.
2. A visor should be placed over the classroom computer to reduce glare.
3. Some light control, such as blinds or translucent shades, should be obtained in the multipurpose room to reduce bright window lighting and glare.

Instructional and Compensatory Strategies

1. Sandra should be allowed to produce assignments on the computer, rather than handwritten ones, when more than a few sentences are required.
2. The educational team should consider subjects in which audiotaped materials may be helpful, particularly those that require sustained reading. The teacher of students with visual impairments will obtain the necessary materials and will work with Sandra on learning to order audiotaped materials.

Services

The teacher of students with visual impairments should work with Sandra for at least an hour each week to help her become efficient in manipulating the monocular, as well as to practice search-and-scanning techniques with unconventional printed material, such as maps and mathematical problems. In addition, an Informal Reading Inventory should be conducted to investigate Sandra's reading speed and error patterns.

Sandra continues to qualify for services as a student with a visual impairment according to the regulations of the Texas State Board of Education.

Functional Vision Assessment and Instruction of Children and Youths with Multiple Disabilities

Jane N. Erin

VIGNETTE

Four-year-old Eric just got his first pair of eyeglasses. When he was younger, ophthalmologists said that it was not possible to tell what he could see, and they doubted that a child with disabilities as severe as Eric's could wear eyeglasses. Recently, Eric's mother found out about Dr. Morton, a local optometrist who had examined many children with disabilities, and took Eric to see him. Dr. Morton used a method called preferential viewing, along with several other procedures, to evaluate Eric's vision. Eric seems more alert and interested in small objects since he learned to wear eyeglasses that Dr. Morton prescribed.

As Eric grows, he will show more interest in his world. He looks at light when the curtains are opened, smiles back at his father's smile, and reaches for the toy truck his brother rolls toward him. Using his vision becomes more exciting as he discovers how much there is around him to be seen.

In many ways, Eric is like most 4-year-old boys. He likes watching *Sesame Street,* eating ice cream, and wrestling on the floor with his older brother and his dog. He does not like bath time or long car rides. Although Eric has physical and mental disabilities, as well as low vision, he is more like other children than he is different from them.

Eric's family and teachers have identified objects Eric sees and uses every day. By adding bright colors and reflective features, they encourage him to notice things around him. For example, the orthopedic device for his foot has bright red happy faces on it, and his spoon has a yellow vinyl handle. At school and at home, he is learning to use vision, and his vision is helping him to learn about his environment.

INTRODUCTION

When children have disabilities in addition to low vision that affect their ability to communicate and to understand the world, the assessment of their vision is a particular challenge. Professionals must become detectives who are alert to subtle behaviors and unexpected clues; they must assemble the facts to solve the mystery of how the children see. Behaviors may occur once and then not again, responses may vary according to levels of arousal and motivation, and vision may be used in one context and not in another. The accurate assessment of vision and the development of instructional procedures that will enable children with multiple disabilities to be active participants in home and community activities are the focus of this chapter.

221

ASSESSMENT AND INSTRUCTION

For children with disabilities in addition to low vision, the assessment must evaluate both their best visual functioning and their typical visual function. Determining a child's best visual functioning is important because the educational team must determine the student's visual capability. Many students with severe disabilities cannot respond to traditional screening and assessment procedures because of their cognitive level or lack of motivation, and even the most practiced clinical low vision specialist may obtain only cursory information during an office visit. Although always of tremendous importance, the careful assessment of vision through observation and interaction is even more critical when a child cannot respond to standard approaches to assessment. To develop an appropriate program and to encourage the use of vision, when appropriate, the educational team must know the child's maximum level of visual efficiency. For example, if Robbie has reached for and picked up a tiny piece of cereal located 18 inches from his eyes, it suggests that he has the visual capacity to locate an object that small at that distance. Even if Robbie does not regularly respond that way, the educational team has determined that he is capable of this response and can work toward shaping and reinforcing it.

With regard to typical visual function, the use of vision by a child with several disabilities can vary greatly according to the nature of the task, the child's physical state, actual changes in brain and eye function, and motivation. For these reasons, single-session assessments will yield information that is not representative of a child's true function. Rather, the assessment should include observations of behaviors that vary according to the following characteristics:

- the child's motivation
- the child's familiarity with people, objects, and settings
- the involvement of others
- the child's physical positioning
- the stimulus level of materials

- the child's use of his or her other senses.

Careful assessment before and during instruction can ensure that the program that is planned provides the best opportunity for mastery.

Undertaking Assessment for Instructional Planning

To determine a child's best visual function and typical visual function, the evaluator must develop an initial assessment that provides a basis for setting instructional goals. The assessment should yield a representative picture of visual skills that includes recommendations for the use of vision or, in the absence of vision, compensatory skills. These recommendations can include specific adaptations needed to improve a student's efficiency in performing tasks, as well as recommendations for instructional procedures to integrate vision into a student's educational activities.

This initial assessment is the functional vision assessment, a narrative description of the child's use of vision, as indicated by his or her behaviors on a variety of tasks. Although there is no standard format, most functional vision assessments include descriptions of the use of vision in near and distance tasks; eye movements; visual field responses; and responses to specific environmental characteristics, such as light and color. The quality of the assessment depends on the objective description of specific behaviors in a variety of situations. Also included in the functional vision assessment are recommendations for instructional procedures and adaptations that form the bridge between the assessment and the development of program goals, as in the following example:

The functional vision assessment for Melanie has identified limitations in her left visual field, and the evaluator has recommended that Melanie should be encouraged to compensate by turning her head slightly to the left. Melanie's goals in the classroom include greeting another person with a smile, eating finger foods independently, and wiping the table with a sponge after snack time. The educational team must consider the implications of Melanie's field loss for the tasks that have been identified as important for her. They may decide that Melanie will be taught to turn her head slightly to the left during these tasks to compensate for the difference in her field, but they may also decide that new tasks will be adapted by placing the materials to the center and right of her visual field. Therefore, when she is learning to eat finger foods, the foods will be placed to her center and right, but once she has mastered the task, they will be placed increasingly to her left to encourage her to turn her head and search. In this case, the educational team has decided to begin by adapting the task but to move toward teaching compensatory visual skills.

Monitoring Progress and Making Changes during the Program

Once the program has been implemented to include adaptations and goals related to a child's use of vision, it is necessary for the child's progress to be monitored. In many cases monitoring will take place through the regular collection of data regarding a specific behavior. To evaluate change, it is important to begin with a clearly measurable goal related to the use of vision or compensation for its absence. For example, it is difficult to assess progress on the goal, "Peter will use his vision more efficiently." It is much easier to assess progress on a measurable goal, such as, "Peter will look at his spoon, presented within 6 inches of his face, before picking it up eight out of ten times."

It is also important to select appropriate data for recording. In the case of Peter and his spoon, it would not be appropriate to record data on how long he looks at his spoon because staring at a spoon for a long period is not realistic or functional. Instead, the data collected here might be percentage data, which provides information about how often he looked at the spoon in rela-

tion to how many times he picked up the spoon. This is a more important piece of information because the educational team wants Peter to look at the spoon every time he picks it up.

Although it may not be practical or necessary to collect data on a particular activity each time a child attempts it, a sampling of data should be recorded at regular intervals, at least weekly for most functional tasks. In this way, a child's progress on a task can be regularly evaluated and the educational team can decide whether to alter a particular objective.

Also during program evaluation, decisions must be made about whether to continue program adaptations. Sometimes when a visual adaptation is made, such as to increase the visibility of a task, team members continue to use it indefinitely. Many adaptations are needed only for short periods, until a student has become competent in a task, as in this example:

> The educational team decides to use shiny tape to highlight Ramona's cup to attract her attention when teaching her to drink, but as time goes on, they remove bits of the tape to make it less noticeable. Eventually, Ramona may search for the cup without any special visual effects. It is important for her to do so, so she can recognize cups that have not been adapted and can drink from cups in a restaurant, while visiting relatives, or in other situations in which an adapted cup is not available. Assessment during program evaluation can make the educational team aware that adaptations are no longer needed.

Many children with severe disabilities have a teacher of students with visual impairments on their educational team, but this teacher acts as a consultant to the classroom staff. Even though this teacher may not work directly with a student on a regular basis, reassessment should be an important part of his or her role. Visiting regularly to evaluate changes in a child's use of vision or mastery of compensatory skills can help give the classroom staff direction with respect to the effectiveness of their instruction. The teacher of students with visual impairments who writes the initial assessment report must be available for continued monitoring of the child's progress and for carrying out recommendations included in the functional vision assessment.

The assessment of vision should be a formative process for the student with visual and other disabilities. Initially, it should identify adaptations and instructional procedures related to vision or compensatory skills, but to be truly effective, there should be a regular plan for monitoring changes in the level of the child's skills, as well as the ongoing need for adaptations related to vision. The following discussion describes specific procedures for assessing vision, particularly during a functional vision assessment conducted to develop the Individualized Education Program (IEP).

APPROACHES TO THE ASSESSMENT OF VISION

The most essential observations of the use of vision take place as the child is using vision in the actual performance of tasks. Watching a child who is eating, dressing, watching television, watering a plant, or setting the table can yield more information than can a game or activity that is developed specifically for the observation of vision.

For example, 7-year-old Amy feeds herself soft foods with an adapted spoon and eats foods with her fingers that are solid enough for her to hold. In watching her at mealtime, the evaluator observes many clues that tell what Amy sees:

- Amy smiled when her child care worker entered the room and smiled at her from about 20 feet away from her.
- Amy reached for her spoon, whether it was placed on her right or left side.
- Amy reached for a piece of potato chip that was less than an inch long and was 24 inches from her eyes on a beige tabletop.
- Amy began to protest when the child care worker put carrots on her plate. Although

she may have smelled the carrots, it appeared that she turned her head toward them before she began crying, which indicated that she recognized them visually.
- Amy blinked when the child care worker brought her bib toward her before the meal.

All these behaviors provide specific information about how Amy sees. To develop a thorough assessment of Amy's vision, the evaluator should first arrange to observe several familiar activities and then plan activities that are designed to demonstrate specific visual behaviors to gather more information. Activities that are specifically planned for visual observation should be both motivating and age appropriate. The objective of these activities is to discover the student's best visual capabilities, which can most likely be done when the child is engaged and motivated.

Gathering Background Information

In conducting a functional vision assessment of a student with visual and multiple disabilities, the evaluator first gathers background information that will allow him or her to select appropriate activities, interpret the child's communicative behaviors, and collect accurate information. The following areas should be reviewed before the evaluator interacts with the child or prepares the assessment report.

Medical Concerns

Many students have chronic medical conditions that influence their ability to use vision. Seizures, which are common, range from brief, almost undetectable moments of inattention through active tonic-clonic seizures. In such cases, students lose visual contact with the environment and some changes in eye movement are noted, including a fixed stare or rolling eye movements. The evaluator should be aware of the nature and appearance of a student's seizure pattern, so that mild seizures can be distinguished from voluntary behaviors.

Many students need medications to manage seizures or to treat other physical conditions. Some medications can have an effect on vision and ocular function; for example, some seizure medications inhibit pupillary function, which may result in light sensitivity or the need for additional lighting. Other medications can affect the child's responsiveness to stimuli, making it important to plan some activities during optimal states of alertness. If it is possible to schedule assessment activities about midway between the administration of medications, a more representative picture of student function can be gained (Kelley, Wedding, & Smiths, 1992).

Other medical conditions can have an impact on responses (Newell, 1982). Changes in the glucose levels of children with diabetes can influence visual function (Newell, 1982). Children with hydrocephaly may show long-term changes in vision based on the efficiency of the shunts inserted in them to maintain normal pressure in the brain, and some may also evidence day-to-day variations in visual function related to intracranial pressure. Students with cerebral palsy will often experience strabismus, either periodically or consistently, and the nature of the strabismus may vary according to the type of cerebral palsy (Harley & Altmeyer, 1982). For these reasons, it is important to review a child's medical records and to be familiar with conditions that may affect visual behavior.

Communication

Gathering information about vision depends, to a great extent, on the evaluator's interpretation of a child's intentional and unintentional communication. A child may use speech to identify and describe objects; gestures to indicate an awareness of objects; or nonspecific communicative behaviors, such as crying or vocalizing, to indicate that he or she likes or dislikes a change in environmental conditions related to vision. The form and function of communication will provide critical information about how a child sees.

The evaluator should consider that all the information about a child's vision will be gathered

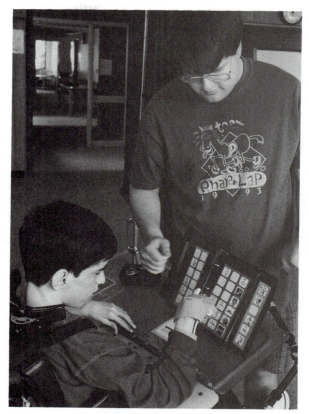

Knowing a child's preferred method of communication, or working with someone who does, is essential for an evaluator.

through two types of communication: vocal sounds and body movements. Vocal sounds may vary from complex speech to cries, coos, and grunts. Even unintentional communication, such as cries or voice sounds, can vary according to what the child sees. The child who suddenly becomes quiet when the window shades are closed is noticing a change in the visual environment, and the evaluator should be alert to this type of vocal response when drawing conclusions about what the child sees, in this case, whether the child is responding to the visual cue or to the sound of the window shades being closed.

Body movements also provide information about what a child sees. These movements can include intentionally communicative movements, such as pointing to a picture or a wanted object, as well as unintentional communicative behaviors, such as moving toward or away from a visual stimulus, turning the head or eyes, and demonstrating reflexive movements, such as a blink. Since an evaluator's conclusions about the vision of a child who does not use language will be based mainly on observations of behavior, it is useful to develop expertise in the observation and documentation of behaviors to draw valid conclusions.

If the evaluator does not regularly work with a child and the child uses a form of communication other than speech, it is best if the primary assessment activities are conducted by someone who knows the child well and understands his or her form of communication, especially if the child uses American Sign Language or an augmentative communication device. It is also necessary if the child communicates nonsymbolically, because regular caregivers will be able to interpret behaviors that express rejection, dislike, preference, and comfort and other behaviors that indicate the child's responses to visual effects in the environment. (For more information on such concepts as intentional, symbolic, and nonsymbolic communication and on forms of communication like augmentative communication, see Huebner, Prickett, Welch, & Joffee [1995].)

If the evaluator wants to try activities or procedures that may be unfamiliar to the child, it is often appropriate to model these procedures first with another person. Many children with additional disabilities become upset by unfamiliar activities, and because they do not have the receptive communication to understand the reason for the new procedures, they may become frightened or resistant. Although most activities during the assessment should be chosen to appeal to a child's interests, some procedures may address a specific visual ability. Procedures, such as the use of a penlight to check pupillary changes or the confrontation test to evaluate field differences, may be more easily carried out after the child watches someone else participating in them, so he or she is assured that the procedures are not uncomfortable. Many students with severe disabilities have undergone injections and other uncomfortable medical procedures, and they may

anticipate a similar experience with an unfamiliar person.

It is important that the evaluator know the child's forms of communication, and be able to use and interpret those forms. If specific alternative forms of communication, such as a communication board, are used, symbols should be identified that can be associated with visual assessment procedures. For example, the symbols for "apple" and "house" that are used in the LEA Symbols and the Lighthouse Flash Card Test can be included to represent those objects, so the child will be familiar with the symbols. Modeling or other approaches should be used to help the child understand procedures that involve unfamiliar materials or activities.

Positioning and Movement

Visual responses can vary according to a child's position in space, distance from the object, and angle of observation. Because students with physical disabilities have limited control over their own positions or movements, providing supportive positions will enhance their visual ability.

For a child who cannot alter his or her body position independently, evaluation and observation should include several different positions, including those in which the child typically spends time. These positions can include supine (on the back), prone (on the stomach), side lying (on the side), independent or supported sitting, and independent or supported standing. The visual limitations and advantages of each position should be considered, in conjunction with an occupational or physical therapist.

Supine Position. The supine position may increase the physical tone and limit the control of many children with severe limitations. It is important that the child be positioned to decrease extension, which often can be done with a soft towel rolled at the base of the head. In this position, the child has limited control over the head and eyes to view events in the environment because the eyes are mainly directed toward the ceiling.

Prone Position. The prone position, which is often supported by a wedge or towel under the upper trunk, offers opportunities for shoulder and arm control and the practice of manipulative skills. In this position, the child may be motivated to move his or her head up and around to gain more information, but the child with limited movement or strength is visually restricted to the surface directly below and in front of him or her. It is easy to vary the viewing distance for students in this position through the use of easels or inclined surfaces.

Side Lying. Side lying allows the child to have mobility in one arm to manipulate objects. It encourages the use of the weaker arm and increased control with the stronger arm, depending on the side on which the child is positioned. Visually, it permits a broader perspective of the environment than either the prone or the supine position, and it gives the child experience seeing the world from another angle other than the one viewed from a vertical position. Children with a field or acuity loss in one eye may experience greater visual limitations if the eye with the field loss is on top in this position.

Sitting. Vertical positioning is desirable because it invites socialization, uses gravity to encourage body and trunk control, and is the position in which people without disabilities spend most of their waking hours. For most students with multiple disabilities, a symmetrical position that aligns the spine is best. If this position requires support through adaptive equipment recommended by a physical therapist, the equipment should be used during the functional vision assessment and a regular caregiver should be involved in positioning the student.

Some students have difficulty maintaining head control in vertical positions. Thus, during the functional vision assessment, the evaluator may want to provide more than the normal amount of head support for some activities to allow the child to concentrate fully on visual information and to maintain a constant visual field.

Children who must exert physical effort to gain and maintain head control may experience a visual environment that changes according to their angle and level of view, and their programs should include at least brief periods in which external support is given to keep the visual environment stable.

Standing. Some students who cannot change positions independently will benefit from supported standing to promote normal organic functions and the development of joints, as well as social interactions. As in sitting, support for head control should be considered because it promotes the use of vision. During supported standing, some students with low vision respond better to visual information that is presented vertically on a magnetic board, computer screen, or felt board, so they do not have to bend their necks and shoulders to observe a table surface at hand level. For sitting and standing, an inclined easel or tray often provides the best compromise between visual access and manual control.

For students who have independent means of mobility, it is important to observe their use of vision both while moving and while performing stationary tasks. Because control of their heads and eyes may vary during movement, many students may evidence less efficiency while moving or may not be able to recognize or select landmarks that they easily recognize when they are in one place. Especially children who have a cortical visual impairment may respond differently to objects in the environment, depending on the movement of the objects and their own bodies.

In addition, for some children with sensory integrative dysfunction, physical activity such as swinging, twirling, or rolling, seems to increase their ability to use vision. This factor should be considered only if it has been discussed with a physical or occupational therapist. However, the use of vision after a normal level of physical activity should be observed for all children.

With respect to positioning and movement, the functional vision assessment should incorporate activities in several situations. The conditions under which the child most effectively uses vision should be noted, as should any changes in visual responses that occur with changes in position or movement.

Temperament and Biobehavioral States

Although all people experience short- and long-term variations in temperament and biobehavioral states, these changes are especially important to consider for students with severe disabilities because they may communicate the times when the students are able to receive and process new experiences, feel comfortable or uncomfortable, and can better integrate information from all the senses. Biobehavioral states were first defined as a range of conditions, from sleeping to being awake to crying in unimpaired infants (Wolff, 1959) and have since been interpreted as strong indicators of the state of the central nervous system (see, for example, Guess et al., 1990). The child's ability to use vision and to seek or respond actively to visual stimuli is likely to be greater in the active states, and the assessment of visual function may be impossible when the child is sleeping or drowsy. Regular patterns of biobehavioral states have been identified in individual students with severe disabilities (Guess et al., 1990), and these variations should be considered in planning observations related to vision.

Variations in temperament can also affect childrens' responses during assessments. A child who is sensitive and easily upset by any change in the environment may not be able to tolerate any interaction with an unfamiliar person or the introduction of any materials that increase the sensation to vision or the other senses. For children who demonstrate unusual behaviors, including extreme aggression or self-abuse, it is important for the evaluator to be aware of the approach to these behaviors that the educational team has decided on. When it is not advisable for an unfamiliar evaluator to work directly with a student, the primary caregiver can conduct specific activities while the evaluator observes.

Individual variations in states of arousal and temperament also support the need for an as-

sessment to be based on observations and activities over several different periods. In this way, there is sufficient opportunity to notice visual variations that accompany physiological fluctuations.

After reviewing background information, the evaluator should have an understanding of the student's individual physical and psychological characteristics. Sidebar 10.1 presents some general questions that an evaluator should consider before observing or interacting with a student.

Assessing Near Vision

The use of near vision may be more functional and therefore easier to assess than distance vision in students who do not walk, crawl, or have other means of mobility. For these children, the immediate world is more meaningful, since they can interact with it, and they will attend more often to objects that are within arm's reach.

The assessment is not a series of structured tasks but, rather, the observation of vision within several contexts, both familiar and unfamiliar. It should never take place in a single session, because factors such as medication, biobehavioral state, and differences in temperament can influence a child's response to the degree that the behaviors may not represent the range of the child's capabilities. Initially, observations should be made of activities that are preferred or highly motivating to the child, although it is also important to observe the child during less preferred functional activities, such as self-care.

Students with multiple disabilities frequently vary their use of vision according to the purpose of an activity. For example, one student may use vision efficiently in a task that involves small, manipulative objects, but may not look at the faces of others during social activities. These variations in the purpose of using vision should also be described in a functional vision report. The following section describes visual behaviors that should be noted during the assessment.

Questions to Consider When Assessing the Vision of a Child with Multiple Disabilities

Communication	Does the child intentionally communicate about what he or she sees? What behaviors give information about the child's vision?
Medical diagnosis	Does the child have a medical condition that may affect vision? If so, how?
Medication	Does the child take medication regularly or occasionally? How does the medication affect his or her vision?
Motivation	What materials does the child prefer for leisure activities? How does the child express his or her preferences?
Physical state	Is the child more alert at some times than at others? When is he or she the most responsive and the least responsive? Does the child demonstrate more visual control after physical activities?
Positioning	What is the child's preferred position? Does the child use vision differently in various positions? Can he or she change body or head positions to alter vision?
Sensory responses	Is the child hypersensitive or hyposensitive to sensory stimuli? Does the child demonstrate unusual sensory responses (such as intense startle, tactile defensiveness, or attraction to strong visual effects)? What is his or her preferred learning mode?
Social interaction	Does the student react positively to unfamiliar people? Does he or she visually or otherwise distinguish between familiar and unfamiliar people? Is the child motivated by social interactions, or does he or she find them aversive?

Ocular Reflexes: Blink and Pupillary Reflex

Blink. Most people blink immediately when a hand is moved toward their faces or across the visual field near their eyes. It is important to keep the fingers apart when evaluating a child's blink reaction because the child may also blink in response to the movement of air caused by the hands. A silent stimulus should be used to evaluate a blink response because blinking to a sound is a normal response that could be confused with a blink to a visual stimulus. If the blink occurs after a delay of several seconds, if it is notable in only one eye, or if it occurs only some of the time, the child may have neurological differences that affect this reflex. If no blink occurs in response to stimuli after several presentations, and there is no compensatory behavior, such as moving the head or shoulders away from the stimuli, blindness is a possibility.

Pupillary Reflex. At some time during the assessment, a moderate light source (for example, a penlight or a sunlit window) can be introduced at 8 to 10 inches from the eyes. Normally, constriction (a decrease in size) of the pupil occurs in both eyes, even if the light source is introduced only to one. When light is withdrawn, the pupils should dilate or increase in size. Also, the two pupils should be equally round. If no constriction and dilation of the pupils occur (fixed pupils), if they occur slowly or spasmodically (hippus), or if they only occur in one eye (Marcus-Gunn syndrome), neurological dysfunction is often the cause. These latter responses imply that the child may be light sensitive or may require increased light to compensate for the inability of the brain to govern pupillary function.

Children who have conditions such as aniridia or coloboma are not good candidates for this type of testing of pupillary reflex. When assessing children who have photophobia, the penlight should be directed toward the forehead, rather than directly into the eye. Pupillary differences in children who have dark irises may be seen by shining the light toward the side of the eyes.

However, normal pupil function does not rule out blindness. The pupils may respond normally to light because they are controlled by sensors that connect with the brain, yet the child may be blind for reasons related to other parts of the eye and brain.

Attention, Identification, and Recognition of Objects

One goal of evaluating near vision is to identify how much detail a child can see. This knowledge is important so that materials for use with the child can be prepared correctly. It can also be determined whether the child should be evaluated by an eye care specialist to check for the presence of a refractive error. Information is gained through observations of the child's behaviors and responses to objects in the environment. During the assessment, the evaluator can present collections of small objects and toys that have been organized and measured beforehand to the child and calculate approximate acuities using the equivalencies presented in Chapter 8. However, what is more important, this activity can provide a basis for identifying what materials a child can easily see during daily activities.

For children who put small objects in their mouths, small edibles can be used to evaluate their responses. The teacher of students with visual impairments should, of course, check with the classroom teacher and parents before presenting any edibles to make sure that the child is allowed to eat them. Raisins, pieces of cereal, miniature marshmallows, breath mints, grapes,

and slices of carrot can be presented against high- and low-contrast surfaces, at various distances, and from the front and the side. In the functional vision assessment, the size and color of each object should be reported, as well as its distance from the child's eyes and the color of the surface on which it is placed.

It is also helpful to evaluate near vision responses with either eye separately, particularly if the child has strabismus or if there is reason to suspect a strong preference for one eye. Covering one eye is aversive for many children, but if they will tolerate it, a mild adhesive patch or cloth patch on a string, purchased at a pharmacy, or a ski cap with one eye left open can be used; some children may prefer to hold a card or hand in front of their eyes for a few seconds. It is important to note whether the child tolerates the covering of either eye better, because if he or she does not protest the covering of one eye, it may indicate that the child does not depend on that eye for visual activities. If the child tolerates the covering of one eye for short periods, his or her performance of activities like finding small objects or putting pennies in a bank can provide information about visual competence using either eye.

Activities for the Observation of Near Vision

Although reading printed letters also requires good visual acuity, many other activities that are part of typical routines require good near point vision. Therefore, it is important to include a variety of activities that require near vision in the functional vision assessment to observe a child's use of near vision in functional contexts. Some common near point activities are these:

◆ spotting small pieces of food on high- and low-contrast surfaces
◆ identifying or sorting coins and putting them in a bank
◆ wiping crumbs from a counter top or floor
◆ responding to photographs of friends or family members

◆ retrieving a dropped button or paper clip
◆ finding a picture of a particular product in a newspaper or magazine advertisement
◆ cleaning a spot from clothing or a tabletop.

Assessing Distance Vision

Formal Procedures

Many children with multiple disabilities cannot respond to typical vision screening procedures because of their mental abilities, communicative difficulties, or attentional problems. The screening procedures presented in Sidebar 10.2 can be helpful in conducting a functional vision assessment. All these procedures, except the rolling balls and preferential viewing (sometimes called preferential looking) procedures, require the child to be able to match or make a choice, which assumes a developmental level of approximately 24 months or higher.

Informal Procedures

The most representative information about distance vision is gained from observations of a student in real situations: attending to light sources or brightly colored objects, turning toward people who move into the field of vision, and responding to a wave or gesture from across the room. Some students can identify objects by pointing or turning toward them on request, such as "Show me the bulletin board. Walk over to the mirror." Others can be encouraged to move toward a desired object, which will indicate that they have recognized it. Placing a cracker or a wind-up toy on the other side of the room while the child is not looking provides an opportunity to notice the distance from which the child spots an object and begins to move toward it.

It is more difficult to evaluate distance vision in students who have no means of mobility and no language system. For these students, head and eye orientation and behavioral changes that indicate that they are interested in an object can provide the best cues.

Activities for the Assessment of Distance Vision

A variety of situations provide the opportunity to observe a student's responses to objects at a distance. The following are among the kinds of responses that can yield information about a student's distance vision:

◆ responses to and imitation of body movements, facial expressions, and hand gestures
◆ interest in moving vehicles, rolling balls, airplanes, and birds
◆ attention to movement and activity outside windows
◆ head and eye movements in large areas, such as grocery stores, malls, sports fields, or theaters
◆ anticipation of obstacles and changes in surfaces when walking.

Activities can be devised to evaluate responses to small objects. For example, small mints, stickers, paper clips, or other tiny objects on contrasting and noncontrasting surfaces can be provided to watch a student's search-and-recognition patterns. Distances between hidden objects and a search point can be measured and marked with tape before the activity begins, so the distances can be estimated.

Evaluating Visual Field Responses

Observations of a child's visual field at near point should also emphasize functional contexts for the use of peripheral and central vision. The point at which a child turns toward a person approaching from either side, a spoonful of food being presented, or a windup toy moving in from the side will indicate whether the child attends equally well from either side and notices objects in all quadrants of the visual field. A teacher's observation of the use of vision in visual fields does not replace a clinical evaluation, but is used to determine how a child is aware of and acts on objects in the visual field.

Screening Techniques for Students with Developmental Disabilities

Preferential Viewing (Preferential Looking)

This technique is based on the assumption that people will attend to a patterned stimulus in preference to a plain one. The procedure can be administered using technological devices that present striped and plain areas or cards that display plain and patterned squares. If the child looks immediately to the patterned side, then it is assumed that he or she can distinguish the stripes of the pattern. When the stripes are so close together that the child does not look at one side more than another, then it is assumed that the child cannot resolve detail at that level of acuity. This procedure is most effective for children who are between two months and two years; children who are developmentally above two years do not attend well to it.

Rolling Balls

This is a subsection of the Sheridan Test for Young Children and Retardates (STYCAR), which consists of styrofoam balls of various sizes. The balls are rolled in front of the child, and the response at 10 feet is noted. This test is appropriate for children who are developmentally below 18 months because it depends on an attentional response. It can also be used informally at various distances to record a child's response to a specific size of ball at a specific distance. Young children are often intrigued by the problem of finding increasingly smaller balls rolled toward them. (Available from Nelson Canada, 1120 Birchmount Road, Scarborough, Ontario M1K #564.)

Miniature Toys

This test, also a subsection of the STYCAR, consists of pairs of small toys: cars, dolls, airplanes, chairs, and several sizes of silverware. Acuities can be estimated on the basis of the child's ability to select the toy that matches one presented 10 feet away. Because it requires matching, it is best for children who are developmentally in the 2–3-year range.

HOTV

HOTV is a 10-foot wall chart that includes four figures: H, O, T, and V. Children do not need to recognize the letters to respond; a card with the four letters on it can be placed in front of them so a pointing response can indicate recognition. Because it requires matching responses to abstract symbols, the HOTV is best for children who are developmentally above 3 years. (Available from Goodlite Company, 1540 Hannah Avenue, Forest Park, IL 60130.)

LEA Symbol Tests

This system includes wall charts, near vision symbol books, contrast sensitivity charts, and training materials that incorporate a circle, square, house, and apple. Responses can be matching or verbal. Tests are highly adaptable for children with language limitations, and are intended for individuals over two years developmentally. (Available from Precision Vision, 745 North Harvard Avenue, Villa Park, IL 60181.)

Parsons Visual Acuity Test

This procedure uses a plus lens to simulate distance vision with cards presented at near point and often encourages attention from individuals (children or adults) who are too distractible to attend at a distance. Behavioral shaping techniques are used to teach the respondent to point to a specific symbol. It is best for individuals who are developmentally above two years because it requires a selecting response.

Structured activities can be tried to document the child's responses to objects in the periphery. One such method is a confrontation test, which is best accomplished by two evaluators, one seated behind and one seated in front of the child. The evaluator who faces the child attempts to engage the child's attention, so the child will continue to face forward. A sticker or a spot of bright color on the nose of the evaluator who is facing the child may help capture the child's interest.

The evaluator seated behind the child presents a small, bright toy or object at the end of a stick. A dark stick less than a quarter-inch wide should be used because it is important that the toy at the tip of the stick, not the stick itself, should be the object that draws the child's attention. From various angles above the child's head, the toy is presented, and the evaluators note the point at which the child's eyes shift from the first evaluator's face to the toy being presented from behind and the contrast between the toy and the background at the point at which the child becomes aware of the toy. It is important for the child to attend again to the evaluator's face before the object is presented from another angle. Langley (1980) suggested another version of this method using a penlight presented at different points on a circle and recording the points of reduced attention.

If only one evaluator is involved, a small mirror can be placed in front of the child and the child can be asked to watch his or her own nose. The evaluator can note the point at which the child turns to one side or the other, using the mirror to check for shifts in gaze. The mirror should be small enough to reflect the child's face but not the stick, the toy, or the arm of the evaluator.

The child's ability to scan an array of objects at near point will also provide information about visual field preferences. Small raisins, pieces of cereal, or coins can be placed on a tray or a tabletop, and the child's search patterns can be observed. Does the child begin by picking up all the objects in the middle? Does the child locate all items in the center and one side but ignore those on the other side? (Field losses on one side often occur among children with unilateral head injuries.) Does the child ignore a cluster of items in the center of the array? (This behavior may indicate a scotoma and the inability to compensate by turning the head.)

As with near vision, opportunities to observe visual field responses at a distance can be found in many natural activities. A child's response to a passing car while riding in an automobile or his or her inclination to watch birds or airplanes can provide evidence of the awareness of objects moving at a distance. Planned activities, such as ball games or flashlight chase games, can allow the evaluator to vary the size, intensity, and contrast effects of the stimulus to gather further information about how readily a child responds to objects moving in and out of his or her visual field. Many children with neurological differences need more time to turn toward a stimulus approaching from the side, so observations of both rapid and slow stimuli should be made to represent variations in the child's response patterns.

Observing Eye Movements and Coordination

Many children with multiple disabilities demonstrate a strabismus or deviation of the eyes because the muscles of the eyes, like those of the rest of the body, vary in tone and tension. When the brain dysfunction causes cerebral palsy, variations in eye muscles may also result. Deviations of gaze may be consistent or may occur only when a child is positioned or moving in a particular way.

Observations of the movements of a child's eyes can be made during activities that require scanning an array of objects or one large object, as well as those that require tracking moving objects. Watching a person walking by, a rolling ball or toy, or a moving car may elicit horizontal tracking movements of the eyes. A bouncing ball, an airplane rising in the sky, or a falling object may stimulate vertical tracking. Vertical tracking may be especially difficult for children with certain types of cerebral palsy, particularly athetosis.

Having a child scan an array of pictures, a store window, or faces of classmates can yield information about whether he or she uses smooth eye movements. Many children with neurological dysfunction have difficulty sustaining horizontal eye movements across the midline, and this difficulty should be noted in a report of visual function. The child who cannot sustain movement across the midline or who moves his or her eyes in a series of irregular movements may benefit from opportunities to practice in real-life and motivating contexts, but many students will never demonstrate completely normal eye movements because of damage to the central nervous system; in these cases, compensatory head movements can be encouraged.

It is also helpful to check convergence responses to determine whether the child uses both eyes equally. It is easy to check these responses by moving a small object on the end of a pencil toward the child's eyes directly in front of the bridge of the nose. At about 4 or 5 inches away, the eyes should turn inward. If one eye seems to turn inward more than another or does not converge at all, it is possible that a strabismus is present, which may mean that the child uses one eye more than the other. Individual assessment of responses in both eyes separately may provide further information.

Eye movements can vary in the level of intentionality. Some eye movements, like a glance toward a sound, are incidental, almost involuntary. Others are directed, as when an adult's voice says, "Look at that bird!" Still others are self-initiated; the child uses them purposefully to seek information or to explore his or her surroundings or react to an object seen incidentally. Thus, it may be useful to record the motivation for a child's eye movements, as well as the child's capabilities.

Testing Responses to Special Visual Effects

Special visual effects can elicit different responses from the child with multiple disabilities. Reactions to lighting can vary from intense interest, as when children flick their fingers before light or gaze into lights, to aversion to lighting, when children avoid even normal light sources. During an assessment, it is helpful to offer a child the opportunity to use or respond to flashlights of different colors and sizes to determine his or her preferences. However, it is important to remember that light sources, such as flashlights, are not instructional tools; rather, they have a functional application only as a means of finding one's way in a darkened environment or lighting a dimly lit task. Watching a flashlight is not a functional goal for a student, and if flashlights or special lighting effects are used in programming, there should be a valid reason for using them.

Responses to color should also be evaluated as part of the functional vision assessment. Children who do not name or identify colors may be able to sort or match objects by color, and those who do not sort or match may show their awareness of color by choosing objects of a contrasting hue from an array of similarly colored objects. This latter procedure can be tried in a controlled situation by presenting two objects of the same color; covering them with a sheet of paper; exposing them again; and, after several presentations, substituting a different colored version of the same object for one that was previously seen. The child's attention will be drawn to the new object because of its color. For this procedure to be reliable, however, the colors chosen should be relatively similar in shade and brightness and the child should have established object permanence.

Perceptual features, such as lighting, color, patterns, and other visual effects, should also be observed in functional tasks. The child who always chooses red and yellow toys, prefers clothing with lively patterns, or seeks dimly lit areas is communicating his or her preferred visual conditions. This information can be used to encourage more functional responses.

The assessment of vision in a child with multiple and visual disabilities requires the sampling of vision during a variety of activities, during

SIDEBAR 10.3

Instruments for the Assessment of Vision of Children with Severe Disabilities

These instruments are appropriate for use in the assessment of vision in children with severe and multiple disabilities, including those who use nonsymbolic communication.

Erhardt Developmental Vision Assessment

This instrument (Erhardt, 1989) to evaluate visual skills was developed by an occupational therapist who focuses on the integration of vision and motor function. It provides a checklist for recording developmental responses and reflexes as they compare to normally developing infants. This information can supplement the results of the functional vision assessment but is not intended as a basis for program development.

Functional Vision Screening Inventory for the Multiple and Severely Handicapped

This instrument (Langley, 1980) includes a short screening procedure, a detailed assessment protocol, suggestions for activities to encourage the use of vision, and a list of related resources. It is a comprehensive document that addresses visual development in individuals whose skills are generally below the developmental age of 2 years.

Individualized Assessment of Visual Efficiency

This instrument (Langley, in press) provides a detailed inventory of visual goals and objectives for children who have developmental delays and visual differences. It is particularly well suited to those who have the visual behaviors associated with cortical visual impairment or delayed visual maturation.

Vision Assessment and Program Manual for Severely Handicapped and/or Deaf-Blind Students

This instrument (Utley et al., 1981) describes behavioral and observational methods of evaluating vision in students with severe disabilities and approaches to integrating visual skills into functional instructional programs.

---

different times, in different settings, and with different people. Several instruments that are valuable for assessing vision among children with additional disabilities are listed in Sidebar 10.3. Although these instruments can support and supplement the assessment process, no one instrument can specify the best assessment process for an individual child. Sidebar 10.4 presents a suggested sequence of steps to be followed in carrying out the functional vision assessment. In addition, a sample report of a functional vision assessment is provided in the appendix to this chapter.

APPROACHES TO INSTRUCTION IN THE USE OF FUNCTIONAL VISION

Selecting Visual Goals

Instruction in the use of vision makes two assumptions regarding learning and vision: that an individual can improve visual efficiency through applied use and practice, and that many tasks can be more efficiently performed through the use of vision. These two assumptions provide a founda-

Steps in Preparing the Functional Vision Assessment

The following procedures should be carried out over an extended period, not on a single day. Although gathering background information and undertaking observation should always be the first procedures, the order of subsequent steps can vary according to the needs of the individual.

1. Gather background information.
   a. Review the student's records.
   b. Interview the family and professionals.

2. Observe the student during at least three daily routines in different environments at different times of the day (for example, during mealtime, dressing, and traveling to class).

3. Interact with the student in a highly motivating activity that involves materials at near point.
   a. Use a variety of materials at different distances.
   b. Use materials against high- and low-contrast backgrounds.
   c. Use materials at various points in the child's visual fields.

4. Interact with the student in a highly motivating activity that involves distance vision.
   a. Use a variety of materials at different distances.
   b. Observe the student's responses to people approaching.
   c. Observe the student's responses to objects moving across his or her visual fields.

5. Conduct formal procedures (when appropriate).
   a. Formal acuity screening procedures.
   b. Blink reflex check.
   c. Pupillary response check.
   d. Convergence check.
   e. Confrontation testing.

6. Carry out follow-up activities to probe areas of inconsistency.

7. Write a report with recommendations for implementing a program.

---

tion for learning for the child with visual and multiple disabilities.

Instructional programming in regard to vision now emphasizes the active use of vision in functional tasks as a means of enabling interaction with the environment, rather than the passive stimulation of vision. The term *vision stimulation* has sometimes been misinterpreted as the presentation of visual stimuli to increase visual ability. For example, the practice of placing a child in a room and presenting blinking lights against shiny surfaces is often assumed to be visually stimulating; however, this is no more a learning experience than the practice of allowing institutionalized adults with developmental disabilities to watch television for hours, as is common in many understaffed institutions. Although the presentation of visual effects may actually enhance the development of neurological and optical structures during the first year or two of life, the presentation of visual material with no expectation of a response will not result in applied learning.

Instructional goals for the use of vision should be selected to improve efficiency in performing tasks and in gaining greater satisfaction in life. Therefore, functional activities are usually the primary contexts for encouraging the use of vision. To enhance the use of vision through direct instruction or consultative support, the teacher of students with visual impairments must be aware of major goals in the child's general education plan.

Functionality

The most important tasks to perform visually are those that are functional, in other words, those that someone would have to perform for a child if the child could not do them independently. Although such tasks as putting on shoes, feeding oneself, or selecting a specific box of cereal can all be performed without vision, since blind individuals routinely carry them out, the use of vision may increase the efficiency in performing them and requires fewer adaptations.

Visual skills that are needed to perform a task are identified and the child's competence in these skills is evaluated using information from the functional vision assessment, as well as from the specific activity. A skill is a specific behavior that is needed in a variety of activities, for example, tracking a moving target or adjusting one's viewing distance. Visual skills should be integrated into activities, as in the program developed for Steven, aged 7.

> Steven has a field loss on his left side because of a head injury, and the educational team identified an important compensatory vision skill for him: turning his head slightly to the left so he can scan the left peripheral field better. That skill, scanning to the left, can be incorporated into several functional tasks to encourage Steven to generalize the skill. It may be practiced during snack time by placing his crackers on his left side; after school, while watching for his bus to approach from his left side; and during a walk with friends, while picking dandelions. Participating in all these are activities that other 7-year-old children do and scanning while doing so helps Steven receive more information with less assistance from others.

Frequency of Use

It is often easier to notice the many activities that students with multiple disabilities cannot do

without considering which tasks they can do. Along with functionality, an important criterion for setting a goal is the frequency of use. Activities that are regular parts of daily routines should take priority over those that are not needed as often, as in the case of Jamie.

> For Jamie, who has a physical disability, it may not be as important to distinguish between objects at a distance as it is to reach for small objects that she sees on the tray in front of her. Being able to reach for what she sees will help her to feed herself finger foods, pick up her own soap and toothbrush, and play with a toy. Because she spends most of her time indoors and does not have an independent means of mobility, Jamie may not use distance viewing skills as often, and the educational team may consider them a lower priority. Although both are important, Jamie and the team will work harder on the near point tasks because she uses those skills more often in her immediate environment.

Active Participation

Finally, skills that encourage the child's active participation usually take priority over more passive responses. Children with multiple disabilities are often accustomed to having things done for them and to them. A vital concept for them to learn is that they can initiate action and act on their environments. Therefore, tasks and activities that involve moving toward, reaching for, or manipulating an object that is seen are usually considered more important than are those that involve only watching. Even though everyone's life includes some activities that are relatively passive, such as watching television or listening to an audiotape, the satisfying aspects of these tasks may be abstract and not meaningful to children with severe disabilities. These children will learn more effectively if the activities provide the opportunity to interact physically with the world they see around them.

Appropriate activities for instruction should be identified by the entire educational team including the child and his or her family. Priorities among the activities will be established according to the parents', student's, and staff's preferences; frequency of occurrence; safety; and social acceptability (Nietupski & Hamre-Nietupski, 1987).

In setting visual goals, the teacher of students with visual impairments should select skills on the basis of the child's visual ability as demonstrated in the functional vision assessment. These skills can be chosen according to whether they are needed to perform functional activities, whether those activities are frequently performed, and whether they encourage active participation by the child. These goals can then be integrated into the child's learning routines.

Integrating Visual Goals into Routines

For most children with multiple disabilities, learning involves routines that are repeated many times so that the child learns to anticipate actions and participate in them. Learning routines are of two types: functional routines for life-relevant activities, such as washing hands, and social or joint action routines for interaction with others, such as turning to see a person who is speaking. Programming for children with multiple disabilities should involve both types of routines, and vision-enhancement activities can be integrated into both.

Once functional learning activities are identified, the teacher of students with visual impairments should observe a student without disabilities carrying out the routines and should identify the "critical visual moment"—the moment when vision is important to perform a step in a routine (Goetz & Gee, 1987). For example, during tooth brushing, a critical visual moment is just before one reaches for the toothbrush in the holder or on the sink. Vision is needed to determine visually where the brush is located and to direct one's reach toward the brush; to do this step tactilely would require more time, although it could be done. Other critical moments in that task may include looking at the toothbrush while applying toothpaste and while placing it under the faucet for rinsing.

At other times in the same task, vision may not be necessary. Most people do not use vision actually to brush their teeth; they may look elsewhere—at a television set, at the face of someone speaking to them, or in a mirror.

Identifying the critical visual moment is important so the use of vision can be prompted and reinforced only at this point in the routine. Sometimes, caregivers assume that better visual efficiency can be achieved by encouraging children to watch the material throughout the entire task. However, it is important to remember that staring at material is not a natural behavior for most tasks and that the sustained use of vision can be an aversive and purposeless experience. Unless the material is unfamiliar and visual examination is motivated by natural curiosity, constant regard is not appropriate for typical functional activities.

Social routines, often called joint-action routines (Carreiro & Townsend, 1987), serve a different purpose from functional routines. The primary goal in these routines is to establish a satisfying interaction among two or more individuals. Unlike functional routines, which are often performed independently when mastered, social routines always require at least two people. Social routines may include games, such as ring-around-the-rosy, for young children, and watching a sports activity for both children and adults. The use of vision in joint-action routines can be considered with respect to how well it supports the objective of interaction. Eye contact, discrimination of gestures, and imitation of facial expressions are pieces of visual information that are critical to interaction. As in functional routines, these behaviors and responses may occur only at specific points during a routine. The times when vision is essential or helpful in a task should be identified before beginning instruction.

In teaching a child to respond to visual signals, one must first decide whether visual information will act as a stimulus, a reinforcer, or both. For example, 10-year-old Patty does not look at her mother's face when her mother calls her name, but she smiles when she hears her name, which indicates that she does experience pleasure related to another person. Patty is prompted to turn toward her mother's face when her mother waves a brightly colored scarf beside her cheek and then is praised for turning to her mother. In this case, vision has been used to produce the response, with the bright scarf acting as a stimulus. Vision is also a reinforcer here because Patty's mother smiles and shakes the scarf when Patty looks. Over time, Patty may begin to turn toward her mother's face on a voice cue alone, and the scarf will no longer be needed or can be replaced by brightly colored earrings, which will continue to attract her attention. She also may be reinforced by her mother's smile, either with or without verbal praise.

In tasks in which a visual effect or object is used to attract attention, two assumptions are made: the child has the physical ability to see the stimulus, and the child wants to look at the stimulus. The second assumption is important to consider with respect to students with multiple disabilities. Many such children do not enjoy highly stimulating visual effects, such as lights or moving reflective stimuli, especially when they show other signs of sensory defensiveness, such as a reluctance to touch moist or sticky substances. If one uses a visual effect to try to gain the attention of a student who dislikes using vision, a response will not be produced, and the student may become less attentive. For such a child, a mild visual effect, along with a strong positive effect from another source of sensory information, can be used until the child begins to accept more intense visual effects. For example, a puff of air can be produced from a brightly colored hair dryer each time Charlie looks toward the dryer. Even though the bright color may not be pleasing, he may begin to tolerate it because it is paired with the puff of air, something he does enjoy.

Learning Skill Clusters

Sometimes behaviors are learned in sequence because the sequences can be applied across many activities. A chain of skills that are normally performed in the same order during many activities is called a skill cluster (for information on

the use of skill clusters in instruction, see Helmstetter, Murphy-Herd, Roberts, & Guess, 1984).

One common skill cluster that involves vision is looking, reaching, and grasping. Some children with central nervous system dysfunction may reach before they look, using vision as a confirming sense, rather than as a way of locating an object before reaching. These students need to be prompted to look and then to reach and grasp during several applied contexts in a day before they may begin to use vision to locate objects before reaching. Some of these contexts are as follows:

- *During mealtime:* Look at finger foods, reach for them, and grasp them.
- *During leisure time:* Look at a desired object, reach for it, and grasp it.
- *While swimming:* Look for a pool toy, reach for it, and grasp it.
- *At bathtime:* Look toward the soap, reach for it, and grasp it.

Another skill cluster is localize, track, and grasp (Helmstetter et al., 1984). It can be used in these contexts:

- *When putting on a coat:* Localize to the name in a cubby, track the coat, and grasp it.
- *When shaking hands with the teacher:* Localize to the name, track the teacher from side to front, grasp his or her hand, and shake it.
- *When taking a book bag from the teacher:* Localize to the name, track the bag, and grasp it.

(For more information on such skills as tracking, see Sidebar 9.2 in Chapter 9.)

Increasing the Use of Vision in Daily Routines

After the educational team has determined which visual goals are important for a student and

<table>
<tr><td colspan="3">

Prompts to Encourage the Use of Vision
</td></tr>
<tr>
<td>Physical prompts</td>
<td colspan="2">Prompts in which the instructor touches the student to facilitate a response

Examples: Touching a student's cheek to move his or her head
Tapping a student's wrist to initiate reaching</td>
</tr>
<tr>
<td>Auditory prompts</td>
<td colspan="2">Prompts in which the instructor creates a sound to encourage a student to respond

Examples: Tapping a shoe on the floor to attract the student's attention
Saying, "Look at the spoon"</td>
</tr>
<tr>
<td>Augmentative visual cues</td>
<td colspan="2">Prompts that increase visual effects to encourage the student to respond

Examples: Shining a flashlight beam to enhance an object
Pointing toward an object</td>
</tr>
<tr>
<td>Time out</td>
<td colspan="2">Prompting by removing the focus object and restoring it when the student looks

Example: Removing a cup and replacing it when the student looks to see where it has gone.</td>
</tr>
</table>

Source: B. Utley, L. Goetz, K. Gee, M. Baldwin, & W. Sailor, *Vision Assessment and Program Manual for Severely Handicapped and/or Deaf-blind Students* (Eric Document Reproduction Service No. ED 250-840) (Reston, VA: Council for Exceptional Children, 1981).

SIDEBAR 10.5

---

where vision is needed, they plan how to increase the use of vision during the performance of tasks. Many students with multiple disabilities do not use vision as often as they might to be efficient during a task. They may not do so because they do not understand that vision can improve their efficiency, because using vision is unpleasant to them, because their neurological characteristics make it difficult to use more than one sense at a time, or because they have not had experiences using vision for a task. In other words, they may avoid using vision so they can more easily process tactile information or attend to sounds they hear.

To encourage a child to use vision, a prompt must be selected to shape the response, and a reinforcer must be present to maintain the response. Prompts can vary according to a child's medium of receptive communication and the strength of guidance that is needed. Utley, Goetz, Gee, Baldwin, and Sailor (1981) identified four types of prompts that can be effective in increasing the use of vision in a task: physical prompts, auditory prompts, augmentative visual cues, and time out (see Sidebar 10.5).

Physical prompts provide the instructor with the most control and, therefore, may be met with resistance or perceived as uncomfortable by a child who is tactilely defensive. However, they may be necessary for a child who is learning a new behavior and who does not respond to auditory prompts. Physical prompts can range from physically guiding a student through the desired movements to touching him or her briefly to signal initiation of the activity.

Auditory prompts, which can be verbal ("Look, Terry!) or nonverbal (tapping a cup on the table), call a child's attention to a stimulus. A verbal prompt assumes that the child understands words as a reference because the sound is not produced from the same source as the object. In other words, when an adult says, "Look, Terry!" the child must understand that the words direct attention to something (a plate? a dog running past?) that is somewhere beyond the speaker's immediate vicinity. Otherwise, the prompt, "Look, Terry" will call attention to the speaker, not to the referent object. If the student does not understand the meaning of words, an auditory prompt originating with the referent itself will be more effective. Such a nonverbal prompt can be created on or with the object being noticed, so it will be more successful for the child who does not understand spoken communication.

Although verbal prompts, such as "Look at the . . .," are routinely used, it is important to remember that these prompts deliver little information for the student whose language is nonsymbolic. Even children who are beginning to use words can be confused by an abstract imperative like "Look!" When directed to "Look with your eyes," one child whom the author knows touched her eyelids with her fingers; she clearly understood the reference to eyes, but had not connected her eyes to the act of looking.

Augmentative visual cues can be used for a child who responds to visual effects to draw attention to materials or to an activity. They also vary in complexity; a child need not understand the reference to attend to a flashlight beam, but pointing will serve as a prompt only if the child understands its referential message.

Time out involves removal of an object when the student does not look toward it. It may be helpful when the student uses touch in preference to vision and when there is evidence that the use of vision may improve the efficiency of a task. When a child begins to search tactilely, the instructor removes the cup or spoon, causing the student to look toward it; when the student looks, the instructor replaces the object immediately, reinforcing the use of vision.

These types of prompts can be used to build the use of vision into activities when students have demonstrated visual ability but do not habitually use it during activities. Once visual attention begins to occur regularly when students are prompted, the prompts should be delivered at intervals and finally not at all. Overprompting or prompting for too long a time can make students dependent on prompts, which makes it more difficult for them to make choices and to generalize.

PROMOTION OF FUNCTIONALITY AND GENERALIZATION

Identifying Functional and Age-appropriate Activities

Vision serves a variety of purposes: It brings information, helps people to know when something is in their pathway, facilitates communication with others, and provides entertainment. Although most activities in life can also be performed tactilely or auditorally, as they are by people who are functionally blind, it is usually more efficient to use vision when it is available. Because vision provides simultaneous and constant information about objects at a distance from the viewer, it allows for a level of anticipation and planning that cannot be gained through the other senses.

Functional and age-appropriate activities should form the basis of instruction for the enhancement of the vision of students with multiple disabilities. A useful perspective can be provided by interviewing students without disabilities about their daily activities. Although some activities, such as reading, may not be appropriate for students with multiple disabilities or developmental delays, other activities may have elements that can be performed with or without adaptations by students with disabilities. Daily routines such as playing with a dog, combing one's hair, or setting the table are real-life activities that involve the use of vision and would be appropriate for students of various ages and abilities.

Although functionality and age-appropriateness are important priorities in identifying tasks to be learned, they should not limit the choices of activities for children who have not yet developed cause-and-effect responses or cannot use objects functionally. For those with profound mental disabilities, the most important priority is to include activities that gain their attention. For example, if a 15-year-old student attends visually to a pinwheel and reaches eagerly for it, he or she should not be prohibited from using it because it is inappropriate for his or her age. Although an effort can be made to locate more age-appropriate objects with similar visual qualities, interacting with the pinwheel can be considered a means of chosen recreation for this student.

Establishing Priorities among Activities

Activities that are selected for instructional consideration may be based on several factors:

The family's preference. Activities that are important to a family should be considered high priorities. A family who wants a child to learn to select matching colors for clothing or to look for toys and put them away in a toy box has identified activities in which vision plays a major role.

The child's preference. Regardless of their functional levels, most children express preferences. Some children with multiple disabilities have preferences, such as an excessive interest in lights or rapidly moving objects, that may not be appropriate. Although such interests should not be encouraged for long periods, they can sometimes be incorporated into functional tasks or brief recreational activities. For example, young children who flick their fingers in front of lights may be interested in cause-and-effect toys with lighted features, and older children may be taught to operate a slide projector.

Frequency of occurrence. The use of vision during activities that are carried out at least once a day should be a primary consideration. Feeding routines, dressing routines, and toileting routines are examples of such activities, and vision can be used to increase the efficiency of some steps in such routines.

Safety. The use of vision to ensure safety, especially in unknown environments, should be a strong consideration in setting instructional priorities. The ability to anticipate visually, to recog-

nize drop-offs and changes in surfaces, and to avoid obstacles are important for the use of vision. For students who do not move independently, the ability to communicate about objects in their way can also be important as they are moved through space.

Social acceptability. The use of vision to reinforce and continue social contacts is also an important area for consideration. Some students with multiple disabilities do not readily seek or engage in interactions. Reinforcing the use of vision may increase the likelihood of their doing so and thus may increase their ability to engage others in meeting their needs.

Generalizing Visual Skills

Students with multiple disabilities may not easily transfer a skill they learn in one context to others. For instance, teaching students to use vision to locate their spoons at mealtime may not mean that they also look for their combs before combing their hair. Therefore, the most important way to ensure the use of vision in functional contexts is to teach it across contexts, in the situations in which it is actually needed.

In some cases, however, more intensive instruction will take place at particular times of the day because of time constraints; for example, the staff at the school may have the time to reinforce the child's use of vision at lunchtime, but the child's parents may not be able to emphasize it at breakfast because of other responsibilities at that time. More intensive instruction may also be given when a student has the cognitive ability to learn a skill at a specific time and then to begin to transfer it; for instance, a child who is learning to recognize numbers may benefit from some specific time to practice that skill, as well as opportunities to recognize numbers in the environment. When increasing generalization is expected, the following guidelines may be considered:

◆ Begin by teaching in familiar contexts and applying the skills in unfamiliar contexts.

- Teach in highly motivating situations and reinforce generalization to less motivating activities.
- Teach with adaptations and prompting and fade prompts and adaptations as mastery occurs.
- Begin by teaching a new skill at school and then work with the family to transfer it to the home.

Usually, generalization should be planned to maintain and extend the use of a student's goals. Goals that have already been mastered should be regularly reassessed, so a student can use vision more efficiently in a variety of tasks.

SUMMARY

Learning related to vision should take place in functional contexts for the student with visual and other disabilities. The assessment of the use of vision in familiar activities, as well as responses evaluated through specifically designed visual tasks, can yield information related to a student's visual strengths and weaknesses. Skills identified during the assessment should be integrated into learning routines, supported with appropriate adaptations and prompting, and generalized across activities. For students with visual and other disabilities, vision can provide the opportunity for greater interaction with their world and an understanding that they can have an effect on activities around them. For these reasons, careful planning for the use of vision by students of all ability levels is important.

ACTIVITIES

With This Chapter and Other Resources

1. In the vignette that opens the chapter, Eric was becoming more involved in his environment as he increased his use of vision. If you were Eric's teacher of students with visual impairments, what recommendations would you make to Eric's bus driver, after-school day care worker, and physical therapist?

2. Develop a program to shape the wearing of eyeglasses by a student who resists them. How would you reinforce the student for keeping the eyeglasses on? How would you increase the time during which the student wears the eyeglasses?

3. Consider the functional vision assessment for Terry that appears in the appendix to this chapter. Write a lesson plan for promoting his use of vision on all sides.

4. Make a list of objects you would use to assess the functional vision of a 17-year-old student with low vision and moderate-to-severe cognitive and physical disabilities who is functioning at approximately 3 years of age.

In the Community

1. Observe a friend or family member eating a meal. Write down the times when he or she uses vision while eating or talking with others. What are the critical visual moments? When does the person track? Scan? Fixate? Observe other routine activities for the same behaviors.

2. Speak with two parents of children who have visual and multiple disabilities. Ask them to describe the ways in which their children use their near and distance functional vision and how the functional vision assessment is used in planning for their children's education, including the development of visual skills.

With a Person with Low Vision

1. Select a young student with multiple and visual disabilities. List the objects the child sees as part of daily routines, such as a cup, a shoe, and a comb. Make another list of objects that the child likes as playthings, such as pinwheels and windup toys. What visual characteristics do the toys have? How can those characteristics be used to gain the child's attention?

2. Observe a student's use of vision when he or she is working with an occupational or physical therapist. Does the student become more

alert? Demonstrate more eye movements? More nystagmus? Use different head and body movements?

From Your Perspective

A significant number of children with multiple disabilities also have visual impairments. What would be the implications for school systems if all children with multiple disabilities received functional vision assessments?

APPENDIX: SAMPLE FUNCTIONAL VISION ASSESSMENT REPORT

Student: Terry Young
Date of birth: December 21, 1988
Evaluator: Valerie Gross, Teacher of Students with Visual Impairments
School: Rodriguez Elementary School
Date of evaluation: April 22, 1995
Date of report: April 27, 1995

BACKGROUND INFORMATION

Medical. Terry, aged 7, receives special education because of multiple disabilities, including left hemiparesis and developmental delays. He was born after 28 weeks gestation and experienced intraventricular hemorrhage and retinopathy of prematurity. An ophthalmological report of September 1, 1994, described Terry's visual acuity as 20/600 in his left eye and light perception in his right eye. With correction, the activity in his left eye is 20/400. Terry takes Dilantin three times daily to control seizures.

Communication and mobility. Terry uses gestures and a few iconic signs to communicate. He responds to simple verbal requests but does not make requests. He uses an adapted walker for routes of less than 50 feet and can move his own wheelchair along longer routes. Terry wears eyeglasses for all activities and actively searches for them when not wearing them. He participates in social interactions that require turn taking and enjoys praise, attention from other people, and opportunities to use sound- and light-producing toys.

FUNCTIONAL VISION OBSERVATION

Eye structure and reflexes. Terry's eyes appear to be aligned except when he looks toward the left, at which time his left eye turns outward. His pupils react normally to changes in light. Occasional nystagmus was apparent during near tasks. Blink responses to a hand moved toward him were immediate and consistent.

Eye preference. Terry positions materials slightly to his left, which supports the medical report of best acuity in this eye. When asked to search for his eyeglasses with either eye covered, Terry located them visually at three feet with his right eye covered and at one foot with his left eye covered.

Near vision. Terry could locate and touch raisins and Goldfish crackers on a noncontrasting table surface at 12–14 inches. He could visually select his toothbrush from two others of different colors at about 18 inches and could locate quarters on a contrasting table top at about 2 feet, but ignored dimes until he found them tactilely. When searching for near objects, he tilted his head slightly to the right. At mealtime, he located his silverware visually. He also located his eyeglasses visually but reached beyond them and corrected his reach. He shifted his gaze from his cup to his plate when he finished drinking and from a sandwich to the face of a classmate at lunchtime.

Distance vision. Terry smiled at familiar adults about 6 feet away. Using his walker, he adjusted his direction to avoid a wastebasket about 5 feet away. When seated on the floor, Terry noticed and turned away from an 8-inch ball rolling toward him at about 5 feet. When asked to travel toward his teacher, who was about 40 feet away, he moved in the direction of another adult until his teacher called his name. His distance vision allows him to avoid large obstacles when traveling, but does not provide him with enough detail to identify people beyond 10 feet.

Visual fields. Terry attended mainly to objects slightly to the left of center. He turned toward a person approaching quietly from the side at about 45 degrees from the center on the left and 30 degrees from the center on the right. When searching visually for raisins on a table, Terry noticed those in the center of his visual fields but ignored those to both the left and right side until a verbal prompt was given.

Color and perception. Terry selected his own red toothbrush and blue cup from an array of others of different colors. He anticipated and reached for objects in space, but sometimes over-reached for objects against low-contrast backgrounds.

RECOMMENDATIONS

1. Since Terry has not been seen by an ophthalmologist for two years, another visit should be scheduled. Valerie Gross will work with Terry's parents to arrange the appointment. It would be helpful to request information about Terry's visual fields during this visit.

2. Terry sees best in situations with high-contrast backgrounds. During tasks that require the discrimination of fine details, a high-contrast background should be provided.

3. An evaluation by an orientation and mobility instructor and inclusion of the O&M instruc-

tor in Terry's educational team may help to address concerns regarding Terry's ability to increase his speed and efficiency of travel and his parent's concerns about Terry traveling at home.

4. Objects should be placed to the left of center for new or challenging tasks, since this placement makes it easier for him to notice them. For easier tasks or those that are highly motivating, objects should be placed in less preferred fields to encourage Terry to search visually.

5. The use of vision should be prompted and reinforced in daily routines that involve the use of objects at near point. These routines include mealtime, toothbrushing, dressing, and others that the IEP team identifies as priorities.

6. Valerie Gross should continue to participate on Terry's educational team to work on encouraging the use of vision during daily routines.

SUMMARY AND ELIGIBILITY STATEMENT

Terry uses vision to accomplish tasks that present sufficient visual contact and stimulus size. He prefers his left eye and easily notices materials larger than 1 inch that are placed to the left of center. When traveling, he avoids objects over a foot long at about 5 feet away. At near point, he can locate objects as small as a raisin (one-third inch) at about a foot. Terry meets the criteria for eligibility as a visually impaired student, as defined by rules of the State Department of Education.

CHAPTER 11

Selection of Learning and Literacy Media for Children and Youths with Low Vision

Alan J. Koenig

VIGNETTE

José is a second grader with Leber's optic atrophy who has 20/300 acuity and 20 degrees of visual field. His parents describe him as an energetic, bright, and curious boy. His regular class teacher reports that although he does well in his oral work, he seems more and more frustrated when asked to do reading and writing assignments in class.

The regular classroom teacher is most concerned about José's reading speed, because José continues to work long after the other children have completed their assignments. When asked to read aloud, José becomes noticeably irritated and even refuses to cooperate. Whereas most children in second grade have an oral reading speed of around 70 words per minute, José reads about 35 words per minute. With regard to writing, José is also slow paced; his classmates tend to finish their workbook pages in 10–15 minutes, but José often takes 30–45 minutes to do so.

The other children receive frequent rest periods from visual work, but José uses these times to continue working. On many occasions, he has missed recess, one of his favorite times of the day, to complete his schoolwork. Many members of the educational team are puzzled over these problems because

the report of José's functional vision evaluation states that he is a "highly efficient" visual learner.

José's parents and teachers, concerned that these difficulties will soon snowball out of control, have discussed whether José should change from print reading to braille reading. However, without an analysis of why he is reading slowly and a sense of his potential to read at a comfortable speed in print, they do not want to switch him to braille as a reading and writing medium. Yet, they also do not want him to be so frustrated that he loses his motivation to learn. To address these crucial issues in José's educational program, the teacher of students with visual impairments, working in conjunction with other members of the educational team, plans to conduct an extensive and deliberate learning media assessment.

INTRODUCTION

As was discussed in Chapter 4, the selection of appropriate literacy media has been a primary educational issue for professionals in the field of visual impairment. Since the passage of legislation in many states to ensure that students who will benefit from reading and writing in braille will have appropriate educational services to develop such skills, professionals in the field have paid much closer attention to systematic and objective procedures for selecting literacy media and have been working to develop guidelines for assessment and processes to guide decisions (Caton, 1994; Koenig & Holbrook, 1989, 1991, 1995; Mangold & Mangold, 1989; Sharpe, McNear, & Bousma, 1995).

Koenig and Holbrook (1989, 1991, 1995) developed a comprehensive process to guide the selection of general learning media and specific literacy media for students with visual impairments that includes detailed procedures in the following essential areas:

- documenting the student's use of sensory channels

- selecting general learning media, including both instructional materials and teaching methods

- selecting the initial literacy medium for beginning formal instruction in reading and writing

- conducting ongoing assessments of the initial decision and determining when to provide instruction in additional literacy tools.

For students with low vision, an additional component of the continuing assessment process is the examination of their reading efficiency in various print media. This evaluation allows the educational team to judge the relative effectiveness of reading in two or more print options, such as large print, regular print with an optical device, or regular print alone. It also provides objective information on fatigue and stamina in print reading. The following discussion briefly describes each of the general areas of the learning media assessment process (see Koenig & Holbrook [1995], for more detailed information on each component, blank forms, and assessment checklists).

OBSERVING THE USE OF SENSORY CHANNELS

The documentation of a student's use of sensory channels is the most basic procedure on which to base a decision on the student's initial literacy medium. This procedure involves sampling a student's behavior in selected settings, noting specific behaviors that he or she demonstrates, and judging whether the student uses vision, touch, or hearing (or any combination) to perform each behavior. After several observations, decisions are made on the student's primary and secondary sensory channels.

Preparing for Observations

To document objectively a student's use of sensory channels, a teacher needs to arrange at least three observations of a student in familiar and unfamiliar settings, structured and unstructured settings, and indoor and outdoor environments. These settings should be selected carefully to make the most efficient use of time. For example, the teacher may choose to observe the student during recess—a familiar, unstructured, outdoor environment. The teacher should also train other members of the educational team, including the parents, to observe the student in other settings, so multiple perspectives can be gained in a variety of environments and activities and various members of the team can help collect data (and, later, participate in the analysis and decision-making processes).

Conducting Observations

During an observation, each discrete behavior that the student demonstrates is recorded in the order in which it occurred. Since this procedure samples the student's behavior, it is important to determine that the behaviors that are noted are truly representative of the entire observation period. If the teacher selectively records behaviors—choosing which to record and not to record—then the resulting profile is not a true sample of the student's behavior. When a student engages in a continuous behavior (such as walking down the hallway or engaging in a self-stimulatory behavior like body rocking), this behavior is recorded once and then the unique behaviors within the continuous behavior are recorded.

After each behavior is recorded, the teacher makes an immediate professional judgment as to whether the student used visual, tactile, or auditory information to perform it. For the later decision on the primary literacy medium, it is important to indicate the primary source of sensory information used in the behavior and the secondary source or sources, if any. If the coding format suggested by Koenig and Holbrook (1995) is used, the primary channel is marked with a box and the secondary channel (or channels) is circled.

Analyzing the Data

After three or more observations are completed, the educational team reviews all the observations and determines the child's primary and secondary sources of sensory information. The primary channel is the one that has been most consistently marked with boxes, and the secondary channel (or channels), with circles. Figure 11.1 presents a coded observation of a fourth-grade student with microphthalmia (see appendix to this chapter for a complete report on this student). If subsequent observations are consistent with this one, then it may be concluded that the child uses vision as the primary sensory channel and hearing and touch as the secondary channels.

Special Considerations

When it is used in an objective and professional manner, the procedure will document the student's use of sensory channels. However, the way in which a student uses his or her sensory channels may not necessarily be the most efficient way to complete tasks. Students tend to use the senses they have been reinforced for using. Those with low vision may be subtly (or even overtly) reinforced for using only vision. The author has observed students with low vision hesitating to explore objects tactilely, perhaps because they perceive that they should "look but not touch," as a result of the overemphasis on the use of vision as part of visual efficiency training. However, to use their vision efficiently, students must learn how to choose which sense or combination of senses is needed to complete a task efficiently.

For example, a preschooler with low vision may be reinforced ("Good looking!") after struggling to locate a favorite toy in a dark closet visually, when a tactile approach may have been more efficient in this situation. Such reinforcement may lead the child to believe that the use of vision is preferable to the use of touch or other senses. Even though it is not the most efficient way to complete the task, the procedure described in this section will document that vision is the primary sensory channel, because it does not yield data on efficiency.

The skillful teacher who notes that the child does not perform some tasks as efficiently as possible during the observation of sensory channels will explore this area through diagnostic teaching during the learning media assessment. For example, the teacher may encourage the child just mentioned to explore the toy closet tactilely to find the desired toy. By giving a student repeated opportunities, encouragement, and reinforcement for using other senses to complete tasks, the team will gain information on the student's *most efficient* primary and secondary sensory channels.

SELECTING GENERAL LEARNING MEDIA

During this phase of the process, the educational team selects general learning media on the basis of a review of information from the observations of the student's use of sensory channels. General learning media include both instructional materials (such as globes, rulers, models, and charts)

Use of Sensory Channels

Student __David Smith__

Setting/Activity __Language Arts class and O&M lesson__

Date __1-25-96__   Observer __Jane Holland__

	Observed Behavior	Sensory Channel		
Class	Located desk	[V]	T	A
	Reached for recorder	[V]	T	A
	Placed disk in disk drive	[V]	T	A
	Turned on computer (switch in back)	V	[T]	A
	Switched on plug-in strip	[V]	(T)	A
	Gathered papers together	[V]	T	A
	Walked to reading circle	[V]	(T)	(A)
	Glanced around room	[V]	T	A
	Put on glasses	[V]	T	A
	Looked at book	[V]	T	A
	Took off glasses	V	[T]	A
	Listened to story	V	T	[A]
	Stared at overhead light	[V]	T	A
	Clapped hands	(V)	(T)	(A)
O&M	Identified parts of cane	[V]	(T)	A
	Located office	[V]	T	A
	Walked in straight line	[V]	T	A
	Waved at friends in hall	[V]	T	A
	Turned corner	[V]	(T)	A
	Looked behind self	[V]	T	A
	Went to office door	[V]	T	A
	Located office number	[V]	T	A
	Shook hands with teacher	[V]	(T)	A
	Examined poster on bulletin board	[V]	T	A
	Located specific room number	[V]	T	A
	Located drinking fountain	[V]	T	A

☐ Probable Primary Channel: __Visual__

○ Probable Secondary Channel(s): __Tactile and auditory__

Figure 11.1. Use of Sensory Channels: Observation Form

Source: A. J. Koenig and M. C. Holbrook, *Learning Media Assessment of Students with Visual Impairments: A Resource Guide for Teachers,* 2d ed. (Austin: Texas School for the Blind and Visually Impaired, 1995).

and teaching methods (such as demonstrations, verbal guidance, and lectures). This process embeds the later decision on literacy media in the broader context of all other learning media.

When choosing general learning media for a student with low vision, the teacher should keep two issues in mind. First, particular attention must be given to the student's use of distance materials and comfort with certain teaching methods. The effective use of distance media, such as chalkboards and overhead projectors, may require preferential seating, the use of distance optical devices, or other strategies for bringing distance information into useful view. Teaching methods, such as demonstrations and gestures, may be outside the viewing distance of the student unless adaptations are made. And facial expressions, which provide many cues to learning, may not be accessible to the student at a "comfortable" working distance. Thus, thorough functional vision and learning media assessments are needed to determine the following:

- the type of information the student receives at given distances
- the adaptations that are necessary to gain access to visual information
- levels of visual comfort
- the student's efficient functional use of vision.

Second, the principle of least restrictive materials (Stratton, 1990) is a valuable framework for selecting general learning media. Simply stated, this principle suggests that materials should be adapted only to the extent necessary for efficient learning. If regular materials can be used in conjunction with environmental adaptations or low vision devices, such an approach is preferable to using specialized materials. Stratton described four stages of learning from instructional materials:

- full learning from the natural environment (the regular colored pictures in a phonics book are used)

- mediation as a way to learn from the environment (the teacher points in the direction of a friend on the playground so a child can use a monocular)
- adaptation as a means to an end (large-type materials are used until the independent use of an optical device is mastered)
- replacement with adapted materials (color labels are placed in the clothing of a child with achromatopsia).

Such an approach prepares the student to live in a world that is largely "unadapted" and highlights the need for even young students with low vision to begin to develop independent strategies for using regular instructional materials, such as regular lined paper. As students progress through school, they will use fewer and fewer specially adapted materials, relying instead on a host of literacy tools, especially optical and nonoptical devices, that give them direct and immediate access to regular instructional media.

CHOOSING THE INITIAL LITERACY MEDIUM

A crucial decision made on behalf of a student with low vision is the initial literacy medium. Given the justified concerns over the appropriateness of assessment procedures used in the past, it is essential that the selection of the initial literacy medium is supported by objective information. Koenig and Holbrook (1989, 1991, 1995) suggested that educational teams gather data in the following areas:

- the student's use of the visual sense for gathering information
- the student's use of the tactile or other senses for gathering information
- the sizes of objects and working distances
- the stability and prognosis of the eye condition
- the influence of additional disabilities on learning to read.

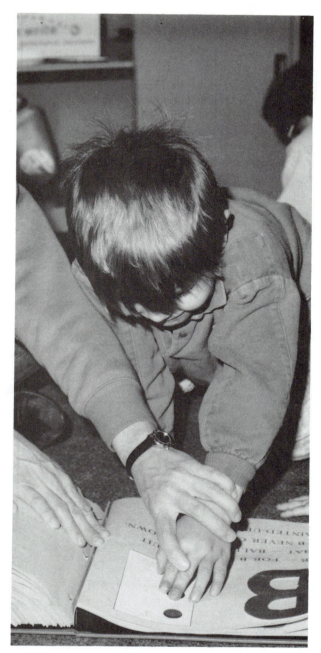

Assessment of a student's use of vision to determine the appropriate literacy medium needs to begin at an early age.

In addition, other information that is specific to the individual student is considered, such as a student's and parents' attitudes toward a certain medium.

Checking Efficient Use of Sensory Information

At this point in the process, the educational team should consider the student's use of vision or touch and other senses to complete a variety of specific tasks, including early literacy events, such as these:

- recognizing others
- initiating the reaching response
- exploring toys or other objects
- discriminating like and different toys or other objects
- identifying objects
- confirming the identity of an object
- using visual-motor and fine motor skills
- showing interest in pictures
- showing interest in books
- showing interest in scribbling or writing
- identifying names or simple words.

Through diagnostic teaching, the student is given both visual and tactile experiences, and the teacher assesses the child's preference for completing tasks with the visual sense or with the tactile and other senses. The gathering of information through diagnostic teaching starts ideally in infancy and is done for a few years, generally until the child enters kindergarten, when it is decided whether the child is ready to enter a conventional literacy program. Educational teams can use Koenig and Holbrook's (1995) assessment checklist to help them make this decision.

To assess the efficiency of various senses in a nonbiased manner, the teacher must provide experiences that are of equal intensity and quality and not reinforce a student more for using one sense than for using another. During this early diagnostic teaching phase, the educational team should seek to stimulate all the senses and provide reinforcement to the student accordingly.

Considering Other Assessment Areas

Although the efficient use of sensory information is important in selecting the initial literacy medium, it must be considered within a larger context. For students with low vision, objective information on the size of objects and the distances at which they are viewed must be paired with other information on the efficient use of vision. For example, if a student is efficient in using visual information but does so at such a close working distance that he or she cannot work for a long time, tactile media may be more efficient. The educational team must consider the implications of combinations of factors and must never make decisions based on isolated pieces of information that are taken out of context.

Also, factors related to the prognosis and stability of the eye condition are crucial in making the initial decision. When a child has a stable eye condition, the educational team can base the initial decision primarily on data about the child's sensory efficiency. When a child has a progressive or unstable eye condition, however, the team may need to focus on the implications of the condition. The educational team must consider both the immediate and the future needs of a student to ensure that meaningful progress is being made toward establishing literacy. Some students with progressive or unstable eye conditions will begin to learn braille reading and writing when their visual efficiency is still high. In such instances, it is essential for the teacher of students with visual impairments to cultivate a positive environment for learning braille and to stress both the present and future value of learning braille.

When students have additional disabilities, the learning media assessment may first emphasize the effective use of instructional time to teach functional literacy skills versus other essential life skills. As the severity of additional disabilities increases, the team is more likely to focus on daily living, social, and employment skills. If it is decided that functional literacy skills will increase a student's independence and are possible to teach, given the student's level of abil-

ity, then essentially the same process is used to decide whether literacy instruction will be offered in print or braille. Koenig and Holbrook (1995) presented guidelines and assessment checklists for selecting learning and literacy media for students with additional disabilities.

Making the Initial Decision

Sometime before the student enters a formal literacy program, the educational team reviews and synthesizes all the objective data that have been gathered, with deliberate care not to take any piece of information out of the context of the entire body of information. Their decision is based on whether the student demonstrates the characteristics of a visual learner who will make efficient use of print or a tactile learner who will make efficient use of braille. (For some characteristics to consider in making this initial decision, see Sidebar 11.1.) In some instances, the team may decide to implement formal reading instruction in both print and braille, use the upcoming semester or year to engage in diagnostic teaching to resolve any lingering questions, and then decide to concentrate on one medium or to continue with both media.

CONTINUING ASSESSMENT OF LITERACY MEDIA

The continuing assessment phase has two purposes: to reassess periodically whether the initial decision on the literacy medium is still appropriate and to address the need for instruction in additional communication skills to expand the student's repertoire of literacy tools. As was noted in the vignette on José at the beginning of the chapter, the educational team was concerned about the appropriateness of the initial literacy medium and, given the time it took for José to complete academic tasks, they decided to expand his repertoire of literacy tools so he would have other options for gaining access to print other than print reading. This vignette highlights the need for the

SIDEBAR 11.1

Characteristics of Students Who May Be Candidates for Print Reading and Braille Reading Programs

Characteristics of a Likely Print Reader

◆ Uses vision efficiently to complete tasks at near distances.

◆ Shows interest in pictures and demonstrates the ability to identify pictures or elements within pictures.

◆ Identifies his or her name in print or understands that print has meaning.

◆ Uses print to perform other prerequisite reading skills.

◆ Has a stable eye condition.

◆ Has an intact central visual field.

◆ Shows steady progress in learning to use his or her vision as necessary to ensure efficient print reading.

◆ Is free of additional disabilities that would interfere with progress in a developmental reading program in print.

Characteristics of a Likely Braille Reader

◆ Shows a preference for exploring the environment tactilely.

◆ Uses the tactile sense efficiently to identify small objects.

◆ Identifies his or her name in braille or understands that braille has meaning.

◆ Uses braille to acquire other prerequisite reading skills.

◆ Has an unstable eye condition or a poor prognosis for retaining his or her current level of vision in the near future.

◆ Has a reduced or nonfunctional central field to the extent that print reading is expected to be inefficient.

◆ Shows steady progress in developing tactile skills that are necessary for efficient braille reading.

◆ Is free of additional disabilities that would interfere with progress in a developmental reading program in braille.

Source: A. J. Koenig and M. C. Holbrook, *Learning Media Assessment of Students with Visual Impairments: A Resource Guide for Teachers* (Austin: Texas School for the Blind and Visually Impaired, 1995).

---

learning media assessment to be ongoing and not to be conducted only at one point in time.

The continuing assessment phase is a safety net that ensures that each student with a visual impairment continues to develop functional literacy skills that he or she needs for independent living and employment. It begins as soon as the initial decision is made and continues throughout the student's schooling. If the educational system has prepared the student to be self-sufficient and to serve as an advocate for himself or herself, the student will take over the process of continually assessing his or her literacy needs and will strive to meet them throughout life.

Components of the Continuing Assessment

To guide the continuing assessment phase, Koenig and Holbrook (1989, 1991, 1995) suggested that at least once a year objective data should be collected and synthesized on the following:

- ophthalmological, optometric, clinical low vision, and functional low vision evaluations, to determine whether there has been a change in the student's visual functioning since the last review

- reading efficiency rates and reading grade levels, to determine whether the student reads with sufficient efficiency to complete academic tasks successfully and comfortably

- academic achievement, to determine whether the student is continuing to make academic progress in his or her current medium or media

- handwriting skills, to determine whether the student is able to read back his or her own handwriting even after a lapse of time and whether handwriting is an effective expressive mode of communication

- the effectiveness of the student's existing repertoire of literacy tools, to determine whether instruction is needed in additional literacy tools to meet the demands of present and future literacy tasks.

Sidebar 11.2 summarizes the five corresponding questions in the continuing assessment phase, possible sources of objective information, and possible actions. Since growth in reading efficiency and achievement are particularly important for students with low vision, these areas are discussed next in greater detail.

Documenting Reading Efficiency

Questions related to reading efficiency and academic achievement focus on the continued appropriateness of print as the primary literacy medium. Members of the educational team gather objective information to document whether the student is completing academic tasks efficiently through print and is making appropriate academic progress within a reasonable time compared to classmates with normal vision.

Data on reading efficiency should be collected in the student's habitual primary reading medium. For example, if the student habitually uses regular print with a 2.5X stand magnifier, testing should occur under this condition. If the student uses print as a secondary reading medium to supplement braille reading and writing, then the use of print reading should be assessed on the basis of how successful the student is in completing those literacy tasks. Under such circumstances, reading efficiency data should be collected in braille, since this is the student's habitual primary reading medium.

Short-term Narrative Reading Rates

Every student's cumulative record should contain a graph that plots annual reading efficiency rates. Sidebar 11.3 (steps 1–7) presents a simple and time-efficient procedure for gathering these data using any commercially available informal reading inventory. The Informal Reading Inventory (Burns & Roe, 1993) is especially useful for this purpose because it contains four parallel passages for kindergarten through 12th grade, as well as formulas for quickly calculating reading rates once the time spent in reading a passage is known. To determine the average rate at which a student reads short-term narrative passages with comprehension, one calculates an average of the reading rates from all passages in which the student comprehended with at least 80 percent accuracy. Collecting reading efficiency data in this manner generally takes 30 to 45 minutes.

Although this procedure is easy and quick to use, the data have specific limitations. First, the rates indicate only reading rates of passages that are shorter than most reading assignments in a classroom. Second, given the short reading time, the rates do not indicate if visual fatigue is a concern for the student. Third, the rates are reflective of only narrative reading materials that are commonly found in basal reading series and literature books.

Long-term Narrative Reading Rates

The first two concerns just mentioned can be addressed by having the student read for a sustained period (such as 20–30 minutes) from a

SIDEBAR 11.2

Components of the Continuing Assessment of Literacy Media

Questions	Sources of Information	Possible Actions
Does available information indicate a change in visual functioning?	◆ Functional vision assessment reports. ◆ Clinical low vision evaluation reports. ◆ Ophthalmological evaluation reports. ◆ Observations of sensory usage.	If yes, consider the impact on the student's current primary literacy medium.
Does the student read at a sufficient rate and with adequate comprehension to complete academic tasks successfully?	◆ Results of an informal reading inventory. ◆ Objective data on reading rate. ◆ Reading rate and comprehension levels in content reading materials. ◆ Feedback from the classroom teacher on the student's level of reading efficiency relative to that of peers. ◆ Feedback from others on the educational team, including the parents. ◆ Objective data on reading in various print media.	If no, explore possible reasons through diagnostic teaching, consider the need to expand literacy tools, and consider the impact on the student's primary medium.
Is the student able to complete academic tasks in the current medium or media successfully and in a reasonable time in comparison with peers with unimpaired vision?	◆ Results of tests on chapters in textbooks and other informal assessment measures. ◆ Grade cards and other feedback from members of the educational team. ◆ Results of achievement tests or state competency examinations. ◆ Observations of the student in the classroom. ◆ Feedback from parents on the amount of time spent in completing homework.	If no, consider the two areas above, especially the need to add additional literacy tools that may increase the student's overall efficiency.
Is the student able to read his or her handwriting and use it as a viable mode of written communication?	◆ Writing samples. ◆ Accuracy of rereading writing samples after time has elapsed.	If no, consider expanding the student's repertoire of writing modes, especially the use of word processing.
Does the student have the repertoire of literacy tools, including the use of technology, to meet his or her current educational needs? To meet his or her future educational and vocational needs?	◆ Checklist of literacy tools to document existing skills and to guide future needs. ◆ Observations of the student using tools. ◆ Feedback from members of the educational team on the student's success in using tools. ◆ Long-range goals to guide the selection of additional tools.	If no, first consider adding literacy tools to meet the student's current needs and then to meet anticipated future needs.

Sources: A. J. Koenig and M. C. Holbrook, "Determining the Reading Medium for Students with Visual Impairments: A Diagnostic Teaching Approach," *Journal of Visual Impairment & Blindness* 83 (1989), pp. 296–302; A. J. Koenig and M. C. Holbrook, "Determining the Reading Medium for Visually Impaired Students via Diagnostic Teaching," *Journal of Visual Impairment & Blindness* 85 (1991), pp. 61–68; and A. J. Koenig and M. C. Holbrook, *Learning Media Assessment of Students with Visual Impairments: A Resource Guide for Teachers* (Austin: Texas School for the Blind and Visually Impaired, 1995).

SIDEBAR 11.3

A Procedure for Documenting Reading Efficiency

1. Select a published informal reading inventory that provides reading passages of increasing grade-level difficulty and that includes at least five comprehension questions for each passage.

2. Prepare the reading passages in the student's primary reading medium.

3. Have the student read the passage orally and/or silently. When reading silently, tell the student to begin reading when you say "start" and to look up at you when he or she is finished. Using a stopwatch, record the time the student spent reading in seconds. (If the student is in the third grade or earlier, data may be collected only on oral reading.)

4. Ask the comprehension questions for each passage and score the student's responses according to criteria provided by the publisher.

5. For each passage in which the student demonstrated at least 80 percent comprehension, count the total number of words. Disregard passages with less than 80 percent comprehension for completing Steps 6 and 7.

6. For each passage with at least 80 percent comprehension, calculate the rate of reading, as follows:

$$\frac{\text{Number of words in passage}}{\text{Number of seconds spent in reading}} \times 60 = \text{words per minute}$$

7. Calculate the average words per minute.

8. Determine the student's independent, instructional, and frustration reading levels. Use this information, along with other data on achievement, to document the student's reading level.

9. Analyze the relationship between the student's reading rate and reading level. Use the quantitative data and other sources of information to determine if the student reads with sufficient comprehension at a sufficient rate to maintain academic progress.

10. If deemed appropriate, judge the student's reading rate in relation to the reading rate of his or her classmates with unimpaired vision. To gather such data, select 10 or more students from the regular classroom and repeat the procedure outlined here. Or use normative data on reading rates, presented in Table 11.1, to make meaningful comparisons.

Source: A. J. Koenig and M. C. Holbrook. *Learning Media Assessment of Students with Visual Impairments: A Resource Guide for Teachers* (Austin: Texas School for the Blind and Visually Impaired, 1995).

lengthy, cohesive passage. Reading materials can be selected from a basal reader or any other book of fiction that is at the student's instructional reading level. A reading rate can be calculated for the first half of the reading episode and another for the second half using the formula in Sidebar 11.3, Step 6. The number of words in each half of the story are counted first. If the reading rate in the second half is significantly slower than the rate in the first, this is one sign of visual fatigue. Some students with low vision may increase their rate of reading in the second half of a reading episode because they have gained a basic knowledge of the story and thus are more efficient at predicting the author's message.

Stamina can also be determined by measuring a student's a reading rates at the beginning and end of the school day and comparing them. Another reading sample could be taken at home during the evening to document the student's reading efficiency during the time the student is expected to complete homework assignments.

Reading Rates with Content Materials

The third concern can be partially addressed by calculating a student's rates of reading the content in textbooks that he or she is expected to read daily. To determine these rates, no instrument is needed other than the textbooks that are used in the classroom.

To gather these data, the teacher selects passages, which have not been read or studied in class, that can be read in about 3 to 5 five minutes from the student's science, social studies, and other textbooks. With the student reading either silently or aloud, the teacher measures the time spent reading with a stopwatch and asks several questions about the content of the passage or asks the student to tell in his or her own words what the passage was about. The level of comprehension is calculated as a percentage of the questions answered correctly or is generally described as, for example, "average" or "adequate." Finally, the rate of reading is calculated by counting the number of words in the passage and applying the formula presented in Sidebar 11.3.

Functional Literacy Tasks

There are many functional reading tasks for which reading efficiency rates cannot be calculated. For example, the location of a specific departure time in a bus schedule is dependent on many factors, such as the person's familiarity with the bus system and accompanying schedule, efficiency in scanning of tabular material, and efficient use of literacy tools to gain access to the printed material. Generally, the individual's timely completion of a given functional literary task to gain the desired information is the ultimate criterion. If a person who seeks a specific departure time for a bus can effectively use a low vision device to locate the desired information and arrive at the bus stop on time, then he or she has demonstrated mastery of this task. However, if it took the person 30 minutes to locate the departure time and he or she then missed the bus, then mastery was not demonstrated. In this instance, an alternative literacy tool, such as phoning the bus company's customer service number, might have been more efficient.

Documenting Reading Achievement

One aspect of the continuing assessment phase is the evaluation of a student's overall academic achievement. Of particular interest to this discussion is achievement in reading and writing. Information on a student's reading achievement can be documented by determining the independent, instructional, and frustration reading levels by following directions given in the informal reading inventory (Step 8 in Sidebar 11.3). However, this information should be viewed only within the context of other data on literacy achievement, such as scores on state or district competency tests, criterion-referenced tests, and appropriately administered standardized achievement tests, the results of curriculum-based assessments, and writing samples.

Administering reading achievement tests in large print, although a typical procedure, does not, by itself, guarantee a nondiscriminatory assessment. A key to nondiscriminatory assessment is to base modifications of testing procedures on findings from the functional vision assessment (see Chapters 9 and 10) and the learning media assessment. Given the concerns about the validity of standardized tests, data from these tests should be used only to supplement many other sources of data from informal instruments; standardized tests should never be the sole source of information on reading achievement for any student with low vision. Duckworth (1993) presented valuable guidelines for the appropriate adaptation of standardized tests for use by students with visual impairments.

Interpreting Data

The interpretation of objective data involves judging whether the student's reading efficiency is appropriate, given his or her present and future academic and vocational demands (Step 9 in Sidebar 11.3) and given the reading rates of peers with unimpaired vision (Step 10). As is indicated in Step 10, the reading rates of peers with unimpaired vision can be gathered either by testing a random sample of students in the same classroom (although this is a time-consuming method) or by using the typical reading rates presented in Table 11.1, which tend to be stable and predictable.

Concerns are continually voiced about the use of standards for students with visual impairments that have been established on the basis of students with unimpaired vision. However, meaningful comparisons provide a general basis for determining the additional time a student with low vision needs to complete reading tasks, as well as partial justification for giving the student additional literacy tools or changing his or her literacy medium.

There is no magic formula for judging whether a student's reading efficiency is "appropriate" or whether the time required to complete academic tasks is "reasonable." Therefore, professional judgment, based on objective findings, is the primary means for making such determinations. The following general guidelines and examples may be helpful in this regard.

Magnitude of the Gap

The magnitude of the gap, if any, should be considered that exists between the reading efficiency rate of a student with low vision and students with unimpaired vision at the same grade level. For example, if a first-grade student with low vision is reading silently at 65 words per minute and others are reading at 81 words per minute, the educational team may consider such a gap to be reasonable. However, the gap between a seventh grader with low vision who is reading silently at 65 words per minute and others who are reading at 180 words per minute is not likely to be considered reasonable. Similarly, with regard to José's oral reading rate of 35 words per minute, the typical minimal oral reading rate for second-grade students with unimpaired vision is 70 words per minute (see Table 11.1), so the gap of 35 words per minute would not be considered reasonable.

Time Requirements

On the basis of a student's documented reading efficiency rate and the typical rate of his or her peers with normal vision, the time required to read a short story of "X" number of words should be considered. For example, to read a typical story of 500 words in the second semester of first grade, a student with low vision reading at 65 words per minute would take about 8 minutes, whereas students with unimpaired vision reading at 81 words per minute would take about 6 minutes. At this grade level, the additional time needed by the student with low vision is reasonable. However, if the first grader with low vision reads at 15 words per minute, it would take about 33 minutes to read the story—27 minutes longer than students with unimpaired vision—a gap that most teachers would consider to be unreasonable for a first grader. On the other hand, if it took a seventh grader with low vision 27 minutes more than students with unimpaired vision to complete a homework assignment, most teachers would consider this gap reasonable.

To apply this guideline to José, it would take about 29 minutes for him to read aloud a story of

Table 11.1. Typical Oral and Silent Reading Rates for Students with Unimpaired Vision (in words per minute)

Grade Level	Minimum Oral Reading Rates	Typical Silent Reading Rates
1	60	less than 81
2	70	82–108
3	90	109–130
4	120	131–147
5	120	148–161
6	150	162–174
7	150	175–185
8		186–197
9		198–209
10		210–224
11		225–240
12		241–255
College		256–333 or more

Sources: Data from Ronald P. Carver, "Silent Reading Rates in Grade Equivalents," *Journal of Reading Behavior* 21 (1989), pp. 158–161; and Frank J. Guszak, *Diagnostic Reading Instruction in the Elementary School*, 3rd ed. (New York: Harper & Row, 1985).

1,000 words (at 35 words per minute), compared to about 14 minutes for his classmates with unimpaired vision (at 70 words per minute), or more than twice as long. When one considers that other reading tasks during the school day may require a similar amount of additional time, the school day would essentially have to be at least doubled to allow José time to complete all the tasks. For a second grader, most teachers would consider this discrepancy to be unreasonable.

Many students with low vision require more time to complete assignments than do their classmates with normal vision, a fact that is likely to extend to employment tasks. Such a situation does not automatically indicate that a change in the literacy medium is appropriate or warranted. Rather, the additional time may be compensated for by adding additional literacy tools, such as audiotaped materials or live readers. However, such tools are only supplements to a primary literacy medium; they are not a substitute for developing basic reading skills in either print or braille.

Yearly Progress in Reading Efficiency

By collecting and graphing reading efficiency rates annually, the educational team can objectively determine whether the student's rates are increasing from year to year. For example, in Figure 11.2, the solid line shows the gains that students with unimpaired vision typically make from grade to grade; the line is essentially linear. The dotted line shows the hypothetical gains made by a student with low vision who truly is progressing in reading efficiency; although the gains do not match those of students with unimpaired vision and the gap increases from year to year, the student with low vision is still progressing steadily.

However, the dashed line shows the hypothetical gains (or lack of gains) by a student who has plateaued in reading efficiency early in elementary school, such as might be the case with José. This student's reading efficiency may have stopped improving for a number of reasons: (1) the quality and intensity of reading instruction may have been inadequate to promote steady gains, (2) changes were not made in the student's educational program to provide instruction in increasing reading efficiency rate, or (3) the student may have reached his or her potential for reading efficiency given his or her visual condition. Regardless of the cause, the resulting gap between the student with low vision illustrated in Figure 11.2 and students with unimpaired vision is not appropriate by any criterion, and the student is at serious risk of entering adulthood without the literacy skills needed for most occupations.

Determining the cause of plateauing requires an extended period of diagnostic teaching, probably by the teacher of students with visual impairments. The general approach is to provide high-quality, intense instruction, using targeted instructional strategies as appropriate (see Chapter

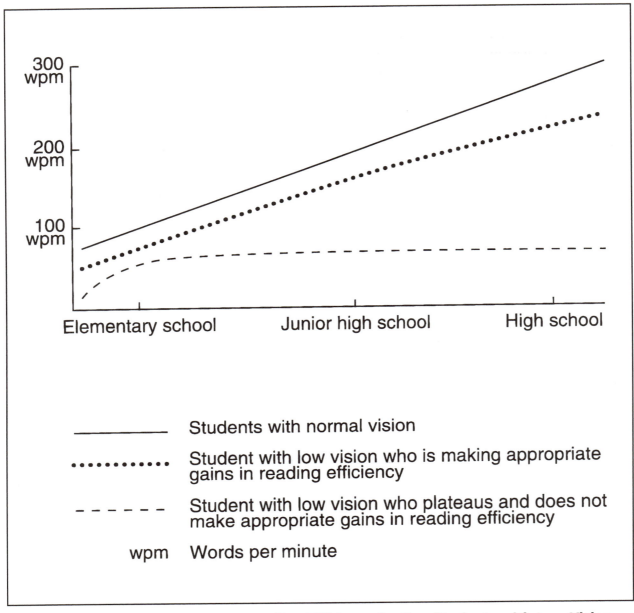

Figure 11.2. Hypothetical Data on Reading Efficiency for Two Students with Low Vision

12), to rule out the instruction as the cause. Team members should not hastily assume that the lack of progress in reading is the result of the student's lack of motivation, family factors, or a "learning disability." Often these excuses are made to justify a student's lack of progress, rather than to address the student's real need: high-quality reading instruction. If a student's reading efficiency and achievement continue to plateau after a period of intense reading instruction, then factors other than instruction may be the cause. Continued diagnostic teaching is then necessary to explore other causes and to determine whether a change in the reading medium is needed.

Stamina and Comfort Level

The objective data on fatigue gained through reading lengthy passages—both in a single session and throughout the day—are one source of information by which the educational team can judge whether the student has sufficient stamina to complete all the required academic tasks with relative comfort throughout the school day and evening. These objective data, however, should be judged within a larger context, including reports from teachers and parents, self-reports by the student, and behavioral observations (such as rubbing the eyes, acting-out behavior, and avoidance of visual tasks). Fatigue is heavily influenced by one's psychological set, which is an important and necessary factor to consider in judging a student's stamina for visual tasks.

A student's level of comfort and general level of pleasure and enjoyment in reading should also be considered. Although these factors obviously cannot be documented objectively, the reflective teacher can use behavioral observations and ongoing interactions with the student to determine them. It is not unusual to hear that a student with low vision simply does not like to read. In such a case, the teacher of students with visual impairments must examine the multitude of influences that may be contributing to this situation. If the student is reading in a print medium that does not offer sufficient comfort for sustained reading, he or she is not likely to find reading pleasurable. Chapter 12 offers suggestions for increasing a student's rate of and stamina in reading print. However, if targeted strategies do not increase a student's comfort in reading, then the educational team must discuss specific changes to be made and actions to be taken to address the student's needs.

Print versus Typical Braille Reading Rates

The issue of which reading efficiency rate in print is considered an acceptable minimum for students with low vision may never be resolved, perhaps because the real issue is the rate that is not considered appropriate and that would therefore justify the introduction of a braille reading and writing program. The latter issue is somewhat easier to address, since typical braille reading rates for school-age students provide some point of reference.

Heinze (1986) suggested that for high school students, a range of 90–120 words per minute in braille reading is typical. Lowenfeld, Abel, and Hatlen (1969) found that the average braille reading rates were 72 and 84 words per minute for fourth-grade students and 116 and 149 words per minute for eighth-grade students who were enrolled in residential schools and local public schools, respectively. Given the greater incidence of multiple disabilities among students who are blind today, Lowenfeld et al.'s estimates may be high.

Clearly, the objective braille reading rates for elementary school students are critical for deciding whether it is appropriate to continue to rely on print as the primary reading medium. Although updated typical rates are needed, a range of 100–125 words per minute seems to be at least a starting point for judging reading efficiency rates in print. If rates are gathered and plotted on a line chart (as was mentioned previously) over the first three to four years of school, a prediction line can be drawn to determine whether a rate of 100–125 words per minute is achievable. Then if the educational team could not be reasonably certain that a student could achieve a print reading rate of 100 to 125 words per minute, they should seriously consider introducing a braille reading and writing program.

Yearly Gains in Reading Achievement

With a variety of data on reading achievement (see Sidebar 11.2), members of the educational team can examine whether the student is making gains in reading achievement and academic achievement in general from year to year to ensure that continual progress is being made. The judgment of progress in reading should be embedded in the larger context of general academic achievement, since the two are likely to be highly correlated.

Making Appropriate Decisions

Interpreting the data on reading skills requires the meaningful interweaving of all information. That is, *a student with low vision should read with sufficient efficiency, stamina, and comfort to complete academic tasks successfully, when compared with peers of similar ability, while making continual gains in reading efficiency and achievement.* One source of information cannot be taken out of context to decide whether print reading should continue to be the appropriate primary literacy medium. For example, a student who simply reads faster from year to year but who does not progress beyond an elementary level of reading achievement, is clearly not making appropriate progress. Nor is a student who makes yearly gains in reading achievement but whose reading rate plateaus early in elementary school.

After critically reviewing the assessment data, the educational team makes decisions to ensure the student's continued development of literacy skills. If the student is making documented progress in reading efficiency and achievement, then the team probably will decide to continue emphasizing print as the primary medium while expanding, as appropriate, the student's repertoire of literacy tools. If the student is not making the desired progress, the team must change the current course of action to address the identified areas of difficulty. Among the many possible decisions are the following:

- continue print as the primary literacy medium and add additional literacy tools, such as audiotaped books and live reader services, to the student's repertoire to supplement print reading and writing
- continue with print as the primary literacy medium but provide targeted and intense reading skills instruction to improve reading efficiency and achievement
- begin instruction in braille reading and writing while continuing to use print and other options to make academic gains until braille becomes either the primary or a secondary literacy medium.

If a student is reading inefficiently in print and is not making appropriate gains in reading achievement, a decision to change the primary literacy medium is not automatically appropriate. The student may lack an appropriate experiential background or specific reading skills, such as decoding or comprehension, or may not have received high-quality reading instruction. In such a case, changing the medium will not eliminate the underlying problems. On the other hand, if the student's progress is hampered or restricted by a literacy medium that does not match his or her sensory functioning, then a deliberate change may indeed be appropriate.

Focusing on Diagnostic Teaching: An Illustration

When conducting the continuing learning media assessment of José, his teacher will explore a variety of factors to determine why his reading rate is not commensurate with his peers. During daily reading lessons, the teacher will analyze José's reading skills, particularly those reading traits and other behaviors that are known to hamper students with low vision, such as the following:

- losing one's place on a line of print
- failing to locate the next line efficiently
- inefficiently changing from one page to the next
- skipping words or punctuation
- mentioning that the size of the image is not sufficient for distinguishing letters or shapes of words
- noting that glare and reflections interfere with the words on the page
- indicating that the position of the materials leads to early fatigue
- needing additional segments of time to resolve and identify images
- finding visual distractions on a page.

When the teacher finds a potential area of difficulty, he or she initiates targeted instruction and then analyzes its effects. For example, if José is found to skip lines while reading, the teacher will document over several days the frequency of line-skipping incidents and then teach José to use a typoscope (a piece of cardboard or other material with a window cut in it equal to the width of one line) to keep his eyes on the appropriate line. During subsequent lessons, the teacher will continue to collect reading samples and calculate José's rate of reading. If the frequency of line-skipping incidents decreases and José's rate of reading increases, then the teacher can conclude that skipping lines is at least partially responsible for his problems in reading efficiency.

If the teacher finds that such strategies do not increase José's rate of reading, he or she may decide to use a targeted instructional strategy to do so. One strategy—called choral reading—is for José to read aloud along with his teacher. At first the teacher reads slightly louder than José and at a slightly faster pace; this "forced pacing" leads to an increased reading rate, and because the teacher is reading louder, José does not feel threatened by not knowing each word. While using this strategy over time, the teacher will regularly calculate José's reading rate to document the effectiveness of the strategy (see Chapter 12 for other strategies).

To identify problems in reading, the diagnostic teacher targets one factor at a time, assesses the impact of instruction, and then continues the instruction if it has proved effective or targets another area. If diagnostic teaching had been used earlier in José's school years, perhaps his difficulties in reading would not have arisen. Providing high-quality reading instruction from the beginning to prevent problems from occurring is the best educational practice.

SELECTING APPROPRIATE PRINT MEDIA

Part of the continuing assessment of students with low vision involves collecting data on read-ing efficiency in various print media, such as regular print, regular print with an optical device, large print, and closed-circuit television (CCTV). The appropriate selection of print media must occur within the context of other sources of information, such as clinical low vision evaluations, ophthalmological evaluations, and the administration of general achievement tests.

Teachers sometimes provide students with large print without objectively documenting its value or efficiency for the students. They may believe that large print is more efficient and less fatiguing for students or can be used at a greater working distance. However, such beliefs are not supported by research. An even more serious problem is that the exclusive provision of large print may actually prevent students from acquiring skills in less restrictive options for gaining access to print, such as the use of optical devices. Given the extensive amount of regular-print materials and the limited amount of large-print materials, the reliance on large print substantially restricts an individual's access to the majority of literacy materials.

Although research has not supported the value of large print for all students with low vision, teachers may be justifiably concerned whether this finding applies to individual students in their caseloads. Therefore, a procedure that helps a teacher make these decisions for individual students is the most appropriate. One such extensive procedure for objectively assessing the relative effectiveness of reading in various print media is the Print Media Assessment Process (PMAP) (Koenig, Layton, & Ross, 1992; Koenig & Ross, 1991). A brief overview and illustration of the process is presented next (see Koenig and Holbrook, [1995], for step-by-step procedures and protocol forms).

Screening Procedure

A screening version of PMAP involves the collection of three sources of data: short-term silent reading, short-term oral reading, and working distance. The teacher selects the media (such as

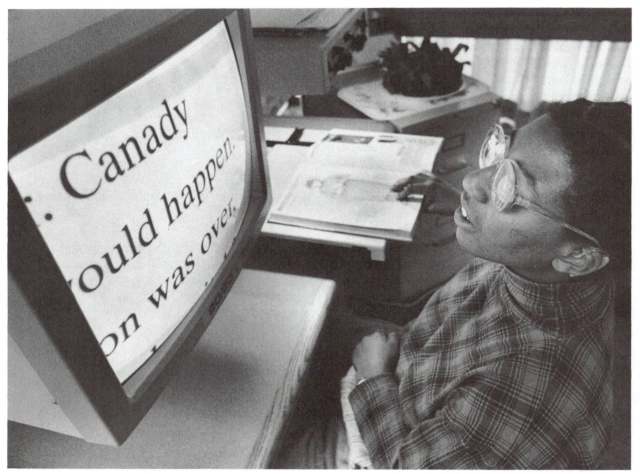

The selection of appropriate print media for a student is the result of the consideration of several factors, such as clinical low vision and ophthalmological evaluations and general achievement test results, in addition to the student's reading efficiency in various media.

regular print with a prescribed optical device and large print) in which a comparison will be made and prepares passages from an informal reading inventory in them. As was mentioned previously, the Informal Reading Inventory (Burns & Roe, 1993) is ideal for this purpose because it contains four parallel passages for kindergarten through 12th grade, two of which can be used for silent reading (one in regular print and the other in large print) and two of which can be used for oral reading. Then actual data are collected using the directions given in Sidebar 11.3, repeating steps 1–7 for each medium in both silent and oral read-

ing. While the student reads each passage, the teacher notes the working distance from the page and, for passages with at least 80 percent comprehension, averages the distances in each medium for oral and silent reading.

After the calculations are completed, the teacher presents the data in tabular form, with data on large print in one column and data on regular print in another column. The educational team then looks for educationally significant differences between figures relating to the two media, relying on their professional judgment because there is no formula for doing so. An educationally significant difference will have an observed effect on day-to-day functioning in the classroom. For example, if a second-grade student reads at 85 words per minute in large print and 80 words per minute in regular print, it is not likely that this difference will have an appreciable effect on his or her daily performance. However, a difference of 80 and 105 words per minute is of sufficient magnitude to be considered educationally significant.

The data on short-term oral and silent reading and working distances can provide initial, cursory evidence of the efficiency of the student in regard to one print medium versus another. When no educationally significant differences can be determined, the team always selects the less restrictive option, such as regular print with an optical device, rather than large print. If additional data are needed, or if the team is concerned about the student's visual stamina while reading, the teacher administers the comprehensive PMAP.

Comprehensive Procedure

In addition to the information collected for the screening, the comprehensive PMAP includes a long-term oral reading task of 20–30 minutes in the literacy media being compared. With these data, an objective measure of fatigue is obtained by comparing the reading rate in the first half of the episode to the rate in the second half in each medium (not across media). An alternate procedure, as was mentioned earlier, is to document fatigue throughout the day by having the student read a lengthy story at the beginning and another at the end of the school day. With this alternate procedure, though, the reading medium is the same for both passages; generally, it is the primary, habitual reading medium. The variable under consideration in this case is the time factor, not the print medium.

Also, a qualitative dimension of reading is gained by analyzing the miscues (or errors) made during oral reading. Miscue analysis looks beyond the simple counting of errors while reading

aloud to analyze qualitatively how the reader constructed meaning. For each miscue in an oral reading sample, the following general questions are asked:

- Is the miscue graphically similar to the actual word in the text?
- Is the miscue contextually acceptable—semantically and syntactically—in the preceding context of the passage?
- Did the student independently self-correct the miscue?

For example, in the sentence, "Mary ran down to the corner store," if the reader substitutes "a" for "the," the meaning of the passage does not change, even though the two words are not graphically similar; thus, the miscue is considered contextually acceptable. Such miscues demonstrate that the student is constructing meaning while reading. However, if the reader substitutes "stove" for "store," the meaning of the passage is disrupted, since "stove" does not make sense in the sentence. If the miscue is self-corrected, though, it shows that the reader knows that the word makes no sense and is attempting to reconstruct the meaning of the passage. The results of a miscue analysis are presented in percentages, which facilitates the comparison of efficiency in various print media. For guidelines for a user-friendly miscue analysis procedure developed by Christie, see Koenig and Holbrook (1995).

A case study presented in Sidebar 11.4 illustrates how the objective PMAP data are interpreted and used to make informed decisions on moving to less restrictive options for gaining access to print. If large print is found to be more efficient than reading with an optical device, for example, this procedure can help the team judge the student's progress toward making more efficient use of the device until the student uses the two options with equal efficiency. The key is to base decisions for print media on objective information, not solely on subjective impressions or unfounded beliefs.

Case Study: Interpretation of PMAP Data on Sarah

BACKGROUND INFORMATION

Sarah, aged 12, is in the sixth grade. She is above grade level in all subjects except mathematics, in which she is at grade level. She has a history of optic atrophy, nystagmus, and photophobia. Sarah's visual condition is considered stable. Her distance visual acuities are 20/200 in both eyes. A screening of her near vision revealed an acuity of 1.6M print at 3 inches. As a result of a recent low vision examination, the eye care specialist prescribed a pair of reading glasses with a 5D add and with yellow tint to reduce glare and photophobia.

To determine whether Sarah was as efficient reading with her newly prescribed reading glasses as reading large print, the comprehensive PMAP was administered. The results were as follows.

Reading Behaviors	Large Print	Regular Print, Tinted Reading Glasses with a 5D Add
Reading rates (in words per minute)		
Oral reading	105	108
First half	104	108
Second half	106	108
Silent reading	144	152
Average working distances (in inches)		
Oral reading	3	3.5
Silent reading	3	3.0
Miscue analysis (in percentages)		
Graphic similarity		
Beginning	89	89
Middle	79	89
End	53	66
Acceptability in context	24	19
Self-correction strategy	13	28

INTERPRETATION OF DATA

Oral reading rates. Sarah read at 105 words per minute (wpm) in large print and 108 wpm in regular print with her tinted reading glasses with a 5D add. These rates are essentially identical, indicating that Sarah read aloud equally as efficiently in large print and regular print.

Fatigue and stamina. During the comprehensive PMAP, Sarah read for 20 minutes in large print from a story in a basal reader and another 20 minutes in regular print from another story in the same reader. Her oral reading rates were then calculated for each half of the reading episode in each medium. An objective measure of fatigue would be reflected by a decrease in her reading rate from the first to the second half of each reading episode in a given medium. However, Sarah read at essentially identical rates—in large print, 104 wpm in the first half and 106 wpm in the second half, and in regular print with her tinted reading glasses with a 5D add, 108 wpm in both halves—so no fatigue was noted. Thus, the results indicate that Sarah experienced no fatigue in either medium and maintained her reading stamina for at least 20 minutes of sustained oral reading.

Average working distance. During oral reading, Sarah read at an average of 3 inches in large print and 3.5 inches in regular print. A slight advantage was noted for reading regular print with

Case Study: Interpretation of PMAP Data on Sarah (continued)

her reading glasses, but it was not of sufficient magnitude to draw any educationally significant conclusions. When reading silently, Sarah used a working distance of 3 inches in both media. Overall, both media afforded the same working distance.

Miscue analysis: Graphic similarity. Graphic similarity refers to how similar the actual text item and the miscue are in overall shape and configuration. Generally, efficient readers tap the most graphic similarity at the beginning, the next most at the end, and the least in the middle. The numbers indicate the percentage of text items and miscue items that were graphically similar in the various positions in the words in both media. A higher percentage in graphic similarity is not necessarily better, however, because it indicates that the reader was relying heavily on graphic information in the text, rather than balancing this information with contextual information (as determined through the "acceptability in context" percentage).

For beginning similarity, 89 percent of Sarah's miscues were similar in both large print and regular print. For middle similarity, 79 percent were graphically similar in large print and 89 percent in regular print. For ending similarity, 53 percent were similar in large print and 66 percent in regular print. Overall, Sarah generally tapped the same amount of graphic information in large print as in regular print, and slightly more graphic information in the middle and ends of words in regular print.

Miscue analysis: Acceptability in context. This number indicates the percentage of miscues that were contextually acceptable and, therefore did not disrupt the meaning of the passage. To be considered acceptable in context for the miscue analysis procedure used in this case study, the miscue had to be both semantically acceptable (it made sense in the sentence) and syntactically acceptable (it conformed to the grammatical patterns of English).

In large print, 24 percent of Sarah's miscues were acceptable in context, and in regular print,

19 percent were acceptable. Thus, there was a slight advantage for large print in that 5 percent more of Sarah's miscues were contextually acceptable.

Miscue analysis: Self-correction strategy. This score indicates the percentage of unacceptable miscues—those that would disrupt the construction of meaning of the passage—that are independently corrected by the reader and hence reveals the reader's monitoring of his or her own reading behavior. Ideally, most of the unacceptable miscues should be self-corrected, although there is some evidence that mature readers may correct miscues silently, not aloud. Note that self-corrections of acceptable miscues are not included in the self-correction strategies because they are considered unnecessary since they do not disrupt the meaning of the story.

Sarah independently corrected 13 percent of the unacceptable miscues in large print and 28 percent in regular print. Her self-correction of 15 percent more unacceptable miscues in regular print indicates an advantage of reading regular print with her 5D reading glasses.

CONCLUSION

When Sarah's profile is examined holistically, it provides convincing evidence that reading regular print with tinted reading glasses with a 5D add was as effective and efficient as reading large print with regular nontinted prescription glasses. Although the school district provides large-print books, Sarah does not like them and prefers to use her tinted reading glasses. Despite attempts by the teacher of students with visual impairments to phase out large-print books, the school district continues to purchase them each year. It is hoped that the objective data gathered for this case study will change this practice.

Source: Reprinted, by permission of the publisher, from A. J. Koenig and M. C. Holbrook, *Learning Media Assessment of Students with Visual Impairments: A Resource Guide for Teachers* (Austin: Texas School for the Blind and Visually Impaired, 1993), pp. 132–135.

DECISIONS ON BRAILLE READING AND WRITING INSTRUCTION

Teaching braille reading and writing to students with low vision is a subject that has been fraught with considerable controversy. However, regardless of the political, philosophical, or other issues under discussion at any given point in time, the focus of instructional planning and programming must be the needs of the individual student. Therefore, decisions on selecting literacy media should always focus on providing students with a variety of skills and tools needed to live and work productively in a competitive society. Koenig and Holbrook (1989) referred to this process as filling a student's toolbox with the tools needed to accomplish given tasks. This analogy allows the team to focus on the ultimate value of any given literacy tool. For students with low vision, all literacy tools should be considered in relation to the tasks that need to be accomplished in school and later in adult life. If braille reading and writing are a useful option for meeting these needs, then serious consideration should be given to including systematic and quality instruction in them in the student's program.

Factors that Influence the Decision

The comprehensive learning media assessment provides the basis for considering, and ultimately recommending and initiating, a braille reading and writing program. When all data have been gathered, analyzed, and interpreted, specific needs of the student will be identified. At that point, the team will decide whether braille reading and writing skills will address one or more of the most important needs. Factors that should influence the ultimate decision may include:

- an objectively determined need to add braille reading and writing as a means of supplementing print
- an objectively determined need to teach braille reading and writing eventually to replace print

- a need to introduce braille reading and writing via diagnostic teaching to determine the student's potential for learning and using braille as an effective literacy medium
- the role of braille reading and writing in accomplishing a specific task or tasks needed for continued progress in school or to facilitate independent living and employment
- the time required to teach braille reading and writing skills relative to other identified needs of the student that need to be met before the student leaves school
- the desire of the student and his or her parents to initiate or continue instruction in braille reading and writing.

Factors that should not influence the decision are easy to identify, since they do not focus on the student's needs. However, they are often the most difficult to address because a multitude of extraneous influences tend to be at work in the team decision-making process. Some factors that should not influence the decision to teach braille reading and writing are as follows:

- administrative considerations, such as the availability of a qualified teacher of students with visual impairments, the available time in the teacher's schedule, or cost factors
- the teacher's level of comfort in teaching braille reading and writing
- the educational team's philosophical or personal biases for or against teaching braille reading and writing to students with low vision
- a child's measured visual acuity or other clinical measures.

The teacher of students with visual impairments plays a key role in ensuring that the team focuses only on the needs of the student and that all decisions are supported by objective information gathered in the comprehensive learning media assessment and functional vision evaluation. The teacher should not allow personal biases to hamper the decision-making process, since to do so is likely to divert the team from considering the student's needs.

Instructional Considerations

When the educational team decides to initiate a braille reading and writing program, the members must then address a number of factors related to instruction. These considerations are addressed here not because they directly influence the decision-making process, but because they constitute additional factors that are likely to be considered during the team meeting.

Primary versus Secondary Medium

The expectations for braille reading and writing instruction should be clearly specified during the team meeting:

- Is the goal to teach braille reading and writing as a primary medium for gaining basic academic literacy skills?

- Is the goal to teach braille reading and writing as a secondary medium to supplement print for establishing another functional literacy tool?

- Is the goal to teach braille reading and writing as a secondary medium with the expectation that at some point it will become the student's primary medium (as is the case with many students with retinitis pigmentosa or other progressive eye conditions)?

The expectations of the ultimate role of braille reading and writing in the student's repertoire of literacy tools will shape the content and intensity of the instruction that is provided. If basic literacy skills are to be established in braille, highly intense and consistent instruction is necessary, as would be expected for establishing basic literacy skills in print. Such intensity and consistency would also be required if the intent is for braille reading and writing ultimately to replace print as the primary literacy medium.

However, if braille is to be used as a functional literacy tool, then instruction will probably target those specific literacy tasks, and the intensity of instruction will be geared to the mastery of those tasks. Although the intensity of instruction may vary from that required for establishing basic literacy skills, consistency should be maintained to foster effective and efficient learning.

Parallel versus Nonparallel Instruction

Another facet of the instructional approach involves the different levels of intensity of instruction in braille and in print for establishing literacy skills. This aspect of decision making is relevant for students who will establish basic academic literacy skills in both print and braille, although it may at first seem to be aligned with the previous discussion on the primary versus secondary medium. Print and braille may be introduced at the same time when beginning reading instruction, with the expectation that similar progress will be made in both media, an approach referred to as *parallel instruction* (Holbrook & Koenig, 1992). In parallel instruction, both print and braille receive equal concentration, and the student is expected to use both to complete literacy tasks and other academic schoolwork.

On the other hand, the team may decide to concentrate efforts in beginning reading on print, emphasizing braille reading and writing to a lesser extent but with the clear expectation that the student will develop basic literacy skills in braille (or vice versa). This instructional approach is called *nonparallel instruction* (Holbrook & Koenig, 1992), since the concentration on print and braille and the focus of instruction are differentiated. Also, the student has established or is establishing basic literacy skills in print, so the focus of instruction is on mastery of the braille code. This approach may be considered for a student with a progressive eye condition (such as retinitis pigmentosa) who probably will retain vision during the elementary school years and will use braille reading and writing as a primary medium in his or her later school years.

If the team has decided that braille reading and writing will be taught as a secondary medium, they will probably choose nonparallel instruction. Given the nature of the decision, the team has decided that print reading and writing will be emphasized in establishing basic literacy skills.

Approach to Designing and Implementing Programs

A skillful teacher of students with visual impairments can use a variety of approaches in designing and implementing an effective instructional program in braille for students with low vision. Holbrook and Koenig (1991) outlined the advantages and disadvantages of using five approaches—basal reader, language experience, whole language, *Patterns* (a basal reading program for beginning readers), and *Read Again* (a braille reading program for persons who learn braille after establishing print reading skills)—as well as their suitability for parallel or nonparallel instruction. A summary of these approaches is presented in Table 11.2. In selecting an approach, the teacher should consider the needs of the individual student, the focus of the instructional program, and whether braille reading will be taught in parallel or nonparallel instruction and then match these factors with his or her philosophy of teaching literacy skills.

Contracted versus Uncontracted Braille

The standard practice for providing braille reading and writing instruction in the United States at this time is to introduce Grade 2 braille contractions in initial reading instruction for students who are functionally blind. If the educational team decides to teach braille reading and writing to a student with low vision, then fully contracted braille is likely to be their choice, given the current teaching practices in this country. Any of the approaches for teaching braille reading and writ-

ing to students who are functionally blind can be considered for teaching students with low vision (see Table 11.2).

Although the standard practice is to introduce contracted braille in initial instruction, the early teaching of uncontracted (Grade 1) braille is gaining some recognition in the field. Troutman (1992) suggested that teaching uncontracted braille is valuable for preventing difficulties that some students encounter, including "those with limited vision who can do some work with large print, but need braille as well" (p. 24). She provides justification for this suggestion based on empirical research and strategies for teaching uncontracted braille.

Teaching uncontracted braille offers some advantages for students with low vision. If braille reading and writing is introduced after a period of print reading instruction (nonparallel instruction), uncontracted braille could be taught with a fairly short amount of intense instruction. Time would have to be spent developing tactile perception and hand movements and teaching the identification of letters. Since this approach allows students to begin to read and write in braille expeditiously, the educational team can determine the future potential benefits of braille for an individual student. If they find that braille is useful to the student in completing literacy tasks, then they can develop a plan for introducing braille contractions.

The adoption of such an approach, however, depends on the availability of uncontracted braille books and materials in a school district. Thus, if the choice is to teach uncontracted braille, the local school district needs to take the responsibility for embossing the student's braille materials because braille production centers in the United States do not routinely produce uncontracted braille materials. Although computer technology offers strategies for embossing uncontracted braille, the school district still needs to commit enough personnel, time, and funds to provide a wealth of materials in uncontracted braille because providing minimal amounts of such materials will not give a student sufficient experience to master uncontracted braille.

Table 11.2. Summary of Selected Instructional Approaches for Teaching Braille Reading to Students with Low Vision

Approach	Advantages	Disadvantages	Type of Instruction[a]
Basal reader	Makes efficient use of instructional time. Is a comprehensive and sequential approach.	Offers no control over the introduction of braille contractions.	Ideal for parallel instruction and useful for nonparallel instruction.
Language experience	Involves no concerns about student's experiential background. Is highly motivating to the student. Is flexible—useful for teaching reading in print and braille.	Offers no control over the introduction of vocabulary and braille contractions. May appear unstructured.	Equally valuable for parallel and nonparallel instruction.
Whole language	Is highly motivating to the student. Offers opportunities for reading and writing activities with classmates with normal vision. Provides student with opportunities to select appropriate tools.	Offers provision of adapted materials. Lacks compatibility with itinerant teaching model.	Ideal for parallel instruction and may be useful for nonparallel instruction.
Patterns	Is a comprehensive program. Offers controlled introduction of vocabulary and contractions. Is not dependent on pictures.	Is incompatible with other approaches. Prevents integration with classmates with unimpaired vision during reading class. Limits reading materials outside of the *Patterns* program.	May be useful for parallel instruction, but of limited usefulness for nonparallel instruction.
Read Again	Is a comprehensive program. Is designed to teach the braille code to individuals with adventitious blindness.	Has age appropriateness restricted to older students. Has beginning exercises that appear contrived.	Useful only for nonparallel instruction.

Source: Based on information in M. C. Holbrook and A. J. Koenig, "Teaching braille reading to students with low vision," *Journal of Visual Impairment & Blindness*, 86, (1992), pp. 44–48.

[a]In parallel instruction, both print and braille reading skills are being developed at the same time and with the same intensity; in nonparallel instruction, basic print reading skills have been established, and braille code skills are being introduced.

Many issues need to be resolved with regard to teaching uncontracted versus contracted braille and teaching braille reading and writing in general to students with low vision. Extensive research is required to replicate Troutman's (1992) findings on teaching uncontracted braille, as well as to determine the value of the various approaches to teaching braille reading and writing to students with low vision. The guiding principle for teachers is to expand their students' options for gaining access to information and never to restrict options by omission or conscious choice.

SUMMARY

The learning media assessment is the key to ensuring that students with visual impairments gain full and meaningful literacy skills. The process of selecting general learning media and specific literacy media begins in infancy and continues throughout the student's school years and, ideally, throughout life. In choosing the initial literacy medium, the educational team gathers objective data on the student's efficiency in using the senses to gain information, preferences for the size of objects and for working distances, the prognosis for the eye condition, and the implications of additional disabilities. This information is then used to match the student's characteristics to a specific literacy medium or a combination of media.

After the initial decision is made, the educational team continually reevaluates it and considers when to add additional literacy tools to the student's repertoire. Best practices indicate that at least once a year, data are gathered and synthesized on visual functioning, reading efficiency, academic achievement, handwriting, and literacy tools. The focus of this continuing assessment phase is to ensure that the student learns to use a variety of literacy tools to meet the demands of present and future environments. For some students with low vision, braille is a valuable option for gaining basic or functional literacy skills.

ACTIVITIES

With This Chapter and Other Resources

1. Using the continuing assessment of literacy media described in this chapter, outline a cohesive and comprehensive plan for the upcoming learning media assessment of José, the student introduced in the vignette that opens this chapter.

2. Read the learning media assessment report in the appendix at the end of this chapter and develop recommendations before you read the ones in the report. Discuss these recommendations with your classmates and compare yours with the ones in the report.

3. Compile a file on various procedures and guidelines that have been developed for selecting appropriate literacy media for students with visual impairments, using the references cited in this chapter as a starting point.

4. A sixth-grade girl who has done well academically is experiencing a vision loss because of uveitis. Reading print has become laborious for her, and it is time to perform a learning media assessment. Role-play a scenario with other classmates acting as the girl and her parents in which you, in the role of the teacher of students with visual impairments, and the parents explain to the girl that you will be conducting an assessment of her learning media needs.

In the Community

1. Discuss with a parent the procedures to be followed in deciding a 3-year-old child's literacy medium.

2. Interview three teachers of students with visual impairments to discuss their guidelines on how to determine whether a student's primary literacy medium should be changed from print to braille and share the guidelines with your classmates.

With a Person with Low Vision

1. Collect reading efficiency data for a student with low vision using an informal reading inventory. Calculate the student's efficiency rate and compare it with rates for students with normal vision in Table 11.1.

2. Observe a student with low vision using the Use of Sensory Channels: Observation Form provided at the end of the chapter. Indicate the student's probable primary and secondary sensory channels.

From Your Perspective

What is needed to resolve the controversy over whether all children who are legally blind should learn to read and write in braille?

APPENDIX A: SAMPLE LEARNING MEDIA ASSESSMENT REPORT

Name: David Smith

Date of birth: July 5, 1984

Age: 11 years

Grade: Fourth

Parents: Tom and Judy Smith

Address: 150 Oak Street

Telephone: 505-332-2345

Examiner: Jane Holland, Teacher of Students with Visual Impairments Spring Valley, TX 72233

Date of evaluation: January 25–26, 1996

Date of report: January 30, 1996

PURPOSE OF ASSESSMENT AND STRATEGIES

The school district requested an independent learning media assessment to provide more comprehensive information on David's learning and literacy media needs. The following assessment strategies were used:

- Observations in integrated language arts class and orientation and mobility (O&M) lesson.

- Interviews with the parent, regular classroom teachers, resource room teacher, teacher of students with visual impairments, diagnostician, physical therapist, and occupational therapy assistant.

- Direct assessment of reading efficiency in print, potential for braille reading, and handwriting.

- Review of selected results of previous assessments and other records.

ASSESSMENT RESULTS

Use of sensory channels. An objective procedure was used to document David's use of sensory channels in natural settings. David was observed on two occasions—a language arts class and an O&M lesson—during which individual behaviors were recorded. For each behavior, the examiner noted if David used visual, tactile, or auditory information; both primary and secondary sources of sensory information were noted.

David used vision as the primary source for gathering sensory information and used touch and hearing as secondary sources. It should be noted, however, that this procedure documents the student's existing approach to tasks, not necessarily the most efficient ones. David uses the sensory channels he has been taught to use and has been reinforced for using.

Visual functioning. The records indicate that David's left eye is anophthalmic and fitted with a prosthesis and that his right eye is microphthalmic with a cataract. His distance acuity is 10/140 (20/280) with correction, and his near acuity is 1M print at 2 cm. Although glaucoma can accompany microphthalmia, there has been no evidence of it to date. The available data suggest that his eye condition is stable. A recent low vision clinic report (dated 7-16-95) indicates that optical devices will not improve his near visual functioning and that his conventional spectacles should be worn for near work. Information on David's visual functioning indicates that there has been no change in functioning that would directly affect decisions on his learning and literacy media.

Reading efficiency. Objective data were collected on David's oral reading rate with comprehension, including both typical reading materials from an informal reading inventory (IRI) and content materials used in the classroom. A summary of the findings is shown in the table that accompanies this report.

The first source of data on reading efficiency was obtained with the *Informal Reading Inventory* by Burns and Roe. David was asked to read

Oral Reading Rates: David Smith

Type of Passage	Mode	Comprehension (percentage)	Rate (words per minute)
First grade from IRI (Form A)	Large print	75	45
Second grade from IRI (Form A)	Large print	75	41
Second grade from IRI (Form D)	Large print	75	44
Second grade from IRI (Form C)	CCTV	88	41
Second grade from SRA (Brown Level)	Regular print	Average	49
Fourth-grade science book	Large print	Average	38
Fourth-grade social studies book	Large print	Average	48

short passages, ranging in length from 113 to 235 words, and then to answer 8 to 10 comprehension questions. The print size ranged from 18- to 24-point type, so all passages are considered large print. One form of the test was administered late on Thursday afternoon, and another form was administered mid-morning on Friday.

To calculate reading efficiency, the examiner included only those passages in which David read with at least 75 percent comprehension. Reading efficiency rates were consistently found at around 45 words per minute (wpm). His working distance was from 1.5 to 2 inches, regardless of whether he wore his glasses. The results of the IRI indicated that David's instructional reading level was at the second grade and that his frustration level was at the third grade. However, a more accurate reading assessment instrument needs to be administered to pinpoint David's reading level more precisely.

David was given an opportunity to practice reading with the CCTV on Thursday afternoon and was given a timed reading test on Friday morning. On Thursday, he was shown how to use the various controls and the tracking table. Initial observations indicated that he was able to scan words presented on the screen visually while moving the table with adequate motor control. He adjusted the letters to about 1 inch in height and read from a distance of 4 inches. David tended to pull the table toward him to advance the reading material, rather than to push it away from himself. This is common for students who are inexperienced in reading with the CCTV. On

Friday, David demonstrated excellent recall on the use of the controls and independently set them according to his preferences. Most notably, he demonstrated much more efficient use of the tracking table by appropriately pushing the table away from him to advance the reading passage. On a timed reading test with the CCTV, David read a second-grade passage at 41 wpm with good comprehension. This reading rate is similar to those obtained in large print. David demonstrated the motor skills necessary to read with the CCTV, and his efficiency will increase with repeated practice and experience.

David was also asked to read short passages (226 and 164 words) from the large-print science and social studies textbooks housed in the classroom. To select a passage from his science book, David independently used the table of contents to locate a familiar passage on birds. He read this passage at 38 wpm and then answered general comprehension questions prepared impromptu by the examiner. His level of comprehension was determined to be average according to the examiner's judgment. In the social studies book, David first answered several questions accurately about Texas geography; for example, he stated that Oklahoma was north of Texas and that the Rio Grande River separated Texas and Mexico. He then read a passage on natural resources in Texas at a rate of 48 wpm with average comprehension.

On two occasions, David was asked to read in regular print. He read a passage estimated to be at the second-grade level from the SRA reading series, printed in approximately 12-point type, at a rate of 49 wpm with adequate comprehension. On another occasion, he was asked to read a paragraph from the regular-print version of the *Weekly Reader*. Although no objective rate was taken, the examiner noted that David read fluently from a passage with poor contrast—black letters on a dark purple background—and responded appropriately to the content of the passage.

Several observations related to David's reading efficiency are noteworthy. First, David appeared deliberately to select when to wear his glasses when reading. No noticeable difference was noted in reading efficiency when his glasses were on or off. Second, there was no appreciable difference in reading efficiency when David read in different sizes of print or with the CCTV. He used some strategies for independently adapting to different print sizes, such as adjusting his working distance and deciding when to use his glasses. Third, he generally tilted the materials while he was reading. When asked if he wished to use a reading stand, David indicated that he did not.

Handwriting. According to information obtained during interviews, David uses keyboarding and dictation as his primary modes of expressive writing. Handwriting was not pursued as a primary mode of writing because of his fine motor difficulties. However, David does use handwriting on a limited basis for completing computation problems in math class.

As part of this assessment, David was asked to write the numbers 1 to 10 and his name. The examiner observed that several numbers and letters did not conform to the standard formations, but were "drawn" to look like them. Given the satisfactory level of fine motor control that David demonstrated, the examiner prepared some primary-style writing-paper lines (solid lines with a dashed line separating them) and then demonstrated a few letter formations for David to imitate. He did so with good accuracy (given no practice) and with direct attention to starting and stopping on the appropriate lines. Such excellent progress in a short instructional session strongly suggests David's potential for developing handwriting skills as an option for expressive communication.

Literacy tools. At present, David primarily uses large print for reading and regular print for some materials (such as the *Weekly Reader*). He uses live readers to an extent, but is not in purposeful control of the reading process. That is, he is not yet directing the live reader to read in a strategic manner to meet a specified purpose. (This skill will develop with instruction and meaningful practice.) For writing, he mainly uses keyboarding with a large-print word-processing program accompanied by the Echo speech synthesizer; he also uses dictation for recording answers. He is currently receiving instruction in touch typing skills, but uses a hunt-and-peck method in the classroom. Objective data collected by the resource room teacher indicated that his writing rates with the two methods are roughly comparable, averaging around 15 to 17 wpm. He sometimes uses handwriting for solving computation problems in math, but not for general expressive writing.

The other members of the educational team asked the examiner to assess David's potential for reading and writing in braille. On both days of the assessment, basic tracking and discrimination activities were presented. On Thursday, David demonstrated rough tracking movements across braille lines, but was generally able to move from the top of the page to the bottom of the page with prompting. On Friday, he demonstrated more efficient tracking movement, so he was presented with two types of discrimination tasks. The first involved tracking lines of actual braille interspersed with full cells, as illustrated here:

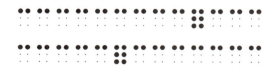

David was directed to track the lines and to indicate when he came to a full cell. He completed this task with good accuracy while demonstrating satisfactory tracking skills. He showed some tendency to want to examine the braille visually, but responded to prompts only to feel the lines. On the second discrimination task, he was presented with sets of braille symbols and was asked to indicate which of the symbols was different in each set. Although he was able to maintain contact with the braille symbols, David was not successful in completing this type of task (which was much more difficult than the previous type). However, one would not be expected to complete such a task without adequate instruction, so this *does not* indicate in any way a lack of potential for braille reading and writing. The level of success demonstrated in tracking and discrimination skills on the first braille task sufficiently indicates David's potential for developing braille reading and writing skills if the educational team determines that these skills are a priority.

One additional note related to braille reading is important. David was observed on both days to apply a great amount of pressure on his fingertips and to have excessive tenseness in his hands. He was able to relax his hands when prompted, but the pressure on the fingertips did not decrease. When this observation was shared later with the physical therapist, she indicated that perhaps the pressure was used as a means of providing stability. She further mentioned that therapy likely would alleviate the excessive pressure. Therefore, the motor difficulties that David experiences should not interfere with his progress in braille reading if such a program is implemented.

SUMMARY OF MAJOR FINDINGS

- ◆ David uses a combination of the visual, auditory, and tactile sensory channels for learning. On the basis of objective documentation, he demonstrated the use of vision as the primary channel and the use of hearing and touch as secondary channels.

- ◆ David's oral reading rates with comprehension were approximately 45 wpm on typical second-grade reading materials and fourth-grade science and social studies passages.

- ◆ At present, David has a limited repertoire of literacy tools for accomplishing reading and writing tasks. His primary reading options are reading large print and using live

readers. His primary writing options are keyboarding and dictation.

- ◆ David demonstrated the motor skills necessary to read with the CCTV and to write in manuscript. Furthermore, he demonstrated a rudimentary level of tracking skills and tactile sensitivity that indicates his potential for learning to read and write in braille.

RECOMMENDATIONS

The following recommendations are offered to the educational team for their consideration in planning an appropriate educational program for David. It is imperative that all team members, including the parents and allied professionals, decide on the priorities for David and then provide the intensity of services required to address these needs. A clear focus and structure for the upcoming school year will ensure that all learning time is used to its maximum benefit.

Expand literacy tools. David needs a variety of options for completing reading and writing tasks. Given a full repertoire of literacy tools, he can then deliberately choose—with instruction and guidance—which option or options will be the most efficient for completing a given task. The following literacy tools should be among the options considered by the educational team:

Reading tools

- ◆ increased use of regular print
- ◆ use of the CCTV
- ◆ use of textbooks on tape
- ◆ directed use of a live reader
- ◆ use of synthetic speech and enlarged print on the computer.

Writing tools

- ◆ use of manuscript writing
- ◆ extended use of touch typing and word processing with Echo and enlarged print on the computer

- use of a live writer (although limited)
- use of a tape recorder for recording answers and notes.

The focus of instruction should be to expand David's options for completing literacy tasks. Reading regular print and using books on audiotape are valuable options for completing certain tasks. David needs to learn that some options are better for certain tasks than are others, but he will not be in a position to make such decisions unless he has a range of options from which to choose. Some essential literacy tools for David are discussed in more detail below.

Teach manuscript handwriting skills. David has the motor ability and the desire to learn handwriting skills. The educational team should consider this a key priority in expanding David's writing options. He will need primary-style writing paper (upper and lower solid lines with a middle dotted line) with sharp contrast and consistent instruction to learn proper letter formations. Since he has been using some writing for math, this may be the best area to focus on initially. He will need to decrease the size of his writing over the upcoming years. For beginning instruction, line widths of about 1 to 1.25 inches will be appropriate.

Teach touch typing skills. The educational team has made a commitment to teach touch typing, and this instruction should be continued and intensified. The hunt-and-peck method is not efficient for anyone, and it is even less efficient for a student with low vision. David will need to continue to use the hunt-and-peck method for some time until he gains sufficient touch typing skills, but a transition should begin as soon as possible to touch typing alone. He will continue to benefit from the auditory feedback provided by a speech synthesizer, as well as the visual information from the enlarged print on the computer screen. The large-print letters on the keyboard should be faded and eventually eliminated as his proficiency in touch typing increases.

Teach the use of the CCTV. David has the motor ability now to make use of the CCTV as an option for reading. Actually, little instruction will be needed because he knows the basics of using the CCTV. The focus should be on providing access to a CCTV and providing practice in its efficient use. To gain efficiency, David will need extended practice in reading continuous text. He needs to learn that he can gain a more comfortable working distance and posture by increasing the size of the letters and moving farther from the screen. If appropriate adjustments are made in the size of letters and distance from the screen, the same retinal image will be gained as with the closer working distance. Consultation with the occupational therapist or physical therapist will help determine the best posture for reading.

Consider the possible role of braille reading and writing in David's repertoire of literacy tools. David has the potential to develop braille reading and writing skills. However, the question is whether it is a priority at this point, and that question can be answered only by the educational team. If David's eye condition remains stable and he develops other efficient options for reading and writing, I believe that braille should be considered as a future option if such a need arises. If his eye condition does not remain stable, or if consistent and targeted instruction does not yield other efficient literacy tools, then braille reading and writing instruction should be given immediate consideration. If it is decided to introduce braille reading and writing, an intensive period must be set aside for instruction (for example, 1 to 1.5 hours daily).

Reconsider the need for abacus instruction. I recommend emphasizing handwriting skills as an avenue for computation. While the abacus is an important option to consider for computation, developing efficiency and accuracy in its use is a long-term process. I think that David has other needs, such as those listed above, that take priority over abacus instruction. Also, I believe that computation on paper can become more efficient more quickly than the use of the abacus; however, it will require consistent and intensive instruction.

Use an experiential, multisensory approach to learning. David has the ability to use all his senses, and he should be given repeated exposure to meaningful experiences in real contexts for learning through all his sensory channels. According to his teachers, a multisensory approach was used throughout the previous school year, and this approach should continue. Students with low vision often miss valuable information because the use of vision alone may provide inadequate or inaccurate information. A multisensory approach to learning will alleviate much of this potential problem. Multisensory experiences must extend beyond the classroom and into the home and community. Using O&M lessons to provide age-appropriate experiences is a meaningful and practical approach to ensure that David gains a wide variety of high-quality life experiences.

Provide sufficient time and services to develop needed skills. After the educational team has delineated and established priorities among the needed literacy tools and other skills, then an appropriate program should be developed that will adequately meet those needs. The team may find that an integrated intermediate school program will not provide sufficient time for intensive instruction. Therefore, time may need to be devoted to the specific teaching of compensatory skills in a more specialized environment. The rationale is that David will then have the repertoire of literacy tools and other skills to benefit meaningfully from an integrated school program. Regardless of the instructional arrangement, sufficient instructional time must be devoted to developing the specialized skills that David will need for independent living and employment.

Provide continuing assessment. The learning media assessment, as well as other assessment processes, are most meaningful when conducted on a continuing basis. David's needs have changed considerably over the past few years; therefore, the instructional program and strategies should change as well. As principles of diagnostic teaching are used to assess emerging skills and changing needs continually, David will benefit the most from all learning experiences.

Use of Sensory Channels: Observation Form

Student _____

Setting/Activity _____

Date _____ Observer _____

Observed Behavior	Sensory Channel		
_____	V	T	A
_____	V	T	A
_____	V	T	A
_____	V	T	A
_____	V	T	A
_____	V	T	A
_____	V	T	A
_____	V	T	A
_____	V	T	A
_____	V	T	A
_____	V	T	A
_____	V	T	A
_____	V	T	A
_____	V	T	A
_____	V	T	A
_____	V	T	A
_____	V	T	A
_____	V	T	A
_____	V	T	A
_____	V	T	A
_____	V	T	A
_____	V	T	A
_____	V	T	A
_____	V	T	A
_____	V	T	A
_____	V	T	A

☐ Probable Primary Channel: _____

◯ Probable Secondary Channel(s): _____

Appendix B. Sample Observation Form for Use of Sensory Channels

Source: A. J. Koenig and M. C. Holbrook, *Learning Media Assessment of Students with Visual Impairments: A Resource Guide for Teachers,* 2nd ed. (Austin: Texas School for the Blind and Visually Impaired, 1993).

Instruction of Literacy Skills to Children and Youths with Low Vision

Alan J. Koenig and Evelyn J. Rex

VIGNETTE

Roseanna, a 17-year-old senior in high school, has congenital nystagmus and a visual acuity of 20/160. She reads at 230 words per minute using her eyeglasses and a 20-diopter hand-held magnifier and takes notes from the chalkboard in class using an 8X handheld monocular. She will attend college in the fall, but during the summer she wanted to find a job, so she could have additional spending money.

Roseanna decided to apply for a position as a secretary at a bank in her community in answer to the bank's advertisement for a high school or college student to fill in for vacationing employees for a six-week period. Roseanna did not expect the bank manager to react negatively when she applied, since he had known her since she was a child. However, during the interview, she learned that he thought she was almost blind and probably could not carry out the tasks of the job. Fortunately, Roseanna kept her wits about her and explained that her literacy skills probably matched those of other applicants and that with her devices, no unreasonable accommodations would be needed for employment. Roseanna got the job and is now several hundred dollars richer and six weeks' more experienced as an employee.

Roseanna's literacy skills did not "just happen."

Early in life, a teacher of students with visual impairments worked closely with her parents at home to ensure that Roseanna was given the essential early literacy experiences that children with unimpaired vision gain incidentally. In elementary school, Roseanna's teachers emphasized the development of efficient, fluent reading skills and stamina. Roseanna did not need a low vision device for reading at first, since regular textbooks for young students are all in large print. As the print sizes of materials decreased in the third and fourth grades, the clinical low vision specialist prescribed a handheld magnifying device. The teacher of students with visual impairments taught Roseanna to use the magnifier to read any print materials she wished to read. As Roseanna moved from elementary school to high school, more emphasis was placed on using literacy skills to accomplish real-life tasks. This instruction included opening and maintaining a checking account for the salary from her summer job.

INTRODUCTION

Teachers of students with visual impairments are responsible for ensuring that students with low vision attain reading and writing skills for learning, living, and working. This process begins in infancy and continues throughout the students' school years. Unless they teach in resource room programs or special schools, teachers of students with visual impairments are generally not the primary teachers of reading and writing, so their role is often to support students in regular classroom programs. If the development of literacy skills is left to chance or if teachers simply assume that such skills will develop "naturally," students with low vision will be at risk of having marginal or no literacy skills and thus will be at a significant disadvantage in school and life. This chapter discusses the factors that influence reading and writing with low vision and presents strategies that teachers of students with visual impairments can use to foster the development of literacy in their students with low vision.

FACTORS THAT INFLUENCE READING AND WRITING WITH LOW VISION

Visual Skills in Reading

In efficient visual reading, the reader fixates on a central point within a group of letters or short words, decodes the information, and then jumps the eyes forward on the line to the next group of letters or words. This process is repeated in successive fixations to the end of the line, after which the eyes quickly find the beginning of the next line. These quick eye fixations, called saccadic movements, occur repeatedly during continuous reading. Efficient readers concentrate on gaining meaning from the text, not on their eye movements.

Reading with low vision also involves saccadic movements, although the efficiency of the movements and the width of the perceptual span differ, depending on the characteristics of the individual and the functional implications of his or her visual impairment. In supporting the development of reading skills, the teacher of students with visual impairments emphasizes the visual portion of the reading process, but in the context of meaningful activities and in a visually comfort-

able and motivating environment. The objective is to make eye movements efficient and automatic. If the reader must attend to eye movements, then attention is diverted from higher-level reading skills, such as comprehension.

If a student's eye movements contribute to inefficient reading, the teacher of students with visual impairments should allow the student ample time to practice reading while concentrating on the use of vision, rather than on new reading skills. The use of nonoptical low vision devices, such as a typoscope (a window cut in a piece of cardboard that is the width of one line), a marker under or above the line (such as a ruler), or one's finger, will decrease the amount of extraneous stimuli from the page and guide the student's eyes to the next appropriate spot on the line. To change lines efficiently, the student can mark the next line to read with a finger. While helping a student to develop skills in eye movements with such strategies, it is preferable to give the student easy reading materials, so less attention is needed for decoding and comprehending. As a student's reading efficiency increases, fewer external strategies and cues will be needed. The method of repeated readings, discussed later, is an ideal strategy for increasing fluency in reading.

To increase comfort in reading and facilitate the development of more efficient eye movements, other modifications of the visual environment are made, when necessary. Appropriate lighting is an essential factor in increasing the contrast and decreasing the glare from reading materials (see Chapter 7). High-gloss desktops and other work surfaces may cause glare that can be alleviated by covering the surfaces with a dark blotter or other material. Other modifications may include the judicious use of acetate filters and book stands.

Whereas the typical saccadic pattern is used in reading narrative text, other eye-movement patterns are used for various types of reading tasks, such as reading a map, finding information in a table or chart, scanning headlines in a newspaper, and locating a word in a dictionary. Finding a word in a dictionary, for example, involves shifting visual fixation from one set of guide words to the next until the right page is found; scanning down the bold-face entries to the correct word; using a saccadic pattern to read the entry, although portions of the entry are usually skimmed to locate the needed information. These visual tasks may be more difficult for a person with low vision and may require more systematic and deliberate instruction.

Visual Skills in Writing

In writing, the individual uses a series of eye fixations around the area in which writing is occurring. Despite the general notion that writing requires visual tracking, such is not the case. Tracking the end of a pencil is both inefficient and unnecessary, and thus it is not helpful to encourage a student with low vision to do so.

An important visual skill for writing (as well as for coloring and drawing) is a combination of eye movements and motor movements, often called visual-motor skills. The precision needed for refined visual-motor skills is heavily influenced by the efficient use of vision. Therefore, children with low vision often need ample practice with appropriate materials and writing tools to refine these skills, which children with normal vision develop automatically and with relative ease.

The key to improving visual-motor skills is to increase contrast and decrease glare, so the student can gain ample practice at a particular task comfortably. The visual environment can be modified by using bold-line pictures, bold-line paper, black felt-tip markers, artists' soft-lead pencils, or white chalk on black construction paper and by adjusting the lighting and the position of materials. Again, the teacher should move to fewer and fewer modifications as the child develops.

Magnification and Reading with Low Vision

Effects on Perceptual Span

Persons with low vision generally need magnification of the text to gain the resolution needed

to read efficiently. As is discussed in detail in Chapter 7, magnification of text can be gained through relative-distance magnification (moving closer to the text), relative-size magnification (making the print larger), angular magnification (enlarging the text optically or making it appear closer to the eye through a lens system), or projection magnification (projecting the image of the text, such as with a closed-circuit television [CCTV]). Although the proper amount of magnification allows the resolution needed for reading, it has an impact on the width of the perceptual span.

The typical perceptual span in mature reading is considered to be 7 to 10 letters. This is the amount of information that an individual can decode and store in short-term memory in one fixation before going on to the next fixation. However, since meaningful information is rarely contained in 7 to 10 letters, readers store a number of "chunks" of this information until they can meaningfully interpret and comprehend the text and then store the chunks of information in long-term memory (Thorndike, 1984).

The width of the perceptual span in reading with low vision depends on the interaction between the size of the letters, the distance from the page, and the intactness of the central visual field. Students with low vision generally need a larger-than-normal print size (or magnification effect) and a closer working distance (the page-to-eye distance) to gain the resolution needed to read efficiently.

However, magnification has an effect on the perceptual span. As the size of letters increases through magnification, the perceptual span decreases. The goal of clinical low vision services is to find the ideal level of magnification and comfortable working distance from the page to optimize the perceptual span. As a student's perceptual span approaches or matches the normal width of 7 to 10 letters, his or her reading rate will increase. If a student is using too much magnification, either because of an inappropriately prescribed optical device or the unnecessary use of large print, then his or her reading rate may suffer.

To ensure that a student is maximizing the interaction between his or her perceptual span and working distance, the teacher of students with visual impairments systematically collects objective data on reading efficiency under various conditions, such as reading large print and reading regular print with an optical device (see Chapter 11 for an objective procedure for documenting this information). Also, the teacher works with the student to explore a comfortable working distance from the page and appropriate head and eye movements. Since studies (Koenig, Layton, & Ross 1992; Koenig & Ross, 1991) have found that students with low vision often read at the same distance from the page, whether they are reading large print, regular print, or regular print with an optical device, students need to be taught strategies for maximizing their reading efficiency by changing their working distance from the page and thereby increasing or decreasing their perceptual span. The goal is to find a comfortable working distance at which the student can sustain efficient reading.

To find a student's comfortable working distance, the teacher of students with visual impairments can ask the student to read at various distances from the page or a stand or handheld magnifying device and then document the differences with objective data, such as reading rates and informal information, such as the student's stated comfort level. It should be noted, however, that the focal distance (page-to-device distance) of a handheld magnifier is a function of the optics of the device and should not change, but that the working distance (page-to-eye distance) may vary.

Since both the focal distance and the working distance of a spectacle-mounted optical device, such as a microscope, do not vary, a student is unable to vary the size of the perceptual span, but uses the textual information surrounding the perceptual span to guide the eyes to the next fixation point. Thus, although the text outside the perceptual span is not readable, it serves a key role in facilitating efficient eye movements and is useful for noting other cues in reading, such as punctuation marks and paragraph indentations. Because

of the value of this information in developing reading skills, Jackson (1973) cautioned against using spectacle-mounted devices with young children that do not allow them to change the working distance. Stand-mounted and handheld magnifiers, which permit the individual to change the working distance, make better use of peripheral cues. For young children, Jackson noted, the use of linear magnification (getting closer to the page) is preferable because they can use their extensive natural accommodative power with closer working distances to gain magnification.

The working distance also affects the level of comfort with the speed and duration of reading. The teacher may continue to emphasize the variation of the perceptual span that is possible with different working distances, but should keep in mind that not all students with low vision can resolve images even at a close range or sustain visual tasks at a functional speed.

Efficient reading with low vision can be viewed as a balancing act. The reader requires magnification to gain the necessary resolution needed to decode words, but has to maximize the working distance to increase the width of the perceptual span. As the magnification increases and the working distance decreases, the perceptual span decreases. The clinical low vision specialist and the teacher of students with visual impairments must work closely with each other and with the student to find the proper amount of magnification and the most comfortable working distance to yield the most efficient reading.

Effects on Visual Fields

The effectiveness of magnification depends to a great extent on the visual field. Persons with full visual fields who simply need the enlargement of text to read more efficiently can gain magnification through any of the methods just mentioned. Magnification strategies that can be used at any time, such as the use of optical devices, put the individual in direct control of gaining visual information from the text.

Persons with central field losses or central scotomas (such as those with macular degeneration) often benefit from the use of magnification, which increases the size of the letters around the central field loss or scotoma but does not magnify the size of the scotoma itself. Those with central scotomas may also benefit from learning a visual technique called eccentric fixation, by which they realign the scotoma, so it is placed above or below what they wish to read (see Chapter 8 for additional information). Because the area outside of the macula provides less clear resolution of the text, magnification will often allow the individual to resolve letters and words while reading.

Persons with restricted central fields caused by extensive peripheral field losses (such as those with advanced retinitis pigmentosa) generally do not benefit from magnification. When only central vision remains, magnification decreases the amount of information within the available central field.

In short, magnification is not always helpful to people with low vision. However, the clinical low vision specialist must consider the amount of magnification needed by the individual to resolve an image when reading. A person may need magnification to gain resolution, and the resulting limit on the perceptual span may be unavoidable.

Effects on Reading Rate

To understand the effect of magnification on a person's reading rate, one must first realize that reading efficiency is influenced by a number of interrelated factors, such as familiarity with information in the text; experiential background; existing decoding, vocabulary skills, and comprehension skills; interest and motivation; stamina and fatigue; intactness of the central field; clarity of the ocular media; and level of magnification. Since many factors interrelate to influence a person's reading rate, it may be more appropriate to address reading efficiency, which encompasses both the reading rate and level of comprehension, and to view the following discussion of the effect of magnification on reading rates in the context of the entire reading process.

Table 12.1. Estimated Reading Rates for Persons with Low Vision under Four Conditions (in words per minute)

Central Field	Ocular Media	
	Clear	Cloudy
Intact	131	95
Loss	39	29

Source: Data from G. E. Legge, G. S. Rubin, D. G. Pelli, M. M. Schleske, A. Luebker, and J. A. Ross, "Understanding Low Vision Reading," *Journal of Visual Impairment & Blindness* 82 (1988), Figure 6, p. 56.

The reading rate is directly influenced by the width of the perceptual span in reading. Mature readers with a perceptual span of 7 to 10 letters read typical print text at about 250 to 300 words per minute. As the width of the perceptual span decreases, the amount of information decoded and sent to the brain for processing also decreases and results in a slower rate of reading. Since the width of the perceptual span decreases when magnification increases as a person with low vision uses the level of magnification needed to resolve letters and words efficiently, his or her reading rate will decrease with the width of the perceptual span.

Little is known about the reading rates of persons with low vision because only a few empirical studies have been conducted. In one study, Legge, Rubin, Pelli, Schleske, Luebker, and Ross (1988) used a statistical procedure to determine the peak reading rates of persons with low vision under four conditions (see Table 12.1). They found that an intact central field is the major factor in efficient reading rates and that clear ocular media are also influential. In a series of case studies on students with low vision, Koenig and Ross (1991) and Koenig et al. (1992) collected objective data on reading rates in various print media. Three observations from this research are noteworthy. First, the reading rates of students with low vision varied widely and did not seem to be a function of age or grade level. Second, students with central field losses demonstrated reading rates near those predicted by Legge et al. Third, the reading rates of individual students were similar across media, regardless of whether the students were reading in large print or in regular print with or without an optical device.

ROLE OF THE TEACHER OF STUDENTS WITH VISUAL IMPAIRMENTS

As was mentioned earlier, the role of the teacher of students with visual impairments depends on the program model in supporting the development of reading and writing skills. Teachers at special schools, as well as those in resource-room programs in public schools, have direct responsibility for providing reading and writing instruction, for teaching disability-specific skills, and for ensuring that the needs of their students with low vision are met. In most public school settings, however, they provide support for regular classroom teachers and supplementary instruction in unique skills, when necessary. The areas of responsibility for teaching disability-specific skills may include the following:

- ensuring that students develop a solid experiential and conceptual basis for literacy
- structuring early literacy experiences in the home so as not to rely solely on incidental experiences
- teaching the efficient use of visual skills in authentic contexts, such as efficient scanning skills to locate words in a dictionary or to interpret a map
- teaching students to interpret pictures of increasing complexity
- teaching students to use optical and non-optical low vision devices
- providing practice to build automatic skills in the use of low vision devices
- providing targeted instruction to increase fluency and stamina in reading

- teaching functional applications of reading and writing skills, if they have not already been taught in the classroom
- arranging the physical environment to maximize the visual learning and increase the comfort of young students
- helping the student assume responsibility for gaining access to print
- providing adapted materials and equipment
- teaching keyboarding and computer word-processing skills if these skills are not part of the early regular curriculum
- teaching a variety of literacy tools for gaining access to print independently, such as using a monocular to take notes from a chalkboard.

For any number of reasons, students with low vision may fall between the cracks of educational programming. Since they seem to be more sighted than blind, their unique needs may not be addressed with the same intensity as may the needs of students who are functionally blind. Regular classroom teachers may not feel the same level of responsibility for students with low vision as for other students, since they believe that the "special" teachers are providing all the assistance these students need. Sometimes, both regular classroom teachers and special teachers think that it is sufficient to give these students large-print books or believe that weak literacy skills are a natural outcome of having low vision and hence do not attempt to use instructional strategies to improve these skills. In some instances, the role of the teacher of students with visual impairments might be misperceived as one of providing tutorial assistance. All of these situations fail to address the unique reading and writing needs of students with low vision.

If teachers of students with visual impairments are not diligent about monitoring the progress of students with low vision, these students may enter adulthood without reading and writing skills because other members of the educational team assumed that someone else was taking care of this instruction and follow-up. Monitoring the students' progress is further complicated by the fact that teachers often ignore the results of tests they give because they believe that the tests are invalid for students with low vision. Therefore, a crucial role of teachers of students with visual impairments is to ensure that the team addresses all the unique needs of students with low vision and that the students are making meaningful progress toward full literacy.

FOSTERING THE GROWTH OF EMERGENT LITERACY

Before the start of formal schooling, young children with normal vision "emerge" naturally into literacy without much or any direct attention from adults, through observing and imitating the functions and uses of literacy in daily life, as described in Chapter 4. Young children with low vision, however, may miss some or most of the opportunities for natural observation and imitation. Therefore, the teacher of students with visual impairments must take direct steps to ensure that a solid foundation for early literacy is established. In this regard, two broad areas require specific attention by parents and teachers of young children with low vision: expanding the range and variety of early life experiences and providing direct exposure to literacy events.

Expanding Early Life Experiences

A rich variety of early life experiences provides the foundation for literacy by helping children to discover the meaning of literacy events, both reading and writing. Lowenfeld (1974) encouraged teachers and parents to emphasize common everyday experiences. Sidebar 12.1 lists some basic examples of experiences that all children need to have early in life.

A role of the teacher of students with visual impairments is to ensure that children receive a variety of high-quality experiences before and during literacy instruction and not assume either that young children with low vision automatically have such experiences or that parents have the sole responsibility for providing them. During the early years, special teachers should work with parents and other members of the educational team—especially orientation and mobility (O&M) instructors, who often provide instruction in the community—to give young children the appropriate experiential base for learning skills that will be meaningful in their lives.

An ideal approach for helping young children have rich learning experiences is the consistent application of Lowenfeld's (1974) principles: using concrete experiences, learning by doing, and providing unified experiences. Although Lowenfeld advocated the use of these special methods for students who are functionally blind, they are equally applicable to students with low vision, who will, however, also use vision to gain information from the world around them. Sidebar 12.2 presents the special methods and their applications for students with low vision. The overriding goal is to engage young children actively in experiences in which they use all their senses to gain information.

Providing Direct Exposure to Literacy Events

Young children typically attempt to read and write because they see their parents and others doing so and because they associate abstract symbols (such as the "Golden Arches" of McDonald's) with meaningful events in their lives. For example, after seeing their parents read a newspaper, young children may pick up a book and imitate this event, perhaps inserting an occasional, "Oh, isn't that interesting!" Or after watching their parents write letters or pay bills, they may scribble something and then "read" back the message aloud. These are important early literacy behaviors that provide an important foundation for later, more conventional literacy skills.

A child with low vision, on the other hand, may miss these important connections. For example, environmental signs, such as the Golden

---

SIDEBAR 12.1

Some Basic Early Experiences for Young Children

HOME EXPERIENCES

- Helping prepare a snack or bake cookies.
- Picking up the morning newspaper.
- Helping stack dishes in the dishwasher.
- Helping rake leaves or plant flowers.
- Picking up clothes or toys.
- Getting the mail from the mail carrier.
- Playing with siblings or friends in the backyard.
- Calling grandmother and grandfather on the telephone.

COMMUNITY EXPERIENCES

- Playing at the city park with siblings and friends.

- Splashing in the wading pool at a public swimming pool.
- Exploring the grocery store and stores at a mall.
- Visiting a farm with animals and machinery.
- Eating at a fast-food and at a formal restaurant.
- Visiting a petting zoo.
- Visiting public places like the post office, fire station, and library.

Source: Alan J. Koenig. "Growing into Literacy," in M. Cay Holbrook (Ed.), *Children with Visual Impairments: A Parents' Guide*, (Bethesda, Md.: Woodbine House, 1996).

Arches, may be outside a child's distance vision range or may speed by while the child is riding in a car to the extent that the information is meaningless. Even at closer distances, a child with low vision may not realize that his or her father is writing a shopping list, although it is clear that something is occurring. For a young child with low vision to gain the same benefits from naturally occurring literacy events, he or she must be actively exposed to and engaged in such events.

A child with low vision is exposed to the Golden Arches by taking the time to stop and actively explore the sign. Most McDonald's restaurants have small versions of the Golden Arches on their entrance and exit signs that children can explore both visually and tactilely to gain accurate information on the characteristics of the signs; they then learn the meaning of the signs by eating at the restaurant. After repeated experiences, they will associate the Golden Arches with eating at McDonald's.

To provide direct experiences in making a shopping list, a parent can place the child in his or her lap and talk through the experience, saying

perhaps, "Let's make a list of things we need at the store. We need lettuce [writes "lettuce"], bread [writes "bread"], and milk [writes "milk"]. What else do we need?" The parent can then encourage the child to name other items and can write whatever the child names on the list. Then to complete the activity (and to make it meaningful), the list is used in the store to help gather the needed items, checking each one off as it is placed in the shopping cart.

Reading aloud to young children is a powerful way to model the use of literacy and is one of the most important factors in their ultimate success in developing literacy skills (Trelease, 1989). For toddlers and preschoolers with low vision, reading aloud by parents and teachers allows young children to engage in a near-point task that is more likely to be within their field of view than many other literacy events. Early books used for reading aloud should have bold, clear, and uncluttered pictures; as the students grows older, books with increasingly more complex pictures can be used. As the book or story is read aloud, time should be taken to examine and enjoy the

SIDEBAR 12.2

Providing Learning Experiences: Principles of Special Methods and Applications for Students with Low Vision

Principles	Applications for Students with Low Vision
Need for concrete experiences	◆ Use real materials for learning activities. ◆ Use scale models to supplement visual information. ◆ Supplement the use of vision with all other sources of sensory information.
Need for learning by doing	◆ Ensure that students participate actively in all aspects of real-life experiences. ◆ Participate in all steps of a sequential activity (such as baking cookies and washing a car). ◆ Supplement the use of vision with all other sources of sensory information.
Need for unifying experiences	◆ Provide instruction in study units to allow the application of skills throughout the day. ◆ Use field trips for learning in real environments. ◆ Ensure that students actively engage in all aspects of an experience and in all steps in a sequential activity. ◆ Use telescopic devices to gain access to objects that are inaccessible to unaided vision (for example, mountain ranges and skyscrapers); pair the use of these devices with a model that can be visually and tactilely explored at a close distance. ◆ Supplement the use of vision with all other sources of sensory information.

pictures on each page. Also, real objects associated with the story should be used to supplement pictures, so a child with low vision has the opportunity to pair tactual information with visual information. For more strategies on reading aloud, the reader is referred to Trelease (1989) and Koenig (1996).

Before a young child starts formal schooling, the teacher of students with visual impairments works with the parents and extended family members, modeling the use of specific strategies, such as those just mentioned, to help them carry out the activities at home. Continued guidance and assessment are needed to ensure that the child is receiving the range of general experiences

and specific literacy experiences that undergird formal literacy instruction.

SUPPORTING THE DEVELOPMENT OF ACADEMIC READING SKILLS

Academic literacy skills are a major focus of instruction in elementary school. As was discussed in Chapter 4, the types of literacy tasks taught to students—reading and responding to stories, reading and interpreting poetry, writing narrative pieces, writing term papers—are fairly unique to school settings. That is, these tasks are not usually the primary literacy tasks performed in everyday

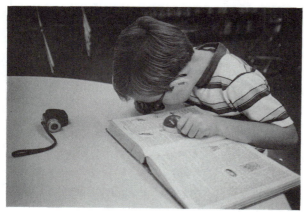

Learning to read and write in school provides the foundation for success and independence in adulthood.

life. Nevertheless, it is universally agreed that the acquisition of basic academic literacy skills is a fundamental goal of schooling. To attain a solid foundation in these skills, students with low vision need a range of instructional and support services, and the teacher of students with visual impairments is ultimately responsible for fostering the development of these skills.

Integrating Nonoptical and Optical Devices

The teacher of students with visual impairments has three broad areas of responsibility in helping students with low vision to become effective and efficient users of low vision devices. First, the teacher guarantees the availability of appropriate devices for reading (see Chapter 7 for a detailed discussion of these devices). This is done by working closely with all members of the educational team, including clinical low vision specialists, to determine a student's needs in reading; matching the student's needs to the nonoptical and optical devices that address those needs; and arranging for the student to obtain the appropriate devices for use both in school and at home. Second, the teacher provides direct instruction of sufficient intensity to allow the student to gain basic mastery of the devices, as well as to practice

using them in appropriate contexts. For example, the teacher may provide initial direct instruction using a stand magnifier for reading and then have the student practice this skill reading leisure books in the classroom (see Chapter 9 for further discussion of teaching the use of low vision devices).

Third, the teacher fosters the student's meaningful integration of the low vision devices in all areas of life. He or she does so by teaching the student to choose the appropriate literacy tool, including such nonvisual strategies as using a live reader, that will help the student complete a given task. The teacher also shows the student real-life applications of the devices in authentic contexts. For example, he or she could prompt the student to use a monocular to read the overhead menu at a fast-food restauraunt during a daily living-skills activity or could prompt the student to position a deposit slip away from glare reflected from a window during a community lesson at the bank.

Round-Robin Reading

Some regular classroom teachers maintain that "round-robin reading" (or having a student read aloud in front of the class) is an important component of the reading program, whereas others undoubtedly have students read aloud simply because it is a "traditional" practice. Regardless of the reason, many students with low vision attend classes in which reading aloud is part of the daily routine.

For students with low vision, reading in general may be a stressful part of the day because it is usually a slower and more laborious activity for them than for their classmates with unimpaired vision. The factors mentioned earlier—field of view, magnification effect, and field restrictions—interact with students' other individual characteristics to influence reading fluency and efficiency. When called on to read aloud, students with low vision are placed in a position of demonstrating to the entire class their different level of reading fluency, as well as their need to look at books in a different way. The emotional impact of this situation can be detrimental to some students' sense of worth, especially as readers.

Although it is tempting simply to exempt a student with low vision from reading aloud, doing so just sets the student further apart from the other students and prevents him or her from developing what some authorities believe is a vital reading skill. A more productive course of action in many cases is for the teacher of students with visual impairments to address the student's difficulty with oral reading by providing additional, targeted practice in reading fluency so the student is better prepared to read aloud and feels more comfortable using an optical or nonoptical device in front of others. In addition, the teacher can help the student practice reading a particular story or rehearse the actual portion that the student will read in class, so he or she is familiar with the vocabulary, plot, and characters, and hence can read aloud with greater confidence and fluency.

Of the four strategies for increasing reading fluency outlined in Sidebar 12.3, repeated readings holds great promise for students with low vision. In repeated readings, the student reads a selected passage again and again until a predetermined criterion level of reading rate is attained. The theory that undergirds this approach—automaticity theory—suggests that as students gain more fluency in reading words aloud in a passage, their attention then shifts to comprehending the meaning of the passage. In Layton's (1993) study of the use of repeated readings with five elementary school students with low vision, the students not only became more fluent in reading practice materials, but generalized this fluency to other reading materials.

The teacher of students with visual impairments can use the time spent practicing reading fluency to develop other unique skills as well. Such sessions can include an introduction to or practice in the use of optical devices, adjusting lighting, using a typoscope, scanning and interpreting of pictures, and so forth. With this integrated approach, the unique skills are always developed in the context of meaningful activities.

Using Targeted Reading Instruction Strategies

A wide range of specific, targeted reading strategies are available for developing or improving reading skills. Although these strategies were developed for use by students with normal vision, when they are applied in a purposeful manner and guided by diagnostic teaching to assess their effectiveness, they are equally valuable for increasing the reading skills of students with low vision. Two such strategies—the language experience approach and the cloze approach—are discussed next.

Language Experience Approach

The language experience approach (LEA) is a straightforward approach that is based directly on actual experiences in which students have engaged, so the concerns about the lack of an experiential base mentioned earlier and in Chapter 4 are alleviated. Teachers can use LEA before students enter kindergarten to give them a "boost" in learning reading skills. The steps in LEA are summarized in Sidebar 12.4.

If students with low vision have some level of formal reading skill before they enter kindergarten, they may concentrate more on other skills needed for success in regular classrooms, such as keeping materials organized, gaining access to the visual information in the classroom and playground, and forming and maintaining social relationships with peers. Although empirical studies on the use of LEA with students with low vision have not been conducted, field experiences provide strong evidence that it is effective when appropriately applied by a skillful teacher.

Cloze Procedure

In the cloze procedure, a meaningful segment of a story is recopied with blanks replacing words of the same length at regular designated intervals. In the classic cloze procedure, every seventh word is replaced by a blank, and the first and last sentences are left intact. Variations on this basic pro-

Strategies for Increasing Reading Fluency

Instructional Strategy	Procedure
Repeated readings	Determine the student's average oral reading rate in the student's preferred medium (or in a medium in which increased fluency is desired). Select short, interesting stories at the student's instructional level that can be read in three to five minutes. Set a criterion goal that the student can easily obtain after three or four rereadings. After the first reading, inform the student of his or her rate. Have the student continue reading the passage and provide feedback on his or her rate until the criterion rate is attained. Begin each session with a new passage. After the student is comfortable reading at the criterion rate, increase it.
Paired reading	Select a classmate who reads faster and more fluently than the student with low vision. Using reading material that is appropriate for each, have the student with low vision read aloud and ask the classmate for help on words, if needed. After the student with low vision has read the passage, ask him or her to retell the story. Then as the classmate reads his or her story aloud, have the student with low vision follow along in the text and retell the story at the end of the passage. In this approach, the classmate provides a model of fluent oral reading.
Choral reading	Select easy reading materials for a pair or a small group of students and have all the students read aloud at the same time, often along with the teacher. The slower students will speed up to match the overall rate of the group. Since no one is "on stage," choral reading provides a comfortable way to increase fluency and confidence.
Echo reading	This approach is similar to choral reading, but the teacher and student read together. Select a period of about 15 minutes to read each day. Use familiar material that is at the student's independent reading level and is of interest to the student. Direct the student to disregard meaning and to slide his or her eyes smoothly across the text without hesitation. The teacher and student hold the book together and read in unison, with the teacher's finger moving simultaneously under the text. At first, the teacher reads slightly louder than the student. Since the teacher sets the pace for reading, he or she gradually increases the student's rate. Also, the teacher reads words with which the student has difficulty, thereby increasing the student's confidence.

Source: Based on S. J. Samuels, "The Method of Repeated Reading," *The Reading Teacher,* 33 (1979); and R. J. Tierney, J. E. Readence, and E. K. Dishner, *Reading Strategies and Practices: A Compendium,* 3d ed. (Boston: Allyn & Bacon, 1990).

SIDEBAR 12.4

General Steps in the Language Experience Approach

1. Arrange an experience for the student or use a naturally occurring one.

2. Have the student tell a story about the experience. Write down the story as the student tells it and watches.

3. Read the story back to the student immediately, pointing to each word.

4. Continue to reread the story with the student over several days or weeks. The student will systematically read more and more of the story independently.

5. Structure appropriate activities around the story, such as

   ◆ Word recognition (for example, place selected words from the story on note cards and review them with the student; have the student find the words in the story).

   ◆ Phonics (for instance, identify a recurring consonant or vowel sound from the story, make up other words that start with the identified sound, and read words with the identified sound).

   ◆ Comprehension (for example, make up a title for the story that expresses its main idea; suggest titles that may be too broad or too narrow for the story).

   ◆ Art activities (for instance, draw pictures or create other works of art that depict the experiences in the story).

---

cedure include omitting every content word or structure word at certain regular designated intervals, providing choices for omitted words, providing a short blank for each letter of omitted words, or providing the first letter of the omitted word. With whatever procedure is used, the student then reads through the story and fills in each blank with a word that makes sense. The cloze procedure fosters growth in comprehension, since students must rely on the meaning of the story to fill in the blanks; no other source of information is available to help them. Although the cloze procedure has not been empirically validated for school-age students with low vision, Watson and Berg (1992) found that it was effective in increasing comprehension and reading skills in older persons with acquired macular degeneration.

Selecting Instructional Strategies

Many similar reading instructional strategies will promote increased reading skills for students with low vision. Therefore, the teacher of students with visual impairments should choose a specific strategy that will meet the targeted needs of an individual student and then assess its effectiveness through diagnostic teaching techniques. If the strategy is yielding objectively determined benefits, it should be continued; otherwise, it should be modified or discontinued. Regular reading specialists are valuable resources for identifying such strategies. In addition, extensive written resources are available; for example, Tierney, Readence, and Dishner (1990) compiled over 80 specific reading instructional strategies that provide a wealth of practical information for the teacher.

Reading instructional strategies developed for children with unimpaired vision are not necessarily invalid for use with children who have low vision, although some may need modification. With an understanding of the effects of low vision on the reading process, the teacher can examine various approaches and make common-sense predictions of their effectiveness, given the characteristics of an individual student and whether modifications are needed. The teacher must examine information from the student's functional vision assessment, learning media assessment, and daily classroom observations to determine the most appropriate modifications to be made.

For example, in using the cloze procedure with a student with low vision, the teacher may need to provide longer blanks and use double or triple spacing to accommodate the size of letters the student uses in writing. In addition, the teacher may use shorter passages or extend the time limit for completing a task to reflect the student's reading rate.

Increasing Speed and Stamina

Students with low vision often read more slowly than do students with unimpaired vision and generally have less stamina for sustaining reading. To accommodate their slower rate of reading and reduced stamina, teachers often have students read fewer materials and for shorter periods. Although this practice would seem to be a reasonable response to the implications of low vision, it actually perpetuates a slow reading rate and reduced stamina. Proficient readers become proficient by reading extensively. If students with low vision do not have ample opportunities to practice reading, they will have greater difficulty developing speed and stamina.

Issues of speed and stamina are often complicated when students are introduced to optical devices. As is true in learning any skill, the initial use of an optical device may make reading slower and more visually demanding because the student must concentrate on the proper use of the device. However, with solid initial instruction and ample opportunities to practice, the student's reading will become increasingly fluent (faster) and his or her stamina will increase.

The teacher of students with visual impairments can use the strategies outlined in Sidebar 12.3 for developing reading fluency to also develop speed and stamina. The ultimate goal is to develop reading efficiency: speed with comprehension. Since some strategies, such as repeated readings, do not emphasize comprehension per se, the teacher may have to provide supplemental instruction in comprehension. Regardless of the methods used to increase speed and stamina, the following general guidelines may be helpful:

- Use easy reading materials that appropriately match the student's experiential background and interests.
- Document the student's reading efficiency rate with the procedure outlined in Chapter 11 and continue to do so annually throughout the school years.
- Determine an objective level of stamina, both within a single session and throughout the school day, using samples that require sustained reading, and supplement this information with interviews with the student, parents, teachers, and others.
- Use objectively gathered baseline data to set reasonable goals for continually increasing rate and stamina to levels of "just manageable difficulty," a general concept for learning suggested by Hobbs (1965).
- Check that the student has demonstrated a consistent and comfortable degree of mastery at a given level before setting the next goal.
- Involve the student directly in setting goals and monitoring the results of instruction.
- Provide feedback to the student on the progress he or she has made in increasing the rate and stamina of reading, using line charts or tables when appropriate.
- Use real opportunities for increasing the student's reading rate and stamina, such as the repeated reading of a passage that the student will later read aloud in a school program.
- Encourage the student to assess continually whether the visual environment is conducive to reading and remind him or her to adjust the lighting, position of reading materials, and other factors to suit individual preferences.

◆ Encourage the student to monitor continually the use of an optical device while reading and to make adjustments, if necessary, in the focal distance, working distance, viewing angle, and so forth.

◆ Teach the student to recognize signs of visual fatigue and offer strategies for dealing with it, such as taking short breaks, changing from reading a text to listening to a recorded version, or shifting his or her physical position.

◆ Teach the student to read for specific purposes: scanning quickly to find needed information, skimming to get the gist of a passage, and studying to understand and remember details.

◆ Encourage the student to read for pleasure, generally with easy reading materials of high motivational value.

When students with low vision do not make steady progress in developing speed and stamina in reading, as determined by objective documentation, the teacher of students with visual impairments must take direct steps to address this problem. The use of diagnostic teaching practices will allow the teacher to determine the factors that are impeding a student's progress. For example, if a student is receiving consistent, high-quality instruction in increasing his or her rate of reading through repeated readings but is not progressing, perhaps the student has an inadequate automatic vocabulary or weak word-recognition skills.

Some students' visual condition (such as a nonfunctional central field) may hinder their progress, and other students may require such a level of magnification to resolve letters and words that a cap is placed on their fields of view, resulting in a slower rate of reading. When a comfortable level of speed and stamina is not readily attainable, then the educational team must add other literacy tools (such as balancing print reading with audiotaped materials and live reader services or introducing braille reading and writing) to the student's repertoire to compensate for the problem. They base their decisions on objective data gathered periodically throughout the school years (see Chapter 11 for a discussion of the continuing assessment phase).

SUPPORTING THE DEVELOPMENT OF ACADEMIC WRITING SKILLS

Nonoptical and Optical Devices

Nonoptical Devices

Typical nonoptical devices or strategies for structuring the visual environment for writing include:

◆ bold-line paper

◆ writing devices, such as felt-tip pens, soft-lead artists' pencils, or ink pens, that provide appropriate contrast between the paper and markings

◆ adjustments in lighting to increase contrast and decrease glare

◆ changes in the position of the writing surface to promote a comfortable posture

◆ software for enlarging visual images on a computer screen.

Many students with low vision can write using nonoptical approaches, but they may need optical devices to reread what they have written.

Optical Devices

The majority of optical devices, such as handheld magnifiers, spectacle-mounted devices, mirror magnifiers, and CCTVs, are useful in writing. However, most stand magnifiers are not useful because a writing instrument cannot be placed under them. The mirror magnifier, however, is an exception, since a pencil or pen is placed in front of it, not under it, and the student can maintain a normal or near-normal writing posture.

The CCTV allows for maximum flexibility in writing because the student can sit upright in front of the monitor and can change the magnification and contrast to suit his or her needs. When teaching a student to write with a CCTV,

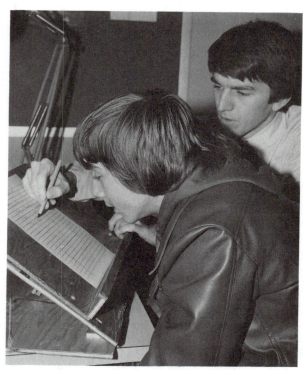

A variety of nonoptical devices, such as bold-line paper and felt-tip pens, are available to help a student with low vision develop writing skills.

the teacher directs the student to look at the monitor and deliberately position the writing device on the paper before writing. Although this procedure gives the student a sense of detachment from the page at first, guidance by the teacher and practice generally yield quick results. The disadvantages of a CCTV, such as its lack of portability and expense, often make other options for writing more attractive. Therefore, the teacher, parents, and the student should consult with the clinical low vision specialist to determine which devices will meet the student's needs and borrow them for use on a trial basis.

Penmanship

Students with low vision may find it more challenging to refine their penmanship than may students with unimpaired vision because re-

duced visual acuity or central field losses influence the development of the fine and coordinated visual-motor skills needed in handwriting. Nevertheless, they can still develop legible handwriting. Thus, the provision of supplementary instruction in penmanship is a legitimate role for the teacher of students with visual impairments.

Manuscript Writing

Students generally learn manuscript writing (printing) before cursive writing. In teaching early manuscript writing, the teacher should use writing paper with bold lines for appropriate contrast and extra width to accommodate the student's level of visual-motor skills; the width of the lines is gradually decreased to normal or near-normal line spacing as the student's writing develops. The writing paper for young students should have a top and bottom solid line with a lighter (but discernible) dotted line between them and a "gutter" (a space for descenders) between the rows that is about half the width of the primary line. These requirements for contrast and width often prevent the use of conventional writing paper with light blue or red lines.

Designing and photocopying writing paper allows the teacher to change the width of lines as the student's needs dictate. Older students can be taught to develop and duplicate their own paper, thereby placing them in control of their writing needs. The goal is to work toward normal line spacing because writing with normal-size letters not only conforms to societal expectation, but provides the student with a greater speed of writing.

Students need to write legibly in an appropriate size to read back their work efficiently. Once they can form letters, it is important that they learn to attend to the meaning of what they are writing and to stay generally on the lines, rather than to concentrate on forming each letter.

In helping a student refine his or her manuscript-writing skills, the teacher should provide verbal guidance or hand-over-hand instruction in starting and stopping on the appropriate solid and dotted lines to form letters. Although placing a pencil on paper may be a conscious effort at first, it will become automatic with instruction and practice. Thus, the goal should be to provide sufficient practice within meaningful writing activities so that both the student and others can easily read what has been written.

Transition to Cursive Writing

Some teachers advocate the introduction of cursive writing earlier for students with low vision than for those with unimpaired vision or at the beginning of penmanship instruction because the letters are connected, and hence the pen or pencil is in contact with the paper most of the time—a factor that is thought to benefit students with low vision. However, some teachers advocate the later introduction of cursive writing, since they believe it is more demanding of the visual-motor system than is manuscript writing. A few teachers advocate the use of cursive writing for some students with low vision only for their signatures. Since there has been no research on whether the early or late introduction of cursive writing is advantageous for students with low vision, the decision on when or if to introduce it must rest with the educational team. A diagnostic teaching approach is useful for ensuring that whatever method is taught will be of maximum benefit to a student.

The D'Nealian approach to penmanship instruction is a possible option for making the transition from manuscript writing to cursive writing. In this approach, the manuscript letters (shown in Figure 12.1) are more curved than the traditional letters and are formed in much the same manner as their later cursive counterparts will be. However, if the D'Nealian approach is not taught in the school district, then the teacher of students with visual impairments must take responsibility for teaching penmanship skills. In such instances, the disadvantages of using the D'Nealian approach likely will outweigh any advantages.

For some students with low vision, the transition from reading manuscript writing to reading cursive writing presents a challenge. The teacher of students with visual impairments should assist students in making this transition by providing practice and sequential experiences until reading of script—including reading script on the chalkboard and written communications from others—becomes more efficient.

Keyboarding Skills

With the proliferation of personal computers, most students learn keyboarding skills in school. However, formal instruction in these skills is generally introduced earlier for students with low vision than for students with normal vision. Therefore, the responsibility for teaching these skills often rests with the teacher of students with visual impairments.

The current trend is to introduce children to computers during the preschool years. Young children with unimpaired vision often start by using the hunt-and-peck method and are taught formal keyboarding skills at some later time in school. Although both computer specialists and typing teachers disagree about the wisdom of introducing young children with unimpaired vision to touch typing or keyboarding, for young children with low vision, these skills should be introduced early and deliberately. The hunt-and-peck method is not an efficient approach, especially for students with low vision.

A computer is much more advantageous for introducing touch keyboarding than is a traditional typewriter, because a typewriter does not allow a student with low vision efficient access to information he or she is typing. The computer can be equipped with a screen-enlargement program and synthetic speech output to allow efficient access to information on the screen and inexpensive keyboarding software programs that permit repeated practice to develop proficiency and even record the student's progress automatically. In addition, nonoptical approaches, such as preferential placement of the monitor (as through a moving arm or shelf) and the adjustment of contrast and illumination, can contribute to a student's comfort.

With basic keyboarding skills, students with

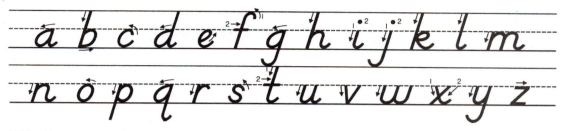

D'Nealian manuscript

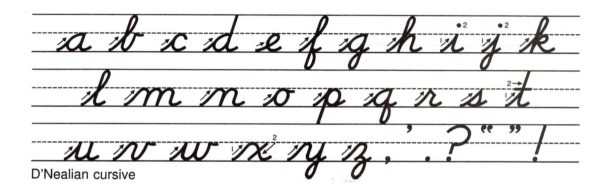

D'Nealian cursive

Figure 12.1. Manuscript Letters and Cursive Letters in the D'Nealian Approach to Writing
Source: Reprinted, by permission of the publisher, from Donald Neal Thurber, *D'Nealian Handwriting, Book 3,* 3d ed. (Glenview, Ill.: Scott Foresman, 1993).

low vision can learn word processing to complete a variety of writing tasks efficiently. Word processing allows the student to use all aspects of the writing process with ease: prewriting, drafting, revising, editing, and publishing. Sidebar 12.5 gives the purpose for each element in the writing process; concerns for students with low vision; and possible strategies, including the use of word processing, for overcoming these concerns. The ease with which a student can produce a clean, readable hard copy in various sizes and fonts of type greatly facilitates communication through writing.

For students with low vision, using computer word processing provides a means of writing that will in all likelihood become more efficient than writing on paper. Also, proficiency in word processing will provide the student with a basic, fun-

damental literacy tool that will enhance later schooling and employment opportunities.

SUPPORTING THE DEVELOPMENT OF FUNCTIONAL LITERACY SKILLS

Functional literacy skills are those that are required to complete everyday tasks, such as reading menus or maps, maintaining a checking account, paying bills, filling out forms, and spotting street signs and house numbers. Two interrelated skills must be addressed in teaching these skills: choosing the specific literacy task and acquiring the means to complete the task.

SIDEBAR 12.5

Elements in the Writing Process with Special Considerations for Students with Low Vision

Element	Purpose	Concerns	Strategies
Prewriting	To generate topics and ideas for writing activities	◆ Possible lack of background experiences	◆ Broaden background experiences using a multisensory approach to learning ◆ Generate ideas on tape or share ideas verbally with others
Drafting	To write down initial ideas and thoughts on paper	◆ Lack of fluency of writing may hamper production of ideas ◆ Difficulty in reading back one's own handwriting ◆ Difficulty in using standard notebook paper	◆ Use computer word processing program ◆ Use pencil with eraser and bold-line paper for drafting ◆ Use low vision devices to enhance the physical environment
Revision	To make content changes in the paper	◆ Problems with fluency may hamper desire to make global changes ◆ Difficulty in reading back one's own handwriting	◆ Use computer word processing program to cut and paste and to make global insertions and deletions
Editing	To make corrections in spelling, capitalization, usage, and style.	◆ Papers written with felt-tipped markers cannot be erased ◆ Difficulty in reading back one's own handwriting	◆ Use computer word processing program to check spelling and to make other editing changes
Publishing	To prepare one's work to be shared with a wider audience	◆ Difficulty of producing a "polished" version of the paper ◆ Difficulty of gaining access to the final published form	◆ Use computer word processing program to create a polished version ◆ Use low vision devices to access the final published form

Source: Information on "Element" and "Purpose" is based on D. J. Leu, Jr. and C. K. Kinzer, *Effective Reading Instruction, K–8,* 2d ed. (New York: Macmillan Publishing, 1991).

Identifying Functional Literacy Tasks

The Inventory of Functional Literacy Tasks in the appendix at the end of this chapter lists some important functional literacy tasks that may serve as a starting point in selecting the types of tasks for instruction. However, it should be noted that functional literacy tasks are specific to the individual, and global statements cannot be made about standard functional literacy curriculum, especially when employment tasks are considered. Children or adults who can read conventional literature are not necessarily able to perform functional literacy tasks; functional literacy can only be assessed and taught with functional literacy tasks.

To gain access to information, a student needs to acquire a variety of efficient literacy tools, including the use of

- regular print with or without optical devices
- large-print materials, such as large-print books and magazines, large print checkbooks, and large-print playing cards
- braille or other tactile reading and writing systems to supplement print reading
- nonoptical devices, such as lighting, line or signature guides, and colored filters
- compensatory techniques, such as repositioning lighting, one's body, or the materials being used
- optical devices to gain access to information at a distance
- electronically controlled print size through CCTVs or computers
- synthesized speech on computers or other technology
- audiotaped materials, electronic textbooks, or live reader services.

To be consistent with the nature of functional literacy, instruction in functional literacy tools should be driven by a student's present and future needs. The following process may be used to explore and select appropriate literacy tools for instruction (Koenig & Holbrook, 1995):

1. Analyze the literacy skills required for present and future educational and vocational tasks.
2. Determine the literacy tools needed to complete such tasks efficiently.
3. Compare the literacy tools that the student needs with those he or she currently uses. Any discrepancies will identify areas of needed instruction.
4. Provide instruction and practice in needed skills before the student actually needs to apply them.
5. Teach the student to engage in this process because his or her future independence will be heavily influenced by this type of self-advocacy (see Chapter 4 for additional information on self-advocacy).

Providing Instruction in Functional Literacy

In teaching functional literacy skills, the teacher has to balance and integrate teaching the literacy task with teaching the literacy tool. In some instances, both the task and tool may be addressed in the same session, but in other cases, the focus may be on only one of the skills (since the other is already mastered). In the first situation, a teacher of students with visual impairments may provide instruction in the use of a handheld magnifier, for example, while introducing a student with low vision to Monopoly, using the motivation to learn a new game as a means of teaching and reinforcing the use of the magnifier. In the second situation, the teacher teaches a student who has mastered a task with one tool, such as reviewing a checking account with a magnifier, to perform this same task using another literacy tool, such as synthesized speech via electronic communications with the bank.

The teacher should ensure that the student is gaining access to information both at near point and at a distance. Since most literacy tasks, such as reading books, writing letters, and checking prices on store items, are accomplished at near point, teachers may tend to emphasize access to near point information. However, much information in the environment is obtained at a distance, such as from a chalkboard, a bathroom scale, or a store sign. Often, instruction in the use of distance-access strategies is most effectively integrated into O&M instruction. As a guiding principle, instruction should be balanced to allow a student to use literacy tools to obtain all available information that is of significance to him or her.

Given the emphasis on disability-specific skills, instruction may be isolated and fragmented and include few applications to real-life tasks. Thus, a student may not make meaningful connections between the isolated skills and their practical uses. To link special skills instruction with functional applications, a teacher may provide instruction in maintaining the proper focal distance and looking through the optical center of a handheld magnifier, for instance, while teaching the student to play a board game, locate telephone numbers in a directory, complete a homework assignment, and so forth.

It is the responsibility of the teacher of students with visual impairments to ensure that all instruction, including special instruction, communication skills, daily living skills, and academic skills, is meaningfully integrated into and throughout a student's life. As was discussed in Chapter 4, such real-world applications are at the heart of functional literacy and are the ultimate goal of literacy instruction.

SUMMARY

In ensuring that students with low vision progress meaningfully in reading and writing instruction, teachers of students with visual impairments are guided by the following principles:

- ◆ understanding the implications of a visual impairment and the effect of magnification on reading and writing and sharing this knowledge with the educational team

- ◆ providing instruction in disability-specific skills to students and consultation to regular classroom teachers
- ◆ giving students ample practice in reading and writing skills so they may develop both solid, academic literacy skills and special skills in applying literacy in real-life situations.

As students progress in school, they develop skills and responsibilities for gaining access to information in print that foster their independence in performing a variety of reading and writing tasks.

ACTIVITIES

With This Chapter and Other Resources

1. Select two short reading passages. Read one with your conventional prescription eyeglasses, if you have them (otherwise with the naked eye), and calculate your rate of reading. Read the other with a spectacle-mounted magnifier and again calculate your rate of reading. Compare the two rates. Discuss the results and your observations of the experiences with your classmates.

2. Select another passage of similar length to the previous ones. Construct a typoscope from a piece of light cardboard that will allow two or three letters to show at one time and that will block the rest of the page. Place the typoscope on the page, read at a normal working distance, and then calculate your rate of reading. Compare this rate to your rate of reading under normal circumstances and share your experiences with your classmates.

3. Choose 8 to 10 specific reading instructional strategies (like those in Sidebar 12.3) that have been developed for students with unimpaired vision and suggest modifications of these strategies that would make them appropriate for use with students with low vision.

4. Read three to five stories in a basal reading series or a literature book that might be used

in a whole language classroom. Determine the essential experience or experiences that would be needed for a young child with low vision to understand the stories.

In the Community

1. Keep a log of the ways in which you use literacy skills throughout the day, both at near point and at a distance. For each use, suggest possible strategies that a person with low vision could use to complete the same tasks.

2. Examine five elevators in public places. Analyze whether the labels are presented in a way that facilitates reading for persons with low vision. Compare the positive and negative features of the various elevators.

With a Person with Low Vision

1. Interview an adult with congenital low vision and discuss his or her development of reading and writing skills; the aspects of these skills that created difficulties, if any; and how these difficulties were solved. Then describe how these skills have affected the individual's current reading and writing skills.

2. Interview a high school student with low vision on his or her use of functional literacy strategies to complete the following tasks:

   ◆ reading the bulletin board,
   ◆ reading maps,
   ◆ taking tests,
   ◆ writing checks at the store,
   ◆ reading signs in the community,
   ◆ reading menus at a restaurant.

Present the results in class and discuss possible approaches to increasing the student's use of functional literacy.

From Your Perspective

What do you consider to be the appropriate role of the teacher of students with visual impairments in teaching literacy skills to students with low vision? In what situations would it be appropriate for the regular classroom teacher to provide primary instruction, and in what situations would it be more appropriate for the teacher of students with visual impairments to do so?

Inventory of Functional Literacy Tasks

Student _____

Review Date _____

School Environment

Mastery	Task	Strategies for Completing the Task
_____	Reading textbooks	_____
_____	Writing term papers	_____
_____	Taking notes in class	_____
_____	Taking closed-book tests	_____
_____	Taking open-book tests	_____
_____	Completing admission and registration forms	_____
_____	Using reference books	_____
_____	Reading periodicals	_____
_____	Reading information on the bulletin board	_____
_____	Completing in-class assignments	_____
_____	Taking general computer courses	_____
_____	Completing science lab exercises	_____
_____	Jotting down assignments	_____
_____	Organizing course materials	_____
_____	_____	_____
_____	_____	_____
_____	_____	_____
_____	_____	_____
_____	_____	_____
_____	_____	_____
_____	_____	_____
_____	_____	_____

(continued on next page)

Appendix. Functional Literacy Skills Inventory

Source: Based on and printed with permission of the publisher, from Alan J. Koenig and Carol Farrenkopf, *Assessment of Braille Literacy Skills (ABLS)* (Houston: Region IV Education Service Center, Department of Special Education, 1994–95).

Inventory of Functional Literacy Tasks (*continued*)

Student _____

Review Date _____

Home Environment

Mastery	Task	Strategies for Completing the Task
_____	Labeling personal items	_____
_____	Paying bills	_____
_____	Maintaining an address and telephone book	_____
_____	Reading a newspaper	_____
_____	Keeping a recipe file	_____
_____	Maintaining a checking account	_____
_____	Reading for pleasure	_____
_____	Using a calendar	_____
_____	Telling time	_____
_____	Writing personal letters	_____
_____	Reading labels on bottles, boxes, and packages	_____
_____	Completing tax returns	_____
_____	Reading mail	_____
_____	Taking phone messages	_____
_____	Reading magazines	_____
_____	Playing games	_____
_____	Sending greeting cards	_____
_____	Reading owner's manuals	_____
_____	_____	_____
_____	_____	_____
_____	_____	_____
_____	_____	_____

(*continued on next page*)

Inventory of Functional Literacy Tasks (*continued*)

Student _____

Review Date _____

Community Environment

Mastery	Task	Strategies for Completing the Task
_____	Reading menus in restaurants	_____
_____	Making shopping lists	_____
_____	Reading street and store signs	_____
_____	Writing directions to a specific locality	_____
_____	Writing checks at the store	_____
_____	Completing deposit slips at the bank	_____
_____	Reading labels on items at the store	_____
_____	Filling out applications	_____
_____	Reading bus schedules	_____
_____	Signing documents	_____
_____	Voting	_____
_____	Making notes for public speaking	_____
_____	Reading maps	_____
_____	Finding restrooms	_____
_____	Reading signs at airport and bus stations	_____
_____	_____	_____
_____	_____	_____
_____	_____	_____
_____	_____	_____
_____	_____	_____
_____	_____	_____

(*continued on next page*)

Inventory of Functional Literacy Tasks (*continued*)

Student _____

Review Date _____

Work Environment

Directions: List the specific functional literacy tasks needed in the student's work-study site or future work environment. Complete inventory as before.

Mastery	Task	Strategies for Completing the Task
_____	_____	_____
_____	_____	_____
_____	_____	_____
_____	_____	_____
_____	_____	_____
_____	_____	_____
_____	_____	_____
_____	_____	_____
_____	_____	_____
_____	_____	_____
_____	_____	_____
_____	_____	_____
_____	_____	_____
_____	_____	_____
_____	_____	_____
_____	_____	_____
_____	_____	_____
_____	_____	_____
_____	_____	_____
_____	_____	_____

CHAPTER 13

Orientation and Mobility for Children and Adults with Low Vision

Audrey J. Smith and Duane R. Geruschat

VIGNETTE

Herb, a 32-year-old salesman in a shoe store, has congenital rubella with 20/400 acuity, a mild hearing impairment, and is able to read the sizes on shoe boxes with his eyes about 1 inch from the boxes. Herb also has a mild cognitive disability that has resulted in his parents being overprotective, even now that he is an adult. Since he started working at the shoe store eight years ago, his parents have taken him to work each day. Now in their mid 70s, they have age-related health problems and worry that Herb will need to quit his job because they can no longer transport him. Herb's mother contacted the state rehabilitation agency and requested that Herb be placed in a job within walking distance of their home.

After a review of Herb's capabilities, the rehabilitation agency determined that orientation and mobility (O&M) services would be beneficial. In fact, it was questioned why such services had not been provided during Herb's educational program before he left school in the 1980s.

Through the rehabilitation agency, an O&M instructor taught Herb how to use visual landmarks along with auditory and tactile cues. The instructor also taught Herb to use a monocular to identify bus numbers and the procedures for using public transportation so he could go back and forth to the shoe store on his own.

The O&M instructor realized that Herb had the potential not only to be a route traveler but to travel to a limited extent in unfamiliar local areas. With his newfound O&M skills, Herb was soon exploring new streets. When printed maps were redrawn and simplified, Herb could use them to find new destinations. Now Herb helps his parents by running errands in their neighborhood and sometimes even in new parts of town.

INTRODUCTION

Mobility is a basic freedom that most individuals take for granted. However, the majority of persons who are blind or have low vision experience problems in mobility. Those with low vision have a different set of mobility challenges from those who are totally blind. This chapter introduces the major components of O&M assessment and training related to the use of functional vision. It can serve as a beginning guide for direct service personnel who are interested in assisting their students or clients to achieve optimal visual functioning for O&M purposes.

Individuals who are totally blind learn to travel independently without visual cues. Independent travel, therefore, does not require vision. However, since the majority of persons with visual impairments do have some amount of usable vision, visual information for them, whether helpful or confusing, is of significance in teaching O&M skills. For those who have congenital or adventitious low vision, learning or relearning how to use visual cues to interpret the environment can augment their O&M skills. The use of vision, even at low levels of acuity, can provide information about landmarks, clues, and maps that assist in orientation, as well as provide advance warning of obstacles and drop-offs.

The effective use of vision (both near and distance) can enable individuals with low vision to be more proactive in daily travel. In many situations, such as finding landmarks or obstacles, determining distance and depth, crossing streets, and negotiating public transportation, training in the effective use of available visual information can increase the efficiency, speed, and pleasure of travel. Although the ability to use vision varies from individual to individual, guided instruction to enhance visual potential and increase efficiency, regardless of the level of visual acuity or degree of restricted fields of view, can be beneficial.

Many of the issues relating to O&M and persons with low vision can be illustrated in the case of John, who is severely visually impaired (20/400 visual acuity with a 10-degree central scotoma caused by diabetic retinopathy). His O&M goal is to travel independently to a large grocery store, where he wishes to purchase a few basic food items. The route is in a familiar neighborhood and involves a four-block walk and crossing two traffic-light–controlled intersections.

Here are some potential problems that this walk may present:

- Glare reflects off traffic lights and signs, causing difficulty in identifying traffic light colors and reading signs as orientation cues.

- The edges of curbs appear to blend into the sidewalk and street, causing difficulty in identifying the exact location and depth of curbs.

- Indoor-to-outdoor lighting changes result in significant decreases in visual ability until the eyes adapt.

- Crowds of people and aisle displays in the store cause John to bump into shoppers and displays.

- Busy and complex intersections cause anxiety and fear about crossing streets.

- New systemic medication taken recently by John results in fluctuating vision.

Although all persons with low vision may not experience all these difficulties all the time, they all will experience some of these problems, to varying degrees, depending on the severity of their visual impairment. In the example, *environmental fluctuations* that were due to the time of day, season of the year, the location, the presence or absence of the sun, the change of lighting from indoors to outdoors (and vice versa), the presence of rain water on sidewalks, and shadows that created false information and obscured important information could have affected travel. *Fluctuating vision*, accompanying systemic conditions such as diabetes or the progressive loss of vision characteristic of retinitis pigmentosa, may further complicate travel. Medications with ocular side effects also cause variations in visual performance. External environmental fluctuations, combined with internal visual fluctuations, contribute to a visual experience that is highly variable and a challenge for both the student and the instructor.

The major difficulties experienced by travelers with low vision include

- adjusting to glare
- adapting to lighting changes
- negotiating drop-offs (stairs and curbs)
- negotiating street crossings
- negotiating changes in terrain

- walking through crowded areas
- bumping into objects and obstacles
- walking in inclement weather
- seeing details (street names and house numbers) during travel.

Many of these challenges are common to persons who are totally blind, as well as to those with low vision. But visual information, available to travelers with low vision, adds a unique dimension to these problems and their solutions. The visual dimension involved in O&M requires a program of assessment and instruction that specifically addresses each person's visual capabilities and skills in the context of O&M.

ASSESSMENT

A suggested approach to an assessment of low vision mobility contains four distinct phases:

1. the review of clinical vision reports
2. the evaluation of functional visual acuities and fields
3. the assessment of the impact of environmental variables
4. the observation of functional vision in a mobility context.

Review of Clinical Vision Reports

Within the field there is general agreement that findings from a clinical assessment of vision do not predict or describe functional visual abilities. Yet, a good clinical assessment, used as a complement to a functional assessment, can provide valuable information for understanding visual functioning and assist in answering the question, "Does this person have 'enough' vision to perform the desired task?"

- The diagnosis of a visual pathology, such as ocular albinism, which may indicate a sen-

sitivity to bright lights, or diabetic retinopathy, which could point to fluctuating vision, can assist the O&M instructor to anticipate specific visual difficulties.

- If the clinical report notes that the person can see 1M print (equivalent to newspaper-size print), it may not mean that he or she can read a newspaper, but it does indicate the capability of resolving (seeing) and discriminating targets that are the size of 1M print under ideal viewing conditions.

- Information on contrast sensitivity provides an even more refined picture of the person's visual ability in regard to various levels of contrast.

- Information on color vision is helpful for deciding which visual skills would be more

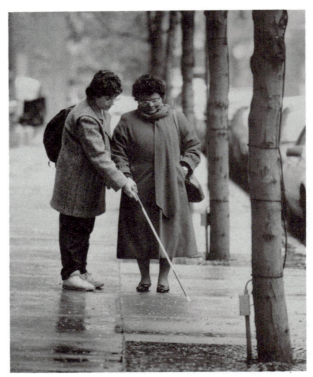

Both assessment and instruction in orientation and mobility need to consider the impact of environmental fluctuations, such as the presence of rain water on a sidewalk or shadows caused by trees, on a person's functional visual abilities.

appropriate for performing a variety of mobility tasks, such as identifying stop signs and traffic lights.

◆ Knowledge of the type and extent of refractive error and type and power of prescribed lenses and low vision devices is also a critical piece of the puzzle in ensuring the best possible visual enhancement.

Clinical measures do not give the complete visual picture. Some persons with low vision may have sufficient visual acuity and fields to interpret a host of visual information, but their visual level of environmental awareness may predispose them to limited visual functioning. These individuals will not learn visual information spontaneously; rather, they must want to be visually aware of the environment and have the motivation to use vision actively. Recognizing that functional vision is highly variable (affected by personality factors, such as motivation; environmental factors, such as lighting; and task requirements, such as speed and distance), the O&M instructor, classroom teacher, or rehabilitation teacher needs to augment clinical information with a holistic set of assessment information that is underscored by the needs and goals of the person being assessed. How these factors affect the level of visual functioning is the focus of the following discussion.

Functional Assessment of Visual Acuity for Mobility

The functional assessment of visual acuity for mobility involves the presentation of a variety of objects or visual tasks at various distances and locations, with the goal of understanding the conditions under which the person can or cannot discriminate objects or perform tasks visually. This assessment should be conducted in both familiar and unfamiliar areas and under different lighting conditions. To achieve the functional goal of the assessment, six pieces of information are necessary:

1. At what distance is the presence of an object first detected (awareness distance)?

2. At what distance is an object first correctly identified (identification distance)?

3. At what distance is the person most comfortable viewing an object (preferred distance)?

4. How does movement or the lack of it affect visual acuity?

5. How do the use of low vision devices and absorptive lenses affect visual acuity?

6. How do environmental variables, such as illumination and contrast, affect visual acuity?

The following sections specify for the practitioner the variables to be assessed in order to obtain the necessary information.

Acuity without Optical Devices

Awareness distance acuity. Assess the person's ability to detect or be aware of the presence of objects or other targets at near (up to 16 inches), intermediate (17 inches to 6 feet), and distance (beyond 6 feet) in a variety of areas, such as the classroom, home, outdoors, and workplace.

Identification distance acuity. Assess the person's ability to identify objects or other targets correctly at the farthest near, intermediate, and distance ranges in a variety of settings.

Preferred distance acuity. Observe and ask questions about the distances at which the person feels comfortable about identifying objects and other targets or performing visual tasks, such as identifying a person or reading a map or bus schedule, the number on a bus, or a street sign. This refined information on acuity includes the person's preferred working distance and the distance at which the person feels more at ease and sure about identifying objects. Vary the targets and settings, since the person's preferred viewing distance may vary with them.

For awareness, identification, and preferred distance acuity, conduct assessments of the person's static and dynamic acuity in different environments, with and without the use of assistive optical devices, to obtain a more complete picture of the person's various levels of visual functioning. This information helps to piece together what is frequently otherwise perceived as a complex, inconsistent puzzle of visual performance.

Static acuity. Assess the person's ability to discriminate and identify a variety of stationary objects while the person is standing or sitting still. For example, determine whether the person can note the presence of a street sign while standing on a street corner.

Dynamic acuity. Assess the ability to discriminate and identify either static or moving objects while the person is moving. For instance, determine whether the person can distinguish signs or taxis from other moving cars while walking. This final measure will provide a more realistic picture of functional acuity in everyday mobility situations.

Acuity with Optical Devices

Assess the effect of distance optical devices and absorptive lenses on the person's visual acuity. Compare the person's identification with and without telescopes, while attempting to increase the range of awareness distance acuity, first with static objects and then with dynamic objects. Also assess whether the use of near devices enhances the person's ability to read maps, menus, telephone directories, and a variety of other reading tasks common to mobility situations.

Functional Assessment of Visual Fields

The functional assessment of visual fields for mobility purposes involves both stationary and moving assessments. Three questions are addressed in this assessment:

1. What is the person's preferred functional visual field while moving?
2. What is the person's stationary visual field?
3. How does movement affect the person's functional visual fields?

Static Visual Field

The person stands still, looking at a stationary object at a distance of 10 to 20 feet. While holding the eyes stationary, the person describes the outermost things he or she sees in the stationary field of vision. This portion of the assessment defines the outer boundaries (superior, inferior, right, or left) of the visual fields. Some or all of the static or potential boundaries of visual fields may be used in dynamic situations, such as mobility.

Dynamic Visual Field

While walking along a route, encourage the person to scan with head and eye movements. Take note of the farthest boundaries (superior, inferior, left, and right) of the dynamic visual field. This information describes the potential range of the person's functional visual field while moving through the environment.

A comparison of the static, dynamic, and preferred visual fields yields a comprehensive view of the functional problems that may need to be addressed through instruction. For mobility purposes, information about the preferred and dynamic functional visual fields is important for understanding which visual pieces of information are available to the person and to what the person is attending. The "puzzle" of what the person is or is not using as visual cues is gradually solved through the assessment process.

Preferred Visual Field

This naturalistic observation describes the visual-field style of the person while he or she moves through the environment. Ask the person to walk along while describing everything he or she sees. Take note of the location (superior, inferior, left, right) of objects the person identifies. The preferred visual field will be the field area in which the person identifies the most objects. For example, a person with constricted visual fields may fix his or her gaze downward and slightly ahead; in this case, the highest frequency of objects identified will be in the inferior visual field. (Record the field by drawing a circle and dividing it into four equal parts. Then mark the circle in the corresponding area each time an object is noted.)

Assessment of Environmental Variables

The environments in which the assessment occurs have a major impact on the person's functional visual performance. In general, the more complex the environment, the lower the proficiency of use of functional vision. Therefore, all statements of a person's functional use of vision should be accompanied by a brief description of the environment in which the findings were obtained. In choosing different environments, the evaluator should consider at least the following variables for their effect on the level and quality of the person's visual functioning.

Indoor or outdoor environment. In general, outdoor environments are more challenging than indoor environments. Note the effect of various weather conditions, as well as changes in visual functioning from one time of the day to another.

Amount of visual clutter (figure-ground). The amount of visual clutter in the environment directly affects the visual performance of a person with low vision. For example, a discount department store is more challenging visually than a small shoe store. Note the effect of areas with varying contrast, as well as any confusion created by visual clutter.

Amount and location of lighting. Is the environment illuminated by incandescent light, fluorescent light, outdoor sunlight, or a combination of lighting? Assess and note the preferred type, amount, and angle of lighting for various tasks. Determine the length of time it takes for the person to adapt when going from shaded to brightly lit areas, and vice versa, and from indoors to outdoors, and vice versa.

Glare. Assess the impact of glare on the person's visual functioning in indoor situations, such as glare from polished or reflective surfaces, and outdoor situations, such as bright sunlight (both direct and off reflected surfaces), as well as glare from the headlights of cars and street lights at night. In addition, assess the helpfulness of hats, visors, and absorptive lenses in decreasing glare and enhancing the person's visual functioning.

Depth perception. Note the person's ability to detect the presence of and negotiate stairs, curbs, and ramps. Even if a person has or can use only one eye at a time, depth can be conceptualized, rather than perceived through binocular vision (stereopsis).

Color cues. Assess the person's ability to discriminate and use different colors or shades as environmental cues, such as traffic lights and the colors of letters on signs. These variables are among the primary ones considered in an initial mobility assessment.

Functional Vision in a Mobility Context

Research (Genensky, Berry, Bikson, & Bikson, 1979; Long, Reiser, & Hill, 1990; Smith, De l'Aune, & Geruschat, 1992) has documented the most frequently occurring critical incidents (common problems) that have an impact on the mobility performance of persons with low vision:

- glare
- changing illumination conditions
- drop-offs (curbs and steps)
- changes in terrain
- street crossings
- collisions with objects and people
- ability to remain oriented.

A variety of other critical incidents affect different people in different ways, depending on the type and amount of vision, environmental setting, and so forth.

One approach to assessing mobility-related capabilities and needs is the critical incidents assessment, in which a person's mobility performance is observed and mobility problems are noted in the order in which they naturally occur in both familiar and unfamiliar areas. The evaluator counts each time the person trips, misses a step or curb, bumps into objects, becomes disoriented, and so forth; tallies the number of each problem; and determines which problems have a higher tally or frequency of occurrence.

The evaluator then establishes clusters of the most frequently occurring mobility problems for the person.

Each occurrence is followed by additional information, such as in which area of the visual field the bumping occurred most frequently; when glare or illumination conditions seemed to cause more problems; whether visual scanning behavior was a factor in the person's becoming disoriented or in making a poor judgment at, say, a street crossing; whether, for example, the person miscued visually, by interpreting a checkered floor pattern as steps, and so forth.

This approach focuses the assessment on the most critical areas observed during the person's performance and hence provides a clear direction for developing specific training techniques to alleviate the identified mobility problems. Any number of short- or long-term mobility situations provide ample opportunities for a critical incidents assessment. For example, a teacher may carefully observe a student during travel to the cafeteria, after asking the student to deliver a message to the main office, or while moving around the playground. Conversely, specific problems exhibited by adults could be observed as they walk about their places of employment or recreational areas. These observations culminate in a picture of the most frequently occurring problems, as well as the visual behavior and environmental variables contributing to them.

The assessment is not complete until two important components have been addressed. The first is the ongoing dialogue and feedback from the person during the assessment. The second is a discussion of the results of the assessment, so the person with low vision has a thorough understanding of his or her functional level of vision and the specific variables that enhance or decrease it.

VISUAL SKILLS FOR MOBILITY

The remaining discussion focuses on the basic visual skills, instructional techniques, and environmental cues commonly experienced during O&M situations. Although the emphasis is on visual skills, it should be noted here that during independent travel, a person incorporates information from all the senses. The recommended approach is to discriminate when vision is or is not useful and to rely on a combination of sensory information, including, when appropriate, the exclusive use of sensory cues other than vision.

The following are some guiding principles for instruction in the use of vision:

◆ Choose targets that are within the person's awareness viewing distance.

◆ Begin with targets at eye level and then generalize to different locations in the visual field.

◆ Begin with high-contrast targets, followed by targets of various levels of contrast.

◆ Begin with simple environments and gradually increase their complexity.

◆ When appropriate, preview the environment through discussion, photographs, slides via rearview screen projection, and so forth. Follow lessons with a review of the visual skills and principles learned.

The purpose of instruction is to change unsystematic visual behavior into an organized and precise visual skills approached. In this chapter, neither entry-level visual skills, such as awareness, attention, and localization (for a discussion of these basic visual skills, see Barraga & Morris, 1980; Smith & Cote, 1982), nor high-level visual skills, such as low vision driving and participating in competitive sports are addressed. In effect, many persons who need to develop low-level visual skills are served in basic vision stimulation programs, and those with relatively high-level visual skills generally do not require extensive intervention from an O&M instructor. In this discussion, three visual skills are discussed: scanning, tracing, and tracking.

Scanning

Scanning is the use of head and eye movements to visually search for and localize a target. Many individuals, even those with normal vision, often exhibit random and unsystematic visual behavior in scanning different environments. Scanning patterns are affected by the type of visual impairment, the purpose of scanning, the location of the target, and the environment in which scanning occurs.

Type of Visual Impairment

Individuals with limited visual acuity generally scan at close distances to obtain critical details, except when they can identify large or high-contrast targets at greater distances. By comparison, persons with constricted visual fields usually scan at greater distances because more information will "fit into" their constricted field of view; if they wait until they are too close to the area or target, only small pieces of the puzzle may be available to them, and they will have to use large head and eye turns to scan systematically.

Purpose of Scanning

Why one scans also defines how one scans. For example, when one scans a new area for general orientation, a systematic pattern of left-to-right and up-to-down visual sweeping of the entire area may be indicated. On the other hand, when one looks for a seat in a familiar classroom, a quick scan up or down each aisle is sufficient.

Location of Target

Knowing or anticipating the location of the target facilitates efficient scanning. For example, horizontal scanning is initially more effective for locating vertical targets, such as the poles of street signs, while vertical scanning up the pole is more effective for locating the horizontal street name sign. The use of steeples and silos for orientation cues require upper-field scanning, whereas locating subway signs is facilitated by eye-level scanning.

Environment

When a person wants to cross a busy urban street, looking for cues, such as the movement of pedestrians and vehicles, or identifying the location and information presented by a traffic signal requires quick and efficient scanning of a complex and rapidly changing environment. At the other extreme, in a quiet rural setting, where few cars or pedestrians are present, a person must scan up and down the street to determine if it is safe to cross. Locating food items in a salad bar requires a horizontal scanning pattern of a small, yet somewhat complex visual area, whereas scanning in a large grocery store for food items requires a variety of horizontal, vertical, and upper-field scanning behaviors. The following examples illustrate an application of factors affecting scanning:

> An adult with low visual acuity wants to find the way from home to a local bank. The targets are visual landmarks along the route (a fire hydrant and a broken sidewalk), and the environment is an urban area. In this situation, it is important for her to scan for pedestrians, intersecting streets, and turning cars and to pay special attention to scanning in various areas of the visual field to detect signs, colors, and building configuration for landmarks that facilitate orientation.

> A child with constricted visual fields veers into a driveway and wishes to relocate the sidewalk. The targets are grasslines, curbs, a street, and a mailbox, and the environment is a small residential neighborhood. In this case, the child needs to scan horizontally while turning from left to right until he or she identifies the sidewalk, shoreline, or street, at which point the child adjusts course to return to the sidewalk. To readjust to his former line of direction, the child then scans left and right to locate a landmark, such as the blue mailbox, which indicates his former direction of travel.

> An individual with low visual acuity wants to cross an intersection. The targets are moving or

turning cars on the parallel and perpendicular streets, traffic lights, and pedestrians, and the environment is a heavily congested urban area. If the traffic light was not discernible, the person would concentrate on cars turning from the parallel street to the left. After beginning to cross, the person would continue to scan periodically to check for turning cars from the left side. On approaching the midpoint of the crossing, her scanning would focus ahead and to the left for turning cars. Scanning for the movement of pedestrians can also facilitate decision making.

Tracing

Tracing—visually following single or multiple stationary lines—helps a person establish, maintain, and reestablish lines of direction. A number of visual lines, such as grasslines, hedge lines, roof lines, overhead fluorescent lights along a hallway, contrasting baseboards, chair molding at waist or shoulder height, or lines along a patterned floor, can serve as tracing cues. The following examples illustrate the usefulness of tracing skills for O&M purposes:

To locate a house on a residential street, a person can visually trace or "trail" a line of hedges until the fourth opening from the corner or trace along the inside grassline until the seventh opening after the first large driveway (or whatever number is appropriate to find a particular house).

After exiting one classroom, a child locates the next one by visually trailing along the right wall, until he or she finds the third inset or recessed doorway.

To locate a particular store along a small business block that is three-quarters of the way down the block and the only store with a red step, a person will attempt to scan down the block and estimate a halfway mark. From there, the person could visually trace along the base of

the building lines, where steps are usually located, until he or she finds the red step.

To establish and maintain orientation while walking along a residential neighborhood, a person with severely reduced visual acuity may intermittently trace a line of trees, parked cars, a grassline, or contrasting curbline to walk in the desired line of travel.

Tracking

Tracking—visually following a moving target—is a useful skill for mobility, especially in congested areas. Individuals with constricted visual fields may be required to compensate with greater head movements to keep targets in their field of view, while those with low visual acuity can use a wider combination of eye and head movements. A variety of tracking skills, illustrated by the following examples, augment O&M decisions:

A person may experience a drop in functional vision on entering a dimly lit restaurant. By following behind and tracking the upper-body movements of his or her companion's light-colored blouse or shirt, the person can anticipate the direction of travel and monitor unexpected turns.

In combination with appropriate scanning, tracking moving cars facilitates safe street crossings, especially in heavily congested business areas. Scanning for and tracking cars perpendicular to one's line of travel helps a person to anticipate approaching intersections, whereas tracking parallel and turning cars helps him or her to effectively judge when to cross.

Tracking the movement of a person walking ahead along a route helps one to anticipate obstacles. For example, a sudden swerving or veering away from a previously established line of direction may forewarn the person with low vision of an impending obstacle, just as the sudden dropping or raising of a person's height may indicate approaching steps.

Tracking the movement of an oncoming bus with a telescope readies the person to detect visually, and then to identify as early as possible, the bus number or route.

ENVIRONMENTAL CUES

The structure and function of the environment in which a person with low vision travels presents both challenges and opportunities. This section describes the general category of environmental cues that, when integrated with the effective use of visual skills, can result in safe and efficient mobility. Often persons with low vision can benefit from learning to attend to cues that travelers with unimpaired vision do not typically use.

Color and Contrast Cues

Color and contrast cues serve as excellent visual prompts for locating objects and destinations and for maintaining or regaining orientation. Even for a person with low visual acuity, color and contrast cues are helpful in interpreting the visual world. Some examples of the use of these cues are as follows:

A person has trouble seeing the details of various types of fruit in the produce section of a supermarket. A quick scan for the color purple eliminates the need to examine each fruit to find grapes. Similarly, scanning down the condiment section for the color red, rather than yellow (mustard) or white (mayonnaise), helps the person to find ketchup.

An upper-field scan to the golden arches of McDonald's could be used as an orientation cue to locate a business two doors away, as opposed to examining one building at a time.

Many information signs in subways are color coded, and following these colored signs may help a person locate or exit from the subway. This technique is particularly useful for those who are unable to read signs.

A person may be unable to discern the colors on a traffic light, but may detect a change in contrast from the middle (yellow) to the top (red) of the light. This contrast cue could be used to facilitate safer crossings at busy intersections.

Distance Perception Cues

Most people with unimpaired vision think of distance vision as being 6 feet or greater. For a person with low vision, a considerable distance may be anywhere from beyond arm's reach to his or her particular awareness distance level. Most people learn about distance through the use of concrete measures, such as rulers and yardsticks, or through practice judging the time it takes to get from one location to another. However, some use additional visual perceptual cues to determine the distance of objects without thinking consciously about them. Instruction in the use of these visual perceptual cues facilitates distance judgment. The following discussion assumes a basic knowledge of positional and distance concepts (for more information on these concepts, see Smith & O'Donnell, 1991).

Familiar and Apparent Size

Familiar-sized objects appear smaller and smaller as their distance from the viewer increases. With two similar-sized objects (such as toy blocks, automobiles, parking meters, or barns), the object that appears larger is closer, and the one that appears smaller is farther away.

Interposition

Interposition also enables a person to judge comparative distance. To determine the distances of two objects the one that is fully visible is closer, and the one partially blocked by the fully visible object is farther away. For example, a child would notice that a sliding board in the playground partially blocks the view of one of the swings in a swing set. This indicates that the swings are farther away than the slide.

Combination of Cues

Combining familiar and apparent-size cues with other visual cues can facilitate quicker decision making. For example, if a teenager is walking in a shopping mall and trying to determine the distance at which a line of people is forming, in addition to noting the apparent size of the people who are congregated in a single position, he or she could glance at the floor and trace along to gage the distance between the crowd and where he or she is standing.

Depth Perception Cues

Depth perception involves judging the relative distance of objects and their spatial relationship to each other. The ability to perceive visual depth is one of the most frequently occurring problems for persons with low vision. Two areas of most concern are stairs and curbs, especially those that go down. The following are examples of alternate cues, used alone or in combination, that can assist a person in detecting stairs and curbs.

Steps

A number of visual signals indicate the presence of stairs or steps, many of them involving judgments and observations about differences in heights, colors, lighting, directions, and sounds.

Slope of a Stair Rail. The person traces the stair railing. If it slopes upward in the field of view, he or she should expect stairs to go up. If the railing slopes downward toward the lower field of view, he or she should expect stairs to go down.

Changes in Position and Height. Persons who gradually become higher or lower indicate up or down stairs, respectively. If one approaches an area and notices that the bottom half (legs or feet) of a person is missing from view, this is a cue that stairs are obscuring the bottom view.

Contrast Color Strips on Edges of Steps. Contrast color strips on the edge of the first or last step, or on all steps, indicate the presence of a drop-off or set of stairs. For some persons with low vision, a strip on each step may be confusing because of the pattern created in the visual field. If the flooring is patterned, contrast strips may be more important because it may be difficult to note the edges of steps when the pattern creates visual clutter.

Broken Shadows. Broken or zigzag shadows of objects such as railings, branches, and poles are indicative of steps, and each break in a shadow denotes a separate step. Although a set of steps may appear as a flat surface or blended ramp to a person with low vision, the presence of broken shadows indicates that steps are present and can signal the need to scan for the presence of a railing. Shadows, particularly intermittent shadows, offer both visual opportunities and visual challenges. For instance, intermittent shadows may help a person with low vision gain information about the presence of objects or cause confusion by masking the presence of small low-lying objects.

Angles at Step Borders. Successive right angles or triangular shapes at the side borders of steps, where the riser and adjoining steps meet, are sometimes visible. These shapes are more evident when the walls adjacent to the steps are of a contrasting color. In addition, they are more discernible if viewed from a side angle, as opposed to a straight-ahead view.

Sound Localization. Any of the aforementioned visual cues (or a combination of them), coupled with an awareness of the change in people's footsteps and voices coming from above or below one's location, represent examples of multisensory cues that signal the presence of stairs.

Curbs

In general, judging the distance between a sidewalk and the street or roadway can help provide an estimate of the depth of a curb.

Contrasting Street Pavement. The macadam, asphalt, or tar on a street are frequently darker than lighter sidewalk pavements, such as cement. This abrupt change in color contrast may signal an approaching curb and street.

Crosswalk Lines. Invariably, the presence of a pair of spaced vertical white, yellow, or blue lines on a road surface indicates a street crossing. Periodically scanning ahead to anticipate the location of these lines forewarns a person of the location of a curb. This cue is particularly helpful when a curb is difficult to discern.

Tires of Parked Cars. The tires of parked cars are partially obscured by a curb. Judging how much of the bottom segment of a tire is "missing" also helps to determine the depth of a curb.

Rural Areas. Rural areas often have less defined spaces for walking, and edges of roads or unpaved areas may present uneven terrain. Checking for changes in grasslines; noting changes in terrain; and identifying landmarks, such as a mailbox or a unique feature of a fence, may assist the traveler in knowing that he or she is approaching a corner. In rural areas, some unique features of the terrain need to be considered, such as cattle guards and low water crossings.

Moving Vehicles Perpendicular to the Line of Travel. A flow of vehicles moving perpendicularly across one's line of travel usually signals the presence of an intersecting street and oncoming curb. A combination of anticipatory visual scanning and auditory cues makes this a readily discernible cue.

End of Grassline and Building Lines. Visually scanning ahead for the end of a grassline or building line may enable a person to anticipate a curb at an intersecting corner. When a sidewalk is broken and the person is unsure whether he or she has reached a driveway, checking for grasslines may be an additional cue.

Contrast Color on Curb Edge. Some regular or blended curb edges are painted yellow or blue to signal their presence. They are found more frequently near public buildings and busy street intersections.

People or Objects at Street Corners. Groups of people who have stopped and are standing together may be waiting for a traffic light to change. This cue, in combination with objects located through visual scanning, such as a stop sign, a traffic light control box, a fire hydrant, or a mailbox, commonly located at street corners, also signals the presence of a curb.

Broken Shadows Cast on Curbs. A curb, like stairs, causes a break in the shadow of an object, such as a light pole or tree branch. The shadow is distorted or broken at the edge of the curb and may be visible even if the presence or depth of the curb is not. Conversely, shadows from trees cast on curbs may be confusing because they darken the sidewalk and street surfaces.

Monocular Vision

The difficulty perceiving depth that is experienced by persons with congenital or acquired monocular disability has been well documented (Schein, 1988; Schiff, 1980; Stevens, 1951). Individuals who function monocularly require additional time for compensatory head movements to obtain more information relative to distance and depth cues. In addition, their reduced peripheral fields cause more difficulty in general mobility situations. It is especially important to teach children with monocular impairment to scan efficiently and to be aware of the environmental cues discussed here before they establish inefficient visual patterns.

OPTICAL DEVICES

No O&M program is complete without an assessment of and instruction in the use of appropriate optical devices. An O&M instructor works with a person with and without optical devices; integrating the use of optical devices in O&M lessons can be essential for obtaining maximum use of visual function. Whether a person is reading a street sign with a monocular or checking a directory in an office building, the use of a telescopic device should not be underestimated. Also valuable is magnification at near point to see maps, timetables, and price tags. Both near and distance optical devices can significantly enhance the efficient use of vision for mobility purposes.

Optical devices and absorptive lenses provide further options for improving the mobility of persons with low vision by increasing their visual acuity and enhancing their visual fields. For example, a person may know the location of a traffic light and have good color perception but may be unable to identify the color of the traffic light because it is beyond his or her visual range. With the use of a telescope, the apparent distance is decreased and the size and brightness of the light are increased, allowing the person to identify the color of the light. For a person with severely constricted visual fields who frequently bumps into objects and people located on the side, the use of a fresnel prism or reversed telescopic system can enhance his or her field of view and, hence, help the person detect these objects and people in the periphery (see Chapter 7 for information on such devices and the following recommended references for instructing people with low vision in the use of optical devices [Berg, Jose, & Carter, 1983; Carter, 1983; J. Ferraro & Jose, 1983; S. Ferraro & J. Ferraro, 1983; Geruschat, 1980; Smith & Geruschat, 1983; Watson, 1980; Watson & Berg, 1983; Wiener & Vopata, 1980]).

SPECIAL CONSIDERATIONS

To be effective, assessment and instructional techniques should take into account a person's unique history. There are numerous background factors to be considered, including such psychosocial considerations as motivation and family support, and such rehabilitation considerations

as the circumstances surrounding the loss of vision and recent versus long-standing visual impairment. However, the age of the person receiving services raises a number of special considerations.

Children

Early intervention programs, such as Head Start, are an accepted best practice to stimulate the development of learning skills in children. This general philosophy of early intervention can be applied to the development of visual skills in children with low vision, for whom early intervention is critical to the achievement of full visual potential. Consistent with this philosophy, early instruction in visual stimulation, body image, concept development, sensory training, and environmental awareness and exposure is recommended. Visual skills do not develop in isolation. To be effective, low vision mobility programs require the integration of all these areas.

Of unique interest to early mobility intervention is the enhancement of distance vision. *Beyond Arm's Reach* (Smith & O'Donnell, 1991), a comprehensive curriculum to develop and enhance distance vision skills, addresses the early intervention needs of children with low vision. It is important to encourage a child's use of distance vision and to provide movement activities, such as running and riding a bike, that incorporate the use of movement with vision, at as early an age as possible.

A mobility question that is frequently asked about children is, "Should I encourage my student to use a cane or to use vision?" In effect, though, this is not an either/or situation. Thus, it may be better to ask, "What combination of vision and cane use best serves my student?" The use of the long cane for mobility purposes complements the use of vision. With this approach, the student is taught to evaluate the quality of all sensory information and to integrate the use of the long cane and vision. For example, the long cane may be used for detecting danger areas, such as steps or curbs, so the child can use vision

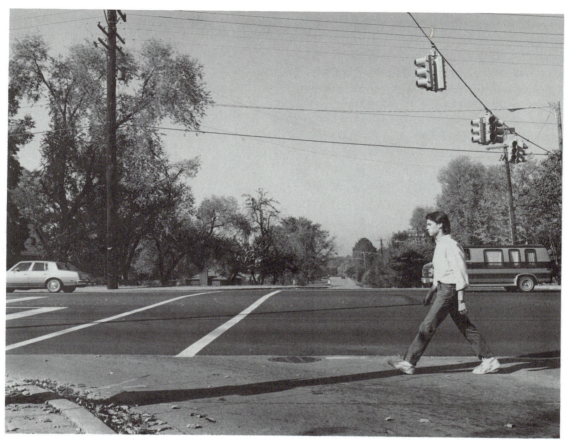

Training in the effective use of visual information and environmental cues can enable a young person with low vision to move about independently and safely.

to locate landmarks and, to anticipate obstacles, as well as for pleasure and aesthetic purposes.

Adults

The long cane is also an effective tool for the adult with low vision. However, some adults with adventitious vision loss may associate long canes with dependence, not independence. Therefore, the challenge for the O&M instructor is to reeducate them, through planned experiences, to see the benefits of combining the use of the long cane and vision for effective mobility, with emphasis on eventual independence.

Many adults with low vision bring to re-

habilitation a long history of unimpaired visual acuity. The advantage of this history is visual memory, visual experiences, and familiarity with a variety of visual concepts. The disadvantage is a habitual visual style that may be resistant to change. For example, a common experience of persons who have recently become visually impaired is the presence of a central blind spot (scotoma). The habitual behavior is to look straight ahead to see clearly, but with the vision loss, adapted viewing to the side, eccentrically, enables a clearer view. Therefore, adults with adventitious low vision frequently require instruction in eccentric viewing techniques, among many other areas of instruction. Instruction for adults generally emphasizes adaptation and the development of new visual strategies. In addition, a person who has a history of unimpaired vision may be frustrated by what appears as an unclear or limited image. This experience may create an emotional challenge to accepting new strategies for determining where he or she is in the environment and how best to use remaining vision for mobility purposes.

SUMMARY

The review of clinical vision reports, assessment of functional visual acuity and fields, evaluation of the impact of environmental variables, and observation of functional vision in a mobility context are critical components of the assessment of low vision mobility. The development of instructional goals and objectives should reflect this information and periodic reviews of assessment information will encourage effective, goal-directed teaching.

Mobility skills can be improved through instruction in the use of vision, and early and continued exposure to systematic instruction offers the best opportunity for maximizing the use of vision for mobility purposes.

The visual environment offers both problems and opportunities for the traveler with low vision. Therefore, professional practice needs to include exposure to and training in situations that could potentially impede or enhance the use of vision for solving mobility problems.

Although the development of visual skills was emphasized, best practice dictates the full incorporation of all available sensory information. Professionals in the field should ultimately help people with low vision discriminate when the use of vision and optical devices is or is not effective for mobility purposes, as well as what combination of sensory information best facilitates decision making.

For low vision mobility programs to be successful, persons with low vision should be active contributors to all aspects of visual assessment and instruction. To ensure that they are, service providers need to recognize and respect the rele-vant and important information that persons with low vision have to offer, encourage their ongoing input, and continually review information and the content of lessons. The implementation of this approach espouses a philosophy of teaching "with," rather than "to" or "at," the person with low vision. Ultimately, this partnership is a philosophy of teaching that better facilitates successful education and rehabilitation.

ACTIVITIES

Using This Chapter and Other Resources

1. In the vignette that opened this chapter, Herb had not received O&M services until recently. He is now able to travel independently, although on a limited basis. If you were his instructor, what would be the next travel goals for him and how would they be established?

2. Develop a lesson plan for explaining the mobility-related functional implications of albinism to a fifth-grade student.

3. Write a transcript of what you might say to obtain O&M services for a client who has the following clinical findings: *diagnosis:* age-related maculopathy; *visual acuity:* 20/220 OU; and *visual field:* 7-degrees central scotoma OU.

4. Role-play with a classmate how a person with low vision who uses a long cane may respond to a passersby who questions whether he or she is "faking blindness."

In the Community

1. Wearing visual distorters of both reduced acuities and constricted visual fields, travel in different environmental settings, noting critical mobility problems and assessing the impact of different environmental variables on your visual functioning. This activity should be completed with a partner who monitors you for safety.

2. Walk a route and identify the landmarks that are important for the following travelers with

low vision: (1) a 12-year-old student with 20/600 visual acuity and full visual fields, (2) a 32-year-old client with 20/40 visual acuity and visual fields restricted to 3 central degrees, (3) a 3-year-old child with albinism, photophobia, nystagmus, 20/200 OU, and light-absorptive lenses.

With a Person with Low Vision

1. Spend some time with two people who have low vision, each with similar etiologies (such as two individuals with albinism or two persons with retinitis pigmentosa). Ask them what travel skills help them and whether they have had O&M instruction. Compare and contrast similarities and differences.

2. Discuss with teenagers who are fully sighted where they go and how they travel. Then hold a similar discussion with teenagers who have low vision. What similarities and differences do you find?

From Your Perspective

There are an insufficient number of O&M instructors in many geographic areas. How might an O&M instructor establish priorities for serving children or adults with low vision?

CHAPTER 14

Adults with Low Vision: Personal, Social, and Independent Living Needs

Karen E. Wolffe

VIGNETTE

Andrea is a woman in her late 30s who lived with her parents until their recent deaths in an automobile accident and now lives alone in the family home. She has no vision in her right eye and reduced acuity in her left eye (20/400) with a 15-degree visual field because of glaucoma. She graduated from high school and, since then, has worked as a substitute receptionist in a local contractor's office. Although the contractor's office is within walking distance of her home, the shops where she buys groceries and takes her dry cleaning are miles away. There is no public transportation, and taxis are expensive. Her neighbor suggested that she call the rehabilitation services agency for help.

Could she receive assistance from the rehabilitation agency? Aren't those services just for people who are unemployed? Of course, without her parents to help her, she, too, could join the ranks of the unemployed. Without them, how could she read all the materials that she used to bring home to her mother? How could she keep up with the house and yard? How could she get to the grocery store, the bank, and the other places she needs to go? How could she handle the utility and tax payments? The more she thought about all her parents had done to help her over the years, the more overwhelmed she felt. Too much had happened in the past few months: she had lost her parents and her freedom to move about in the community, and she could even lose her job.

When Andrea called her state's separate rehabilitation agency for individuals who are blind or visually impaired to inquire about services, she spoke to a rehabilitation counselor, who suggested that she should come to the local field office to complete an application. Andrea asked directions to the office and was pleased to discover that it was in a location with which she was familiar. She also scheduled an appointment with the rehabilitation counselor, who would help her complete the application and advised her to bring documentation of her disability to determine her eligibility. To receive services, Andrea was told, federal law requires that a person must have a documented disability and that rehabilitation services could reasonably be expected to result in employment. She mentioned her job as a substitute receptionist and said that she really needed assistance with the household responsibilities her parents had managed before they died. The counselor again encouraged her to come to the office to determine what services might help her maintain her independence, as well as her job. Andrea decided to see for herself and phoned the taxi company to reserve a taxi for her trip to the office.

On the day of her appointment with the rehabilitation counselor, Andrea was pleased to meet a woman close to her own age. She and the counselor talked about Andrea's current situation and what the agency might do to assist her. Andrea discovered that the agency would send a rehabilitation teacher to her home to evaluate her need for the services of a teacher, to provide some immediate help with her new household responsibilities, and to suggest some adaptive tools and techniques to help her at home and on the job.

INTRODUCTION

Although living with impaired vision can be time consuming and difficult on occasion, life with low vision can be pursued successfully, with dignity and satisfaction. This chapter discusses the personal-social skills and independent living skills that are essential for adults with low vision, as well as the rehabilitation services that are available to them in the United States and Canada. (Issues related specifically to employment are covered in Chapter 15.) The following sections present information about the personal-social (or interpersonal) skills and self-advocacy skills that can help persons with low vision lead a successful, fulfilling life.

PERSONAL-SOCIAL SKILLS

A variety of personal and social issues may arise for the individual who is visually impaired. One of the common side effects of low vision is social isolation. Some adults with adventitious low vision withdraw socially because they are unsure of themselves and of how others will react to them now that they can no longer see as well as they did in the past. They may be concerned about whether they have applied their makeup properly or shaved completely. They may be embarrassed to say they cannot read a menu or admit that they

can no longer drive. Since adults who experience a sudden loss of vision are unlikely to know compensatory techniques for managing their daily lives, unless they have been referred for rehabilitation services, it is understandable that many individuals with low vision may be concerned about their appearance or ability to travel safely and efficiently. Such factors may contribute to anxiety, frustration, and sometimes depression. Rehabilitation services may include teaching home and personal management techniques, adaptive communication skills, orientation and mobility, counseling and guidance, or other service as needed to enhance independent living and employability.

In addition, various relationships of adults who lose their vision may be adversely affected by role reversals or changes. Suddenly, a spouse or a parent may have to assume full responsibility for transporting the individual with low vision and other members of the family when, in the past, driving was a shared responsibility. Or, a family member may have to assist the person with low vision to read bill statements and to write checks to pay bills, when in the past the person had full responsibility for such a chore. Besides the change in roles that an acquired visual impairment may cause, the person with low vision may have less privacy than before the visual impairment and may find it worrisome having to rely on others for help. These changes can strain relationships until appropriate adjustments are made.

Similar issues often arise for many individuals who are born with low vision. Many people with congenital low vision are raised in families and communities in which they are the only persons with a visual impairment. As a consequence, other people, particularly family members, may do things for them that they are capable of doing for themselves. This behavior may result in dependence on others and learned helplessness. People who develop learned helplessness believe they have no control over what happens to them. They tend, therefore, to be passive and demoralized (Monbeck, 1973; Scott, 1969; Seligman, 1990). In addition, the self-esteem of persons with low vision may be adversely affected by others' treating them as if they can do little and expecting little from them.

Many individuals with low vision struggle with issues related to fitting into groups in which others are able to drive or to engage in sports or other activities that require good vision. A complicating issue for some visually impaired people is that they often look as if they are fully sighted, and thus others do not understand their visual limitations. Therefore, it is important for them to be reminded that they are more like other people than they are different from them. (These and various other psychosocial issues are explored in Chapter 2.)

Social and Leisure Skills

Like everyone else, adults with low vision benefit from developing a healthy sense of who they are. They need to be encouraged to think of what they have to offer and what others have to offer them. In addition, they need supportive feedback concerning their behaviors—what is working for them socially and what is not—and their strengths, particularly their strengths in interacting with others and the impact of their behaviors on others. They also need to know about visual cues they may miss and the significance of those visual cues, especially visual cues that are related to social messages, such as a wink, a nod, a smile, a leer, a wave, or a pointed finger.

For adults with low vision, as for adults with unimpaired vision, a key to success in social situations is to interact with and treat others as they would wish others to treat them. Since giving to others is one way to foster social success and life satisfaction, involvement in community life is both socially and personally beneficial. Thus, some individuals with low vision contribute to their communities through volunteer work, engaging in the same range of activities that others in the community participate in: scouting, religious activities, voter registration, assisting at balloting booths, coaching Little League teams, cleaning up neighborhood parks, and so forth.

A significant psychosocial issue that many people with low vision face is whether to discuss their visual impairments and with whom. This decision is an individual one, and the person with low vision must choose whether to do so and the way that feels most comfortable to him or her. However, it is important to realize the consequences of one's decision. On the one hand, if a person chooses not to tell others about a visual impairment, he or she risks appearing awkward in situations in which his or her vision is not adequate to accomplish visually demanding tasks. On the other hand, if a person chooses to tell, he or she risks being treated differently—often either as a helpless person or as an extraordinarily heroic person. For this reason, the middle ground—revealing one's condition to acquaintances, friends, and relatives but not revealing it to the general public—is considered the safest by many people. When an adult with low vision decides it is important to reveal the fact of his or her visual impairment, one way in which to do so is to talk about what can be seen and not focus on medical terminology or jargon that the average person may find confusing (for a detailed discussion of these issues, see Chapter 2).

Persons with low vision who pursue a variety of recreational activities can have their access to leisure skills facilitated by using modified materials, like jumbo-size playing cards or playing cards with both large-print and braille markings. Also, many popular games, such as Scrabble, Monopoly, checkers, chess, dominoes, backgammon, and bingo, are available in accessible formats from adaptive equipment vendors (see the Resources section at the back of this book). Most of the vendors that carry adaptive games stock large-print crossword and other puzzle books, too. In addition, they may carry television-screen enlargers and large-button adapters for television remote controls. Many persons with low vision and the professionals who work with them may focus on the ability to participate in leisure activities, which helps promote and refine social skills and encourages relationship building. Helping individuals with low vision obtain adapted materials and learn adapted techniques for pursuing their interests is a vital contribution to this process (see Ludwig, Luxton, & Attmore, 1988).

Strategies for Fostering Self-Advocacy Skills

In general, people who feel competent and in control of their lives are better able to stand up for what they want and need than are those who feel incompetent or out of control. By teaching and reinforcing skills for performing daily chores like taking care of one's home and family or techniques for expressing oneself and communicating with others, service providers help adults with low vision exercise control over their lives. By helping people with low vision to learn to live independently and hold down jobs, raise families, and actively participate in the community, they promote their clients' sense of competence and self-esteem.

Successful outcomes are achieved when service providers allow individuals with low vision to identify their problems and develop strategies for resolving them. Thus, it is essential for adults with low vision to be involved in any goal-setting and teaching processes because they need to make decisions about what they will do and where they will do it and when and experience and deal with the natural consequences of their decisions. Therefore, counselors, teachers, caregivers, and other members of the rehabilitation team need to listen closely to what persons with low vision want and not assume they know what is best.

Clients may need some assistance in gaining access to resources, as well as in understanding the array of choices and techniques that are available. However, it is important for service providers to recognize that no one solution or technique is appropriate for everyone and that only the individual with low vision can decide which choice in the array will work best for him or her. Hence, providers of services need to generate multiple ideas or strategies and let their clients pick the ones that suit them best. This technique encourages problem solving, which builds self-confidence.

In addition, various resources are available for persons striving to develop an increased sense of self-worth. Seligman's work on learned optimism (1990) is useful for anyone who is struggling with issues of low self-esteem or poor self-image. In addition, numerous books written by and about people who are blind or visually impaired may provide insight to someone in a similar situation (see, for example, Charles & Ritz, 1978; Flax, 1993; Jahoda, 1993; Ringgold, 1991; Sullivan, 1980; Tuttle, 1984).

Finally, adults with low vision may find it helpful to join a support group in which they can meet others who have similar impairments. Among the numerous support groups available are those for anyone with low vision (such as the Council of Citizens with Low Vision International) and those for people with specific syndromes or diseases (diabetes, albinism, retinitis pigmentosa, Usher's syndrome, and age-related macular degeneration, for example). Talking with people who have developed organizational systems and alternative methods for doing things often helps reassure someone who feels helpless or who lacks confidence. In addition, many people who have hereditary conditions may find it helpful to meet with others who have experienced the difficult decisions associated with genetic counseling. The Resources section of this book lists a range of organizations that may be contacted.

INDEPENDENT LIVING SKILLS

People with unimpaired vision unconsciously depend on their sight for processing information about the world around them and for managing their daily affairs. When an adult experiences a significant loss of vision, everyday tasks, such as personal care and home management; reading, writing, and calculating; and getting around in the community, and the requisite abilities to perform these tasks may pose a significant challenge. Thus, the person must learn new techniques for performing common tasks like doing laundry,

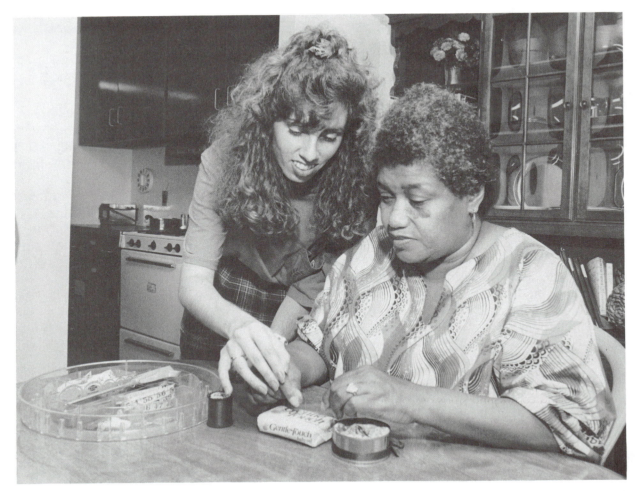

Adults who experience vision loss can learn a variety of adaptive techniques for accomplishing the tasks of daily living efficiently.

preparing meals, and taking care of personal needs, as well as learn how to acquire and use adaptive equipment to process information in order to remain as independent as possible.

A rehabilitation teacher can provide guidance and instruction in independent living skills and, together with other members of the rehabilitation team, can help the person with low vision and his or her family cope with the new set of circumstances in which they find themselves. The roles and responsibilities of rehabilitation teachers and other rehabilitation professionals are discussed later in this chapter.

For adults with congenital low vision, the sit-uation is often somewhat different. Many adults who have grown up with a visual impairment have learned compensatory skills in home and personal management and communication skills either on their own or through service providers in school and rehabilitation settings. However, due to a variety of circumstances, such as previously overprotective family environments, individuals with a congenital vision impairment frequently need to learn these skills as adults. The following sections present information about the independent living skills that benefit adults with low vision and environmental adaptations that are helpful (see Sidebar 14.1 for a summary).

SIDEBAR 14.1

Environmental Adaptations and Skills

A great number of environmental adaptations and skills can be used by people with low vision for independent living. The following list provides a sample.

FOOD PREPARATION

◆ placing fluorescent lights under kitchen cabinets for additional light on counter tops

◆ using different-colored cutting boards to increase contrast: light-colored boards for dark foods and dark-colored for light foods

◆ placing colored mats or trays under clear glass mixing bowls to increase contrast

◆ using Good Grips measuring cups and spoons: white and black sets to provide contrast with colored dots on handles to differentiate size

◆ placing contrasting strips of Contac Paper on the refrigerator to provide contrast when pouring liquids into a clear glass

◆ placing colored or tactile markings on the controls of a stove, oven, microwave oven, and small appliances

◆ reorganizing kitchen cabinets to reduce the need for labeling

◆ using large-print or tactile markings for canned, packaged, and frozen foods

◆ using large-print or tape-recorded recipes

◆ using visual and nonvisual techniques for determining doneness of food

◆ using visual and tactile techniques for measuring, cutting foods (knife skills), and using the stove or oven safely

◆ using visual and tactile techniques for grocery shopping.

PERSONAL CARE

◆ using tactile techniques for applying makeup

◆ caring for a prosthetic eye

◆ using large-print or tactile labels to match similar-colored clothing

◆ using large-print or tactile labels for medication containers

◆ using adaptive equipment for filling insulin syringes

◆ using adaptive equipment for monitoring blood glucose levels.

HOME MANAGEMENT

◆ using adaptive techniques for cleaning and repairing clothing (for example, marking stains with a safety pin, threading a needle, and pairing socks with Socks-Locks)

◆ using adaptive techniques for house cleaning (such as using overlapping patterns and dividing a room into small sections)

◆ using contrast and lighting to increase visibility in dangerous areas (for instance, removing throw rugs, putting a contrasting cover on a hassock and contrasting no-slip strips on top and bottom steps, and increasing lighting in stairwells and shower stalls)

◆ labeling cleaning supplies in large-print or tactile codes

◆ using adaptive techniques for minor home repairs (such as changing fuses)

◆ using adaptive techniques for yard work.

COMMUNICATION

◆ using supplemental lighting and glare control for visual reading

---

Environmental Adaptations and Skills (continued)

- using low vision devices for reading

- learning or improving typing or keyboarding skills

- using library services (for large-print books and Talking Books)

- using an audiotape recorder

- using handwriting aids (bold-tip markers; bold-line paper; and signature, letter, envelope, and check guides)

- reading and writing in braille

- using adaptive time pieces (large-print, braille, or talking watches, clocks, and calendars)

- using adaptive calculators (large-print or speech output)

- learning adaptive techniques for managing money (identifying coins and currency, using check-writing guides and large-print checks, paying bills by telephone)

- using community information resources (radio reading information services, descriptive video, newspapers on telephone)

- using adaptive techniques for telephoning (large-print or tactile dials and writing and recording a personal telephone-address book)

- using computers with screen enlargement and speech or braille output.

LEISURE ACTIVITIES

- using adaptive techniques for crafts (such as knitting, crocheting, and sewing)

- using adaptive techniques for hobbies (for example, woodworking, fishing, and stamp collecting)

- using adaptive techniques and resources for sports (beep softball, goalball, golf, and the like) and adapted games (playing cards and board games)

- joining community social groups (such as senior citizens' centers and church groups).

JUDY C. MATSUOKA
University of Arkansas at Little Rock

Home and Personal Management Skills

Home and personal management skills, sometimes referred to as daily living skills or activities of daily living, are necessary for taking care of one's living space and person. Home management tasks include housekeeping (dusting, vacuuming, sweeping, mopping, and washing and drying dishes and clothes), planning and preparing meals, shopping, managing money, and performing light home-maintenance chores (changing light bulbs or washers, tightening loose door handles, replacing appliance parts, and the like). Personal management tasks include grooming and hygiene activities like washing and bathing, taking care of fingernails and hair, and shaving.

Labeling and Identifying Objects

Depending on the amount of usable vision a person has, he or she may require large-print or tactile labels to identify and locate objects. Personal care items, for example, may need to be marked in such a way that the person can tell the difference between shampoo and body lotion or aspirins and vitamins. If items are not marked and the person's vision is not acute enough to discern visual differences, another strategy will need to be used, like discriminating among similar items according to smell, color, or size. Also, the person with low vision will find it useful and important to get in the habit of returning things to specific places, so he or she can find them easily.

Appliances such as the stove, oven, microwave, dishwasher, and clothes washer and dryer, as well as the thermostat or other household controls, may need to be marked in large print or with colored tape so the settings can be adjusted properly. If the person with low vision also has diabetes or some other chronic health impairment that affects tactile sensitivity, markings may need to have a rougher texture than colored tape offers. In such instances, Velcro markings may prove easier for the person to discriminate. Some common household items, like telephones, timers, and temperature gauges, can be purchased with enlarged numbers. Articles of clothing may also need to be labeled so that outfits are not mismatched or sorted improperly for laundering. Another alternative is to tie or otherwise connect items, such as like-colored socks or stockings for laundering. Some people circumvent difficulties in this area by buying socks that are all the same color.

In the kitchen, it may be necessary to have measuring cups and spoons with large-print, raised, or colored markings and large-print or recorded recipe books. However, some cooks prefer to read regular-print cookbooks with low vision devices. Food stuffs and cooking supplies can all be organized and labeled to facilitate the preparation of meals. It is just a matter of what methods work best for each individual (see, for example, Dickman, 1983; Ringgold, 1991).

Finding Resources: Adaptive Tools and Techniques

There are numerous commercial vendors of appliances and adaptive tools for individuals with low vision, many of which are listed in the *AFB Directory of Services for Blind and Visually Impaired Persons in the United States and Canada* (American Foundation for the Blind, 1993) and Yeadon's (1988) *International Low Vision Direc-*

tory. An excellent way to see and experiment with the latest items is to attend a local or regional conference of a consumer organization like the American Council of the Blind (ACB) or the National Federation of the Blind (NFB) or a meeting of professionals, such as the Association for Education and Rehabilitation of the Blind and Visually Impaired (AER) (see Resources).

Various books describe alternative techniques in home and personal management for individuals with low vision (Dickman, 1983; Ringgold, 1991; Smith, 1984; Yeadon, 1974; Younger & Sardegna (1991, 1994). In addition, curricula and texts for teaching independent living skills to students (see Loumiet & Levack, 1993) and rehabilitation professionals (see Ponchillia & Ponchillia, 1996) have information applicable to teaching young adults with low vision.

Communication Skills

For individuals with low vision, reading and writing may require the use of low vision devices or compensatory skills. Although oral communication is not obviously or directly affected by vision, low vision has an indirect effect because of the person's diminished ability to read the facial expressions and body language of others. However, a variety of techniques can be used for enhancing communication skills in adults with low vision.

Depending on the degree of their visual impairments, people with low vision can effect written communication for themselves and others in a number of ways. Some people may be able to read regular print by using corrective lenses, magnifiers, or a closed-circuit television (CCTV). Others may be able to read typewritten or printed materials but may have difficulty with handwritten materials, particularly cursive script. (If a person is unable to read handwritten materials independently, he or she may benefit from the services of a fully sighted reader.) Often, a reading stand will prove helpful (see Chapters 7 and 8; see also Jose, 1983). Paper with bold dark lines or raised lines and dark pens or bold-line markers can make it easier to write clearly and without running into previous sentences. Bold-line paper and typoscopes (pieces of cardboard or other material with a window cut in to allow viewing of lines of print on a page), separately or in combination, can contribute to the clarity of reading. In addition, large-print calendars, address books, and other organizers, as well as electronic devices, can be obtained for noting addresses, phone numbers, and appointments.

With current technology, people with low vision can use computers efficiently and effectively. Screen-enlargement software allows users to see what is displayed on the screen more easily, and speech programs and speech synthesizers provide access to screen information via spoken output. The combination of a screen-enlargement program and a speech program may be useful to some people for word processing and for constructing databases and spreadsheets. Adaptive software is useful for both personal and business applications. Antiglare screen filters are especially helpful to computer users with low vision. People who already have some degree of computer expertise may not need specific training for learning the adaptive software programs for screen enlargement or audio output. However, those who are just learning to use computers will in all likelihood need some additional training.

To assess adults' most efficient and effective means of gaining access to print, it is important to determine their reading and writing needs. Do they want or need to be able to read newspapers, blueprints, recipes, or notes from loved ones? Will they be reading at work, at home, and in shops or to drive or travel in the community? Or do they have special reading demands? What is more important to them: accuracy or speed? Once reading needs have been pinpointed, it will be necessary to evaluate different low vision devices and environmental modifications to determine the best options. Communication needs and the willingness to work with adaptations and appliances vary from individual to individual. (See Chapter 8 for more information on procedures for assessing appropriate options.) However, a variety of resources providing information on assistive reading and other devices for people with low vision

are available (National Library Service [NLS] for the Blind and Physically Handicapped, 1993).

Orientation and Mobility

One of the major challenges that a person with low vision faces may be diminished mobility. Depending on the severity of his or her visual impairment, the person may or may not be able to drive or walk safely unassisted in unfamiliar environments. Mobility devices and techniques can be taught to increase an individual's safety while traveling. The first priority is to be certain that the individual feels comfortable moving around in his or her house and neighborhood. Family members should be advised not to move furniture or leave objects lying about that could be hazardous without first notifying the person with low vision. Changes in lighting and contrasts in color may make moving about the house easier. For example, a dark coffee table on a light-colored rug will be more visible than will a dark table on a dark rug. Likewise, placing white place mats on a dark tablecloth or brightly colored flowers on a dark table will help the person identify objects.

An evaluation of which, if any, traveling devices may be of use should be conducted as soon as possible by an orientation and mobility (O&M) instructor (see Chapter 13). Devices such as telescopes, may be useful for reading signs and the like while traveling outdoors. It is sometimes recommended that persons with limited vision carry white canes so motorists and pedestrians recognize that they are visually impaired. However, many people with low vision still have good travel vision and do not think that it is necessary to carry canes. Still others can see sufficiently to travel without assistance during the day but have difficulty traveling at night because of poor night vision and thus may need to carry both canes and flashlights. In short, whether to use a cane or any other travel device is a personal decision. Adults make such decisions on the basis of various considerations, such as their level of comfort with the tools and their immediate needs.

REHABILITATION SERVICES

What happens when an adult receives rehabilitation services varies from state to state in the United States and from province to province in Canada. However, in the United States, the eligibility criteria are that an individual must have a documented disability that constitutes or results in a substantial impediment to employment and can benefit in terms of an employment outcome from vocational rehabilitation services. In this country, rehabilitation services are provided by the states through a state-federal system administered by the Rehabilitation Services Administration of the U.S. Department of Education. Criteria for eligibility for some services vary from state to state, depending on funding sources.

In Canada, most rehabilitation services for adults with low vision are provided by the Canadian National Institute for the Blind (CNIB). CNIB is a private, nonprofit organization that serves individuals who are blind or visually impaired from birth until death. Its only criterion for services is the presence of a visual impairment. Although there is a national rehabilitation agency, Vocational Rehabilitation Services of the Ministry of Skills, Training and Labour, its responsibility is to oversee the integration of all people with disabilities into the labor force, and its presence varies from province to province. The national agency will often contract for services from CNIB to assist current and prospective workers with low vision. Its eligibility criteria are that an individual must be disabled and aged 16 years or older.

There is some variation in the roles that rehabilitation counselors and rehabilitation teachers play in the United States and Canada. For example, in the United States the rehabilitation counselor is frequently a case manager who represents the state agency in the implementation of the Individualized Written Rehabilitation Program (IWRP), mandated by the 1992 amendments to the Rehabilitation Act of 1973 (P.L. 102-569), which is agreed to by the client and the counselor. (See Chapter 15 for additional information.) The situation in Canada differs from province to province. In some provinces, the case management responsibilities rotate among members of a multidisciplinary team. The team may include rehabilitation counselors, daily living skills teachers (or rehabilitation teachers), low vision specialists, O&M instructors, social workers, and others. In other provinces, case management is the sole responsibility of the rehabilitation counselor.

In both countries, services are provided in homes, in rehabilitation centers, in local community facilities, or in agency offices. CNIB provides low vision evaluations and assistive technology assessments, demonstrations, and, frequently, equipment on loan (called "loaner equipment"). However, the acquisition of equipment or low vision devices is the responsibility of the client. Clients with vocational potential can request fiscal support for equipment from the office of vocational rehabilitation services. If funding is not available through public assistance offices, the client can approach charity organizations or pay for the equipment outright.

Most state rehabilitation offices in the United States either contract out for low vision and technology evaluations or send clients to the agencies' center-based programs. Rehabilitation counselors can typically assist financially when low vision devices or equipment are necessary for employment. However, the amount of money available for such purchases varies from state to state, as does access to technology evaluations, loaner equipment, and training on adaptive equipment.

Overall, the roles and responsibilities of rehabilitation counselors and rehabilitation teachers in the United States and Canada are remarkably similar. The following sections describe these roles and responsibilities (for a summary, see Sidebars 14.2 and 14.3), as well as related services provided or contracted by rehabilitation agencies.

Rehabilitation Counseling

In general, rehabilitation counselors are responsible for determining eligibility for services, pro-

Roles and Responsibilities of Rehabilitation Counselors

SIDEBAR 14.2

Rehabilitation counselors are employed by state rehabilitation agencies, nonprofit agencies, and federal rehabilitation agencies serving veterans. They typically serve as case managers and play a multifaceted role on the rehabilitation team, performing the following functions and services: review of referral, intake, assessment, determination of eligibility, development and implementation of the Individualized Written Rehabilitation Program (IWRP), counseling and guidance, coordination of services, job placement and follow-up, and postemployment services. These responsibilities require various competencies:

- awareness of disabling conditions
- knowledge of alternative skills, low vision

devices, adapted appliances, and technology for work accommodations

- understanding of legislation regarding vocational rehabilitation and disability rights
- personal- and career-counseling skills
- ability to perform vocational assessments, job-development activities, and work-site analyses
- case management skills
- job placement and follow-up techniques.

JUDY C. MATSUOKA
University of Arkansas at Little Rock

viding counseling and guidance, doing case management, and coordinating services for people with low vision. They are also responsible for job development and overseeing clients' job seeking efforts. They negotiate contracts between the rehabilitation agency and individual clients (IWRPs in the United States or Individualized Program Plans [IPPs] in Canada). An IWRP documents an individual's vocational goal, spells out the services and equipment to be provided by the agency and the funds the agency will expend, and describes the client's contribution. The client's contribution may be a commitment to look for work, participate in a training program, or pay for all or part of the bill for equipment or specialized vocational training.

In Canada, most clients are referred for rehabilitation services by ophthalmologists or optometrists, whereas in the United States, clients are more likely to apply for services directly. Rehabilitation counselors are typically the first point of contact for people who want rehabilitation services. They provide information about what an agency can and cannot do to facilitate

independent living and employment. As case managers, they are responsible for contracting and paying for services and equipment that clients need and want. However, it is important to understand that most rehabilitation services are not automatically provided free of charge or at reduced rates; rather, clients must meet criteria for economic need that are established by the agencies. The only services that are typically provided free of charge, regardless of economic need, are counseling and guidance, information and referral, and tests needed to determine eligibility.

Once a person has been determined eligible for services, the counselor will develop an IWRP with him or her. If a client needs assistance with independent living skills or communication skills, the counselor typically will refer him or her to a rehabilitation teacher or a rehabilitation center. However, not all public agencies provide rehabilitation teaching services or have access to their own rehabilitation center. Generic agencies, which provide rehabilitation services to people with different kinds of disabilities and do not offer

SIDEBAR 14.3

Roles and Responsibilities of Rehabilitation Teachers

Rehabilitation teachers are employed by state rehabilitation agencies, nonprofit agencies, and federal rehabilitation agencies serving veterans. Although they usually work with rehabilitation counselors who serve as case managers, they may act as case managers for clients with homemaking goals or adults served by federally funded programs, such as Title VII, Chapter 2 (Independent Living Services for Older Individuals Who Are Blind).

Because rehabilitation teachers work with individuals at all stages of the rehabilitation process, they may be expected to perform the following job functions specific to low vision:

1. Conduct a functional evaluation of the person's visual abilities in the home, school, or workplace.

2. Discuss the person's specific needs for improved visual functioning and counsel the person about his or her visual condition and realistic expectations for the outcome of low vision services.

3. Refer the person to a low vision clinician or an eye care provider (ophthalmologist or optometrist).

4. Give the low vision clinician or eye care provider information on the person's perceived needs and observed level of visual functioning.

5. Review the findings of the clinical low vision examination with the person.

6. Review the use of any recommended optical devices and environmental adaptations with the person, help him or her to practice using the devices, and provide adjustment counseling until the person is comfortable using the devices or environmental modifications.

7. Provide feedback to the low vision clinician or eye care provider for a reevaluation or follow-up of the prescribed devices.

8. If acting as a case manager, process the necessary paperwork to arrange for and authorize payment of the low vision examination and prescribed devices.

9. Teach adaptive independent living skills and suggest environmental adaptations, working with the person to develop techniques that are safe, efficient, and effective using low vision and integrating the use of the other senses, such as touch and hearing.

JUDY C. MATSUOKA
University of Arkansas at Little Rock

---

specific services to individuals who are blind or visually impaired, do not usually have rehabilitation teacher services. In such instances, rehabilitation teaching services are frequently provided by private, nonprofit agencies to people who are blind or visually impaired.

Although there are training programs for rehabilitation counselors throughout the United States and Canada, there is no credential specific to counselors for persons who are visually impaired, as there is for teachers. In the United States, national certification, the Certified Rehabilitation Counselor, is awarded to rehabilitation counselors who meet standards established by the Commission on Rehabilitation Counselor Certification. In addition, many states have legal requirements governing the licensure of professional counselors that may stipulate the required credentials for rehabilitation counselors. Also, many rehabilitation agencies provide in-service training in blindness-specific skills for counselors who work for them.

Rehabilitation Teaching

Rehabilitation teachers deliver a variety of both in-home and on-the-job services to rehabilitation clients with low vision that range from teaching rudimentary independent living skills to teaching communication skills. Among the various kinds of instruction and assistance they provide is visiting a client's home and marking appliances and other objects with large-print or braille labels to help make the person's daily life run more smoothly. They explain services that are available through national resources like NLS, the Hadley School for the Blind, and Recording for the Blind and Dyslexic, and encourage clients to use local resources and become involved in community-based support groups. They primarily teach clients techniques for performing home and personal management, using adaptive tools and low vision devices, and refining alternative communication skills. In short, especially for people who are experiencing progressive decreases in visual acuity or who have undergone a traumatic vision loss, the services of rehabilitation teachers help individuals to be independent and continue to live at home.

Rehabilitation teachers work directly with individuals in a variety of ways. A large number of rehabilitation teachers are blind or have low vision, and they need to elicit information from their clients in different ways than do their colleagues with normal vision. For the most part, they obtain information directly from their clients by asking open-ended questions and confirm their initial impressions through a sighted driver or family member who is present during an evaluation. For example, a blind rehabilitation teacher may begin an interview by saying to the client, "Tell me a little bit about how and what you can see." If the client reports no difficulty with travel vision, but a family member mentions numerous close calls, the rehabilitation teacher knows from the conflicting information that this is an area that will have to be investigated further.

Both sighted and blind teachers often carry materials, such as colored construction paper; bold-lined paper, notes written in different sizes and styles of print, samples of large-print magazines, checks, and playing cards, sheets of acetate and paint samples or fabric squares in different colors, and the like, to use for evaluating clients' vision; incandescent light bulbs of various wattages, as well as screw-in fluorescent bulbs and halogen bulbs to demonstrate different types of illumination; and colored place mats and plates, typoscopes, colored filters, and so forth for demonstrating the effects of contrast manipulation. Using an evaluation kit with materials like those described and labeled with braille, a blind rehabilitation teacher can ascertain a great deal about what a client with low vision can see. If a client reports seeing blank places on a sheet of bold-lined paper, it is likely that he or she has scotomas in the visual field. Similarly, if a client says that a sheet with a yellow square drawn on it or with light blue lines on a white background is blank, the teacher knows that the client cannot discriminate subtle color differences on a white background. Some teachers take manipulatives, like rubberized shape puzzles, as well as static materials, and ask a client to work with the materials to see whether he or she uses vision or touch to perform a task. (Putting a puzzle together also demonstrates to a teacher how well a client follows directions, how quickly the task can be accomplished, which hand is dominant, and a wealth of other information.)

A blind or visually impaired rehabilitation teacher can also use an overhead transparency of a near point reading card to estimate print sizes, which a volunteer fully sighted reader can provide and which can then be brailled or put into large print. The teacher may have a client read print samples while he or she reads along from a braille or large-print script to monitor accuracy. Furthermore, the teacher can measure reading distance with a tactilely marked tape measure. He or she can monitor the client's posture, head position, and head movements by lightly placing a hand on the back of the client's neck or upper back and can physically monitor the client's hand position while using an optical device to determine whether the client has hand tremors and consistently lifts the device from the page.

In addition to the use of evaluation materials, a teacher who is blind or has low vision may wear a particular outfit and ask a client to describe it to determine what the client is seeing. All rehabilitation teachers should ask clients with low vision what their concerns are and what assistance they would like from them. If a client has not had a low vision evaluation recently, the rehabilitation teacher will usually recommend one, especially if there is any evidence of usable vision.

To prepare for a clinical low vision evaluation, rehabilitation teachers usually perform a functional low vision assessment with the individual (see Sidebar 14.4 for the steps involved) and share the results with evaluators at the low vision clinic. They also often help clients put together packets of materials from home (utility bills, bank statements, letters from family and friends, the family Bible, favorite magazines, and so forth) to take to the low vision clinic for use during the evaluation. Whenever possible, they accompany their clients to their low vision evaluations, both to provide support and to learn as much as possible about what the clients can see.

Rehabilitation teachers play a primary role in teaching adults the skills they need to maintain their independence: communication skills, home and personal management skills, and basic O&M skills. They also provide a great deal of informal counseling. Because rehabilitation teachers go into clients' homes and are frequently more available than are counselors, they often work with clients on self-esteem issues and adjustment to disability. If clients need more intense instruction in activities of daily living than can be offered by a field teacher, they may be referred to a center-based program or encouraged to enroll in a distance education course through the Hadley School for the Blind (see Resources).

A primary concern for clients who have low vision is how best to use their remaining vision. Teachers spend considerable time with clients on techniques for using vision effectively. They show individuals how to scan; how to use background colors to discriminate, templates for filling out checks, or a typoscope to focus on a single line of print at a time; how a sheet of yellow acetate over a page can enhance print; how to minimize glare; and how to use lighting to maximize the ability to see materials while performing tasks. Following low vision evaluations, rehabilitation teachers work with persons who have received low vision devices to help them understand how to use the devices in everyday activities and in natural, rather than clinical, environments. They may also provide nonprescription low vision devices like halogen lamps, reading stands, and visors.

With clients who have additional medical problems, such as diabetes or high blood pressure, teachers may often work on techniques for maintaining medical regimens. For example, many medication management systems, which rely on plastic day-by-day pill holders, can be fitted with large-print and braille demarcations. In addition, pill holders with programmable timers and alarms to indicate when an individual needs to take a pill can be obtained, as can devices that allow a person with low vision to halve a pill or crush a pill accurately. Also, devices designed specifically for persons with diabetes enable a person to draw a single dose of insulin, guide a needle, and read blood glucose levels without good vision. Rehabilitation teachers not only help clients obtain such devices, but they also provide instruction and support in their use.

Rehabilitation teacher services tend to be more individualized than are rehabilitation counselor services because the caseloads of rehabilitation teachers are in general smaller than are those of counselors. Overall, counselors are the case managers, whereas teachers are the providers of direct services in the rehabilitation service system. Teachers often provide clients with relatively inexpensive tools, such as large-print watches or large-print timers, but more expensive tools, such as computer equipment or optical devices, must be approved and ordered through counselors. Counselors and teachers work as a team, each keeping the other informed of a shared client's progress and needs.

There are undergraduate and graduate university-based training programs in rehabilitation teaching with adults with visual impair-

Steps in a Rehabilitation Teacher's Functional Low Vision Assessment

1. Review the client's records to determine the cause, severity, prognosis, and treatment of the visual condition.

2. Interview the client to ascertain the level of his or her understanding about the cause of the visual condition, the course of treatment, and its prognosis.

3. Determine if low vision clinical services have been recently delivered. If so, what was the outcome? What follow-up services were delivered or are still needed? Is the client still using any previously prescribed devices?

4. Ascertain the client's expectations and motivation for the clinical low vision examination and any anticipated low vision devices and discuss whether the client's expectations are realistic.

5. Determine the impact of environmental factors on the client's visual functioning by manipulating illlumination, contrast, and glare during assessment activities and introductory teaching activities.

6. Determine the tasks the client needs to do and the working distance, special equipment, speed, accuracy, and duration for performing them.

7. Assess the client's visual functioning in terms of near vision, intermediate vision, distance vision, color, contrast sensitivity, peripheral field, central field, duration, fatigue, accuracy, and motivation, and his or her problem-solving abilities while performing various tasks, as in the following examples:

   ◆ Ask the client to locate a given item in his or her environment. Observe his or her viewing distance, visual behaviors (head tilt, scanning, squinting), and problem-solving abilities.

   ◆ To evaluate the client's near vision, have the client read print samples (such as labels on cans and medicine bottles, utility bills, currency, pages in a telephone directory, and own handwriting), thread a needle, and fill a syringe. Note the smallest size of detail seen or print read, effect of changes in the intensity and angle of illumination and contrast, preferred working distance, use of optical devices, and use of nonoptical devices (such as a reading stand or clipboard).

   ◆ To assess the client's intermediate distance, have the client pour liquids, dial a telephone, identify money, and measure ingredients. Observe the viewing distance, effect of changes in illumination and contrast, use of low vision devices, and use of tactile auditory cues.

   ◆ To evaluate the client's distance vision, ask the client to locate specific canned goods on a shelf and read a wall clock. Observe the viewing distance, effect of changes in illumination and contrast, and use of low vision devices.

   ◆ To assess the client's color vision, have the client identify colors of threads, clothing, or pictures on canned goods. Observe the effect of changes in illumination on the client's color vision.

   ◆ Evaluate the client's use of eccentric viewing (fixation, scanning, tracking) if he or she has a central field loss.

   ◆ Observe the visual scanning and tracking of the client who has a peripheral field loss.

JUDY C. MATSUOKA
University of Arkansas at Little Rock

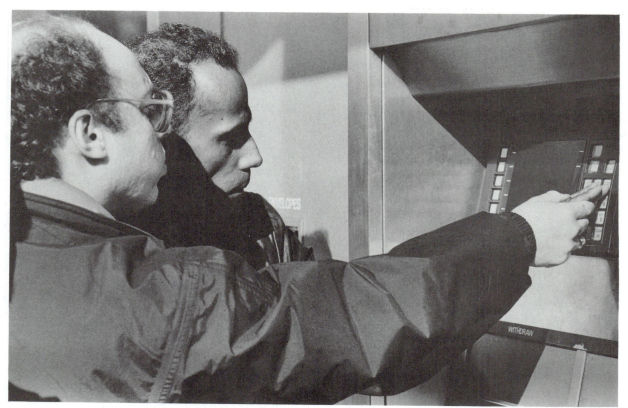

Training an individual with adaptive methods and materials can often be more effectively done in a natural, instead of a clinical, environment.

ments. In addition, AER grants certification to individuals with demonstrable skills in rehabilitation teaching and the requisite education and experience. To receive AER certification, rehabilitation teachers must have their supervisors attest to their teaching abilities. However, not all rehabilitation agencies require AER certification or university-based training for rehabilitation teaching; many state and private agencies train their rehabilitation teachers in-house.

Related Services

Related rehabilitation services include almost anything relevant to the IWRP, including a low vision evaluation, O&M training, a technology evaluation and training, occupational or physical therapy, psychological or career counseling, psychological or vocational assessment, and occupational training. Although most related services are provided by private contractors outside the rehabilitation system, these services are sometimes offered at rehabilitation centers. All related services that a rehabilitation agency pays for must be approved by a rehabilitation counselor.

In reviewing the needs of individuals with low vision, an important question to ask is, what are the consequences of not referring a person with low vision for rehabilitation services in a timely manner? In addition to a particular need remaining unmet, the individual may experience a serious loss of self-confidence and self-esteem. Without intervention from rehabilitation counselors and teachers, many adults with low vision are unaware of the full range of activities being performed by visually impaired individuals, and their functional skills in areas like personal care, communication skills, and mobility may diminish. Circumstances like these can often lead to a loss of motivation to live and work independently, which in turn presents a threat to an individual's self-esteem and confidence.

By providing effective services when they are needed, rehabilitation professionals can play a critical role in helping persons with low vision continue to lead independent lives and achieve desired goals.

SUMMARY

Many adults who lose their vision are often filled with fear and anxiety about the future and have to learn or relearn various tasks to make life more manageable. Likewise, adults with congenital low vision may find that they would prefer to perform tasks for themselves that family members, friends, and teachers did for them when they were children. They, too, discover tasks that have to be learned or relearned.

In addition, individuals with low vision may frequently discover that resources have to be found for acquiring and learning to use adaptive equipment and low vision devices. However, because no two individuals with low vision have the same needs or interests, it is important for a service provider to inform an individual of what is available, show him or her the myriad adaptive devices that may be helpful, and have the person decide what will work best for him or her.

People who experience a vision loss may isolate themselves without intentionally doing so. In such cases, many persons benefit from being helped to reach out to and make contact with others. Since staying involved or getting involved in activities can frequently be therapeutic, many adults will find it valuable to evaluate their interests and find others who have similar ones. Making people aware of community activities and local support groups can be helpful in integrating them into the community. Suggesting that they consider participating in support groups for people with low vision or for those with the same or similar eye conditions as theirs can help them realize they are not alone.

Rehabilitation services can provide adults with low vision with the knowledge and resources they need to lead successful, productive lives. Rehabilitation teachers teach individuals the skills and techniques they need to perform home and personal management tasks and to express themselves and communicate with others. Rehabilitation counselors help coordinate services and facilitate the career-exploration and job-seeking process. As members of the rehabilitation team, they can help individuals develop skills for managing everyday affairs, exploring vocational options, and increasing their sense of competence and self-esteem.

ACTIVITIES

With This Chapter and Other Resources

1. In the vignette that opens this chapter, Andrea had concerns about managing her household chores and maintaining her job following the deaths of her parents. Consider what it may be like for Andrea to suddenly have household and personal tasks for which she has never had responsibility. Describe the emotional factors a rehabilitation teacher or counselor may need to consider when providing services for Andrea.

2. Using low vision simulators, perform an activity of daily living, such as vacuuming or washing dishes. Record the details of your experience, and consider whether you could increase your efficiency in performing the task with a different method or by using a device. Consider trying the same activity over time under different circumstances, such as in a darkened room or at twilight, or with different simulators. Record your impressions for future reference.

3. Compare the roles and functions of a rehabilitation counselor and a rehabilitation

teacher. If you decided to work with adult clients, which of these professions would be a better match with what you are looking for, with regard to services provided, location for work, and amount and type of involvement with individuals with visual impairments? Choose one profession and write a letter that could be sent to a prospective employer explaining why you are suited for a particular job.

4. Consider two adults, one with a congenital visual impairment and the other with an acquired visual impairment. They are both in their early 20s, have similar levels of visual function and education, and are being overprotected by their families. How might a rehabilitation counselor work in the same or different ways with these individuals and their families? Write a plan of action as if both adults were in your caseload.

In the Community

1. Visit a large discount store, such as Walmart or K-Mart, and list 20 to 35 items that may be helpful to an individual with low vision. For each item, briefly describe how it can be beneficial to someone with low vision. Be creative.

2. Make arrangements through your local rehabilitation agency to meet and observe the work of a rehabilitation teacher with adult clients. Explain your purpose and what safeguards you will make to ensure confidentiality. Ask the rehabilitation teacher about the professional preparation he or she received, the techniques he or she has devised for working with clients with low vision, the kinds of devices or appliances he or she routinely uses and recommends, and the specific challenges that rehabilitation teachers face in providing services. You may also want to ask the rehabilitation teacher for advice about considering a career in rehabilitation teaching.

With a Person with Low Vision

1. Identify a common household task for which a person with low vision would use an adaptation. Consider different options that may be used to complete the task. Then arrange to observe an adult completing the task. Inquire how the person determined which of the available options would be the most efficient or preferred method for completing the task. Also ask if other options had been considered.

2. Interview two adults who have received rehabilitation services because of their visual impairments. Discuss the qualities in their rehabilitation counselors and teachers that facilitated or hindered their progress in reaching their vocational and personal objectives. Write a summary of both interviews.

From Your Perspective

If services to persons with low vision were reduced in your area because of a shortage of personnel or budget cuts, what criteria might you use to determine which adults with low vision should receive services? Consider such factors as employability, age, congenital or adventitious low vision, and cognitive level.

CHAPTER 15

Employment Considerations for Adults with Low Vision

J. Elton Moore and Karen E. Wolffe

VIGNETTE

Everything was falling into place for Heraldo. He had just had his 25th birthday; he was offered an accounting job at a prestigious company in the Northeast, where he and his wife had hoped to move; and he and his wife had had their first child. While he and his family were driving to visit his wife's parents, however, Heraldo's world fell apart. A drunk driver missed a stop sign and crashed into Heraldo's side of the car. Heraldo was severely injured. After two weeks in the hospital, Heraldo went home. His right eye had been enucleated, and he had lost considerable vision in the other eye, so that his visual acuity was now about 20/400, and the ophthalmologist did not think there was much hope of regaining normal vision in that eye.

Heraldo thought that he could not return to accounting, and he was beginning to feel that he would never be able to offer his family what he had planned. His wife, who had quit her job when their baby was born, suggested that she should get a job and that Heraldo could stay home and care for the baby. However, this was not the best solution for Heraldo; he needed to get back to work. Heraldo's ophthalmologist suggested that he contact the local office of the state commission for the blind. Although this suggestion did not seem correct either, since Heraldo was not really blind, he had to do something. Therefore, he made an appointment to see a rehabilitation counselor at the commission for the blind.

The rehabilitation counselor told Heraldo that many adults who become visually impaired or blind can retrain for various occupations or return to their former occupation. Heraldo was offered various options for equipment that would help him to return to his accounting job. He found that a combination of a computer with a screen-enlargement software package and a closed-circuit television (CCTV) was the most efficient way for him to carry out his job duties. He also received orientation and mobility (O&M) services, and soon he and his wife decided that it would be helpful for them to move closer to his place of employment so that he could use public transportation.

Heraldo found the solutions for traveling and reading his job tasks to be the easiest part of adjusting to his visual condition. He experienced several bouts of depression, which added much stress to his family and placed him at risk of losing his job. Over the next year and a half, his rehabilitation counselor provided emotional support, referred him for personal counseling, and helped him to see that his ability to perform his job was an encouraging factor in his recovery.

INTRODUCTION

Work is an essential part of the lives of most adults. Holding a job provides the means to support oneself and one's family; to engage in a regular, predictable daily routine; and to experience work satisfaction and self-esteem. People with low vision are no different from people with normal vision in the value they ascribe to being contributing members of society (Salomone & Paige, 1984); as Neff (1985, p. 6) noted, "to be able to work in a work-oriented society is to be like others." Schmidt (1989) clearly showed that workers with visual impairments are represented in all areas of the labor force, both in Canada and in the United States.

Previous chapters have described the challenges and adjustments individuals with low vision may undergo in education, social experiences, and many daily activities. Persons with congenital visual impairments or adventitious visual impairments are also concerned about their ability to obtain or maintain gainful employment. It is widely agreed that unemployment and underemployment are major problems for men and women who have low vision. Kirchner and Peterson (1988) estimated that fewer than one-third of the working-age visually impaired population in the United States is in the labor force.

The substantial, chronic high rate of unemployment among people with severe visual impairments is a serious concern. Genensky, Berry, Bikson, and Bikson (1979) found that 90 percent of people with low vision believed their visual problems affected the kinds of jobs they could obtain, and more than 50 percent of those who had stopped working reported that they did so because of their visual problems. Although new laws have been passed and new technology has become available since that study, the impact of low vision on the beliefs of many individuals with low vision about maintaining employment seem not to have changed over time.

For persons with low vision to be competitively employed, three sets of conditions must occur simultaneously. First, jobs must be available. Second, persons with low vision must be willing and able to work. Third, persons with low vision and employers must know about each other and be willing to establish a relationship (Institute on Rehabilitation Issues, 1975).

Rehabilitation services can help an individual determine appropriate career goals, develop job-seeking skills, and acquire adaptive tools and skills for obtaining employment. Through a series of interviews, assessment instruments to determine aptitudes and preferences, technology evaluations, and a market analysis of job openings, a rehabilitation counselor can provide options and directions for a client to consider.

CRITERIA FOR ELIGIBILITY FOR VOCATIONAL REHABILITATION

Vocational rehabilitation services are not mandated for every person with a disability. Eligibility criteria, which may vary from state to state, are in general based on the following criteria:

- ◆ The individual must have a documented physical or mental disability that constitutes or results in a substantial impediment to employment.
- ◆ The individual can benefit from vocational rehabilitation services in terms of preparing for, engaging in, or retaining gainful employment.
- ◆ The individual requires vocational rehabilitation services to prepare for, enter, engage in, or retain gainful employment.

According to these criteria, persons whose disabilities do not pose a barrier to employment, those whose disabilities are deemed too severe to have a reasonable expectation of benefiting from rehabilitation services, and those who lack vocational goals may be denied vocational rehabilitation services. These persons may be eligible for rehabilitation teaching services and financial assistance through Title VII, Chapter 2 (Independent Living Services for Older Individuals Who Are Blind) of the Rehabilitation Act or from private organizations and groups. Limited financial assistance for clinical low vision examinations may be available from private health insurance, Medicare, or Medicaid.

Services that are paid for or provided by a vocational rehabilitation agency must support the vocational goal stated in the person's Individualized Written Rehabilitation Program (IWRP). Financial assistance, including payments for clinical low vision examinations, optical devices, adaptive tools, and related services, is provided only to clients who can demonstrate financial need, as established by the states in which they reside. For example, a person whose vocational goal is to become a paralegal may receive a clinical low vision examination, paid for with vocational rehabilitation funds, to ascertain whether optical devices would improve his or her ability to carry out the tasks of his or her job and to live independently. However, only prescribed devices that support the vocational goal may be paid for with vocational rehabilitation funds and only if the client meets the test of financial need.

Thus, although a telescope might improve a client's distance vision to 20/30, it would not be purchased for a client who wanted it for watching television, but it might be purchased for a client who would use it to read signs in a law library to find materials related to a case or to read street signs to find his or her way to and from work. Similarly, a telescope might be purchased for a client on a fixed income who would use it to read signs in a supermarket while independently doing the family's grocery shopping, if the client was designated the primary homemaker in the household, which is considered a viable vocational goal.

ECOLOGICAL EVALUATION

The assessment of a person's visual functioning at the work site, including the use of vision, is known as an environmental evaluation. It is a multifaceted process involving clinical and on-site assessment of vision, assessment of the work environment and the demands of the tasks, and evaluation of the individual's ability to perform to the standards set by management on the job. The sequence of all the steps of this assessment process is not static, but is highly dependent on the status of the person in the rehabilitation process.

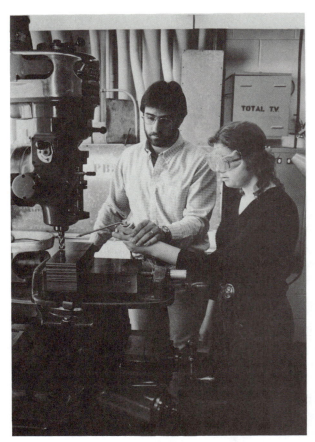

In an environmental evaluation, a rehabilitation counselor assesses an individual's visual functioning at the work site.

Rehabilitation counselors may initially evaluate the visual demands of a job to determine the characteristics of individuals who may be suited for particular occupations or job placements. When working with individuals with low vision, they may evaluate the visual demands of a specific job and the functional vision of a prospective job candidate simultaneously. These functional assessments may lead to referrals for clinical low vision evaluations to determine the feasibility of low vision devices and modifications at the job site. Following such assessments and with the use of any prescribed devices or modifications of tasks, an on-sight evaluation of functional abilities reinforces the capabilities of the individual to perform the job.

The following sections detail the kinds of information an evaluator needs to collect during observations for an ecological evaluation of an adult with low vision. A vocational evaluation is frequently a service purchased or contracted for by a rehabilitation counselor. The evaluation might be performed by an evaluator at a private rehabilitation center, or, in some of the larger rehabilitation agencies, the evaluation might be performed at the agency's rehabilitation center or by an outreach evaluation team. The Vocational Evaluation and Work Adjustment Association (VEWAA) certifies vocational evaluators; however, not all evaluators working in rehabilitation agencies are certified. Certified evaluators have been through a course of training that includes basic rehabilitation philosophy, information about medical and psychological ramifications of disabling conditions, and specialized training in the use and interpretation of vocational testing materials.

Vocational Considerations

The most critical set of questions with regard to an adult with low vision in the workplace is how the person learns a new task—through sight, touch, or hearing. If the person uses all three modalities or some combination, which is primary, which is secondary, and which is tertiary?

If the person uses vision as the primary means of gathering new information, does he or she use optical devices to enhance vision? If so, what kind of low vision devices are used and under what circumstances? Does the person use low vision devices competently? An evaluator will note the fluidity, efficiency, and frequency with which the individual uses low vision devices and will determine whether the person has experimented with other devices at work.

It is also important to note the person's stamina, or how long he or she can use vision. Does the person's stamina fluctuate and if so, what causes it to fluctuate? (For example, the blood sugar levels of people with diabetes and hypoglycemia have a direct effect on their stamina.) It is equally important to notice whether the person can consistently rely on his or her vision to provide critical information.

For a worker with low vision who uses a computer, an evaluator will note the type of contrast the worker prefers (black on white, white on black, yellow on blue, or some other color combination.) The evaluator will also determine the effect of illumination on the person's ability to perform tasks. Does the person have difficulty accommodating when moving from a brightly lit area to a darker area? Can the person see better in areas that are lit with incandescent or fluorescent light bulbs? Has the person tried halogen lighting? Is the individual's posture awkward because he or she needs to be closer than normal to materials in order to work? If so, how long can he or she maintain such a position?

If the individual with low vision relies on kinesthetic or tactile cues for processing information, how are those cues picked up? Would the person benefit from a combination of tactile and visual cues? For example, would it be helpful to mark key buttons or switches with locator dots, Velcro, or other types of tactile cues? Is the individual's sense of touch reliable for information processing?

It is also important to find out how the person sees best. Does the individual see only what is directly in front or to the side of him or her? Does the person see best while appearing to an observer to look up or down or to the side? Will a visor or tinted lenses help the person see? Could the individual benefit from a reading stand or an editor's table? Many devices that provide considerable help to readers with low vision are inexpensive, and the evaluator needs to experiment with them in environments where the individual will be using them. Two excellent sources of information about assistive devices for people who are blind or visually impaired are *Assistive Devices for Reading* by the National Library Service for the Blind and Physically Handicapped (1993) and *Solutions* by Espinola and Croft (1992). The latter book covers such items as speech and braille output devices that are used by people with low vision and those who are blind, but it does not include information on equipment that is specific to people with low vision.

Mobility Considerations

The evaluator will have to determine a number of things with regard to the person's mobility. First, how does the individual get to and from work—by public transportation, by walking, or by riding with another worker? Is he or she consistently on time, early, or late? If the person drives, can he or she drive during rush hour, inclement weather, or at night? What is the worker's backup plan in the event that the usual method of transportation becomes disrupted?

Second, how does the person navigate between the parking lot or drop-off site into the work environment (with or without sighted assistance, with or without a cane or another mobility tool, and with or without optical devices)? What kind of mobility skills does the person demonstrate (fluid movement, stumbling, groping, or jerky movement)? What kind of orientation skills does the person demonstrate (easily finds a destination, overshoots sidewalks or entryways, consistently identifies landmarks, solves orientation problems)?

Third, at the work station, is the individual able to orient to the work space: that is, to put away things he or she has carried in, find tools, find and read instructions or notes, easily move from space to space (desk to desk, to telephone or office equipment, desk to rest room, desk to snack area or cafeteria), retrieve things as needed, and exit without difficulty (in both routine and emergency situations)? Since consistency is essential, a single observation is rarely adequate for evaluating mobility skills in the workplace. Rather, it is necessary to observe a person on different days of the week, at different times of the day, and in different areas of the workplace.

OBTAINING EMPLOYMENT

Researchers and rehabilitation professionals have considered the underlying reasons for the high rates of unemployment and underemployment of persons with low vision and have suggested a number of causes, including the following:

- negative attitudes of employers toward people with visual impairments
- lack of employment and employment-related skills
- lack of motivation for employment
- government-generated work disincentives, such as entitlement programs that provide welfare or disability benefits
- lack of housing and family supports
- lack of transportation
- lack of access to information.

It is important for rehabilitation professionals to have a good understanding of the difficulties faced by persons with low vision who have never worked, as well as of those who need to find ways to keep their jobs or find new ones. With this information, counselors are better able to help persons with low vision decide where and how they wish to be employed. Support should be offered in the framework of a counseling relationship that is focused on meeting the challenges of public attitudes, altering self-concepts, increasing employers' knowledge of visual impairment, and undergoing career planning and vocational preparation.

A rehabilitation team, consisting of such professionals as rehabilitation counselors, rehabilitation teachers, O&M instructors, ophthalmologists, optometrists, job-placement and job-development specialists, work-evaluation specialists, social workers, psychologists, and rehabilitation engineers, may assist in the process. The rehabilitation counselor must act as a synthesizer and liaison (a case manager), carefully incorporating and balancing information about the individual, the employer, the job, and the impact of any potential modifications.

Although the rehabilitation counselor may provide and coordinate a variety of services to assist the person with low vision to become gainfully employed, the client needs to be an active participant in implementing the rehabilitation plan by making meaningful and informed choices about vocational goals and objectives and ultimately by finding a job. It is preferable for the client to take an active role in finding his or her own job, rather than simply to accept a placement offered by a counselor for many reasons, primary among them the sense of self-esteem and satisfaction derived from doing so.

Each country has its own laws, services, and processes for adults who need assistance with employment owing to a disability. The system operating in the United States is used as a basis for this chapter (see employment-related legislation in Sidebar 15.1). Readers in other countries are encouraged to consider whether the process described is applicable to other locales and whether instituting similar systems would help or hinder persons with low vision who need to seek or retain employment.

Implementing the IWRP

The Individualized Written Rehabilitation Program (IWRP) is basically a contract between a person with low vision and the rehabilitation agency. (See the appendix to this chapter for a sample IWRP.) Before the IWRP is developed, the rehabilitation agency must determine that the individual is eligible for vocational rehabilitation services. According to U.S. law, this determination must be made within 60 days after the individual has submitted an application, unless an extended evaluation is required or exceptional or unforeseen circumstances beyond the agency's control preclude the agency from completing the determination within the prescribed time. The person involved must agree that an extension of time is warranted.

Once the applicant has been determined eligible for services, the IWRP is jointly developed, agreed on, and signed by the person with low vision (or, a parent, guardian, family member, advocate, or another authorized representative, if appropriate) and a rehabilitation counselor. The IWRP is designed to delineate the services needed to achieve the employment objective of the individual, consistent with his or her unique strengths, resources, priorities, concerns, and abilities. The IWRP includes the long-term rehabilitation goal and intermediate objectives related to the attainment of the vocational goal. It also contains a list of the specific vocational rehabilitation services to be provided and the projected dates for their initiation and completion, as well as the delineation of any specific rehabilitation technology services and an assessment of any expected postemployment services that may be required (such as a change in optical devices or medication for progressive eye conditions).

The 1992 amendments to the Rehabilitation Act of 1973 (P.L. 102-569) now require a statement on the IWRP in the words of the individual (or, if appropriate, the parent, guardian, or another authorized representative) describing how the person was informed about and was involved in choosing among the alternative goals, objectives, services, and entities providing services. Since the policy of many agencies is to train individuals for entry-level jobs, it is important for an individual to select his or her vocational objective carefully when developing the IWRP. For example, an eligible person whose vocational objective is to be an elementary school teacher may request support for undergraduate and graduate training through the doctoral level but be granted support only for undergraduate education since that is all that is required to teach in most elementary schools. However, if the person's vocational objective is to teach special education at the college level, support for training through the doctoral level may well be required and support for such training would probably be provided.

The rehabilitation counselor is required to furnish a copy of the IWRP and any amendments to the client or an authorized representative. The IWRP is signed by the individual and reviewed annually. An example of a completed IWRP for Heraldo, who was introduced at the beginning of this chapter, is in the appendix to this chapter.

Each applicant or individual served by the state rehabilitation agency has the right to appeal

SIDEBAR 15.1

Highlights of Federal Rehabilitation Legislation Related to Persons with Low Vision

Title	Year	Purpose
P.L. 74-732: the Randolph-Sheppard Act	1936	Enabled persons who were classified as legally blind to operate vending facilities on federal property.
P.L. 75-739: the Wagner-O'Day Act	1938	Made it mandatory for the federal government to purchase designated products from industries for persons who are blind.
P.L. 78-113: the Bardon-LaFollette Act	1943	Provided the first federal-state rehabilitation support services for persons who were blind.
P.L. 92-28: the Javits-Wagner-O'Day Act	1971	Extended the law to cover industries that employ persons with severe disabilities other than blindness and provided paid staff for the President's Committee for Purchase from People Who Are Blind or Severely Disabled.
P.L. 93-112: the Rehabilitation Act of 1973	1973	Introduced the Individualized Written Rehabilitation Program (IWRP) and postemployment services and established a priority of services to persons meeting the federal definition of severely handicapped, established client assistance pilot projects, mandated consumer involvement in state agency policy development activities, and prohibited discrimination against persons with disabilities in federally funded programs (Sections 501-504).
P.L. 93-651: the Rehabilitation Act Amendments of 1974	1974	Strengthened the Randolph-Sheppard Act (referred to as the Randolph-Sheppard Act Amendments of 1974) and provided for the convening of a White House conference on "handicapped individuals."
P.L. 98-221: the Rehabilitation Act Amendments of 1984	1984	Established client assistance programs in each state and required the use of qualified personnel in training programs.
P.L. 99-506: the Rehabilitation Act Amendments of 1986	1986	Established supported employment as an acceptable goal for rehabilitation services and included rehabilitation engineering services in vocational rehabilitation services.

Highlights of Federal Rehabilitation Legislation (continued)

P.L. 100-407: the Technology-Related Assistance for Individuals with Disabilities Act of 1988	1988	Provided financial assistance to states in developing and implementing a consumer-responsive statewide program of technology-related assistance for individuals of all ages with disabilities.
P.L. 101-476: the Individuals with Disabilities Education Act (IDEA)	1990	Required schools to provide transition services to all students with disabilities.
P.L. 101-336: the Americans with Disabilities Act of 1990	1990	Prohibited any covered entity from discriminating against a qualified individual with a disability with regard to job application procedures; the hiring, advancement, or discharge of employees; compensation, job training, and other terms, conditions, and privileges of employment.
P.L. 102-52: the Rehabilitation Act Amendments of 1991	1991	Made technical amendments to the Act as amended and extended the Act for one year.
P.L. 102-569: the Rehabilitation Act Amendments of 1992	1992	Created rehabilitation advisory councils and provided funding for braille training projects.
P.L. 103-73: the Rehabilitation Act Amendments of 1993	1993	Made technical amendments to the act and clarified the role of the State Rehabilitation Advisory Council.

Source: Adapted from R. M. Parker and E. M. Szymanski (Eds.), *Rehabilitation Counseling—Basics and Beyond* (Austin, TX: PRO-ED, 1992).

any decision by the agency, such as the denial of software to enlarge print on a computer, to an impartial hearing officer. Each state is required to inform all clients and applicants of all available benefits under the Rehabilitation Act through the Client Assistance Program (CAP). If a person with low vision who is not legally blind is refused services by the rehabilitation agency, he or she should contact the state CAP, which will assist him or her in obtaining services by pursuing legal, administrative, or other appropriate remedies to ensure that the person's rights are protected and to facilitate his or her access to the services funded under the Rehabilitation Act.

Using Strategies for Identifying Jobs

The key to obtaining employment is for the person with low vision to identify jobs that meet his or her needs, desires, abilities, and values. The rehabilitation counselor can help the client identify appropriate jobs by encouraging him or her to go through the processes of self-analysis, job analysis, and discrepancy analysis, as described in the sections that follow. Identifying jobs or job clusters necessitates making matches between the job seeker and the work that is available. All job seekers, including those with low vision, need to consider both their strengths and weaknesses in order to select jobs that challenge them, for which they are qualified, and in which they can perform adequately. Following the identification of jobs or job clusters, the client will need to tailor his or her application to the identified jobs and begin the actual search for employment.

Self-Analysis

To identify the best possible match between job seeker and job, adults with low vision need to examine closely their interests, abilities, values, and liabilities and to document their thoughts in writing or by audiotaping them. They should be encouraged to identify at least 10 interests, 10 abilities, 10 values, and 2 or 3 liabilities. It is important to capture clients' perceptions of their liabilities to understand what they consider barriers to their employment. They should draw from all areas of their lives, not just aspects that they perceive to be work related. Often, skills and interests that are honed through leisure or domestic activities can be transferred to work. Although counselors can provide some insights and the extent to which vision is demanded in particular jobs, clients should be encouraged whenever possible to investigate jobs for themselves to make sure that they have adequate vision to perform the required tasks.

Usually, people can identify their interests and abilities with minimal assistance from a counselor and encouragement to think broadly. However, they often need help to identify their values, and the counselor may need to provide them with lists of values, such as health, wealth, fame, security, freedom, family living, independence, recognition, religion, adventure, creativity, craftsmanship, and orderliness, pointing out that these are just examples and that the lists are not inclusive. Once clients have identified their values, they should be asked to put them in rank order to identify priorities.

Clients should also be encouraged to consider how others view them. Rehabilitation counselors and teachers can provide feedback to adults with low vision, as can families, friends, and significant others. Clients may need some guidance about the most useful questions to ask, for example: What do you see as my greatest strengths or talents? What do you like most about my work efforts? Would you hire me for a job in your company? Why or why not? Sometimes feedback from others reinforces areas of strength, which can be included in the interests or abilities section, and sometimes it highlights areas of need or weaknesses, which can be incorporated into the liabilities section. It is important to remind clients to be aware when they solicit feedback from others that others see them differently than they see themselves and that those differences may or may not be important.

Two excellent resources that may facilitate clients' self-analysis are *What Color Is Your Parachute?* by Bolles (1995) and *Take Charge* by Rabby and Croft (1989). Both books, which are available in print, on cassette, and in braille, contain exercises to help an individual think about personal attributes and their relationship to employment. In addition, they provide general information on job seeking and extensive lists of relevant resources that can be used throughout the job-search process.

Job Analysis

Job analysis involves extensive research by the job seeker. The client starts by determining an occupational cluster (for example, business) or the titles of three or four jobs (for example, retail clerk, cashier, and buyer) that are of interest to him or her. Then the client needs to read about these jobs in books that provide generic information on occupations, such as the *Dictionary of Occupational Titles* (U.S. Department of Labor, 1991), available in print and on disk; the *Occupational Outlook Handbook* (U.S. Department of Labor, 1994b), available in print and on cassette; and the *Guide to Occupational Exploration* (U.S. Department of Labor, 1994a), available in print and on disk. From these broad information sources, the client can retrieve the following information:

- general job duties
- education required to perform the job
- physical demands of the job
- kinds of environments in which the job is performed
- labor market forecasts related to the job
- salary predictions.

The generic information retrieved from these resources should be written down or audiotaped in an organized fashion, as should any questions the client may have. Two pertinent questions may be these: Could someone with low vision perform the job? and Does such a job actually exist in the client's community?

The client can obtain answers to his or her specific questions by interviewing people who perform a particular job or a closely related one. During such an interview, the client can find out how the person acquired the position, what kind of education or training was required, what job or jobs the person held before this one, the hiring process in the firm where the job exists, if anyone with low vision has ever performed the job in the firm, and if anyone with low vision is currently employed by the firm.

Although the client may want to record (in writing or on audiotape) an information interview, he or she should know that some people are not comfortable with verbatim recording and should be prepared for the possibility his or her request will be rejected. Ideally, the client will be able to interview a person with low vision who is performing the job of interest. To find such people, the client can contact the American Foundation for the Blind (AFB) Careers and Technology Information Bank (CTIB) (see Resources at the back of this book). CTIB maintains a database of adults with visual impairments who are working in a variety of jobs across the country and refers callers to those with similar eye conditions who are performing specific jobs of interest.

Two other excellent sources of information about workers with visual impairments are the American Council of the Blind's Council of Citizens with Low Vision International and the Job Opportunities for the Blind Project of the National Federation of the Blind (for information on these organizations, see this book's Resources section and AFB, 1993). Two additional books that may be of help to the client are *Career Perspectives* by Attmore (1990) and *Jobs to Be Proud of* by Kendrick (1993). Both books contain interviews with workers who are blind or have low vision and can shed some light on how these workers are able to perform their jobs.

Discrepancy Analysis

Once the client has completed the self-analysis and three or four job analyses, he or she needs to conduct a discrepancy analysis, comparing the self-analysis and the job analyses to determine where they match up and where they differ. For example, if the client is a high school graduate and a job requires a college degree, there is a discrepancy between what is required and what the client has. If the client has the interest and ability to attend college, this is a discrepancy that can be remedied. On the other hand, if the client does not want to attend college or is unable to do so, then this discrepancy would stop him or her from pursuing that particular job.

The rehabilitation counselor can help the adult with low vision analyze the discrepancies to determine whether they can be remedied. If the differences can be remedied, the individual and the counselor can develop a step-by-step plan to do so. It is important to note that discrepancies can often be remedied by job modifications or accommodations, as well as by skills enhancement or training. If the differences cannot be remedied, the individual may want to determine whether there are related jobs that he or she can research in lieu of the job that has been ruled out.

Finding and Applying for Positions

Once clients have an idea of the job in which they wish to be employed, they may or may not know how to identify positions that are available. They may not have personal contacts through which they can hear news of an opening and may need visual assistance in searching through newspapers or other postings for potential jobs. Counselors often have access to listings of job lines that local companies use to disseminate information about openings that can also be helpful to job seekers. Also, a rehabilitation counselor may be helpful as a member of the client's network, providing information about job leads while the person searches independently for a job or helping to negotiate a placement if the client is unable to obtain a job independently.

Submitting an Application

Once a position has been identified, the job seeker must submit an application. If the person has adequate vision to complete an application independently, he or she should do so; then, the application should be carefully proofread by the individual or a trusted friend, relative, or service provider. If the person does not have adequate vision to fill out a form, he or she needs to obtain aid from someone with better vision. It is important to find a helper whose assistance can be depended on for accuracy and legibility, because no matter who fills out the application, it is a reflection on the job seeker who submits it. A properly completed application that shows how the individual is qualified for the position of interest is usually the only way to get to the next step in the job-seeking process: the interview. However, it is important that the application accurately reflect the job seeker's ability. If the form is filled out perfectly and everything is spelled correctly and the job seeker is a poor speller without any understanding of how to fill out a form, during the interview the employer may come to feel that the applicant was misrepresented on paper. Whoever fills out the application must use common sense and rely on the client to guide the process.

Interviewing

Interviewing tends to be anxiety provoking for all job seekers, with or without disabilities. For people with low vision, there are several consider-

ations that relate specifically to their disability. The first is the initial impression they make on potential employers. Can they maintain eye contact with interviewers? Can they put interviewers at ease if they have atypical eye movements, an involuntary twitch, or unusual physical features? How will they adapt to potentially uncomfortable visual situations that may occur if they are facing a window with glare or an interviewer with a patterned jacket or dress that causes visual discomfort?

The second consideration is how to establish a friendly rapport with an interviewer without the visual cues that fully sighted job candidates are able to use. For example, a fully sighted job candidate may be able to see trophies on an interviewer's credenza, recognize them as bowling trophies, and use that insight to start a conversation with the interviewer about bowling. A job seeker with low vision has to rely on information culled from co-workers or gathered in the course of conversation with the interviewer to generate this type of helpful small talk.

The third consideration is for the job seeker with low vision to answer any questions that relate to his or her disability and to inform the interviewer how he or she will perform the essential elements (critical tasks) of the job. It is important for the individual to remember that most interviewers will have little, if any, insights into what it means to have low vision. They may assume that the job seeker cannot function with visual cues at all, or, conversely, that he or she can capture the same visual cues as a normally sighted person. In this regard, adults with low vision should be encouraged to develop what may be called functional disability statements, which focus on what they can and cannot see, how they compensate for the limitations of low vision, what their prognosis is (if favorable, what they do to preserve and enhance their available vision; if not favorable, how they manage now and how they will manage in the future with alternative techniques), and what services are available to them (rehabilitation services, O&M services, public and private transportation alternatives, low vision specialists, and so forth).

Functional disability statements to employers should avoid medical jargon or rehabilitation terminology; all descriptors should be in lay terms. The following is an example of such a statement:

I have had difficulty with my vision since I was born. Perhaps you've noticed that I cannot control my eye movements as you do. I honestly do not notice it myself because it's always been this way. I can see to read regular print with my reading glasses. I hold the paper a bit closer than you would, perhaps, but I have no difficulty reading for prolonged periods. In fact, I read throughout my academic career using these same glasses. I do have difficulty when things are far away or are not clearly written, for instance, on a chalkboard menu in a restaurant. However, if there is enough light and contrast, I can even read a chalkboard menu with my telescope. Would you like to see my telescope? Please feel free to ask me any questions you have concerning my vision. I'm comfortable describing what I can see.

Some of the critical points to cover in a functional disability statement or during an interview are these:

◆ related experiences that demonstrate competencies required for the job
◆ how one gains access to print materials
◆ information on visual abilities and needs
◆ safety concerns relevant to the work environment
◆ avocational interests, such as photography, painting, or sports, that demonstrate skills that are transferable to the job
◆ how one's interests and abilities match the job description
◆ how one will get to and from work (hired driver, bus, carpool, driving oneself).

In addition to preparing to address disability-specific concerns as just described, a job seeker should be prepared to answer open-ended questions, like "Will you please tell me a little bit about yourself?" In such circumstances, the interviewee's response should in general be no more than two minutes and should focus on background indicators of stability, reliability, and the desire to work as a part of a team. An interviewee will also want to give at least three good reasons why he or she should get the job and should try to have at least one job-related question. Before a job seeker leaves an interview, he or she should find out the next step in the hiring process. Finally, successful job candidates often follow up on their interviews with a thank you note or a phone call.

Clients often want to know what is legal for an interviewer to ask in job interviews. It is not legal to ask if a job candidate has a visual disability or if there is something wrong with an applicant's eyes. It is legal to ask if the applicant can perform the essential functions of a job. For example, if a client applies for a job as a pizza delivery person, it is within the employer's rights to ask if the applicant can drive because driving is an essential element in a job description for a delivery person. However, if the same job candidate applies for a position cooking pizza or taking pizza orders, then the employer cannot legally ask about the applicant's driving ability.

Although most employers are aware of the rules concerning legal interviewing questions, some will either be unaware or are unconcerned. If an applicant is asked a question that he or she believes to be illegal, a decision needs to be made about whether or not to answer. In some instances, the individual might have a strong desire to obtain that particular job and might decide to answer the question, regardless of its illegality. However, the person might decide that an environment in which such questions are deemed acceptable does not bode well for the future and choose not to respond.

ON THE JOB

Use of Vision and Other Senses

An individual's use of vision and other senses may help or hinder his or her performance of a given task. The efficient use of low vision is greatly affected by such situational and environmental factors as artificial lighting, the size and distance of objects, spatial organization, changes in natural room lighting owing to weather conditions, the time of day, color, and contrast. Appropriate illumination and sufficient contrast are especially crucial to the efficient use of low vision in the workplace.

There is a pressing need to develop procedures and methods to assess the functional vision of individuals with low vision and the visual demands of their jobs. The identification of the visual demands of an individual's work environment can help a clinical low vision specialist determine which low vision devices will increase the person's visual functioning in the workplace.

The Work Environment Visual Demands Report (WEVD) (Graves, Maxson, & McCan, 1987) is one instrument that is used to analyze the visual demands of a job. Designed for use with a computer software package, the WEVD can be used in educational or vocational training settings. According to Graves, Maxson, and McCan, the WEVD is most useful with persons who have had a recent onset of visual impairment or recent changes in the severity of the visual impairment. Workers who have long-standing visual impairments would benefit most from the use of this protocol when job tasks change or their current low vision devices are not meeting their needs. For an example of a completed WEVD, see Figure 15.1.

In addition to the use of vision in the workplace, it is also important to remember that nonvisual modifications, such as auditory or tactile adaptations, can increase work efficiency. Such modifications may include the use of synthetic speech on computers, audiotaped materials, braille materials, and tactile guides.

Adaptations and Accommodations in the Workplace

This section describes the visual modifications, modifications in job tasks, and modifications at the job site that may constitute reasonable accommodations for employees with low vision. Sidebar 15.2 describes similar modifications for selected jobs.

Visual Modifications

To address appropriate visual modifications, consideration must be given to standard corrections, low vision devices, and the match between specific devices and the tasks to be performed. In regard to standard optical corrections, a person who receives a prescription for standard corrections but does not have it filled or who does not have eyeglasses repaired when needed may be compromised in completing his or her job tasks. Although not all individuals with low vision benefit from standard corrections, those who can need to understand the relationship between their prescription and the performance of their jobs. For example, a person who needs thick lenses and debates whether to wear them while working as a receptionist must realize that without them, he or she may make errors in such activities as recognizing customers, reading telephone numbers, or conveying written messages to others. In contrast, with the lenses, he or she may well be able to work at a level commensurate with that of his or her fully sighted co-workers. If the worker feels that the lenses are too unattractive to wear in the position, he or she can look into the feasibility of alternatives, such as obtaining tinted lenses, wearing contact lenses and a less thick pair of spectacles, or wearing the eyeglasses only when absolutely necessary and using other compensatory skills to perform routine functions.

Those who cannot benefit from standard corrections may benefit from using low vision devices. Appropriate low vision devices, both optical and nonoptical, should be matched to the individual's visual and physical condition, personal preferences, and the demands of a specific job. For example, a storekeeper with hand tremors may need a stand magnifier or spectacle-mounted device, rather than a handheld magnifier. However, a pharmacist who needs a longer working distance may benefit from a handheld

Work Environment Visual Demands Report

Name: ___Heraldo A. Gomez___   Job title: ___Accounting Clerk___

Social security no.: ___000-00-6044___   Job activity no. 1: ___Calculator___

Age: ___27___

Lighting
- Ceiling light—Direction: Left of subject
- Task lighting—Direction: Front of subject
- Task lighting—Type: Cool, white fluorescent light
- Size of illumination area: Length = 060", width = 060", height = 096"

Primary Display: Vertical Measurements
- Primary working sight line = 06 inches
- Display object is below horizontal sight line
- Primary horizontal sight line = 06 inches

Primary Display: Lateral Measurements
- Distance to center = 006 inches

Measurements of Sitting Work Area
- Work surface height: 29 inches
- Primary display height: 30 inches
- Secondary display height: 30 inches
- Eye height of worker: 44 inches

Types of Displays
- Printed and forms tasks
  8-10-point (1–1.5M) clear print with good contrast
  8-9-point print (1M) regular book print
  7-8-point newspaper print
  4-5-point (.08M) want ads, telephone directories
  Maps
  Typed originals
  Typed second and successive carbons
  Colored forms
- Handwritten tasks
  Ballpoint pen
  No ruled paper
- Copied tasks
  Xerograph
- Other displays

Work Devices
- Reading and writing often used (20 percent to 50 percent of the time)
- Calculator often used (20 percent to 50 percent of the time)

Characteristics of Visual Displays
- Color of visual display: white
- Percentage of reflectance: 10 percent

Environmental Factors Surrounding the Visual Display
- Visual indicators are uniformly aligned
- Visual indicators are in the same position for standard functioning

Mobility Requirements
- The client must move from one work area to another to perform tasks.
- It is necessary for the client to use corridors.
- There are likely to be nonfixed (moving) objects in the work path.
- Nonfixed obstacles in the work path are below the horizontal sight line.
- Obstacles have poor contrast.

Flexibility of the Workplace
- The workplace is adaptable for:
  Ceiling supplemental lighting
  Wall supplemental lighting
  Task supplemental lighting
  Stand-type magnifier
  Clamp-on magnifier.
- Range within which a task can be performed:
  Minimum distance = 06 inches
  Maximum distance = 06 inches
- Distance from the worker's eyes to the display is adaptable.
- The workplace is adaptable for a CCTV or computer-access technology.

Figure 15.1. Sample Work Environment Visual Demands Report

Some Possible Job Adaptations for Workers with Low Vision

SIDEBAR 15.2

CASHIER-CHECKER

The tasks include itemizing and totaling customers' purchases in a grocery or department store and operating a cash register. The individual's vision must be sufficient to review price sheets, read price charges and listings of items on sale, identify the special keys on a cash register, and read the cash register receipt. The person must also be able to collect cash, checks, or credit-card purchases from customers and to make change for cash transactions. Adaptive equipment may include binocular spectacles, special lighting, and a handheld magnifier.

CARPENTER

The tasks include reading blueprints and sketches and building plans and using carpenters' hand tools and power tools. Adaptive equipment may include a large-print tape measure, a handheld magnifier or an illuminated stand magnifier, light-absorptive lenses with side shields and a visor or cap if the person has problems with glare or bright sunlight.

PRESCHOOL TEACHER

The tasks include teaching personal hygiene, music, art, and literature to children aged 3–5.

Adaptive equipment may include a CCTV, a gooseneck lamp with fluorescent lighting, and a pocket magnifier. The teacher may also use large-type or color-coded labels on printed materials and miniblinds to control light and glare.

BANK LOAN OFFICER

The tasks include interviewing applicants and obtaining specified financial information for placement on loan applications. A variety of optical and nonoptical devices could be used, including a CCTV, reading stand, magnification software for computers, color-coded labels on printed material, templates for positioning work, and other adaptive tools as required.

CUSTODIAN

The tasks include keeping the premises of an apartment house, office building, or other commercial or institutional building in a clean and orderly condition. Various modified tools or precision instruments can be used to maintain furnaces, air conditioners, or boilers, as well as guides for tools, templates for positioning work, and color-coded handles for tools. Magnification devices may prove helpful for reading labels on chemicals or cleaning solutions.

---

device and may be fatigued by a spectacle-mounted device. A musician or other performing artist may wish to explore various levels of tinted contact lenses to reduce glare from intense spotlights. Ideally, matches such as these will be made as part of the comprehensive clinical low vision evaluation. Nevertheless, it should be noted that the demands of the job may change, thereby requiring a reexamination and further prescription of low vision devices to accommodate those changes.

An individual's failure to use optical devices and other compensatory strategies or tendency to be overly dependent on others to complete job assignments may diminish others' perceptions of his or her competence and may limit future job opportunities and advancement. Such circumstances may be a concern for some adults who have congenital visual impairments and for whom reduced school assignments and the overuse of sighted helpers may have resulted in unrealistic expectations of the amount of work that is typically required in school and in employment. Adults with fluctuating vision, as is common with diabetic retinopathy, need to have multiple strategies for obtaining and conveying information to

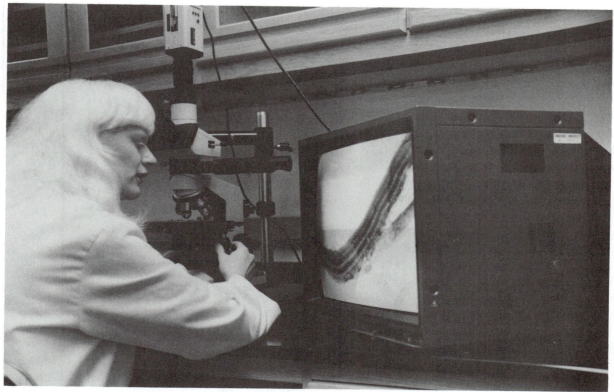

A variety of accommodations in the workplace can be made for individuals with low vision. Here, a closed-circuit television is attached to a microscope to allow a scientist with low vision to look at a specimen under the microscope.

match the visual changes they may experience throughout the day or workweek. In general, attempting to hide a visual impairment, rather than using compensatory strategies, is likely to hinder a person's job performance.

Modifications of Job Tasks

Reasonable accommodations in the workplace may include making existing facilities readily accessible to and usable by people with disabilities, restructuring the job through part-time or modified work schedules, reassigning an individual to a vacant position, acquiring or modifying equipment or devices, adjusting or modifying examinations, adapting policies, and providing qualified readers or drivers. Modifications of job tasks are one type of reasonable accommodation. In such

a modification, the person completes the tasks required of a job in a different way, but the outcome is the same. For example, a teacher who is bothered by glare or bright sunlight may exchange playground duty with a colleague for additional indoor lunchroom duty, thus completing the ancillary teaching duties required of all teachers. Or a nurse who has difficulty reading a standard thermometer may consider using a digital thermometer to accomplish the same task.

Modifications of the Job Site

As Scadden (1991) pointed out, work-site modifications involve environmental changes to an individual's work station or workplace to make it more functional, comfortable, and convenient. Such modifications must be tailored to specific occupations, and what is considered a reasonable modification in one job may not be considered a reasonable accommodation in another. For example, a person with low vision who applies for a bartender's job could be accommodated by the placement of large-print labels on beverage bottles or through the use of special lighting. However, a person with low vision who applies for a job as a waitress or waiter in an exclusive nightclub may face more of a challenge. The nightclub may maintain dim lighting to create an intimate setting and lower its lights even further during its floor show; an applicant who requests bright lighting as an accommodation to take orders may not be easily accommodated because it could affect the nature of the business operation.

The key components of any decision about job-site modifications or accommodations should be the worker's efficiency, a nonintrusive design, and cost effectiveness (Bradfield & Tucker, 1988). The logical result of such an assessment is the modification of the work site or an individual's skills.

Job Retention

Because of the way an employer may react to an employee's visual impairment, some people try to hide their visual problems from their existing employers. However, hiding one's visual impairment may have detrimental effects, such as a delay in seeking medical treatment, decreased job performance, lowered self-esteem, increased anxiety on the job, and a failure to find alternative strategies to accomplish tasks in a timely way. As a result, the person may lose his or her job.

If an employee with low vision experiences a further loss of vision, it is critical to attend to the consequences of it immediately. A rehabilitation agency can work with the person to help him or her retain employment. A rehabilitation counselor, rehabilitation teacher, O&M instructor, or adaptive technology expert may be able to come to the work site and make suggestions for job-site modifications or adaptive equipment and can analyze the current job and suggest ways to restructure the job tasks or identify ways in which

the employee could share tasks with other employees to get the work done.

However, there are times when an acquired visual impairment precludes an individual from retaining his or her current job, such as a bus driver, a camera operator at a television station, or a surgeon. In such cases, it is necessary to determine how a person's interests and abilities may lead to new employment through retraining. For example, a bus driver may chose to teach a defensive driving course or become a dispatcher in the company for which he or she was once driving. Whenever possible, it behooves job seekers with acquired visual disabilities to capitalize on their transferable job skills.

Knowing when to try to keep a job and when to retrain for a new occupation is often difficult. One should not assume that if a person can visually "handle" a job, even with visual fatigue and discomfort, he or she should maintain it. Alternative employment may result in a more successful adjustment to low vision. A rehabilitation counselor is one of the first resources not only for help in retaining a job or retraining for a new one, but for helping a person decide in which direction to go. For example, a person who can function at a minimal level with new optical devices may be concerned that retraining will be costly and cause an interruption in family income for too long a time and hence may prolong a difficult work situation. A rehabilitation counselor may be able to alleviate some of these concerns and suggest additional options or new directions.

FUTURE ISSUES

At a 1995 meeting convened by AFB, rehabilitation professionals, consumer advocates, business leaders, and representatives of federal agencies met to explore future issues related to the employment of individuals who are blind or who have low vision (Johnson, 1995). The following are 10 of the major issues and action-related goals they identified as critical to enhanced employment opportunities for people with visual disabilities:

◆ promote greater access to technology with regard to its availability, skills training, and access to visual displays

◆ ensure that job seekers with low vision have core employment skills and ongoing follow-up services

◆ improve society's attitudes to and awareness of the capabilities and achievements of workers with low vision

◆ promote the acquisition of career information and work behaviors for children with low vision

◆ encourage risk taking and educate individuals with low vision about the changing labor market, so they can make informed career decisions

◆ emphasize the importance of personnel preparation programs to meet the demand for rehabilitation workers with credentials and skills to work effectively with adults with low vision

◆ redirect rehabilitation systems to emphasize integration, independence, and employment, rather than the delivery of services

◆ improve communication linkages between rehabilitation agencies and consumer organizations

◆ obtain adequate funding for job-development and job-placement programs

◆ maintain accurate and current information about the requirements of employment in a dynamic labor market.

It is to be hoped that these goals will be incorporated into a national agenda on rehabilitation and will direct service efforts into the twenty-first century.

SUMMARY

Work is an activity that is central to the lives of millions of adults, including adults with low vi-sion. With few exceptions, individuals with low vision can perform the same jobs and engage in the same occupations as do people with normal vision. Holding a job provides the means to support oneself and one's family, to engage in a predictable daily routine, and to experience job satisfaction and self-esteem. Rehabilitation professionals working with visually impaired adults need to take into account the overall level of functioning of each individual, the rehabilitation goals, and the formal and informal supports that are available in the community. When the functional impact of low vision is addressed, adults with low vision can maintain independent, productive lifestyles that include gainful employment.

ACTIVITIES

With This Chapter and Other Resources

1. In the vignette that opens this chapter, Heraldo had to modify his approach to perform his job tasks, but he was able to remain in the same occupation. Discuss why you believe retaining employment, rather than retraining for a new occupation, may have been a good or poor decision for Heraldo.

2. Using a form from a vocational rehabilitation agency that is used in your area, develop an IWRP for a 28-year-old woman with 5/200 visual acuity as a result of an infection that affected both eyes. The woman needs a variety of optical devices and sighted readers to obtain employment as a teacher's aide.

3. Develop a transcript of an interview between a vocational rehabilitation counselor and a 20-year-old college student who has congenital low vision and who has never been employed. The vocational rehabilitation counselor plans to encourage the college student to obtain summer employment, although the student is being told by his parents that he does not need to work because of transportation difficulties.

4. Identify the job-site accommodations and modifications that may be needed for a 50-year-old dairy farmer with glaucoma who has lost all but 10 degrees of his peripheral vision.

In the Community

1. Identify the various agencies or groups in your community from which an individual with low vision may receive financial assistance to purchase a personal computer and large-print software. Find out and record the groups' eligibility criteria, amount of assistance available annually, and assistance that has been provided before. These resources could include the state vocational rehabilitation agency, nonprofit organizations like a local Lions Club or a local chapter of Delta Gamma, which provide services to visually impaired persons, and so forth.

2. Interview three employers in your community, including the manager of a hardware store, a head librarian, and the owner of a landscaping company. Ask them whether they would be willing to hire employees with low vision and about the various job tasks that their employees perform. Then describe what accommodations may be made for an employee with low vision.

With a Person with Low Vision

1. Interview two persons with adventitious low vision, one who retained his or her original job and one who retrained for a new occupation. Discuss how they came to their decisions about employment. Also detail the job accommodations necessary in both cases and who furnished any adaptive equipment needed by the workers.

2. Role play and record (audiotape or videotape) a job interview with a young adult. Include how the person will complete an application, adjust to the interview environment if it is visually uncomfortable, and describe his or her visual functioning to the interviewer.

From Your Perspective

What needs to be done to reduce the unemployment rate among individuals with low vision to a level that is comparable to that of the general population?

Commission for the Blind
Individualized Written Rehabilitation Program

Client's name Heraldo A. Gomez   _____ Extended evaluation

Agency representative John D. Thomas   __X__ Initial rehabilitation program

Case number 12345   _____ Major program revision

_____ Independent living program

This Is Your Rehabilitation Program

Part 1. Vocational Goal Accountant   **D.O.T. No.** _____

Part 2. Date of Program Initiation _____ **Date That Goal Is Expected to Be Reached** _____

Part 3. Major Steps Needed to Reach the Goal (Numbered intermediate objectives and dates of expected completion)

1. Heraldo will follow the instructions of his ophthalmologist to maintain maximum visual acuity and overcome functional limitations.

2. Heraldo will obtain assistive technology needed to function as an accountant.

3. Heraldo will learn to use his CCTV in an effective and efficient manner.

4. Heraldo will actively participate in a mental health treatment program for his depression.

5. Heraldo will acquire orientation and mobility (O&M) skills needed to travel safely to and from work and in his community at large.

6. Heraldo will come to work on time and will carry out his assigned accounting responsibilities in a timely and effective manner.

(continued on next page)

Appendix. Sample Individualized Written Rehabilitation Program

Individualized Written Rehabilitation Program (*continued*)

Part 4: Services Necessary to Reach Objectives

Client's Name Heraldo A. Gomez **Case Number** 12345

Objective Number	Services Necessary to Reach Objectives	Starting Date	Ending Date	Resources/Provider	Rate (Amount per hour)	Total Cost	Progress Review[a]
1.	Clinical low vision examination and treatment as required.			Vocational Rehabilitation for the Blind			
2.	Purchase a CCTV and personal computer with magnification software for use in performing accounting duties.			Vocational Rehabilitation for the Blind Local Lions Club			
3.	Training in the use of adaptive equipment at the local rehabilitation center.			Vocational Rehabilitation for the Blind			
4.	Guidance and counseling as needed.			Vocational Rehabilitation for the Blind and regional mental health center			
5.	O&M training at the local rehabilitation center.			Vocational Rehabilitation for the Blind			
6.	Public transportation services.			Metro Handilift			

Note: (The counselor should complete this section on the basis of scheduled reviews)

[a] *Periodic Progress Review: Please record a cross reference to the case file for each periodic review.*

(continued on next page)

Individualized Written Rehabilitation Program (*continued*)

Client's Name ___Heraldo A. Gomez___   **Case Number** ___12345___

Part 5. Comparable Benefits and Services

The local Lions Club will be used to obtain partial payment for the purchase of a CCTV. The local handilift van service will be used to provide transportation to and from work. Heraldo will use his health insurance for follow-up visits to the ophthalmologist.

Part 6. Specific Responsibilities of the Client and Agency Representative

The client agrees to keep all appointments and to cooperate with the vocational rehabilitation counselor in completing his rehabilitation program. The counselor, in turn, will work closely with the local Lions Club and the handilift transportation service to coordinate the purchase of a CCTV and make arrangements for transportation to and from work.

Part 7. Progress Will Be Evaluated by (list by numbered intermediate objects. Note: Status 06 must be evaluated at least every 90 days).

1. Eye examination report from the low vision clinic.

2. Evaluation report from the assistive technology specialist with regard to which personal computer and adaptive software is recommended for purchase.

3. Monthly facility progress reports that reflect the client's progress in learning to use his adaptive hardware and software.

4. Weekly meetings of the client and the vocational rehabilitation counselor and monthly progress reports from the regional mental health center.

5. Monthly progress report from the O&M instructor.

6. Periodic contact with the employer regarding the client's work performance.

(*continued on next page*)

Individualized Written Rehabilitation Program (*continued*)

Client's Name   <u>Heraldo A. Gomez</u>   Case Number   <u>12345</u>

Part 8. Statement in client's, parent's, guardian's, or representative's own words of how he or she participated in formulating his or her program:

_____	_____	_____	_____
Client	**Date**	**Agency Representative**	**Date**

Part 9. Program Annual Progress Reviews: (Includes 06 cases at 12 months)

The client and agency representative have reviewed and discussed the program and agree on the program, the progress being made, and program changes, if any. See case-record entry for details.

_____	_____	_____	_____ (first review)
Client	**Date**	**Agency Representative**	**Date**
_____	_____	_____	_____ (second review)
Client	**Date**	**Agency Representative**	**Date**
_____	_____	_____	_____ (third review)
Client	**Date**	**Agency Representative**	**Date**

Older Adults with Low Vision

Gale R. Watson

VIGNETTE

Lillian Thomas, a 70-year-old widow who developed age-related macular degeneration in both eyes one year ago, had cataract extractions and lens implants in both eyes five years ago, but has no other major health problems. After the death of her husband 10 years ago, she moved from the large, old home in which she raised her children to a small apartment in a Victorian house that has been converted into apartments. She has lived in the same small town all of her life, and because of the proximity to downtown, is able to walk to do her errands; she never learned to drive. Mrs. Thomas's youngest daughter lives nearby with her family and is the main source of support for her mother, driving her to physicians' appointments and to the beauty shop once a week.

"Miss Lil," as she is known, has been a homemaker most of her life, except for brief years as a salesclerk after her children were grown and married. She is renowned among family and friends as a great cook, especially for her cakes and candies. Miss Lil's social life revolves around her family, church, and two senior citizens' clubs. Having lived a quiet life as a wife and mother, she enjoys traveling with the clubs and participating in their social activities.

Miss Lil's vision loss has caused some changes in her life that have not been pleasant. Because she lost detail vision, she can no longer read the Bible, recipes in cookbooks, or newspapers. In addition, she is unable to write checks; balance her checkbook; sew, even to make repairs; or knit. She feels that her housework may not be up to her usual standards and she can no longer do her own shopping at the corner grocery store. She is unable to recognize faces and feels that friends and acquaintances think she is "stuck up" when she does not acknowledge them on the street until they speak to her. She misses the ability to see the minister in church and the face of her granddaughter, also named Lil, who sings in the choir. Generally, she says that she is "missing out on life."

Several incidents have shaken her confidence in her ability to live independently. She tripped over a curb she did not see and fell, breaking her wrist. A few weeks later, she did not see that the gas flame was lit on the stove, and the sleeve of her housecoat caught on fire while she was cooking, causing a nasty burn on her arm. With both arms injured, she had to stay with her daughter until she recovered. Miss Lil and her children have begun to discuss whether she should give up her apartment and live with one of them permanently or consider entering a retirement home.

Miss Lil's daughter has made sure that her mother has more light, replacing ceiling lights with stronger bulbs and adding fluorescent lighting in the kitchen over the stove and sink. She bought her mother a flexible-arm magnifying light that is not helpful for reading, except newspaper headlines, but does help for sewing. Miss Lil and her daughter asked the ophthalmologist what could be done to help her see better, and the ophthalmologist replied that she should "go home and learn to live with it."

Miss Lil is confused about what to do. Formerly active, she reports that some days it is all she can do to get dressed and make some toast and tea, which may be all that she eats. She loves her independence and the freedom of having her own apartment, yet is worried about what the future will hold. She does not want to inconvenience her children, nor does she want them to worry about her. She is concerned about her fixed income and is fearful of "living too long" and having her money run out, which would make her totally dependent.

Through a friend in one of the senior citizens' clubs, Miss Lil heard about the low vision service at Mid-Town Services for the Blind. She wants to see better, to read, and to take care of her apartment again, but she is hesitant to apply for this service. If the service is worthwhile, would her ophthalmologist not have told her about it? What if it is just a waste of her meager money? She does not want her children to think she is foolish, grasping at "miracles" that do not exist. And besides, this is a service for persons who are blind, and she knows she is not blind. Will people think she is blind if she goes there?

INTRODUCTION

The difficulties and challenges that Miss Lil is confronting in the vignette that opens this chapter are faced by many other older people. Elderly persons represent the fastest-growing segment of the population of individuals with visual impairments in industrialized countries. This chapter discusses the normal age-related changes and most prevalent visual impairments associated with aging. It includes information for rehabilitation professionals on preparing an elderly person to benefit from a clinical low vision evaluation and how to perform an environmental evaluation for an elderly person; provide environmental modifications; and teach the use of visual skills, low vision devices, and environmental cues to en-

hance the use of vision. It also emphasizes the importance of teamwork to provide a full scope of services to elderly persons, and the importance of support by family members and caregivers to maximize coping, adjustments, and independence.

DEMOGRAPHICS

As was noted in Chapter 1, there were approximately 4 million persons with severe visual impairments in the United States as of 1990 (Nelson & Dimitrova, 1993). This estimate is low because it does not include persons in institutions, such as nursing homes. Estimates of the number of people with visual impairments per 1,000 persons demonstrates the dramatic increase in visual impairments with age. Nelson and Dimitrova estimated that 6.07 per 1,000 persons aged 0 to 54, but 104.1 in 1,000 persons aged 55 to 84 and 210.6 per 1,000 persons aged 85 and older were visually impaired in 1990.

The most prevalent age-related causes of visual impairment in this country are macular degeneration, diabetic retinopathy, glaucoma, and cataracts (Tielsch, Sommer, Witt, Katz, & Royall, 1990). In addition, visual impairment is commonly related to other health impairments. Approximately 60 percent of persons with visual impairments who are not institutionalized have one or more additional impairments, including the loss of hearing; impaired mobility; decreased energy and stamina from respiratory and heart diseases; cognitive changes resulting from stroke or dementia; and chronic illness, such as failure of the endocrine system, which leads to diabetes and myxedema. Vision loss has been ranked third, behind arthritis and heart disease, among the most common chronic conditions that require persons who are elderly to have assistance with activities of daily living. Because approximately 90 percent of people with visual impairments have useful vision, low vision devices and rehabilitation services offer opportunities to enhance their visual and general functional capacity.

AGING AND LOSS OF VISION

Age-related Changes in Vision

The physiological and perceptual aspects of age-related vision changes were summarized by Morgan (1993) as follows:

- the skin around the eyes becomes looser and the eyelids become baggier

- there is a general loss of muscle tone and elasticity around the eyes leading to ectropion (turning out of the eyelids), entropion (turning inward of the eyelids), age-related ptosis (drooping of the eyelids), and enophthalmos (displacement of the eyeball back in the socket)

- the tear film decreases in volume, causing dry eyes, or there may be insufficient drainage of tears, causing tears to run

- the sclera is less elastic, and fat deposits develop; the sclera becomes yellowed as it becomes thinner, and the uvea shows through and adds a bluish tinge

- the cornea thins and flattens, it loses luster, and there is increased light scatter after the age of 75

- corneal sensitivity decreases with age, which might facilitate the wearing of contact lenses, but also makes accidental scratching of the cornea easier

- the corneal shape changes, resulting in a different axis of astigmatism;

- the average refractive state becomes more hyperopic with age; myopia is often associated with incipient cataracts;

- the volume of the anterior chamber decreases with age, caused by the growth of the lens

- the lens becomes more yellow with age and absorbs more light, significantly changing the amount and quality of light reaching the retina

- accommodation decreases, caused by the hardening of the lens and by the change of muscle tone

- the vitreous becomes more liquefied, causing floaters to become more visible

- the vitreous may detach from the retina after the age of 60, but is not normally visually threatening

- the retina becomes narrower, hardens, and becomes less flexible

- metabolic by-products begin to collect in the retinal pigment epithelium, decreasing its ability to clear these by-products from the retina

- the photoreceptor density decreases with age, and other retinal cell layers become disordered

- visual acuity declines modestly beyond age 60, measured by high-contrast acuity charts; larger losses are seen with low-contrast charts, and when tested under decreased illumination, due to the changes in pupil size, lens, and retina

- the amount of light reaching the back of the eye decreases (the amount of light for an 80-year-old is at least 10 times lower than that of a 25-year-old)

- the ability to adapt to darkness is significantly slowed with age, and the time to adapt to changing environments from light to dim and from dim to light (such as from going from outdoors into a movie theater or from a restaurant to outdoors) is increased due to changes in the pupil size, lens, and retina

- the ability to recover from glare or visual sensitivity from bright lights worsens after age 50 due to lens and retinal changes

- the ability to see rapid flicker worsens with age

- there is a decrease in sensitivity to movement and figure-ground organization

- the size of the peripheral visual field decreases slowly with age so that the useful field of view for elderly adults is diminished when compared to younger counterparts, even when clinical peripheral field measures are unchanged.

For an illustration of the most common functional effects of age-related vision changes, see Figure 16.1.

Age-related Cognitive Changes

Age does not limit the potential to benefit from vision rehabilitation services. As Aiex (1987, p. 283) stated, "Although cognitive changes occur with age, the present consensus among researchers is that while short term memory ability decreases with age, there are few changes in long term ability and the basic intellectual abilities remain intact." In a study of perceptual training for persons with low vision, Bross and White (1986) concluded that age and the severity of visual impairments do not limit the potential for successful intervention. Watson, Wright, and De l'Aune (1992) studied the reading comprehension of older adults with low vision and found that some readers scored at the 17th-grade-level equivalent of a standardized reading evaluation, the highest possible score for adults, despite slow reading rates.

Most Prevalent Age-related Causes of Low Vision

As already indicated, macular degeneration, diabetic retinopathy, glaucoma, and cataracts are the most common age-related causes of visual impairment in the United States. For an illustration of the impact on vision of these age-related visual impairments, see Figure 16.2 (for additional information, see Chapter 6).

Age-related Macular Degeneration

In 1993, the National Advisory Eye Council estimated that of the 33.9 million people who will be 65 or older in 1995, approximately 1.7 million will have some visual impairment as a result of age-related macular degeneration (ARMD), with approximately 100,000 experiencing a rapid loss of vision due to subretinal neovascularization. The prevalence of ARMD is greater for women (Ferris, 1982) and it accounts for almost 45 percent of all low vision (National Advisory Eye Council, 1993). This condition is the leading cause of new visual impairment, and its incidence increases with age. The end result of ARMD is usually a dense scotoma. At present, only two known treatments hold promise for its amelioration or prevention: taking dietary zinc, which has been associated with a slowing of the loss of visual acuity after ARMD is manifest (Newsome, Swartz, Leone, Elston, & Miller, 1988), and protecting the eyes from blue, violet, and ultraviolet (UV) radiation by using absorptive lenses, which has also been suggested as a preventive (Goodlaw, 1991).

Diabetic Retinopathy

Diabetic retinopathy progresses more rapidly in older persons with diabetes, but fewer older persons than younger persons with diabetes develop proliferative retinopathy. Early detection and treatment is especially important for older people with diabetes before the disease causes an acceleration of atherosclerosis, which can lead to stroke and coronary disease (Cockburn, 1993).

Proliferative retinopathy can cause large fluctuations in vision that are sometimes reversible, and fluctuations can occur dramatically from day to day. Older persons with diabetes may need help identifying tasks for which vision is useful and those for which nonvisual techniques are more efficient.

Glaucoma

Advanced age is a factor that predisposes people to optic nerve damage, and older persons with glaucoma tend to show signs of losses in their visual fields before changes in the optic disk can be detected (Cockburn, 1993). Furthermore, African-Americans are at risk for glaucoma at a rate that is about five times greater than that for Caucasians. The rates for blindness among African-Americans due to glaucoma are six times greater than for Caucasians (National Advisory Eye Council, 1993). Because night blindness and increased susceptibility to glare are functional implications of advanced glaucoma, elderly people may be reluctant to travel alone outside their homes.

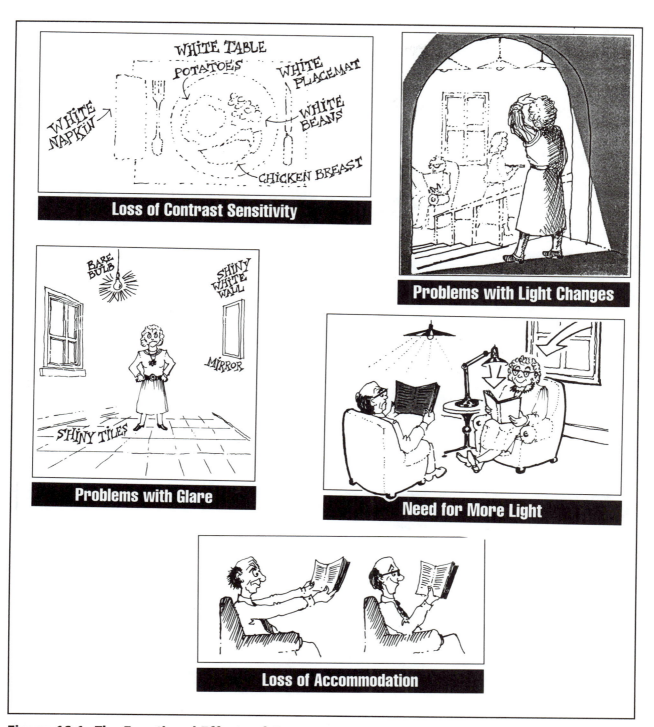

Figure 16.1. The Functional Effects of Common Causes of Age-related Vision Loss

Source: Reprinted, by permission of the publisher, from M. Duffy and M. Believeau-Tobey (Eds.), *New Independence! for Older Persons with Vision Loss in Long-Term Care Facilities* (Mohegan Lake, NY: AWARE, 1992).

Cataracts

Cataract surgery is the most common major surgical procedure performed for persons over age 65 who receive Medicare (Straatsma, Foos, Horwitz, et al., l985). In one study, cataract surgery with lens implantation resulted in a visual acuity of 20/40 or better in 88 percent of the cases (Straatsma, Foos, Horowitz, et al., 1985). In another study (Applegate et al., 1987), cataract surgery and lens implants were associated with improved objective and subjective measures of function in activities of daily living, as well as improved levels of vision.

Research has also found a strong relationship between exposure to UV light and the development of cataracts (Taylor et al., 1988), which has led to the recommendation that all people should wear UV filtration lenses from a young age to avoid developing cataracts (Goodlaw, 1991). Although studies (see, for example, Ham, 1983) have suggested that blue light may lead to the development of cataracts and macular degeneration, controlled clinical studies on this topic have yet to be conducted.

ADAPTATIONS OF FUNCTIONAL AND CLINICAL EVALUATIONS

Rosenbloom (1993) suggested five principles of low vision care of older adults:

- distinguish the effects of aging from disease
- see the older individual as a whole person
- use a team approach
- emphasize the person's goals
- improve the person's quality of life by facilitating independence and goal-directed activity.

In clinical low vision services, certain aspects of the examination sequence will need to be adapted to accommodate these principles.

Case History Interview

Every effort should be made to maintain the dignity of the elderly person with low vision. The individual should be addressed by his or her title and last name, unless permission is given to use his or her first name. The person's history should be taken in a direct interview, if possible, and family members, other caregivers, and professionals should provide supplemental information that complements the personal history. Multiple sessions may be necessary to minimize fatigue or to diminish the problems created by health difficulties. To lessen the duration of the first visit, basic information can be obtained in a preexamination telephone interview with the individual.

Since the clinical low vision process requires a great deal of energy and concentration by the elderly person, it is guided by his or her personal goals for rehabilitation. Therefore, conflicting goals of the individual and his or her family members or friends may need to be carefully negotiated. For example, if the person wishes to continue to live independently but family members consider this goal to be unrealistic, the professional may suggest that the elderly person and family visit other elderly persons with low vision who live independently to learn how they manage their situations.

As the interview unfolds, the team approach to low vision care may become more and more important in relation to goal-setting. For example, an individual with multiple reading needs may require a reading specialist; if the same person also has multiple traveling needs, an orientation and mobility instructor will be added to the team. Furthermore, the low vision professional may find that he or she has to educate the client and assist in the setting of realistic goals. In addition, since most low vision interventions are task specific, goals should be stated as specifically as possible. However, an individual may state a particular goal because of his or her assumption that the ability to perform one task means that all visual tasks are achievable. For example, the person may state that his or her goal is to "read," thinking

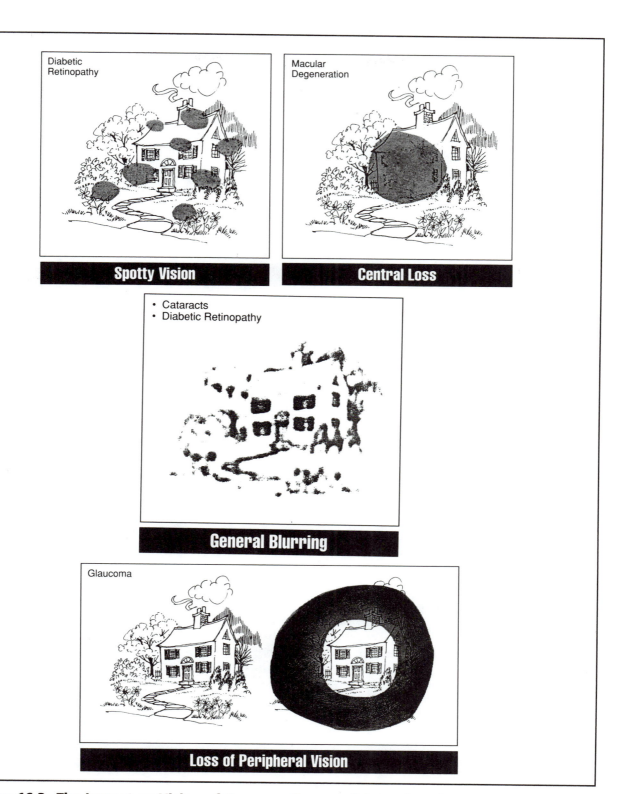

Figure 16.2. The Impact on Vision of Common Causes of Age-related Vision Loss

Source: Reprinted, by permission of the publisher, from M. Duffy and M. Beliveau-Tobey (Eds.), *New Independence! for Older Persons with Vision Loss in Long-Term Care Facilities* (Mohegan Lake, NJ: AWARE, 1992).

SIDEBAR 16.1

Common Goals of Elderly Persons for Low Vision Rehabilitation

◆ Reading
1. Continuous text (newspapers, magazines, and books)
2. Spot reading (materials such as bills, letters, prices, phone numbers, labels, and recipes)

◆ Writing
1. Short-term tasks (including signing one's name and writing checks, notes, grocery lists, and telephone numbers)
2. Long-term tasks (such as writing letters and filling in address books)

◆ Seeing a clock and watch

◆ Dialing telephone numbers

◆ Using appliances with numbers and dials

◆ Identifying the colors and condition of clothing

◆ Cooking safely and efficiently

◆ Completing personal grooming (such as caring for the hair, shaving, applying makeup, and cutting nails)

◆ Seeing faces and recognizing people

◆ Enjoying hobbies (such as games, card playing, woodworking, sewing, and needlework)

◆ Watching television

◆ Moving safely in various environments
1. Within one's residence (such as on stairs and in entryways)
2. Within the neighborhood (such as at a supermarket, church, social club, and street crossings)

that if it is possible to see small letters, it will be possible to see everything he or she was once able to see. When the person discovers that it may be impossible to watch television or recognize faces with a low vision device used for reading, the first reaction may be one of dismay. With further conversation, it is possible to help the person to define goals that more completely express personal priorities for using vision. Some commonly expressed goals of elderly persons for using vision are presented in Sidebar 16.1.

Functional Vision Assessment

Whenever possible, the functional assessment should take place in the older person's daily environment. The person's specific goals will guide the functional assessment to discover the size and distance of targets and the visual skills that will be required to identify them. The functional assessment can also uncover the need to address additional goals and the need for a separate, more comprehensive environmental assessment and provision of modifications. Performance of the assessment in the elderly person's environment provides ongoing opportunities to educate the individual and his or her relatives and friends about vision and rehabilitation. The functional assessment should include evaluations of these factors:

◆ The person's *functional visual acuities* at various distances and under different lighting conditions. The distance at which the person identifies items should be noted for such common objects as labels on food cans, the television screen, indoor and outdoor signs, facial details, and printed materials.

◆ The person's *functional visual fields*, including the person's location of everyday objects and perception of information in the upper, lower, and side fields and for near, intermediate, and distance views. This evaluation should be conducted in both the static and the dynamic modes, in both indoor and outdoor settings, and under different lighting and weather conditions. It should also include the individual's use of visual fields when directed to look at a specific target and when gathering incidental information.

◆ The person's ability to discriminate and identify the *color and contrast* of a variety of materials and objects under various figure-ground and lighting conditions. Older adults may have more difficulty with color and contrast for such tasks as identifying photographs; discriminating dark and pastel colors; and visually identifying textures, such as vinyl and stone flooring.

◆ The person's *ocular motor skills*, including fixation, localization, scanning, tracing, tracking objects, and reading materials. Older adults who acquire low vision later in life must relearn these skills using different body, head, and eye postures.

◆ *Lighting*, including the type, amount, position, and angle of light sources used while performing tasks. The lighting assessment should evaluate the amount of glare and the effects of glare experienced in different settings; the time it takes to adapt from indoor to outdoor lighting, and vice versa; and the effect of absorptive lenses and nonoptical techniques for eliminating glare and decreasing the adaptation time.

◆ The person's use of a combination of *visual and nonvisual cues* to detect a variety of objects, landmarks, depth (such as, slopes, steps, curbs), glass doorways, differences in terrain, and so forth. The older adult may have additional problems in this area because of other physical and sensory problems (such as neuropathy, impaired balance, and reduced reaction time). Falls for elderly persons are especially devastating, since bones may break more easily and recovery from breaks takes longer.

◆ The person's *demonstrated use of vision* to perform specific tasks that constitute his or her goals. Each goal should be evaluated separately to determine which visual skills are required to accomplish it and whether the person exhibits these visual skills, both without and with optical and nonoptical devices.

Ideally, the functional vision assessment is completed by a team of rehabilitation professionals, clinicians, and other professionals. However, for elderly persons, it is usually conducted by a rehabilitation teacher, an orientation and mobility (O&M) instructor, or another professional from the field of visual impairment. As low vision services increasingly are provided by hospitals and comprehensive outpatient rehabilitation facilities, a part of or all the functional vision assessment may be performed by other professionals, such as occupational therapists. Whichever professionals ultimately conduct these assessments, they should be well versed and experienced in the following:

◆ basic optics of the eye

◆ the causes and functional implications of visual impairments

◆ lenses and low vision devices

◆ methods of observing and evaluating individual visual skills for activities of daily living

◆ basic sighted guide and O&M techniques

◆ assessment of reading

◆ basic techniques of assessing and using optical devices, nonoptical devices, adaptive equipment, electronic devices, and computers

◆ assessment of the environments in which elderly people travel or are occupied.

If the professional who conducts the assessment is also a rehabilitation instructor, he or she must also be knowledgeable and experienced in

- ◆ teaching visual skills for activities of daily living with and without optical devices, nonoptical devices, electronic devices, and other adaptive devices
- ◆ conducting task analyses
- ◆ teaching basic O&M techniques
- ◆ teaching basic techniques of reading with low vision devices
- ◆ using techniques that do not require the use of vision for performing activities of daily living when vision is not the safest, most efficient, or preferred modality.

Clinical Low Vision Evaluation

To provide the best low vision services to older adults, the clinical low vision specialist should be flexible and be able to adapt to a variety of different environments, schedules, and communication styles. The conventional pattern of the low vision evaluation should be followed. For many older adults, especially those in long-term-care facilities (such as nursing homes), careful refraction and updating of conventional spectacles may significantly improve their vision.

Because of the growing trend of providing low vision services for older adults as part of outpatient hospital services, comprehensive outpatient rehabilitation facilities, long-term-care facilities, and clients' homes, it is often necessary to conduct low vision evaluations in these settings. In each setting, it is crucial to have an appropriate contact person to arrange schedules and to provide information to the low vision team. Mancil (1993) discussed the following considerations related to these nontraditional settings.

Nursing Homes

The common age-related visual impairments are usually seen among the 5 percent of the elderly population who reside in nursing homes. However, few nursing home residents receive vision care. For example, Snyder, Beliveau, Yeadon, and Aston (1986) found that 70 percent of the 2,000 nursing homes they surveyed had no policy for screening their residents' vision. Morse, O'Connell, and Finklestein (1988) found that there was no difference in the referral rate for vision services for nursing home residents between those who complained about their vision, and those who did not. Newell and Walser (1985) found that only 11 percent of residents in 19 nursing homes had had eye examinations in the last two years. In a nursing home that does provide vision services, the low vision team will adopt the medical model that prevails in these facilities. To increase the effectiveness of low vision care, it is vital to work closely with the social work staff of the home, as well as families and friends of the residents. Providing information about vision and visual impairments to the nursing home staff is one of the most critical factors in assisting and encouraging residents to use their vision (Beliveau, Yeadon, & Aston, 1986).

Hospitals

Outpatient facilities in private hospitals are increasing their services to elderly persons, including low vision rehabilitation services. Low vision care is routinely provided to elderly veterans in the hospital system of the U.S. Department of Veterans Affairs (VA). VA Blind Rehabilitation Centers provide up to 16 weeks of rehabilitation, including low vision services, to legally blind veterans; VA Blind Rehabilitation Clinics provide services for veterans with multiple disabilities, including visual impairments; and Visual Impairment Centers to Optimize Remaining Sight provide low vision services to veterans with low vision who are not legally blind; and optometric outpatient clinics in VA medical centers routinely provide low vision services. In addition, many colleges of optometry provide outpatient low vision services.

Community Service Agencies

The Older Americans Act mandates the provision of supportive community services for older adults through State Units on Aging and Area Agencies on Aging, which were created under the auspices of the Administration on Aging, a branch of the U.S. Department of Health and Human Services (Ficke, 1985). Examples of community agencies that provide such services are senior citizens' centers, nutrition centers, senior clubs, adult day care centers, and senior rehabilitation centers. Information about these centers may be obtained from the local Area Agencies on Aging.

Private Residential Settings

Almost 71 percent of the long-term-care population reside in the community (DeSylvia & Williams, 1989). Most frail elderly persons who require care are living at home with family members, not in long-term-care facilities (AARP, 1991), and many elderly people are living in senior residential retirement and congregate living centers. Interactions with family members and caregivers is essential in these situations, so they understand the sometimes inconsistent and variable nature of visual impairments and can provide assistance that will help older adults achieve their goals for vision rehabilitation.

Rehabilitation Centers

Because stroke is another common medical condition among elderly people that necessitates rehabilitation, it is important that the low vision team work closely with professionals who diagnose, treat, and rehabilitate elderly persons' cerebrovascular accidents, including physicians and occupational and physical therapists. Rehabilitation centers may be located in hospital centers or in separate facilities.

Orientation to New Settings

Four basic techniques can be used to orient an older person to any type or size of room or area:

using a starting-ending point, compass directions, a clock face, and landmarks and cues. Some clients may be able to use all these techniques, and some may need only one or two. Clients should not be rushed in gaining orientation, but should be allowed the time they need to explore and to memorize where objects are in relation to each other. Teaching family members these techniques may be helpful when their older relatives encounter new environments.

Using a Starting-Ending Point

Begin at one starting-ending place in the room, such as the door. Have the person reach out and feel both sides of the doorway and then describe the contents of the room. While leading the person using the sighted guide technique, have him or her trail and visually and tactilely identify features. Use simple names for the walls that incorporate some feature (for example, the wall to the right is the bed wall, and the wall opposite is the window wall). Give the person plenty of time to explore the furniture and features of the room. Next, go back to the starting point and explore the room in the opposite direction. Then go to the opposite wall of the starting point. Continue moving back and forth across the room using different walls as the starting and ending points. Use visual features to identify landmarks in the room that will assist in orientation. For example, note the position of the bed by mentioning the contrast of a dark wood door to a lighter wall or a brightly colored bedspread. Ask the person to give verbal feedback when identifying the visual landmarks to ensure that he or she sees them.

Using Compass Directions

Using the same starting points as in the foregoing example, use compass directions (north, south, east, and west) to name the four walls of the room, instead of the bed wall, window wall, and so forth. Proceed as in the first example, using compass directions to find and name locations in the room.

Using a Clock Face

Some persons may have used the clock face to orient themselves in other situations and will be comfortable and familiar using this analogy to orient themselves to an unfamiliar area. Pretending that the entire room is a clock face, familiar objects in the room can be located at certain numbers on the clock. For example, the door is at 12 o'clock, the bed at 3 o'clock, the television set is at 6 o'clock, the bathroom door is at 9 o'clock, and so forth. Proceed as in the first example, using the clock settings to locate and talk about objects in the room.

Using Landmarks and Clues

Familiar landmarks and clues can be used for orientation to a new environment. For example, the smell of food can be used as an indication that the person is near the dining room of a facility, and the large, red soft drink machine with an audible hum can mark the end of the hall and the location of the elevator in a hotel. Help the older person to use as many senses as possible to identify landmarks and clues. When negotiating an unfamiliar environment, notice which landmarks and clues are useful in that environment and ask the older person what he or she notices that may help him or her remember how to return.

VISION REHABILITATION

The functional vision assessment and clinical evaluation should culminate in an Individualized Written Vision Rehabilitation Plan (IWVRP) that summarizes the information obtained in the evaluations in clearly stated goals and objectives that are developed by the low vision team and the elderly person. A sample IWVRP, based on the vignette that opened this chapter, is presented as an appendix to this chapter. The implementation of the IWVRP should emphasize an educational process using the principles of andragogy, or teaching adults, that incorporates the older person's values, beliefs, attitudes, and life experiences. An understanding of relevant cultural issues and inclusion of family members and support systems into all aspects of the functional and clinical evaluations increase the chances for greater success.

Principles of Andragogy

According to Knowles (1984), the principles of the andragogical model are as follows.

Using Self-directed Learning

The adult learner is capable of taking responsibility for and directing his or her own learning. It is often tempting for an instructor to think that the adult learner "should" appreciate the improvement in vision and independence that is possible through rehabilitation or to try to impose his or her will on the learner. However, only the learner can decide whether the level of benefit and required effort meets his or her priorities.

Placing an Emphasis on Experience

Adults enter the learning process with a greater breadth and a different quality of experience than do youths and are the richest resources for each other. Thus, in adult education, emphasis is placed on experiential techniques and on individualized lesson plans, such as learning contracts. The downside of this situation is that some adults bring to the learning experience preconceptions about reality, prejudices, and defensiveness about their past ways of thinking and doing. For example, some older people with low vision may think that the loss of visual function is an inevitable part of the aging process for which nothing can be done. Some may misunderstand the rehabilitation aspects of low vision and expect low vision devices to restore their vision to 20/20 detail with full visual fields. When low vision rehabilitation is unable to meet these expectations, they may fail to appreciate the small gains of being able to function independently, but with more effort. To overcome these problems, instructors must devise strategies for helping people become more knowledgeable and open-minded. In addition to demonstrating low vision devices and instruction, they may also encourage their clients to join peer support groups or undergo short-term counseling and involve their clients' relatives as much as possible.

Increasing Motivation

Adult learners are ready to learn when they have a need to know or do something to perform more effectively in some aspect of their lives. Adults do not learn primarily for the sake of learning, but to perform a task, solve a problem, or live in a more satisfying way. The motivation to learn must come from them, but the instructor can increase or awaken this motivation by exposing adult clients to more effective role models and provide diagnostic experiences in which they can assess the gaps between their present and desired functioning. Working-age adults respond to some external motivators—a better job or a salary increase, for example—but older adults are more likely to respond to internal motivators—self-esteem, recognition, independence, a better quality of life, greater self-confidence, and self-actualization.

Creating a Climate for Learning

Knowles (1984) recommended using a one-on-one or small-group approach, rather than lecturing. Furthermore, the setting should be comfortable and conducive to learning. It should include good lighting adapted for low vision; sufficient ventilation; comfortable chairs that support the back, legs, feet, and arms; and a nonsmoking area; appropriate breaks and refreshments should also be provided. The characteristics of a psychological climate conducive to adult learning are mutual respect, collaboration, and trust; supportiveness, openness and authenticity, and pleasure.

Establishing Goals and Measuring Outcomes

In low vision rehabilitation, older persons designate their own goals for independent functioning or a better quality of life, and the entire rehabilitation process builds on these needs. At times, they may need some guidance because they may not know what rehabilitation strategies are possible. In such cases, checklists of daily activities or performance assessment systems can be used to negotiate between felt needs and ascribed needs. Objectives in the form of observable, measurable competencies that reflect a person's needs should be written by both the person and the instructor, so the person can identify the gaps between what he or she knows and can accomplish and what can be anticipated following instruction.

It would be a mistake for the clinical low vision specialist to prescribe optical devices and leave it to the elderly person to find uses for them; rather, strategies to help the person maximize methods to accomplish his or her objectives should be explored. For example, a person who wants to use an optical device for reading may need to consider setting up a "reading corner" in the home, with a comfortable chair; appropriate lighting; and nonoptical devices, such as colored filters, typoscopes, and a reading stand, to make reading as easy as possible. Or, some elderly persons in a retirement community may decide to meet together to practice with their low vision devices.

The elderly person needs to use both qualitative and quantitative measures of outcomes to be actively involved in evaluating his or her learning. For example, in addition to measuring the ability to read smaller print and increased reading duration, the person may also evaluate his or her comfort and satisfaction with reading following low vision services.

Knowles (1984) recommended the use of a learning contract (or IWVRP) to assist in implementing the adragogical model. In such a contract, the person first translates a diagnosed learning need into a learning objective that describes the end behavior to be achieved. Next, he or she identifies, with the instructor's help, the most effective resources and strategies for accomplishing each objective. Then, the person specifies what evidence will be collected to indicate the extent to which each objective was accomplished and how this evidence will be judged or validated. The IWVRP in the appendix to this chapter demonstrates the use of these principles.

Evaluation of Low Vision Devices

Following the functional vision assessment and the clinical low vision evaluation, the older person and the instructor assess the usefulness of various low vision devices for that person. McIlwaine, Bell, and Dutton (1991) found that the successful use of low vision devices was related to the intensity of the instructional program, and Nilsson (1990) concluded that specialized training in visual skills and low vision devices improved the abilities of elderly individuals with low vision.

Essential Principles

The instructor gives the older person the opportunity to develop appropriate visual skills; learn the benefits and limitations of low vision devices; and apply the principles of color, illumination, and contrast that make the environment as conducive as possible to the use of vision. It is often important to help caregivers and relatives understand how vision and low vision devices assist the older person to accomplish visual tasks, so they can give the person social support for the use of vision. If possible, pertinent low vision devices should be loaned to the person, so he or she can try them at home to see if they are beneficial in daily activities.

The instructor estimates the scope and duration of instruction required to meet the stated goals; presents the devices tactilely and visually; and describes uses, advantages, and limitations of the devices. Limitations, such as a small field of view, speed smear (objects seem to move faster as they are magnified), initial nausea, and decreased visual acuity with prisms, can be daunting. Older persons may need reassurance that instruction and practice can overcome these initial difficulties and that the use of devices can become automatic. Tradeoffs between the limitations of devices and the individual's ability to fulfill personal goals must be discussed.

Special Considerations for Older Persons

Some aspects of instruction in the use of vision and low vision devices are particularly important when working with elderly persons with low vision. First, because of the potentially devastating consequences of falling, the instructor must be certain to address safety issues to prevent falls that are related to using low vision devices. Thus, older people should be cautioned never to stand up or walk while wearing spectacle-mounted magnifiers, since the blurred image may cause them to fall or trip. Those who use telescopes should be cautioned not to walk while viewing through the telescopic lenses, but should stop to spot and then resume walking while using unaided vision or standard-correction lenses.

Second, nausea, dizziness, and other aspects of motion sickness are common side effects of using magnification. Motion sickness is the body's reaction to confusing signals between the eyes and the equilibrium system; the eyes perceive motion, but the body is still. To reduce the feelings of nausea while reading, the older person must be instructed to keep practice sessions short in the beginning, to sit before picking up lenses, to have reading materials readily available when donning magnification lenses, and not to look up or around the room when looking through the lenses. The person should scan a page by slowly moving the page to the left and reading the line, then moving the page to the right to pick up the next line. As soon as nausea or dizziness become evident, he or she should stop reading until the feeling passes. Some older people report that eating soda crackers helps, and some have found it helpful to use a cardboard cut-out inside their lenses that allows for a small central field of view and completely blocks peripheral vision. Gradually, the person should be able to increase the sessions by a few minutes at a time. If the feelings of nausea or dizziness do not subside, the low vision team may want to explore the use of another type of device.

Third, hand tremors may be severe enough that the person cannot maintain focus with handheld magnifiers or telescopes. In such a

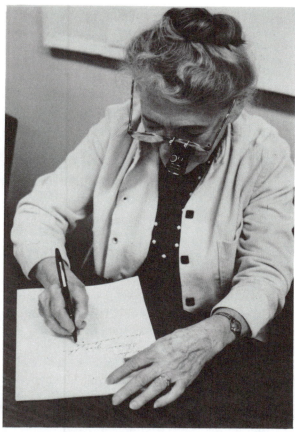

Older adults with low vision may experience symptoms, such as hand tremors, that may preclude them from using handheld devices. In such cases, spectacle-mounted devices may be more useful.

case, the low vision team may want to explore the use of spectacle-mounted devices.

Fourth, postural support is an important consideration with elderly persons. Because of the prevalence of back and neck pain, as well as limited stamina, the instructor should keep the elderly person as comfortable as possible. He or she should provide a chair with a supporting back, head rest, and arms; a cushion for lumbar and/or cervical support; and, for a short person, a footstool for relief from lower-back and leg pain. The lamp should have a flexible arm, so it can be positioned to maximize its use without the person having to bend toward the light. A reading stand on a flexible arm will also allow the person

to sit comfortably and keep the reading material at the proper focal distance.

Fifth, instructional periods should be kept short—about 30 minutes—with frequent brief rests, snacks, and extra time for practice. Most elderly persons will say when they have had enough. However, the instructor should watch for signs that the session should end, such as slumped shoulders, deep sighs, tearfulness, or gesturing or speaking nervously, that indicate that the person is tired or frustrated that the device is not providing more help.

Sixth, at times, older persons may resent instruction and view it as a reminder of the body's deterioration. They may respond emotionally, rather than discuss problems associated with the instructional approach or physical fatigue. The wise instructor will encourage the person to verbalize his or her feelings, acknowledge this expression of emotion, and offer clear but brief support.

Finally, most elderly persons need two to three times more light than do younger persons, but some are extremely sensitive to light. Before flooding the instructional area with light, ask the person what kind of lighting he or she uses at home. Begin by trying to duplicate that light and then increase the level or type of lighting, if necessary. Consider the use of a variety of illumination controls, such as lamps with flexible arms, rheostats, colored filters, typoscopes, side and top shields for glasses, and tinted lenses. Some elderly people may find a combination of different kinds of light, such as incandescent, fluorescent, and sodium vapor, useful. Bright sunlight is full-spectrum light and may be the best for some people. The person's chair should be positioned so the light is shining over the shoulder of the better-seeing eye onto the target to be illuminated, not into the person's face.

Instruction in the Use of Low Vision Devices

The sequence of instruction in low vision devices covers the use of:

◆ visual skills without a low vision device

◆ visual skills with a low vision device

◆ vision and low vision devices for individualized functional tasks that lead to the achievement of stated goals.

Use of Visual Skills without a Device

Instruction in the use of visual skills without devices includes fixation, spotting, localization, scanning, tracing, and tracking. Individuals with ARMD may require additional instruction in the development and maintenance of fixation using eccentric viewing.

Eccentric viewing refers to the use of a parafoveal area for fixation, following the loss of foveal functioning with ARMD (for a review of eccentric viewing and its instruction, see Backman & Inde, 1976; Maplesden, 1984; Watson & Berg, 1984; Wright & Watson, 1995). The resulting damage to the macula results in a scotoma that may be absolute, in which case there is no remaining vision, or relative, in which case some vision may be perceived, but it is cloudy or smoky. Most adults with ARMD have one or more strongly preferred eccentric viewing positions, and some will have one direction that functions for detail vision (closer to the fovea) and another for distance vision (a wider field of view). (See Chapter 8 for additional information.) To elicit the direction of eccentric viewing for general use, the instructor asks the person to look at his or her face using the better eye, covering the other eye with the cupped palm. The instructor's face should be about 2½ feet away and evenly illuminated, with no shadows or bright spots. The instructor's request to look at his or her face generally elicits one of the following responses:

◆ The person will immediately turn his or her eye or head to see the instructor's face eccentrically, will describe what part of the instructor's face or the surrounding area is "missing" or "unclear," and will verbalize what happens if the eye is shifted so he or she is looking "directly" at the instructor's face (the face becomes unclear or appears to be missing).

◆ The person will move the eye rapidly in darting eye movements. In this case, the person is not able to identify a strongly preferred eccentric viewing direction; rather, he or she is constantly shifting his or her field of view and is unable to notice that the scotoma or blind spot is interfering with the ability to see. If the person responds this way, the instructor may wish to instruct him or her in developing eccentric viewing skills.

Use of Visual Skills with a Device

Instruction in the use of visual skills with a low vision device includes integrating unaided abilities with the unique demands of the device, such as maintaining the focal distance or focusing the device, and adjusting eye and head movements to compensate for a restricted field of view. If the individual is using eccentric viewing, the instructor assures that the device and the way it is used allows the person to maximize his or her visual field and acuity in the eccentric position.

These skills are initially demonstrated in a setting that the instructor may have manipulated to provide illumination control, nonoptical devices, and targets that lead to initial success with the device. Frustration is minimized when the instructor assigns tasks to teach visual skills at the person's level of understanding and functioning and gradually increases the difficulty of tasks when the person demonstrates proficiency at lower levels of complexity. Proficiency in goal-related tasks may require extensive instruction and the use of additional nonoptical devices and environmental modifications.

Follow-up Issues

Most low vision services are provided in center-based facilities (American Foundation for the Blind, 1993), a practice that ignores an important element in the elderly person's rehabilitation—

the home environment. A number of clinicians have suggested that home follow-up services are essential (Fagerstrom, 1971; Farrar, 1971; Rusalem, 1972). As Quillman and Goodrich (1979, p. 37) noted, "It is something of a paradox that most low vision clinics strive hard to provide aids and services to clients, but spend little or no time and energy in finding out if the aids and services have helped [them]."

Although many practitioners have stressed the importance of follow-up (Faye, 1984; Jose, 1983; Silver & Thomsitt, 1977), few facilities provide such services. Nevertheless, follow-up studies have reported that 45 to 87 percent of the adults who are prescribed low vision devices continue to use them after they complete low vision services (Faye, 1970; Jackson, Silver, & Archer, 1986; Sanderson, Cumming, & Polkinghorne, 1986; Skejskal, Zahn, & Van Dollen, 1987). However, there is little information on precisely which low vision devices are not used after they are recommended. Clinical information from low vision professionals indicates that devices are rejected for the following reasons:

- deterioration of vision
- declining health
- inability to adjust to the device because of such factors as a small field of view and a narrow depth of focus
- inadequate training and/or practice
- a change in goals for seeing that may require a different device
- differences in the ergonomics of the low vision clinic and the home setting, such as different lighting and seating and the need for a reading stand and filters
- dizziness or nausea when first using the device
- competing priorities for time
- psychosocial reasons, including depression or anxiety; censure by family members or friends for using the device; cosmesis; possible vulnerability, especially as a potential crime victim; and fear of losing

support from those on whom one depends for help in daily activities.

Various factors, including age, family structure, intelligence and education levels, and environment, have been studied in isolation to determine whether they affect people's success or failure with low vision devices (Mancil, 1986). Lighting is one environmental factor that can present a significant problem to the elderly person with low vision for both near and distance tasks (Rosenberg, 1984). Although proper lighting with minimum glare is used in clinical settings, a person is often not given information about duplicating this lighting at home. Without proper lighting at home, the prescribed low vision device that worked in the clinical setting may not work at home. Elderly people are sometimes unaware that their difficulties in using devices are related to improper lighting in their homes and may stop using the devices because of frustration.

Hall, Bailey, Kekelis, Raasch, and Goodrich's (1987) survey of the use of telescopes by elderly veterans with low vision and a matched control group of nonveterans found that the telescopes were used for the tasks for which they were prescribed and that weather and lighting affected the users' abilities to travel independently and to use the devices. In addition, the veterans used their telescopes more often and for more tasks than did the nonveterans.

Reading with Low Vision Devices

Visual impairments that affect the central visual field and cloud the media, such as ARMD and cataracts, inhibit reading more than do visual impairments that restrict only the peripheral fields. Because ARMD and cataracts are the most prevalent causes of visual impairments and reading is central to maintaining independence, most elderly persons who receive low vision services state that reading is their primary goal for rehabilitation. Since cataracts are successfully remediated by surgery in most cases, ARMD is the most prevalent cause of reading problems for older people with low vision. For this reason, and because reading is a task that lends itself to testing, most research on low vision has focused on reading by elderly people with low vision. Studies have determined the following with respect to the reading problems of older people with ARMD:

- People with ARMD can develop consistent eccentric fixation (Timberlake, Mainster, Pelli, Auglier, Essock, & Arend, 1986; Whittaker, Bud, & Cummings, 1988) and can fixate successive words in a reading task (Cummings, Whittaker, Watson, & Bud, 1985).

- People with ARMD may continue to read accurately, but their rate of reading is severely inhibited by the size of their scotomas—the larger the scotoma, the slower the rate of reading (Cummings et al., 1985).

- Poor control of gaze or unstable fixation may contribute to the significantly slower reading rate (25 to 30 words per minute) of persons with ARMD compared to those with other ocular disorders (Baldasare & Watson, 1986; Kirscher & Meissen, 1983; Legge, Rubin, Pelli, & Schleske, 1985; Rayner & Bertera, 1979).

- In clinical low vision practice, the rate of reading is sometimes used as a measure of reading performance and the basis of predictive judgments about reading potential. This practice is based on studies of the reading rates by individuals who are normally sighted, which have found that a slow rate of reading is highly correlated with difficulties in comprehension (Shankweiler & Liberman, 1982; Stanovich, 1980). Baldasare and Watson (1986) postulated that a slow rate of reading is also responsible for difficulties in comprehension for persons with ARMD. However, Legge, Ross, Maxwell, and Luebker (1989) found that a reduction in the reading rate alone did not reduce comprehension for persons with low vision. In addition, Watson et al.'s (1992) study of the reading comprehension of individuals with macular degeneration found the following:

- Macular loss may severely disrupt the comprehension of some people with visual impairments and the restoration of visual skills (the ability to identify symbols and words accurately) does not necessarily restore comprehension.

- The rate and accuracy of reading are not predictive of comprehension, or of the potential of regaining comprehension, since in the treatment group, comprehension improved while the rate and accuracy of reading remained stable.

- The instruction in comprehension strategies that a reading specialist provided to the treatment group was associated with a significant gain in comprehension scores compared to that of the control group.

- Age does not limit the potential benefit of instruction and practice in reading because improvement in reading occurred in persons of various ages.

- Practice in reading leveled printed exercises is an effective rehabilitation technique.

On the basis of the evidence, one cannot assume that among older people, a visual impairment that slows reading will also impede comprehension. In those with ARMD who have good visual skills and cognitive abilities, the visual requirements for good comprehension may be met by the visual requirements for a slow reading rate. For skilled readers, low vision appears to create an information "bottleneck" that slows the transmission of information from the printed page to the language centers of the brain. Once they get past the bottleneck, they may process information normally.

These findings are based on elderly readers who continued to read using low vision devices. However, because there have been no controlled follow-up studies on the use of low vision devices for reading, it is not known why some elderly persons with low vision continue to read with their devices and some do not. Elderly persons frequently tell low vision professionals, "It's just not like it used to be." Thus, some of them may not be able to adapt to the precise focal distance or the reduced field of view of the low vision device or to master the precise eye movements required to maintain eccentric viewing. Others may be self-conscious about being seen using the device or embarrassed that their vision is so impaired that they need to use a device. Still others may think that the energy required to practice and still read slowly is just not worth the investment or they have family members or friends read to them or take care of bills, so reading is no longer a necessity.

Successful readers who use optical devices seem to have one thing in common: They will go to great lengths to continue reading. For example, when a well-known activist for the Gray Panthers (an advocacy organization of elderly persons) came for an appointment at a low vision clinic, she demonstrated her present reading paraphernalia: a bifocal and two low-powered magnifiers that she held together in front of her bifocal. With this awkward arrangement, she continued to read several daily newspapers and several professional journals. She asked, "Can you improve on this setup? I can't lecture from my notes because I have to hold all these devices at the same time!" It had never occurred to her to stop reading. With low vision services, she learned to use and was comfortable with half-eye eyeglasses and a pair of small spectacle-mounted telescopes for reading and lecturing.

Driving with Low Vision

Studies have investigated elderly drivers and drivers with low vision, but there is little information directly related to the driving habits and abilities of elderly drivers with low vision. Therefore, information about elderly drivers with low vision must be extrapolated from two types of research. Owsley, Sloane, Ball, Roenker, and Bruni (1991) studied the driving of elderly persons with and without low vision in Alabama using state reports of the frequency of accidents and citations as a measure of driving ability. After collecting data from subjects on measures of eye health, visual acuity, contrast sensitivity, disability glare, stereopsis, color discrimination, visual field sensitivity, visual attention, mental status, and driving habits, they found that a measure of visual attention called useful field of view (UFOV) and mental status were the strongest predictors of accidents. UFOV refers to the extent of the visual field needed for a specific visual task; the size of the UFOV is different from the size of the visual field, as determined by clinical perimetry, and is typically smaller than the area of visual sensitivity (Ball, Owsley, & Beard, 1990). The study found that subjects with severe problems with central vision (such as ARMD) or the ocular media (such as cataracts) avoided difficult driving situations, including driving at night, driving in heavy traffic, driving on freeways, making left turns, and driving in situations in which glare was a problem. However, neither the composite score on driving avoidance nor the eye-health ratings was related to the frequency of accidents or the number of citations on the state record. Therefore, it seems that elderly persons with low vision seem to limit their driving to avoid dangerous situations and hence that their eye-health status is unrelated to the number of accidents in which they are involved.

ACCESSIBLE ENVIRONMENTS FOR ELDERLY PEOPLE WITH LOW VISION

Environmental Evaluations and Modifications

An environmental evaluation for an elderly person with low vision should address the components listed in Sidebar 16.2. The goal should be to allow the person to develop a wide repertoire of skills and options for completing tasks that will allow for maximum flexibility, safety, and efficiency. Sometimes an elderly person will not notice when a situation is unsafe or will be hesitant

SIDEBAR 16.2

Steps in an Environmental Evaluation

1. Identify the tasks that the person wishes to perform in a particular environment.

2. Identify the characteristics of the important targets that the person must see to complete these tasks.

   ◆ Size

   ◆ Distance from the eye

   ◆ Color

   ◆ Contrast

   ◆ Figure-ground

   ◆ Angle of viewing

   ◆ Illumination.

3. Modify the targets, if necessary, to make them more visible.

   ◆ Increase their size

   ◆ Decrease their distance from the eyes

   ◆ Increase the hue or saturation of the color or change it to a more visible color

   ◆ Provide more contrast

   ◆ Decrease the "busyness" of the background, so the target is more visible

   ◆ Provide illumination controls.

---

to learn to use a new adaptation. For example, if the person has always felt uncomfortable using a flight of stairs with a patterned carpet, then he or she may at first be hesitant to try a new adaptation, such as placing stripes on the top and bottom steps to mark the boundaries of the stairs. Four ways to make the environment more visible are (1) to change the perceived or real size of objects and images, (2) to improve lighting, (3) to increase the contrast, and (4) to use clear, bright colors.

Changing the Perceived Size

Any type of visual impairment that results in the loss of visual acuity or constriction of the visual fields requires changing the perceived size of objects. An object or image can be enlarged in several ways:

   ◆ *Making the object larger:* Use large-print phone dials, make labels in large print, and so on.

   ◆ *Moving closer to the object:* Move closer to the television set, clock face, signs, friends, and so forth.

   ◆ *Using an optical device:* Use a magnifier, a pair of binoculars, or another type of optical device to enlarge the image and make it easier to see.

If the older person has a visual condition, such as glaucoma, that results in restricted visual fields, the person can sometimes see an object more clearly if he or she moves away from it to get more of it in his or her visual field. Imagine looking at a television screen through a soda straw; if one sits close to it, one can see only a portion of it, but if one sits farther away, one can see more of the screen.

Improving the Lighting

As was mentioned earlier, most older people need two to three times more light than younger persons, but those with impairments of the lens or cornea (such as cataracts or keratoconus) are more sensitive to light. The problem is to get enough light to support the use of vision without creating glare. Most forms of light can be managed by the way the light is spread out and screened.

Fluorescent Lighting. This type of light is used a great deal, especially in homes. It spreads out evenly and is inexpensive and energy efficient. But fluorescent lighting also provides less contrast because it is an even light and produces fewer shadows. Furthermore, because it is harsh and flickers, it may be bothersome to older persons with low vision and may cause headaches and eye strain. Coverings or shades over the fluorescent bulbs can help, as can mounting the lights with a covering that bounces the light off the ceiling or walls before it hits the eyes.

Incandescent Lighting. Incandescent lighting is easier to direct, provides more contrast, and creates more shadows. Shadows can be beneficial when they highlight a target, such as the triangular shadow that is created on the side of a step that indicates the height and depth of the step. But shadows can be dangerous when they obscure targets; for example, the shadow created by a building can obscure the curb adjacent to the outside sidewalk, causing the elderly person with low vision to trip or fall.

Certain types of incandescent fixtures, such as those that suspend one lightbulb from the ceiling, can cause pinpoint glare or pools of light within relative darkness in a room or hall. The solution to these problems is to position several incandescent fixtures in a room to create more even light throughout the room and to use lamp shades to cut down on the pinpoints of light. Incandescent lamps are good for near work, such as reading, sewing, or other hobbies because the light can be directed to create bright light directly on the task and can be shaded to keep the bright light from going directly into the eyes.

High-intensity bulbs used in tensor lamps may be incandescent or halogen. Tensor lamps are usually positioned close to the page and direct a smaller pool of light than do regular lamps. Halogen bulbs use the glow of charged halogen gas, as well as the incandescent filament, to create a brighter light; they give more light in the blue end of the spectrum and are brighter.

Studies are exploring the benefits of an incandescent bulb mixed with neodymium oxide for individuals with low vision. This bulb emits fewer ultraviolet and infrared rays, and there is a sharp drop in the emission of yellow light. The effect is a more vivid "true" color, similar to sunlight, so contrast is increased.

Incandescent and fluorescent lighting can be combined to take advantage of both types. The fluorescent light can be used for general lighting in a room and the incandescent light used for near tasks.

Sunlight. Although sunlight is bright and natural, but neither flickers nor is harsh, it is not easy to control and can cause shadows that can make it difficult or painful for older persons to adjust to sudden changes in lighting when they enter or leave such places as patios and sunporches and can reduce their already limited vision. Bright lighting in sunny areas can be controlled by using lattices, blinds, or sheer panel curtains that reduce sunlight, but do not cut it off completely, or older people can wear sunglasses or hats with visors that limit the amount of light entering their eyes.

Glare. Glare is caused by bright light reflecting from shiny surfaces (such as highly polished floors, metal objects, mirrors, and tiled or enameled floors and walls) or when certain types of visual impairments cause light entering the eye to "bounce around," rather than to come into focus. Brightly lit bathrooms are prone to glare, which is worse when they are entered from a dark environment. Some suggestions for reducing glare are to install dimmer switches; to clean but not polish floors and other surfaces; to use carpets and wallpaper instead of tile or enamel paint on walls and floors; and to wear sunglasses, a hat with a large brim, or a visor or to carry an umbrella in places where glare is unavoidable.

Light-Dark Adaptation. Most older persons have difficulty traveling from bright areas to dim ones because the mechanisms that allow people to adapt quickly to changing light no longer work with the same efficiency. Persons who have severely restricted fields, such as those with advanced glaucoma, become functionally blind in dim lighting. Avoiding light-dark areas in the environment will be helpful. When these light-dark areas are unavoidable, the older adult might not be able to see clearly for a period of time until the usual adjustment is made.

Increasing Contrast

Light-dark contrast is produced by the amount of light that is reflected from different surfaces (a light object is brighter than a dark one). This difference in contrast makes objects that contrast with the background easier to see. Therefore, providing an area of dark background and an area of light background in the bathroom, kitchen, and bedroom can help a person more easily identify his or her possessions. For example, if the person's comb and brush are a light color, they may be kept on a dark colored tray, and marking the edges of stairs or steps (especially the top and bottom steps) with contrasting tape makes them more visible.

Using Color

The ability to identify color diminishes with age, and certain types of visual impairments cause problems with color discrimination. However, the use of color in the environment can be helpful if the colors are bright. White or yellow on black is the most visible. Pink, powder blue, and light aqua are usually less distinguishable for persons who are elderly, and dark brown, navy blue, and dark grays tend to blend together.

Specific Applications

This section presents examples of how the instructor or person with low vision can apply the four ways of modifying the environment in each room of a person's home, as well as the yard. In addition to visual modifications, it includes tips on organizing these rooms and suggests modifications that use the other senses. Since each older person has individual needs, it may be necessary to experiment to find the environmental solutions that work best.

Modifying the Bedroom

◆ Lighting should be evenly spread throughout the room, with no bright spots or dark areas.

◆ An incandescent flexible-arm lamp should be used for near tasks, such as reading or sewing. Position the lamp so the light shines over the shoulder on the same side as the better-seeing eye on to the object to be seen, not in the person's face. Experiment with the person to find the best position.

◆ Furniture should contrast in color and shade with the walls, and the edges of the floor and of furniture should be marked with contrasting tape, so the person can avoid tripping or bumping his or her shins.

◆ Wall sockets, light switches, eyeglass cases, and other objects should be marked with contrasting tape or stripes of tape to make them more visible.

◆ Mirrors should be placed where they will not create the illusion of another room or another person in the room or reflect a lightbulb.

◆ Black felt-tip pens and paper with bold lines will help the person write notes that he or she can read later.

◆ Large-print books, a phone with large-print dials or buttons, and large numerals on a clock will be easier to see.

◆ Medications should be marked and organized in specific ways, and directions on medicine bottles should be enlarged to make them easier to find and take.

◆ The room should be organized to help the person predict where items are in the room. If furniture or personal items must be moved, make sure the person is familiar with their new location.

◆ To reduce visual clutter, solid color should be substituted for busy prints on the bedspread, sheets, and an upholstered chair that make it difficult to see items placed on

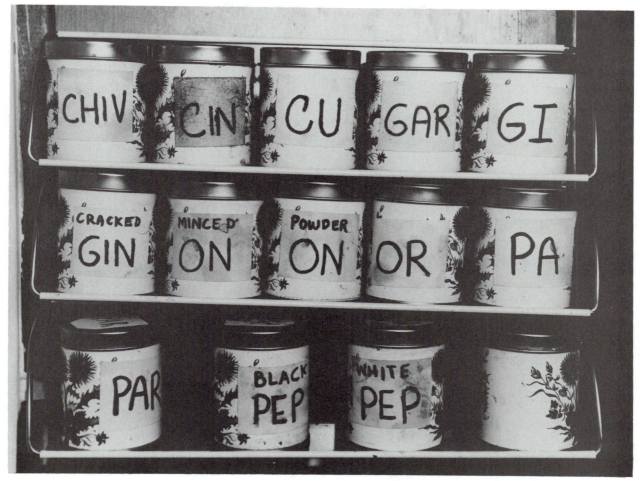

Making modifications at home for an older individual with low vision does not have to be costly. Sometimes, adaptations may be as simple as adjusting lighting around the house or attaching large-print labels to often-used items.

them. Other areas of visual clutter should be reduced by organizing them or simplifying the background.

♦ Doors to the bedroom, adjoining bathroom, and closets should always be left completely open or completely closed because a half-open door could be a safety hazard, and visitors should be reminded of this practice.

Modifying the Kitchen

♦ Lighting should be spread out evenly throughout the room.

♦ Each work station, such as the area over the sink, the stove top, the chopping block, should have its own light source.

♦ There should be areas of light and dark on counter tops and walls to provide contrast when chopping, pouring, and assembling ingredients for a recipe.

♦ The instructor and person should experiment with organizing foods, containers, and dishes, so each item is easier to find using visual and tactile cues. Many items inthe kitchen have a distinctive odor that can also be used for organizing.

- Glassware should be colored or have a pattern, so it is easier to see.
- Dials on often-used temperature settings, lines on measuring cups, and timers should be marked with colored tape.
- Recipes should be rewritten in large print and enclosed in a spiral-bound notebook.
- Mount a reading stand that can be swiveled on a counter too, so recipes will be at the correct height and focal distance for cooking.
- A telephone should have large-print dials or buttons, and commonly called phone numbers should be programmed in speed dial or written in large print.

Modifying the Bathroom

- Lighting should be spread evenly throughout the room; a dimmer switch may be helpful.
- Rugs on the floor and wallpaper will cut down on glare.
- Toothbrushes, cups, and bottles should be brightly colored and in different colors, to make them easier to see.
- One wall should be in a light color and one wall should be in a dark color to assist the person to complete tasks. For example, it is easier to put white toothpaste on a toothbrush against a dark background, and dark bottles or cans stand out better against a light background.
- If the person has light hair, the wall behind the mirror should be dark, and if the person has dark hair, the wall should be light, so the outline of the hair is easier to see and comb.

Modifying the Hallway and Stairway

- Lighting in hallways and on stairs should be bright and spread evenly; if there are pools of light with dark areas, the person may have difficulty adapting visually.

- Walls and steps should be free of clutter, trash cans, and other unnecessary items.
- The edge of each step, (or of the top and bottom steps) should be marked with contrasting tape to make the edges easier to see.

Modifying the Dining Room

- The color of furniture should contrast the color of the floor and walls, and the color of the table and chairs should contrast. Providing contrast will make it easier to see the path between the table and wall and to find a chair. Tablecloths should also be in lighter or darker colors than the walls and should be in solid colors to avoid visual clutter.
- Reflective surfaces, such as mirrors and waxed floors, and bright sunlight from windows should be minimized.
- Food, dishes, and the tabletop should contrast with each other. Light dishes and dark place mats should be used for dark colored food, and dark dishes and light place mats should be used for light colored food.
- Plants, including those in hanging pots, should be placed out of the person's path of travel.

Modifying the Living Room

- Lighting should be bright and evenly distributed throughout the room, lighting fixtures, such as crystal lanterns, sconces, or chandeliers, that provide little overall light and create bright spots and shadows should be avoided.
- The door frames should be in a color that contrasts with the wall color.
- Light colored upholstery should be used for a room with a dark carpet, and dark colored upholstery should be used for a room with a light carpet.
- Space should be provided for the person to move closer to the television screen or sug-

gest that the person buy a large-screen television. The individual may prefer to use optical devices for viewing television.

- An older person's color vision changes when he or she is working on crafts that require the identification of colors, so work surfaces should have contrasting backgrounds.

- The person should use large-print or tactile playing cards.

- The person should use a flexible-arm lamp for auxiliary lighting for crafts, reading, and sewing.

- Encourage the person to obtain large-print books and newspapers at the public library or regional library for blind persons.

- Furniture in conversation areas should be arranged so people can sit closer to or farther away from each other, to help the person see faces as well as possible. Sitting areas in which one person's back is to a sunny window should be avoided.

- Chairs should not have legs that extend outward, since they are a safety hazard.

- A glass door should be marked with decals at eye level, so the person will know if it is open or closed.

Modifying the Garden and Backyard

- The person should wear sunglasses, a large-brimmed hat, or a visor (or a combination of them) to protect his or her eyes from glare.

- Garden paths should contrast with the ground.

- Shrubs and trees should be pruned to eliminate overhanging branches on walks.

- Outdoor furniture should be placed on firm, level surfaces.

- Outdoor furniture should be in a color that contrasts with the surroundings.

PSYCHOLOGICAL CONSIDERATIONS

Psychological Adaptation

Older people's reactions to the development of visual impairments later in life can vary considerably. The way that any individual copes with any loss may be predictive of the way that he or she deals with changes in vision. Thus, it is not possible or productive to use stereotypical beliefs about how an older person will adjust to diminished vision.

Overbury, Greig, and West (1982) found that psychological factors play a significant role in the successful use of low vision devices; for example, when a person with low vision perceived that his or her visual impairment was causing a greater change in lifestyle and/or when the person's anxiety level increased, the use of low vision devices decreased. However, Wheatley (1987) found that although the level of stress increased as an elderly person's vision worsened, there was no relationship between stressful life events and the continued use of low vision devices.

Anxiety and depression are common psychological reactions to the onset of visual impairment, and there are two schools of thought on the timing of rehabilitation intervention for individuals who manifest these reactions. Some rehabilitation professionals subscribe to a "loss theory" of psychological adjustment, such as Carroll (1961) proposed. Others subscribe to a theory that such depression and anxiety are related to a person's perceptions of the negative stereotypes about visual impairment and a lack of confidence and motivation to attempt rehabilitation (Dodds, 1989; Dodds, Bailey, Pearson, and Yates, 1991), but that if rehabilitation is successful, the person's depression and anxiety should be reduced.

Watson, Wright, De l'Aune, and Sweison (1991) administered the Mini-Mult, a 71-item subset of the Minnesota Multiphasic Personality Inventory to persons with ARMD and identified three types of potential clients. The largest group, labeled "normal," should benefit from straightforward rehabilitation programs. The second-largest group, labeled "neurotic," may need more attention and positive reinforcement during rehabilitation and may benefit from short-term counseling to explore some of the maladaptive belief systems they may have. The smallest group, labeled "psychotic," shows signs of more intense psychological distress and should be referred to a mental health professional as part of the rehabilitation process.

The low vision professional will be able to determine whether an elderly person with low vision requires psychological intervention by observing his or her behavior and by listening carefully to what he or she says. Individuals who are experiencing psychological distress may cry; yell; sigh deeply and constantly; speak in a low tone or a monotone; frown or show other signs of sadness and distress, such as rolling their eyes, looking frightened or lost, slumping their shoulders, and jumpiness; and exhibit tactile defensiveness. They may manifest cognitive problems, such as appearing unable to follow a conversation or to repeat directions, or may worry about seemingly inconsequential problems that appear to be unrelated to low vision services.

In all situations of psychological distress, it is important that the instructor remain calm and offer comfort if the distress is acute. If talking briefly about the emotions being exhibited does not allow the person to continue with the evaluation or instruction, the instructor should end the session and attend to the individual's psychological needs more completely. If necessary, the instructor should refer the person for mental health counseling or inform the person's relatives and suggest that they or the instructor consult with or take the person to a mental health professional to determine the extent of the problem and how it can be remediated.

There is no reason that an elderly person who is under the care of a mental health professional should not receive low vision services, provided that the mental health professional is a member of the low vision team. If the evaluation and instruction are carefully controlled to maximize success, the results can provide a tremendous psychological boost. In addition, peer counseling and self-help groups of people with low vision can provide emotional support for all persons who are experiencing vision loss.

Family and Social Support

It is difficult for some older people to express how they are experiencing their visual impairments; for example, a person with cataracts may see well in some instances, but worse if the lighting or reflective surfaces cause glare. Furthermore, elderly people and their family members may misunderstand the ability to see under some circumstances and the failure to see under others. For example, the relatives of a person with constricted visual fields may accuse the person of faking his or her visual impairment to get attention when the individual is able to pick up a dime off the floor, but bumps into a chair or a partially opened door. One elderly woman was able to read her church bulletin when exiting the church into the bright sunlight; thinking that her visual impairment had diminished, she was crushed when she could not read the same print at home.

Visual impairment is experienced by the entire family or caregiving system, not just by the older person, and both social and psychological concerns must be addressed. The loss of vision by one family member can disrupt roles in the family, create economic demands, and add stress when tasks previously performed by the older adult must be performed by someone else. On the one hand, spouses and other family members can reinforce what the person with low vision is learning and can help him or her make the necessary changes in lifestyle. On the other hand, they can be detrimental to the person's adjustment if their expectations are in conflict with the person's visual abilities or goals.

A dramatic example of differences in the functional implications of low vision and dementia is as follows: The family of an elderly woman with cataracts, ARMD, and Alzheimer's disease were at a family reunion when the elderly woman asked one of her daughters, "Who is that woman?" "That woman" was another daughter who was standing facing her mother with her back to a sunny window. The second daughter's facial features had disappeared in the glare, and her mother did not recognize her. That daughter thought that her mother's dementia had progressed, and she burst into tears at the thought that her mother no longer recognized her. Another astute family member asked the daughter to stand facing her mother in the opposite direction, with the sun illuminating her face, rather than obscuring it, whereupon her mother exclaimed, "Well, where have you been?" For the family members who understand the functional implications of visual impairment, it is easier to understand the behavior of their elders with low vision.

In addition to the support of family members, neighbors, and friends, the elderly person with low vision may benefit from a social support group with others who share similar visual impairments. Support groups may be found through multiservice agencies for persons who are visually impaired or may be started by senior citizen's centers or other groups. Two books that were written for older people with low vision and that may lend support are *Out of the Corner of My Eye* (Ringgold, 1991) and *Making Life More Livable* (Dickman, 1983). The first was written by a woman with ARMD, and the second features aging persons as models to demonstrate coping strategies for persons with low vision.

Psychosocial Factors in the Use of Devices and Technology

Even with the best efforts of the low vision rehabilitation team, elderly people often reject low vision devices and technology for a variety of reasons. First, as do other device users, an elderly person may reject a device because it draws attention to the person and marks him or her as different. Second, a person may reject a device, such as a handheld magnifier, because its perceived unattractiveness outweighs the benefits, but find a mirror magnifier, which does not "look" like a low vision device, to be more accept-

able. Third, as was mentioned earlier, a person may not use a device in unsafe neighborhoods because the device may "target" the user as being more vulnerable to criminals.

The low vision team must be open and flexible in discussing all aspects of the device and how the user perceives it. Sometimes modification of the prescription, such as replacing a full-size monocular with a ring telescope that fits in the palm of the hand, can ease the difficulty. At other times, the user may need to weigh the benefits of the device against its negative aspects and try it out at home or among friends to determine whether he or she can get used to it.

SUMMARY

Elderly individuals with low vision can maximize their remaining vision through a variety of mechanisms, including increasing their visual skills, using low vision devices, enhancing the visibility of the environment, using other senses to gather information, and using cognitive skills to supplement vision. Family members and caregivers can help elderly people adjust to their visual impairments by understanding the sometimes contradictory nature of common age-related visual impairments, providing social support, and modifying the home environment and supporting the relearning of visual skills and the use of low vision devices to increase their relatives' independence. Since older people with low vision are at risk for other impairments, a team of professionals should work closely together to optimize the use of vision.

ACTIVITIES

With This Chapter and Other Resources

1. Write a letter to Miss Lil, introduced in the vignette that opens this chapter, to explain the services she might receive through the Mid-Town Services for the Blind. Be sure to

address her concerns about visiting the agency.

2. The family of a 90-year-old woman with cataracts and glaucoma, as well as Alzheimer's disease, is having a difficult time understanding which of her functional difficulties are related to her visual impairments and which are related to her cognitive problems. What professionals should be involved in the rehabilitation team? What information can you provide about functional vision that would be helpful to the team? What questions would you ask the family to learn about its concerns?

3. An 80-year-old man with ARMD is interested in learning to cook, clean house, and shop following the death of his wife. His vision is 20/200 in both eyes. He has been evaluated in a low vision clinic and has been prescribed a handheld magnifier that allows him to recognize small print, a monocular that allows him to recognize the 20/40 line on an acuity chart, and nonoptical devices (a reading stand, typoscope, yellow acetate filters, and a flexible-arm lamp). Write a vision rehabilitation plan for the man's functional assessment and instruction in the use of his vision unaided and with his low vision devices for the activities he wants to pursue.

4. Select a lesson you have prepared for another chapter in this book that teaches a child or young adult a new visual skill. How could the lesson be changed for a 92-year-old woman who needs to learn the skills, but who has hand tremors?

In the Community

1. Conduct an environmental assessment of your home as if a 60-year-old man with diabetic retinopathy (who can no longer see the headlines in a newspaper but can see to choose from among different cereal boxes on a shelf) was going to live there. Recommend the modifications that would allow the man to function as independently as possible.

2. Visit a nursing home in your community and look for environmental modifications that may assist residents who have low vision. What additional recommendations can you make to facilitate the residents' orientation and mobility?

With a Person with Low Vision

1. Go to a grocery store or a department store with an elderly person with low vision. Observe what helps or hinders the person's visual functioning inside the store. What can the store do to provide its customers with low vision the ability to shop with greater ease?

2. Assist an older person who is learning to use an optical device for reading. Consider the efficiency and comfort of using the device. Is the person now able to read the sizes and types of print for which the device was prescribed?

From Your Perspective

What changes will need to take place so more elderly people with low vision receive the rehabilitation services that can benefit them?

Individualized Written Vision Rehabilitation Plan

Learner Name   Mrs. Lillian Thomas   Record Number   00481

I understand that I will receive individual vision rehabilitation lessons in my home and/or other locations.
(specify: home, grocery store, lv service   )

My objectives for vision rehabilitation are:

   reading Bible, recipes, newspaper, prices on grocery or shopping labels

   sewing (buttons, repairs)

   recognizing faces

   seeing grocery aisle signs

   writing checks, balance checkbook

The low vision devices I will be using are:

optical:

   4X microscope

   4X pocket hand held magnifier

   4X monocular

   +8 half-eyes

   chest magnifier

non-optical:

   checkwriting guide, glare tamer, High Marks, reading stand, colored filters,

   typoscope

I will know that I have succeeded when I can:

   read continuous text for 15 minutes

   write checks and balancing checkbook

   recognize faces in church

   read grocery aisle signs and prices in store

   sew on a button and mend a torn hem

I agree to have lessons   one   time(s) a week for   45   minutes each. I agree to keep appointments unless there is an emergency, illness or prior commitment. If I need to cancel a lesson, I will notify my instructor as soon as possible. If my instructor needs to cancel, I will be contacted immediately. I understand that I will need to practice using my vision and low vision devices daily for   20   minutes, and I agree to do this unless I have an emergency or illness.

(continued on next page)

Appendix. Sample Individualized Written Vision Rehabilitation Plan

Individualized Written Vision Rehabilitation Plan (*continued*)

My instructor, my eye care specialist and my social worker and I have reviewed the attached checklist outlining my plan of services. I understand that this list cannot be changed without my approval. My progress can be reviewed at my request. If I am not making progress, not using learned skills, or not doing assigned practice, lessons will end. I may request an administrative review if I do not agree with decisions concerning my program.

We estimate that I will learn these skills by ___October 15, 1997___ (date). When I have learned these skills, I may decide to pursue other skills, or stop vision rehabilitation at this time.

Participation of my family and/or utilization of other resources:

My daughter will participate in the first two training sessions in order to reinforce practice at home. I will be referred for orientation and mobility instruction and rehabilitation teaching instruction at the Mid-Town Services for the Blind. Funding for my program will be sought from Medicare. The LV Therapist will provide an in-home environmental assessment and make recommendations for modifications. I am considering whether I want to join the Older Adults with Low Vision Support Group.

This vision rehabilitation plan has been developed with my full participation and may be revised with my consent on the basis of changing circumstances and/or new information.

Learner _____   Eye Care Specialist _____

Instructor _____

Social Worker _____   Date: _____

(*continued on next page*)

Individualized Written Vision Rehabilitation Plan (*continued*)

This section to be finished when services are completed:

I received individualized vision rehabilitation services in home and/or other locations.

The instructor and I reviewed the plan to determine my plan for services. I learned to use the following low vision devices:

optical:

4X microscope

4X pocket hand held magnifier

4X monocular

+8 half-eyes

chest magnifier

non-optical:

checkwriting guide, glare tamer, High Marks, reading stand, colored filters, typoscope

I learned to use these devices for the following objectives:

reading Bible, recipes, newspaper, prices on grocery or shopping labels

sewing (buttons, repairs)

recognizing faces

seeing grocery aisle signs

writing checks, balancing checkbook

My ability to complete these tasks is (circle):

Satisfactory   Somewhat satisfactory   Not satisfactory

I had the following participation of my family and/or utilization of other resources:

My daughter participated in the first two training sessions. I received orientation and mobility instruction and an environmental assessment at home; rehabilitation teaching instruction was provided at the Mid-Town Services. Partial funding for my program was obtained from Medicare. I have joined the Older Adults with Low Vision Support Group and am now Treasurer.

(*continued on next page*)

Individualized Written Vision Rehabilitation Plan (*continued*)

I understand the other services may be helpful to me if my vision changes and the low vision devices I am presently using are not helpful. I understand that the low vision services will provide follow-up by calling me or visiting me to check on my progress within six months. If I have any difficulty with my low vision devices or using vision, I will contact <u> Janice Cannon </u> at <u> 404-447-2304 </u>.
                                                   (name)   (number)

Learner _____   Eye Care Specialist _____

Instructor _____

Social Worker _____   Date _____

PART FOUR

Changing Perspectives

CHAPTER 17

Low Vision: A History in Progress

Gregory L. Goodrich and Virginia M. Sowell

VIGNETTE

Anita was born in 1915 with congenital cataracts. She lived in Cleveland, and she learned to read large print (36-point type) using the Clear Type reading series in elementary school. In 1928, when Anita was 13, her parents moved to another state, and she was sent to a residential school for children who were blind, where she was taught to read braille. For Anita, both media were beneficial because she could read headlines in newspapers in print and use braille for school work and leisure reading.

As an adult, Anita married, had a child, and did assembly work in a factory. She was widowed during World War II. When she moved to New York City in 1955 to be close to relatives, she went to one of the first low vision clinics, and with special magnifiers, Anita found that she could read standard print. She found a job as a receptionist, answering phones and doing light typing. Anita considered her salary sufficient for her family, but more important, she thought that her vision was not as much of a hindrance as it had been in the past.

In 1957, Anita's grandson, John, was born with congenital cataracts in another state. In the early 1960s, he was placed in sight conservation classes, where he was taught to read large print and was given frequent rest periods. Anita wondered if her experience with magnifiers could help John and why his teachers did not also teach him to read braille or

to use magnifiers. John was fortunate to have Anita as his grandmother. She not only provided emotional support for John as he was growing up but asked the right questions, which resulted in John's receiving a clinical low vision evaluation and an appropriate education.

INTRODUCTION

The field of low vision came into being early in this century because people needed specialized services to meet their specific needs—needs that were not always the same as those of people who were blind or who had correctable visual impairments. This chapter presents a history of the field, based on written accounts of low vision services and the experiences of the authors and their colleagues. Although the history recorded here is relatively brief, it is a rich one that has brought together professionals who received their training in a variety of disciplines in the sciences and human services.

Early in the 20th century, the group identified as "partially sighted" were primarily children, and a few pioneers in special education began to develop programs to meet their needs. Such programs gradually became more prevalent because they were more effective in generating self-reliance and independence than were attempts to teach these children the adaptive skills that well served children who were blind. The number of visually impaired children increased in the second half of the century because of advances in medical care that dramatically improved infant survival rates, but these children had an increased risk of having other disabilities in addition to low vision.

Before World War II, there were no low vision programs for adults with visual impairments and probably little demand for such services, simply because there were few adults with adventitious visual impairments—most such impairments affect older people, and life expectancy in the United States was less than age 65. After World War II, life expectancies increased dramatically, leading to a greater number of adults with severe acquired low vision.

With the increasing numbers of children and adults with low vision, professionals had a greater interest in and devoted more time to meeting the unique needs of this population. Over time, they began to work cooperatively and to learn from each other. In today's system of delivering low vision services, it is sometimes difficult to imagine separate efforts that often pulled individuals with low vision in various directions. This chapter describes five stages of development that contributed to the high quality of services that are available today in more and more locations throughout the world. Sidebar 17.1 provides a time line of developments in the field of low vision from the late 1200s to the present.

STAGE 1: BEFORE THE 1950s

People with low vision were not included in the few references to blindness in the classical literature, such as the biblical story of the conversion of the Apostle Paul, the Greek tragedies, or the works of John Milton and Theresa von Paradis. Whether these writings accurately described the characteristics of people who were visually impaired at that time, knowledge of and services for individuals with low vision developed much later in history than did services for people who were totally blind. In fact, the first services for persons with low vision developed in agencies specializing in services for people who were totally blind.

Early Educational Services

Before the 20th century, distinctions between the educational experiences of children who had low vision and those who were functionally blind did not exist. Children with low vision were taught to read and write in braille and were often fitted with aprons to cover their hands and arms or high collars so they could not read braille with their eyes (Burritt, 1916). In some cases, teachers were told to dim the lights in classrooms to discourage the use of the eyes when reading braille.

In the early 1900s, astute observers in Europe and the United States recognized that children with low vision needed to be educated differently from children who were functionally blind (Hathaway, 1943/1959). James Kerr, the first medical director of the London (England) School Board, included a survey of the visual status of all children in the district in a general school health program. An ophthalmologist, Bishop Harman, found that many of the children covered by this survey had high myopia (nearsightedness) and could see items that were close to their eyes. Kerr reported these results to the Second International Congress of School Hygiene in 1907 and proposed that these children had educational needs that were different from those of children who were totally blind.

In 1908, the London County Council formed the first class in the world for children with low vision, called the Myope School, to differentiate it from schools for children who were blind. In this class, children with low vision did some oral and other nonvisual work with sighted children in the regular school, but they were not supposed to use their vision for reading and writing because they might damage their eyes. A sign over the door of the school read: "Reading and Writing Shall Not Enter Here." Later, large letters were used on chalkboards and enlarged materials were produced with rubber stamps (Hathaway, 1943/1959).

Time Line of Developments in Low Vision

1270   Marco Polo discovers elderly Chinese people using magnifying glasses for reading.

1784   Benjamin Franklin invents bifocal lenses.

1897   Charles Prentice invents the typoscope.

1907   First issue of *Outlook for the Blind* published (later renamed the *New Outlook for the Blind* and, still later, the *Journal of Visual Impairment and Blindness*).

1908   The London County Council institutes the Myope School, the world's first class for children with low vision.

1909   Edward Allen, director of the Perkins Institute, visits the Myope School in London.

1910   M. von Rodgin publishes the first paper on telescopic and microscopic spectacles.

The Clear Type Publishing Company produces a series of 36-point books.

1913   In Roxbury, Massachusetts, Edward Allen starts the first U.S. class for children with low vision called the "defective eyesight class."

Robert Irwin establishes a "conservation-of-vision" class at The Waverly School in Cleveland.

1914   Robert Irwin researches the use of large type and recommends 36-point clearface font.

C. Usher's article on the inheritance of retinitis pigmentosa is published.

1915   The term *sight saving* is coined by the National Society for the Prevention of Blindness.

1916   Olin Burritt, president of the American Association of Instructors of the Blind, attacks the use of aprons and high collars to prevent children with low vision from using their eyes.

1922   P. Baunschwig reports on the use of prisms to aid persons with hemianopsia.

1924   Ophthalmologist Jules Stein and a colleague report on the use of telescopic spectacles at a meeting of the American Medical Association (AMA).

1925   The first specialized university program in the United States to prepare teachers of partially sighted students is instituted at the University of Cincinnati.

1930   Ophthalmologists report that use of vision does not further harm vision of people who are partially sighted

The first issue of the *Sight Saving Review* is published.

1934   Report of the Committee of Inquiry into Problems Relating to Partially Sighted Children, London, is issued.

The AMA defines *legal blindness*.

1935   William Feinbloom's article, "Introduction to the Principles and Practice of Sub-normal Vision Correction," is published.

1938   William Feinbloom reports on 500 low vision cases in the *American Journal of Optometry and Archives of the American Academy of Optometry*.

1940   *Manual on the Use of the Standard Classification of Causes of Blindness* (edited by C. E. Kerby) is published by AFB and the National Society for the Prevention of Blindness.

1942   The American Optometric Association establishes the Department of Visual Adaptation and Rehabilitation.

Time Line of Developments in Low Vision (continued)

Alfred Kestenbaum, a physician, develops the microlense, a simple reading device.

1943   The first textbook on children with low vision, *Education and Health of the Partially Sighted Child,* by Winifred Hathaway, is published.

1947   The American Printing House for the Blind begins the regular publication of large-print books.

1948   M. B. Bender and H. L. Teuber's paper, "Spatial Organization in Visual Perception after Brain Injury" is published.

1953   The first low vision clinics open at the New York Lighthouse and Industrial Home for the Blind.

1954   The first exhibition of low vision aids is organized for the International Congress of Ophthalmologists.

National Aid to the Visually Handicapped, a private organization organized solely to produce large-type textbooks for school-age children, is founded in San Francisco.

1955   Berthold Lowenfeld, an innovative educator of children who are blind and partially sighted, publishes on the psychological problems of children with low vision.

1956   Louise Sloan and A. Habel publish a method for rating and prescribing low vision aids.

1956   The Subnormal Vision Clinic (later called the Low Vision Center) is established at the Maryland Workshop for the Blind.

1957   The Industrial Home for the Blind reports on its optical aids service and defines the basic model for what has become the standard low vision service.

Richard Hoover, an ophthalmologist, presents the functional definitions of blindness.

E. C. Atkinson reports in the *Lancet* on what was probably the first newspaper for people with low vision.

1958   The American Optometric Association establishes the Department of Vision Care of the Aging.

The American Academy of Optometry creates the Prentice Medal to recognize scientists who have significantly advanced knowledge in visual science.

1959   The American Optometric Association establishes the Committee on Aid to the Partially Sighted.

Howard Lewis, an optometrist, reports on a survey of institutions serving the "partially blind."

1960   William Ludlam, an optometrist, reports on the contact lens telescope.

1961   Gerald Fonda evaluates telescopic spectacles for mobility.

1963   Natalie Barraga studies the increased visual behavior of children and develops a visual efficiency scale and sequential learning activities and materials for training children with low vision.

1965   S. C. Ashcroft, Carol Halliday, and Natalie Barraga replicate Barraga's original study on visual efficiency.

Time Line of Developments in Low Vision (continued)

Gerald Fonda's book, *Management of the Patient with Subnormal Vision,* is published.

1966   Conference on Aid to the Visually Limited is held in the United States.

1967   AFB sponsors the Geriatric Blindness Conference.

Ruth Holmes replicates Barraga's (1963) study and reports on visual efficiency training of adolescents with low vision.

1969   Samuel Genensky, a mathematician with low vision, and his colleagues at Rand Corporation in Santa Monica, California, report on their development of the CCTV.

1970   Natalie Barraga's *Teacher's Guide for the Development of Visual Learning Abilities and Utilization of Low Vision,* including the Visual Efficiency Scale, is published by the American Printing House for the Blind.

Loyal Apple and Marianne May's paper on distance vision and perceptual training is published. Apple, though totally blind, advocates vision rehabilitation services for veterans with low vision and helps form the Low Vision Division of the American Association of Workers for the Blind.

The U.S. Office of Education sponsors a Low Vision Conference.

The National Accreditation Council of Agencies Serving the Visually Handicapped publishes standards for producing reading materials for blind and visually impaired persons.

D. R. Korb's article on preparing visually impaired drivers is published.

Eleanor E. Faye's book, *The Low Vision Patient: Clinical Experience with Adults and Children,* is published.

1971   Virginia Bishop's textbook, *Teaching the Visually Limited Child,* is published.

1972   The Low Vision Diplomate program, chaired by Edwin Mehr, is established by the American Academy of Optometry.

Western Michigan University institutes the first required course on low vision as part of its program for preparing O&M personnel.

The Clinical Low Vision Society begins to hold meetings, allowing ophthalmologists and optometrists to discuss topics of mutual interest.

1973   The U.S. Rehabilitation Services Administration sponsors the conference on low vision titled "Services of the Decade of the 70's."

Ophthalmologist Elliot Berson and his colleagues introduce the Pocketscope, a night-vision aid.

Berthold Lowenfeld's book, *The Visually Handicapped Child in School,* is published.

1974   Audrey Smith demonstrates vision stimulation for mobility in her videotape, *Consider Me Seeing.*

The European register of research on visual impairment, by John Gill, is published.

1975   The American Association of Workers for the Blind forms its Low Vision Division.

The American Academy of Ophthalmology forms its Low Vision Society.

The Veterans Administration sponsors the Low Vision Mobility Conference.

Time Line of Developments in Low Vision (continued)

Edwin Mehr and Alan Freid's book, *Low Vision Care,* is published.

In Sweden, Krister Inde and Örjan Bäckman's book, *Visual Training with Optical Aids,* is published.

Eleanor E. Faye and Clare Hood's book *Low Vision,* is published.

1976   Judith Holcomb and Gregory Goodrich's article demonstrates the ability to teach eccentric viewing to older people.

Chris Johnson proposes the "two visual system" theory, which has had a profound effect on the field of low vision.

Health and Safety Associates sponsors the National Conference on Telescopic Devices and Driving.

Ian Bailey and Jan Lovie propose new design standards for visual acuity charts.

The AMA and the American Association of Motor Vehicle Administrators sponsor a conference on telescopic devices and driving.

Large-print calculators become available.

1977   AFB conducts and publishes a survey of low vision clinics.

The U.S. Rehabilitation Services Administration sponsors the Sensory Deficits and Aids Workshop.

The American Academy of Optometry establishes its Low Vision Section, chaired by Randall Jose.

New Outlook for the Blind is renamed the *Journal of Visual Impairment & Blindness.*

1978   The Low Vision Conference is held at the University of Uppsala, Sweden.

Geof Arden proposes contrast sensitivity testing in cases of visual disturbance.

1979   Michael Tobin and his colleagues publish the *Look and Think* book and teachers' handbook in England.

The American Academy of Ophthalmology establishes the Low Vision Committee.

1980   The first Low Vision Ahead Conference is sponsored by the Association for the Blind, Melbourne, Australia.

Robert "Dee" Quillman's *Low Vision Training Manual* is published.

The National Society to Prevent Blindness publishes *Vision Problems in the U.S.*

Ophthalmologist Michael Marmor and his colleagues develop the Wide Angle Mobility Light.

1981   The World Health Organization sponsors a meeting, The Use of Residual Vision by Visually Disabled Persons.

The National Accreditation Council of Agencies Serving the Visually Handicapped establishes standards for low vision services.

In a letter to the editors of the *New England Journal of Medicine,* DeWitt Stetten, a physician, reports his personal difficulty, after developing age-related macular degeneration, in finding low vision services even at the National Eye Institute. This letter led to several actions by ophthalmologists to inform patients of rehabilitation services.

Time Line of Developments in Low Vision (continued)

1982   George Timberlake and his colleagues report on retinal localization of scotoma by scanning laser ophthalmoscopy.

The Electrical Council and the Partially Sighted Society of London report on lighting and low vision.

Olga Overbury and her colleagues report on the psychodynamics of low vision.

Optometrists James Maron and Ian Bailey report on visual factors and mobility performance. Optometrist Jan Lovie-Kitchin and her colleagues in Australia publish *Senile Macular Degeneration.*

The North American Conference on Visually Handicapped Infants and Preschool Children is held.

1983   The *Rehabilitation Optometry Journal* (later renamed the *Journal of Vision Rehabilitation*) is founded by Randall Jose.

Understanding Low Vision, edited by Randall Jose, is published.

Anne Corn's theoretical model of visual functioning for persons with low vision is published.

Vision Research: A National Plan: 1983–87, published by the National Eye Institute, includes a panel on low vision.

Optometrist Steven Whitaker and his colleagues develop the Pepper test of reading skills.

The Pennsylvania College of Optometry offers a master's degree in low vision rehabilitation.

1984   Ian Bailey and Amanda Hall publish the University of California, Berkeley, preferential looking test for infants.

Guidelines for the Production of Materials in Large Type is published by the National Society for the Prevention of Blindness.

Laurence Gardner and Anne Corn's position paper, *Low Vision: Topics of Concern,* is adopted by the Division on Visual Handicaps of the Council for Exceptional Children.

John Gill's first *International Survey of Aids for the Visually Disabled* is published.

Allen Ginsberg's first widely available contrast sensitivity test is published.

Microcomputers become widely used aids for people with low vision.

Dennis Kelleher's personal view of driving with bioptics is published.

David Reagan and his colleagues publish a low-contrast letter acuity chart.

The Royal National Institute for the Blind publishes a demographic study of the visually disabled population in Great Britain.

1985   Corinne Kirchner and her colleagues' first resource guide, *Data on Blindness and Visual Impairment in the U.S.,* is published.

Gordon Legge's first article in widely cited series of psychophysical studies on reading and visual impairment is published.

1986   The Asilomar International Low Vision Conference, sponsored by AFB, is held in Califo...

The Low Vision Conference is held in Waterloo, Canada (University of Waterloo)

Time Line of Developments in Low Vision (continued)

Alfred Rosenbloom publishes *Vision and Aging: General and Clinical Perspectives.*

Geraldine T. Scholl's *Foundations of Education for Blind and Visually Handicapped Children and Youth* is published.

1987   The Conference on Low Vision and Aging is held in Washington, DC.

1988   The International Low Vision Conference, sponsored by AFB, is held in Beverly Hills, California.
The first issue of *Integracion,* a journal on visual impairment and blindness, is published in Spain.

1989   David Loshin and R. D. Juday's article demonstrates spatial remapping.

1990   The conference on AIDS and Low Vision, sponsored by AFB, is held in San Francisco.

The second Low Vision Ahead conference, sponsored by the Association for the Blind, is held in Melbourne, Australia.

The first edition of *Low Vision—The Reference,* a computerized database of the low vision literature, edited by Gregory Goodrich and Randall Jose, is published.

1991   Laurence Gardner and Anne Corn's revised position paper, *Low Vision: Topics of Concern* is ratified by the Division on Visual Handicaps, Council for Exceptional Children.

Paul Freeman and Randall Jose publish *The Art and Practice of Low Vision*

1992   The Americans with Disabilities Act is signed into law.

The World Health Organization holds a Consultation on the Management of Low Vision in Children in Bangkok, Thailand.

Division 7 (Low Vision) of the Association for the Education and Rehabilitation of the Blind and Visually Impaired (AER) publishes a Code of Ethics, Standards of Professional Behavior, and a Body of Knowledge in low vision.

1993   The International Low Vision Conference, sponsored by Visio and the University of Groningen, is held in Groningen, the Netherlands.

The American Academy of Ophthalmology establishes the Shared Interest Group for Low Vision.

1994   The National Eye Institute's Low Vision and ITS Rehabilitation Panel notes that the term *legal blindness* is "an old-fashioned concept, rooted in the premise that vision much below normal is useless."

Rodney Nowakowski publishes *Primary Low Vision Care.*

1995   Joint Commission on Allied Health Personnel in Ophthalmology publishes criteria for subspecialty of Assisting in Low Vision.

1996   *Journal of Videology* begins publication.

International Society of Low Vision Research and Rehabilitation holds its first business meeting.

Vision 96, The International Low Vision Conference hosted by the Organization Nacional de Ciegos Españoles is held in Madrid, Spain.

The notion that the sight of children with low vision needed to be conserved was widely promoted by the National Society to Prevent Blindness (NSPB), which was organized in 1908. A basic tenet of this organization was that children with low vision risked a further loss of sight by using their vision, and in 1915, NSPB coined the term *sight saving* to emphasize this focus on the conservation of sight (Koestler, 1976).

In 1909, Edward E. Allen, director of the Perkins Institute in the United States, visited the Myope School to find ways to alleviate some of the problems of educating children with low vision alongside those who were functionally blind. He had observed that children with low vision often served as guides for those with no vision, felt unrealistically superior, and thought that many of the rules for the safety of students who were totally blind were unnecessary for them. Acting on these observations, Allen was instrumental in starting a class for children with low vision in Roxbury, Massachusetts, in April 1913. This first class of its kind in the United States was called the "defective eyesight class," and the Perkins Institute supplied funds for the materials that were used (Hathaway, 1943/1959; Merry, 1933).

In 1913, Robert B. Irwin, director of special classes for children who were blind in Cleveland, suggested that children with low vision should be separated from those with no vision and that special materials should be developed for them (Koestler, 1976). Therefore, he established a "conservation-of-vision" class at the Waverly School in Cleveland, the second program for children with low vision in the United States. At this school, children with low vision were educated with children with normal vision as much as possible (Hathaway, 1943/1959; Merry, 1933). Irwin was instrumental in promoting the use of a 36-point clearface font with children in the special classes in 1914, and the Clear Type Publishing Company began printing children's books in this font size. Irwin later researched the issue of type faces and decided that 24-point Caslon boldface was preferable (Hathaway, 1943/1959).

As schools began to question the inclusion of children with low vision in schools for the blind, professional organizations began to address the issue. In his president's address to the American Association of Instructors of the Blind (AAIB) in 1916, Olin Burritt attacked the use of aprons and high collars to prevent children from using their eyes and stated that children with low vision should be educated in local schools with specially trained teachers. He added that children who live in rural school districts should be educated in residential schools but should be given "eye-instruction."

Special university programs were instituted in the 1920s, when the NSPB drew up a minimum schedule of courses for the preparation of teachers of children with low vision. The first program, introduced at the University of Cincinnati in 1925, included 30 hours of instruction in methods and materials, observation and practice teaching, and anatomy and physiology of the eye (Hathaway, 1943/1959). In 1943, the first textbook on children with low vision, by Hathaway (1943/1959), was published. In 1947, the American Printing House for the Blind (APH) began to publish textbooks in large type for school-children.

By the end of the 1940s, some 17 or 18 residential schools for the blind had established specially equipped classrooms for children with low vision (Koestler, 1976). In spite of the controversy surrounding low vision, the early decades of this century proved to be too early for widespread change. The principle of sight conservation, as well as sight-conservation classes, prevailed in the majority of public schools.

Roots of Vision Rehabilitation

Perhaps the first documented use of low vision devices occurred when Marco Polo visited China in 1270 and discovered that older people used magnifying glasses to read. During this period, Roger Bacon advanced the concept that contact lenses could be used for magnification (Stein & Slatt, 1995). In 1784, Benjamin Franklin developed bifocal lenses (Scholl, 1986), and in 1897,

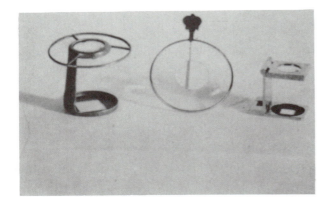

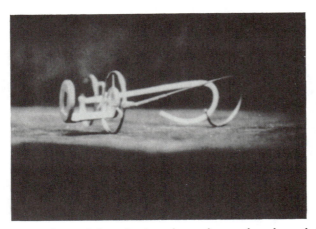

Many low vision devices have been developed since the 1200s, when magnifying glasses were already in use in China. These are some early examples of low vision devices.

Charles Prentice invented the typoscope—a piece of black paper with a viewing window cut in it—for reducing glare and keeping one's place while reading (Prentice & Mehr, 1969).

Low vision devices have been discussed in the optometric and ophthalmological literature since 1910. In that year, Rodgin (1910) published the first professional article on the use of telescopic and microscopic lenses to help those with impaired vision use their vision better. Jules Stein, an ophthalmologist, reported on the benefits of telescopic devices at a meeting of the American Medical Association (AMA) in 1924 (Stein & Gradle, 1924, 1977). Anne Sullivan Macy endorsed the telescopic spectacles, stating, "I never knew there was so much in the world to see." By 1930, ophthalmologists reported that using impaired vision would not further harm the eyes (Scholl, 1986).

In 1934, the AMA defined *legal blindness*, thus separating, in the minds of many, those who had low vision from those who were truly blind (Scholl, 1986). In the Social Security Act of 1935, adults who met the criteria for legal blindness were considered eligible for services and benefits for "the blind," and children were eligible for specialized materials, entrance to schools for the blind, and so forth.

During the mid-1930s, William Feinbloom, an optometrist and psychologist, began to develop optical devices to enhance the use of vision by persons with low vision. Feinbloom was arguably the most influential of the early founders of low vision services and invented numerous low vision devices (Feinbloom, 1931, 1935).

A pioneer in the use of optical devices, Alfred Kestenbaum, a Viennese physician, found that a patient with macular degeneration used magnification to read. In 1942, he designed a simple reading device, called the microlens (or microglass), which used small-diameter high-plus lenses; the small diameter was used to minimize aberrations (Sloan, 1977). Kestenbaum was also an early advocate of the use of magnifying lenses for some patients (Kestenbaum, 1953).

Before the 1950s, uncorrectable visual impairments were considered the province of physicians (typically ophthalmologists), and the only option for a person who wanted to improve his or her "residual" vision was surgery (Hellinger, 1967). Ophthalmologists were generally not comfortable with people who had low vision because conditions that caused low vision, like those that caused total blindness, were not treatable medically, and thus these people represented a "failure" of the medical system. Robert Bowers (personal communication, 1993) noted that "since blindness was seen as a failure by the professionals, they were uneasy with individuals who had less than the magic 20/200 visual acuity."

STAGE 2: 1950s TO 1970s

The first modern stage in the development of the field of low vision began in the early 1950s and lasted until the mid-1970s. In this stage, each professional discipline developed a knowledge base relevant to treating people with low vision. Gradually, the emphasis on sight saving in educational programs was replaced by the view that the vision of children with partial sight was not a fixed quantity that could be used up. Optometrists were learning to prescribe optical devices, discovering which optical features were important for low vision devices, and developing reliable clinical measurements in low vision care, and both ophthalmologists and optometrists were beginning to develop successful (albeit limited) low vision practices.

Educational Programs' Focus on the Use of Vision

In the 1950s, the trend toward including children with low vision in public schools began to accelerate (Hanninen, 1979), and educators began to look for new ways of working with these children (Ashcroft, 1963). During this stage, educators were experimenting to determine educationally sound methods for teaching children with low vision to use their visual potential, rather than to "conserve" their sight. In 1954, National Aid to the Visually Handicapped—the first national organization devoted solely to producing large-print books for people with low vision—was started in San Francisco when a mother noted the need to provide large-type textbooks for her son.

In the 1960s, Barraga (1964) developed a visual efficiency scale and a set of sequential learning activities and materials designed to develop "visual efficiency" in children with low vision; her dissertation research was a turning point in the way many educators viewed these children's use of vision. Ashcroft, Halliday, and Barraga (1965) replicated the original study and found the same results, as did Holmes' (1967) replication of the study with adolescents. These three studies were responsible for the major shift in the focus of instruction. In 1970, APH published Barraga's Visual Efficiency Scale and teacher's guide. (Barraga and Morris's, 1980, *Program to Develop Efficiency in Visual Functioning* was a revision of Barraga's earlier work.)

A federal survey in 1960 showed that more than half the children in public school classes for children with visual impairments read large print, as did 29 percent of those in residential schools (Koestler, 1976). Jan, Freeman, and Scott (1977) criticized large-print books as being "generally oversized, heavy, and cumbersome" and lacking in color and interest to children. However, large-print books continued to be used widely in school programs.

Orientation and mobility (O&M) instructors were just beginning to recognize that children with low vision could benefit from their services and that techniques could be developed to enhance these children's visual functioning. Smith's (1974) classic videotape, *Consider Me Seeing*, so titled because a child spontaneously used this phrase in the videotape, was issued. Smith, an O&M instructor, was an early influential advocate of low vision instruction.

Growth of Vision Rehabilitation

Although the development of low vision services for adults has generally trailed the development of low vision services for children, major advances were made during this stage. Lens systems and clinical techniques to enhance the visual function of adults with low vision were not developed until the mid-1950s (Scholl, 1986).

Before 1955, the most commonly prescribed low vision optical device for reading was the telescopic loupe (Sloan, 1977). From 1955 on, however, the number and variety of low vision devices expanded rapidly, thanks, in large part, to the work of such pioneers as Gerald Fonda, Louise Sloan, George Hellinger, and Feinbloom (Bier, 1970; Fonda, 1965). Hellinger (1967, p. 297), noted that from the early 1950s to the mid-1960s, "a virtual revolution has taken place in vision rehabilitation" for adults.

In 1953, the first low vision clinics for adults and children opened in New York at the New York Association for the Blind, under the direction of Fonda, and the Industrial Home for the Blind established a low vision service under the direction of Hellinger (Faye, 1970). In 1955, Fonda, who has been credited with coining the term *low vision*, published a report of his clinical experience with 200 patients with low vision. In 1957, the Industrial Home for the Blind published a survey of its first 500 cases, using a model of rehabilitation services that was the forerunner of modern low vision services and the interdisciplinary team. Optical aid clinics quickly gained acceptance in the 1950s and were approved by the federal government as a component of the vocational rehabilitation program in 1957 (Apple, Apple, & Blasch, 1980).

By the late 1950s, the U.S. Veterans Administration (VA) began to develop low vision services (Goodrich, 1991) and rapidly assumed a leadership role in promoting the development of low vision services, training, and devices, a role that it continues to play today. In rehabilitation settings, such as the VA's Hines Blind Center, O&M techniques that had so dramatically improved travel for veterans who were newly blind were being adapted to the emerging population of veterans with low vision.

The emergence of perceptual psychology also influenced the development of low vision services. The work of Kohler (1964), for example, demonstrated that one could learn to adapt to inverting prisms (prisms that visually turned the world upside-down) and thus provided support for the view that adults who became partially sighted later in life might also relearn visual function by adapting to a degraded retinal image or scanning with a constricted visual field. The ability to relearn visual function was a necessary tenet for the establishment of low vision services, since without this visual perceptual capacity, vision rehabilitation would not be possible. Other perceptual psychologists, notably Eleanor and J. J. Gibson and their students (see Gibson, 1991), were exploring the development of vision and constructing a theory of visual perception. Their work contributed to the understanding of the role of developmental factors and learning in low vision and of normal visual perception.

In 1956, Sloan and Habel published a method for rating and prescribing low vision devices. Sloan, a psychologist, was an early advocate of low vision, as well as for the systematization of low vision testing and devices.

In the late 1950s, Potts, Volk, and, West (1959) proposed a radical departure from conventional optical devices: the use of a closed-circuit television system (CCTV) as an improved reading device. However, it was not until almost a decade later that Samuel Genensky, a mathematician at the Rand Corporation in Santa Monica, California, and his colleagues developed the first commercially viable low vision CCTV system (Genensky, Baran, Moshin, & Steingold, 1969). Genensky, who had low vision, developed the CCTV primarily to improve his own reading abilities; however its unparalleled ability to improve reading performance led to its almost immediate widespread use in educational and vocational settings and later for avocational pursuits.

A 1966 survey by the Chicago Lighthouse for the Blind reported that 68 percent of the persons who were referred for low vision services benefited from optical devices (Rosenbloom, 1966). This and similar surveys supported the view that low vision devices were helpful in a majority of cases, but they also raised concerns about why almost a third of the clients did not benefit. Clinical practice in low vision clinics followed the interdisciplinary team model and promoted the need for additional research. This research quickly demonstrated the increasing benefit of low vision services; for example, later follow-up studies of CCTVs demonstrated that 87 percent of the persons for whom these devices were prescribed were still using them four years later (see Goodrich, Mehr, & Darling, 1980).

Contributions of Professional Organizations and the Literature

In the 1970s important roles were played by three professional organizations: the Low Vision Section of the American Academy of Optometry, the Low Vision Division of the American Association of Workers for the Blind, and the Low Vision Clinical Society of the American Academy of Ophthalmology. These groups actively solicited papers and panels on low vision for presentation at their annual conferences, which came to be critical forums on topics specific to low vision.

In 1972, the American Academy of Optometry established the Low Vision Diplomate program, with Edwin Mehr as its first chair. Mehr was an influential low vision clinician and researcher at the time, and his private practice was one of the first in the United States. Mehr and his wife, psychologist Helen Mehr, advocated the incorporation of psychosocial considerations in low vision care (Mehr & Mehr, 1969).

Members of the three organizations debated on a wide variety of topics, including the value of newly developed low vision devices; the appropriate role of each profession in the low vision team; and whether visual function could be retrained and, if so, how. The leaders in these organizations included Feinbloom, Fonda, Eleanor Faye, Hellinger, Alfred Rosenbloom, Mehr, and Randall Jose, among many others. All promoted a low vision ethic that no device or idea should be accepted on faith, but that research must prove its value and clinical practice must show its validity. Effectiveness in research and clinical practice and the promotion of the functional nature of vision were the touchstones of these three organizations.

A number of influential books were published in this period, including Fonda's (1965) and Faye's (1970) textbooks. Faye was the most influential ophthalmologist in low vision and took the lead in advocating for advancement of low vision, the education of ophthalmologists, and the development of high standards of low vision practice. In addition, Mehr and Freid (1975) wrote a textbook for optometrists, and Bishop (1971) wrote the first textbook for special educators since Hathaway's (1943/1959) original book almost 30 years earlier.

This second stage, then, was characterized by professionals learning about low vision within their own disciplines. It was a time when a population that had been relatively ignored began to receive professional attention by a few pioneers in each discipline.

STAGE 3: MID-1970s TO MID-1980s

During Stage 3, from the mid-1970s to the mid-1980s, professionals in the field sought to develop a team approach to low vision care, knowing that each discipline alone could not offer a person with low vision what a multidisciplinary team could provide. Although the foundation for this stage was laid in 1957 at the Industrial Home for the Blind, it was not until the late 1970s that each discipline had sufficient expertise and a sufficient number of experienced low vision professionals to make a meaningful contribution to the team approach. The growth in low vision services were "driven, in large part," by the demagraphic imperative of the aging population" (Rosenbloom & Goodrich, 1990).

Growth of Educational Programs

The passage of the Education for All Handicapped Children Act (P.L. 94-142) in 1975 forever changed the landscape of special education. Since then, children with low vision have increasingly been educated in public school settings. Multidisciplinary teams became important components of the Individualized Education Programs for children and youths. Educators were beginning to research such topics as print media and optical devices, exploring ways to work with children with multiple disabilities, and developing theories of visual functioning. To do so, they needed to learn about the work of other disciplines and services.

Expansion of Vision Rehabilitation Services

In rehabilitation settings, the optometrist's low vision evaluation and prescription were sought before an individual's potential to work on a job that required visual functioning was determined. Low vision programs at The Lighthouse in New York; the School of Optometry at the University of California, Berkeley; and VA facilities were actively publishing studies on low vision and creating a science of low vision care. Technology also came to play a major role, with the introduction of CCTVs, which are now standard fixtures in both special education and vision rehabilitation programs.

By 1975, low vision was recognized as an international field. Much of the credit for this recognition goes to the work of Inde and Bäckman (1975), whose book was a seminal publication that advocated for a structured, coherent rehabilitation program that would combine vision training and the use of optical devices within the interdisciplinary team model. Quillman (1980) expanded on the development of training materials in a book that is still widely used. Interest in low vision mobility was heightened by the 1975 VA sponsored Low Vision Mobility Conference held at Western Michigan University (Apple & Blasch, 1976), which integrated orientation and mobility instructors into the low vision team.

The publication of Inde and Bäckman's book coincided with the publication of two articles that reinforced the exciting new view of visual function. Johnson's (1976) article on the relevance to low vision of the theory of two visual systems states that the visual system is composed of two distinct sensory perceptual systems: one system for localization (the so-called where system) and one system for identification (the so-called what system). This was an exciting theory because it differentiated visual perception anatomically and functionally. Holcomb and Goodrich's article (1976) demonstrated that eccentric viewing could be taught to older people who lost central vision and that the function of the "what" system could be taken over by the "where" system, thus validating an important premise of vision rehabilitation. According to this premise, the visual perceptual system is plastic and retains its plasticity throughout the lifespan; thus adults, like children, can learn to use remaining areas of their visual fields to perform functions that are usually associated with the damaged areas.

During the 1980s, refinements continued to be made in both near and distance devices, and great strides were made in creating technology to give persons with low vision access to microcomputers. Conventional low vision reading devices allowed many people with low vision to use computers, however persons with lower levels of visual function benefited from a large-print computer-access program (McGillivray, 1994). Large-print access programs are usually software programs that enlarge computer print and display it in black and white, color, or reversed polarity, depending on the needs of the individual. In the late 1980s, some eight large-print computer programs were available.

During this stage, the American Foundation for the Blind (AFB) established the position of national consultant in low vision, a prominent position, both nationally and within the organization. In 1977, the name of AFB's journal, *New Outlook for the Blind* was changed to the *Journal of Visual Impairment & Blindness,* to include persons with low vision in the journal's identity. In 1983, the field benefited from such publications as Jose's book, which became a mainstay of professionals in educational and rehabilitation settings, and by the introduction of the *Rehabilitation Optometry Journal,* which was devoted to vision rehabilitation. In 1984, Gardner and Corn's position paper, which promoted the use of optical devices and the judicious use of large-print materials by children with low vision, was adopted by the Council for Exceptional Children's Division for the Visually Handicapped.

Professional preparation programs in universities also began to change their curricula in response to the growth of low vision programs. In 1972, Western Michigan University became the first university-based O&M program to require a course in low vision mobility (Apple, Apple, & Blasch, 1980). This practice was soon adopted by virtually all O&M and rehabilitation teacher preparation programs. However, even today, university curricula in O&M and rehabilitation teaching place more emphasis on techniques for rehabilitating persons who are blind than on techniques for rehabilitating persons with low vision. In response to the need for greater depth in personnel preparation, the Pennsylvania College of Optometry founded its master's program in vision rehabilitation in 1983. That this program is still the only degree program in vision rehabilitation highlights the need for additional educational opportunities.

STAGE 4: MID-1980s TO MID-1990s

In the mid-1980s, Stage 4 began to emerge, characterized by movement beyond each profession's areas of expertise to the collective provision of services for those with low vision. Thus, professionals of each discipline learned the selected philosophies, skills, and techniques of associated disciplines and how to incorporate them into a comprehensive low vision plan. For example, more educators and rehabilitation teachers began to learn how to read prescriptions for optical devices and to see the relationship among a child's or adult's visual functioning, a prescription, and the task at hand. Optometrists began to learn about the skills of educators in assessing children with multiple disabilities in addition to low vision. Optometrists learned from such disciplines as O&M; for example, by using sighted guide techniques, they became better able to provide assistance and security to their patients who enter their offices and attempt to locate the examining chairs. Rehabilitation professionals developed expertise in taking clinicians' prescriptions and incorporating them into training programs that would give clients the opportunity to relearn to use their visual abilities. Furthermore, microcomputer technology adapted for computer users with low vision attracted personnel who were skilled in assistive technology. These developments expanded the breadth of the interdisciplinary team and created exciting new educational, vocational, and avocational opportunities for people with low vision.

The field of low vision also struggled with such ethical questions as who should prescribe low vision devices and whether persons with low vision should be granted driver's licenses. Practical concerns arose as well: Which profession had responsibility for persons with low vision, or did the responsibility shift among practitioners, depending on the clients' needs and progress? To help answer these questions, conferences were held and special projects were initiated with the explicit goal of bringing various professionals together, so they could learn from each other and mutually increase their expertise and cooperative abilities. In 1986, the first International Low Vision Conference to be held in the United States, sponsored by AFB, was held in California. As a result, professionals learned new combinations of skills that resulted in better direct services, as well as better-designed research projects, which, in turn, fostered better care.

During this period, approximately 35 teacher preparation programs and 14 O&M programs, based in universities, were preparing professionals to work with children with low vision. These preparation programs included courses in visual assessment, low vision devices, and other topics that were not available in the early days of instruction.

The use of low vision devices and standard-size print materials for children with low vision was advocated primarily by Corn (1990). Corn's article highlights a controversy that arose in special education over the relative benefits of producing large-print materials for children with low vision or of training children to use low vision devices. Large-print books were criticized because relatively few titles were available and such materials might stigmatize the children who used them. Although large-print books were beneficial in the past, in an era in which low vision devices were well known, readily available, and less costly than specialty printings of large-print books, their continued use was considered questionable.

In 1991, the Division for the Visually Handicapped of the Council for Exceptional Children ratified Gardner and Corn's (1991) revised position paper advocating the use of optical devices

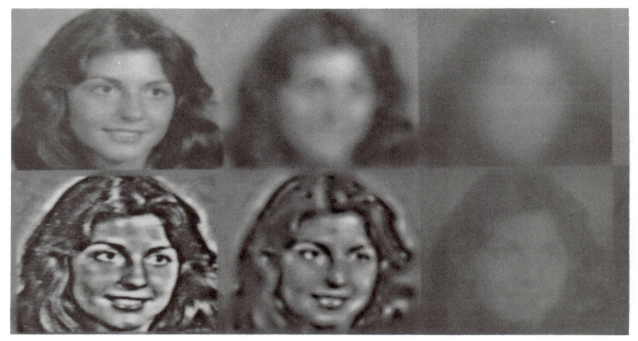

Among the many advances that have taken place in computer technology for persons with low vision is the enhancement of images, shown here in the bottom row.

to provide print access to children with low vision. The main premise of this paper was that "properly prescribed optical devices are essential for maximizing a child's visual function" (p. 6). Corn and Koenig (1991) wrote that the use of large print was a restrictive approach to the visual environment and called for a national effort to give all children with low vision the opportunity to be evaluated for the use of optical devices.

Microcomputer technology showed promise in constructing low vision devices tailored to the needs of the individual. Even with CCTV technology, clinicians had little ability to improve the image presented to the person with low vision. Computer technology could take a video image and modify it in interesting ways and then display it to the person. Peli, Arend, and Timberlake (1986) demonstrated that the enhancement of selected frequencies of an image could improve functional vision for such activities as reading and facial recognition (see also Peli, Goldstein, Young, Trempe, & Buzney, 1991). A few years later, Loshin and Juday (1989) demonstrated spatial re-

mapping, a technique with the potential to extract information that would fall within the borders of a scotoma and remap it so that the information would be presented to surrounding, functional areas of the retina. Neither technique is as yet available in a low vision device, but developmental work continues (Massof & Rickman, 1992). Although these microcomputer-controlled low vision devices are still in their infancy, they hold a greater potential of revolutionizing low vision services than did the video technology of the 1970s.

STAGE 5: THE PRESENT

The field of low vision is currently in its fifth stage of development, in which each profession needs the other professions' literature and all are finding common ground by publishing across professional disciplines. For example, the *Journal of Visual Impairment & Blindness* publishes articles by authors from a variety of disciplines. Of major significance is that the field of low vision has generated its own multidisciplinary publication, the *Journal of Vision Rehabilitation* (founded in 1983 as the *Rehabilitation Optometry Journal*).

Interdisciplinary efforts are also being demonstrated in conferences, guest lectures, university curricula, and research projects. Each year, over 350 works on low vision are published. A review of *Low Vision—The Reference* (Goodrich & Jose, 1993), a comprehensive bibliography of the field, shows that rehabilitation and special education journals account for about 25 percent of the publications; optometry and ophthalmology journals account for about 30 percent; and journals from such diverse professions as psychology, education, computer science, and engineering, account for about 40 percent.

In 1993, the International Conference in Low Vision brought together over 600 professionals from 60 countries. At that conference, held in the Netherlands, the International Society for Low Vision Research and Rehabilitation, whose purpose is to further research and rehabilitation of persons with low vision worldwide, was formed.

The authors believe that this stage will launch the field of low vision into the new century. Professionals will need to work together and find the strength, unity, and purpose to become proponents and advocates not only for each other, but especially for people with low vision.

SUMMARY

Advances in the education of children with low vision began early in this century, but widespread improvements have occurred largely since the 1950s. Services for adults with low vision, which have developed since the 1950s, were largely driven by the rapid growth in the number of visually impaired elderly people caused by the longer lifespan of persons in the United States. Clinical experience and research since the 1960s have provided a basis for using instructional programs with persons who have low vision. University programs for preparing specialized teachers developed across the country, as did programs for pre-

paring O&M instructors and rehabilitation teachers for adults with low vision. The most effective services to children and adults with severe visual impairments are those that use the multidisciplinary model, the application of which has become widespread.

As a result of the increased attention to the individual needs of people with low vision, services have evolved into a discipline with strong focus on assessment and training of visual function. Instead of sight saving, the emphasis is now on the optimum use of functional vision, which has been further advanced by new optical devices and the application of video and computer technology. These historical gains have resulted in unprecedented opportunities for people with low vision, yet many challenges remain. One can only hope that a history written 40 years from now will be able to report as much progress.

ACTIVITIES

With This Chapter and Other Resources

1. Briefly compare the evolution of services for children and for adults with low vision, using Anita and John from the vignette that opens this chapter to illustrate various points.

2. Prepare a brief presentation on the history of optical devices to help an association for the blind that is putting together a museum display of optical devices to open its new low vision clinic.

3. Consider how changes in educational practices, attitudes toward persons with disabilities, and medical practices have paralleled the development of low vision services. How have these changes facilitated the evolution of services?

4. Read one of the classic journal articles or books written before 1950. Compare the recommended practices at the time the article or book was written with current practices.

In the Community

1. Interview a clinical low vision specialist who has provided services for at least 20 years. Ask

about changes that have occurred in the philosophy of services, advances in optical devices, and challenges to the field.

2. Contact agencies that provide services to persons with low vision in your community. Determine the length of time the various agencies have been in operation and how their services have changed over time.

With a Person with Low Vision

1. Interview an elderly person with congenital low vision and ask about the educational practices that were used by teachers when he or she was in school.

2. Interview an elderly person who acquired low vision during early adulthood and inquire about the rehabilitation practices that were used during that time.

From Your Perspective

In what ways can a knowledge of history help shape the future quality and availability of low vision services?

CHAPTER **18**

What the Future May Hold

Alan J. Koenig and Anne L. Corn

VIGNETTE

Jim, a planet cartographer on a space station, has a family history of macular degeneration. With his parents and grandparents, the disease began well into their 90s, but with a life expectancy in the 24th century of 120 years, the 90s is no time to start having visual problems without doing something about them. Jim's grandfather had a device which was invented in the 22nd century, implanted behind his eyeball, that boosted the impulses sent to his brain, so the central scotoma could virtually be ignored. Jim's father had an injection of Xonbjk-42, which helped his retina to produce new cells in the macula while the diseased macula was "digested" by the pigment epithelial layer of the retina. Jim just hit his 98th birthday, and in a routine physical examination, he was told that he was developing macular degeneration.

Jim asked his physician, "Is it time for the injection?"

"You have a choice," his physician replied. "I can give you the injection, which will help your retina create more cone cells, or I can just exchange your eye for an eye that can be replicated from your DNA pattern and then reconnect your optic nerve with an NAC (Nerve Array Connector). Either way, you'll be out of here in about 1 hour and 20 minutes."

Jim thought about his choices for a few moments and then chose to have the injection. The other method was just too new for him, and the NAC had only been invented two years before.

INTRODUCTION

The vignette that opens this chapter implies that by the twenty-fourth century, the functional implications of low vision that are due to macular degeneration will be eliminated. If the reader finds remnants of *Star Trek: The Next Generation* in this vignette, he or she is correct, since both authors of this chapter are enthusiasts of that television series. However, the seriousness of macular degeneration in the twentieth century cannot be discarded with a fantasy, and the implications of the medical and optical research that is now being done cannot be overestimated. Advances in technology will not cure the world, though its promise is ever present.

Indeed, the first generation of the Low Vision Enhancement System, a head-borne device that electronically enlarges images at a distance, as though the individual has a head-borne closed-circuit television (CCTV), has been developed by researchers at Johns Hopkins University. Researchers have also developed devices that enhance contrast through electronic filtering and use image remapping techniques that "can change spatial relationships as well as the position of objects within the field by reassigning the

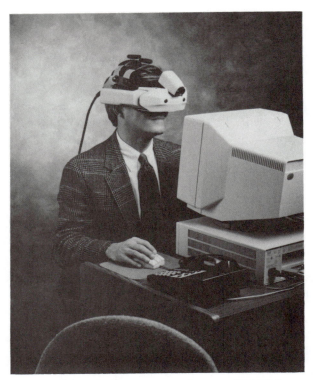

A Low Vision Enhancement System (LVES) functions much like a head-borne closed-circuit television and can be used for near, intermediate, and distance vision tasks. In the future, this device and others will perhaps be readily available to people with low vision.

location of each pixel [on a video display]" (Loshin, 1993, p. 20).

Researchers at Vanderbilt University are studying the regeneration of retinal cells in goldfish that regrow their own retinal tissue after being injected with retina-destroying substances (M. Powers, personal communication, February 1995). In Israel, researchers are recovering visual responses in injured optic nerves of rats by treating them with transglutaminase (Eitan et al., 1994).

If medical and optical advances progress as the authors hope they will, then a text such as this will no longer be necessary, nor will professions that evolve from the need to provide educational, vocational, and vision rehabilitation services to people with low vision. Until that time arrives,

however, it is prudent to prepare, at least for the next 50 years, so children and adults with low vision can become successful and competent. The authors hope that the future holds medical advances, advanced technology, the provision of better services, and a better understanding of low vision by people with low vision and the society in which they live. This chapter revisits some of the children and adults presented in the vignettes of the previous chapters and suggests what they could experience in the twenty-first century. It concludes by presenting the authors' thoughts on future research.

Most of the information presented in this chapter, especially the discussion of the future of people in the vignettes, is purely fictional. Although the predictions are based on the direction of medical, technological, and other advances, no one can know with certainty what the future will bring. Therefore, these perspectives on the future are offered to promote creative thinking on what may eventually be common and practical solutions to the needs of people with low vision.

PERSPECTIVES FOR THE FUTURE

Medical Advances

Medical researchers have different approaches to solving the effects of low vision. Whereas some researchers are seeking new ways to regenerate living tissue, others are looking more specifically at the genetic components that alter the effect and progress of malformations and hereditary degenerative diseases or are seeking approaches that will prevent, circumvent, or provide a cure for a pathology. What effects would such medical advances have on John and Bjorn (discussed in Chapter 3) and Jenny (discussed in Chapter 2)?

John

John, who had lost all but light perception because of retinitis pigmentosa (RP) by the time he was 38, received a call from a medical center in 2032 requesting his participation in the first human trials of retinal replacement therapy. He was both apprehensive and excited about participating in the trials, since he had finally come to grips with his blindness and was truly content with his work, his family, and his life experience. After much thought about his experiences in losing vision, John decided to participate in this research because it might alleviate the anguish that teenagers with RP undergo knowing that their retinas are slowly degenerating.

Bjorn

A middle-aged father of three, Bjorn had aniridia and used a variety of light-absorptive lenses. In 2010, medical researchers teamed up with biomedical engineers to develop an artificial iris that could adapt to changes in light, and a high-tech company had developed a new microchip that, though intended for a new space station's light-filtering system, was the answer to Bjorn's light-gathering problems. When Bjorn received a call to try out the new artificial iris, he thought about how wonderful it would be to discard his numerous light-absorptive filters. Although he knew that his visual acuity would probably remain the same, he thought that he might be able to function more comfortably and even enjoy playing golf outdoors on bright, sunny days. Although the malformation of his anterior segment was still present, Bjorn was also concerned about developing glaucoma and vision loss.

Jenny

As a child with congenital nystagmus and cataracts, Jenny wore thick tinted lenses. When she was 18, she received an intraocular lens implant. In 2015 a new contact lens was developed that truly stopped the apparent oscillations of her eyes. Jenny uses optical devices that fit into her eyeglasses without any cosmetic detraction. In her late 40s, she is still struggling with feelings of inadequacy. Medical science alleviated her visual challenges, but it could not eliminate the effects of her earlier emotional hurts. Although Jenny is successful in her career and in her family life, she still feels as though she has to hide the feelings she has about her medical condition.

Technological Advances

At the start of the twenty-first century, the information superhighway propelled this society into a period of new technological advances that were barely even imaginable in the 1990s. Although in the year 2016 many people react to these advances with awe and amazement, believing that technology has the potential to expand opportunities, others regard them with great skepticism, doubting that technology will solve all life's problems. For people with low vision, technology has solved some of the functional problems of low vision, and they look to the future for optical-technological devices to alleviate or reduce the problems that medical science and existing low vision devices have not solved. What changes would technological advances make in the lives of Billy (Chapter 7), Miss Lil (Chapter 16), and Herb (Chapter 13).

Billy

Armed with a magnifier and a telescope obtained in a clinical low vision evaluation, Billy, who had optic nerve atrophy, was ready to tackle academics in his sixth-grade class. Twenty years later, he is an architect. Although his optical devices had been efficient for learning through high school and college, architecture presents new visual demands that require more precision and a greater need to see larger, magnified areas at a glance. The CCTVs of the twentieth century could have helped him with these needs. However, because of recent advances in technology Billy wears eyeglasses that are near vision magnifiers that electronically enlarge and accommodate to the distance from the page, so his view of architectural plans are more easily seen.

Miss Lil

Twenty years after Miss Lil, then age 70, went to her first clinical low vision evaluation, she is now cooking, reading the Bible, and seeing the faces of her great-great-grandchildren. Image remapping has become commonplace for individuals with macular degeneration, and the devices fit neatly in the temples of a conventional pair of eye-glasses. At age 70 Miss Lil commented that she was "missing out on life" because of her low vision. Today, however, she complains more about her arthritis than anything else. During her weekly volunteer hours at a senior citizens center, she has become friendly with Joe Lewis, who is totally blind and plays cards, cooks for himself, and enjoys his great-great-grandchildren. She has come to realize that although she was fortunate to regain much of her functional visual abilities through advances in technology, her life could have become as rich and fulfilled as that of her newfound friend.

Herb

After Herb learned to use his new orientation and mobility (O&M) skills to get around the city, he was able to retain his job at the shoe store and to help his parents with their errands. Herb explored much of his local community. However, with his cognitive disability, he was cautious about going into areas where sighted assistance was not readily available.

On his 52nd birthday, Herb's sister presented him with a TechnoMap, a new device that would expand his potential for traveling in unfamiliar areas. Herb had benefited from simplified maps, and his sister had programmed the characteristics of maps that Herb would be able to understand into the TechnoMap. Through a satellite link, Herb was now able to record his destination, hit a button, and receive both verbal and simplified map instructions on how to proceed. Herb's sister had hopes that with his new confidence in mobility and his new TechnoMap, he will feel freer to travel to friends' houses and have more companionship.

Provision of Services

By the beginning of the twenty-first century, low vision services were a recognized part of the medical, educational, and rehabilitation programs offered to people with disabilities. Legal definitions of blindness no longer were used, and functional assessments guided the provision of education, rehabilitation, and clinical services for persons with low vision. By 2010, philosophical views on educational programming practices, such as full inclusion, had been replaced by a shared view that all program options have equal merit and status when appropriate matches are made between the needs of the students and the services that meet those needs. Rehabilitation services had developed into a more cohesive system so that all individuals who need services to enter gainful employment received them.

With strides in integrating the education and rehabilitation systems, transition services had been defined and coordinated to allow more efficient transitions from school to work. As a result, the unemployment rate among persons with low vision is steadily approaching the rate for the general public. The elderly population with low vision has swelled to the extent that they are now seen as a political force. Organizations that address the needs of senior citizens have taken proactive measures to ensure that services are provided and the public understands the needs of persons with low vision. How have these developments affected the circumstances of José (Chapter 11) and Tracy (Chapter 9)?

José

As a child José read so slowly that his teacher of children with visual impairments conducted a learning media assessment (LMA) to determine why his reading was at such a low rate of speed and whether print was efficient for his learning needs. The results of his LMA indicated that with targeted reading instruction to gain fluency while using his optical device, he had the potential to attain a more normal reading speed. By the time José was in high school, he was silently reading 210 words per minute.

As a state senator, José now has a great deal of reading to do, as well as many speeches to deliver. He still experiences visual fatigue after about 30 minutes of continuous print reading. Given that much of his communication now occurs through telecommunications, he can balance what he reads in hard copy with what he obtains through synthesized speech from his computer. While on a trip to a small community in Newfoundland, José lost the case containing his portable speech synthesizer and optical devices. His host said there was no problem—the local low vision clinic would be able to replace these devices. "How wonderful!" José commented, "When I was a boy, we had to travel several hundred miles to get an optical device that could help me read."

Tracy

As a new teacher of students with visual impairments, Tracy developed a list of students whom it was necessary for her to see at the beginning of the first week of school—students who were blind and those with multiple disabilities. When she saw Andrew, a student with low vision, he was upset that Tracy had not addressed his needs at the beginning of the week. Tracy then reconsidered her priority list of students.

Tracy recalled this incident years later when she was interviewing a new teacher of students with visual impairments. She recalled how teachers at the turn of the century had fought to reduce their caseloads and how students with low vision in her school district began to receive time commensurate with their individual needs, so she did not just have to give them large-print books and consult with them once a month. The new teacher asked Tracy whether she could work with any low vision students who were just becoming visually efficient. Tracy thought how nice it was to hear the enthusiasm of someone who was prepared to see the needs of children with low vision as a high priority in her teaching.

Acceptance by Self and Society

Although medical advances, technological advances, and better services have had a great impact on the lives of those with low vision, the personal and societal struggles experienced by individuals have not been totally alleviated. It is now easier to be "in the middle" between sightedness and blindness and is less burdensome to

"see" small details or to "see" around scotomas. This progress has reduced the significance of low vision in the lives of many people and has resulted in more opportunities to function easily with vision. However, self-esteem comes from a feeling of self-worth, and acceptance by society comes from a genuine understanding of differences from others.

In 2022, strides have been made in including people with low vision and other disabilities in society without regard to their differences. Parents of children with low vision are more assured that their children will be accepted, and older adults, whose low vision is acquired, know that the visual effects of aging need not stifle a vibrant life or hamper their ability to fulfill their desire to enjoy vision. These societal changes have influenced the lives of Carol (Chapter 1) and Roseanna (Chapter 12).

Carol

Carol became aware of low vision when she was covering a story on the winter Olympics for her newspaper. Although her research allowed her to delve into the various issues involved in the impact of low vision on the lives of those she interviewed, she concluded her story with a continued sense of confusion and fuzziness. On the positive side, her article resulted in a dramatic increase in the number of referrals to a local low vision clinic and rehabilitation agency.

Over the next several years, Carol covered a host of other interesting societal dilemmas and issues and rarely had time to reconsider her research on low vision. However, she occasionally saw persons with low vision using optical devices and was pleased to think that her story may have influenced the lives of those who were successfully using those devices. At the least, she had increased her knowledge of low vision and knew what the devices were and how they were used.

It was not until the year 2022 when Carol renewed her interest in low vision. In that year, her elderly father began to experience the effects of an age-related visual impairment. When Carol once again began researching the topic of low vision, this time for personal reasons, she was thrilled to come across the fourth edition of *Foundations of Low Vision: Clinical and Functional Perspectives.* Carol felt a sense of comfort as she read the various chapters, noting the many innovations and improvements in medical and clinical services. She also was reassured that society's understanding of low vision was allowing a more nurturing environment in which persons with low vision could develop a sense of self-acceptance and self-esteem.

A few weeks later as she was shopping for shirts with her father at a busy mall, she overheard a clerk say to him, "We have a portable low vision device if you would like to read washing instructions or price tags." Carol was thinking about the excellent accommodations that the store was making when her father responded, "No thank you, I have one with me, but it's good to know your store cares about people with low vision."

Roseanna

When Roseanna, who has congenital nystagmus, was in high school, she was enjoying the benefits of having a summer job at a bank. Among those exquisite pleasures of getting a weekly paycheck were her ability to write checks to purchase the latest fashions for the upcoming school year and to buy new romance novels to read in the evenings. She also dreamed of going to college to pursue a career as a high school drama teacher.

After several "leads" in college plays, one of the professors asked Roseanna if she would like an introduction to a talent agent. Roseanna was elated at this prospect, but considered, as she had in the past, how it would look for her to use her optical devices while auditioning for parts. She had always been a self-advocate, such as when she dealt with the bank manager; however, she did not think she could take the rejections that would come when a director would see her need for various devices.

After she declined the offer, the professor invited the talent agent to see Roseanna in a play at the college; the agent was impressed by her performance and took her on as a client. After three years on Broadway, Roseanna was approached to be in a situation comedy on television. When the television director learned of Roseanna's low vision, he thought that rewriting the part to include her low vision was not only a reasonable accommodation but a real-life trait to convey in the character. Now people in the general public have an accurate media portrayal of a person with low vision that will allow them to gain a better understanding of low vision.

RESEARCH AND DEVELOPMENT NEEDS

Some of the progress reported in this chapter, although fictitious, includes advances in medicine, technology, and professional training and service delivery. To arrive at these and other hoped-for advances, further research and the implementation of its findings are needed, as are societal change and opportunities to participate in that change. Therefore, the authors propose the following directions for professionals in the field:

- Establish low vision as a human condition that warrants public attention.
- Continue and increase personal involvement in the preparation of new professionals in low vision.
- Conduct further interdisciplinary work and break down the political and professional biases that currently exist.
- Ensure that funding of services will be readily available to address the needs that are identified.
- Continue to do research to keep pace with and improve the scientific knowledge base on the functional use of vision, technological developments, provision of services, medical knowledge, and the psychosocial impact of low vision.

SUMMARY

Jim, in this chapter's vignette, did not have to deal with the effects of low vision. By the twenty-fourth century regenerated parts of the eye and boosts to the optic nerve were readily available. This chapter presented futuristic, fictitious scenarios of the situations of some people introduced in the vignettes in the various chapters of this book. Pushing our thoughts into the next decades and stating boldly what we hope for people with low vision can only expand our goals and allow us to develop creative solutions that may help us achieve these goals.

ACTIVITIES

With This Chapter and Other Resources

1. Jim, in the vignette that opens this chapter, did not have to cope with having low vision. If a person who is 50 years old has congenital low vision, why might he or she choose not to alleviate the visual condition?

2. Select two vignettes that were not discussed in this chapter. For each vignette, project what might happen to the character.

3. Think about a new device that will assist persons with low vision. Describe the characteristics of the device even if it does not seem plausible at this time.

4. Write a letter to the editors and/or authors of this text, describing your personal and professional beliefs about low vision. Feel free to add any suggestions that you may have for improving this textbook.

In the Community

1. Interview a medical researcher who is interested in ophthalmology. Ask how he or she is attempting to alleviate some of the medical conditions that create low vision.

2. Plan a project to effect changes in society's acceptance of people with low vision.

With a Person with Low Vision

1. Discuss with a person with low vision how his or her life could change if told that there was an experimental program to alleviate his or her low vision.

2. Ask a child with low vision to help you invent a new optical device that would help him or her in school.

From Your Perspective

Will there come a time when so few people will have low vision because of advances in medicine and technology that those who cannot be helped will face new societal challenges? What have we learned from the past that would help us address such challenges?

EPILOGUE

The authors of the chapters of this book have presented many of the challenges facing children and adults who have low vision and have tried to challenge both new and experienced professionals to address these needs in appropriate and ethical ways. It is hoped that their messages have encouraged the view that people with low vision are members of an identified population who have unique needs and experiences and that they also have needs and experiences similar to those of people who are blind and people who are normally sighted.

Services are designed based on the beliefs of professionals about low vision. If professionals believe that those who have low vision should be called "blind," then they may imply to these persons that they should not attempt, for example, to obtain low vision driver's licenses with or without bioptic telescopic devices. If they believe that those who have low vision have minimal needs compared to those who are "truly blind," then they may provide services only when the needs of those who are blind are fully addressed.

Just as it is important to empower people who are functionally blind with the skills developed for their needs, it is important to empower those with low vision with the skills developed to help them benefit from learning to use the visual environment and to feel comfortable and confident as persons with low vision. To ensure that appropriate services are provided, it is necessary to be-lieve that persons with low vision have unique rights to services.

The following Bill of Rights for Persons with Low Vision was first proposed at the 1993 International Conference on Low Vision held in Groningen, the Netherlands (Corn, 1994). It is understood that once opportunities are presented, individuals with low vision have the right to determine whether these opportunities are within their best interests. For example, if a person chooses not to accept a low vision service and feels more comfortable functioning as a person who is blind, that choice should be respected. Therefore, the following rights are offered as a guide the development and delivery of low vision services:

1. to receive medical care and early referral for clinical low vision evaluations, education, and rehabilitation services

2. to have access to the normal visual environment

3. to be free from ridicule and discrimination based on low vision

4. to develop an identity as a sighted person who has low vision

5. to have one's needs related to having low vision considered valid

6. to choose whether to use vision and/or other approaches for task completion

7. to receive services from professionals with competencies and interest in low vision care

8. to have one's visual capabilities comprehensively and accurately described

9. to have visual function considered more important than clinical measures for receiving devices and instruction

10. to receive devices and instruction based on scientific evidence and individualized assessment

11. to receive state-of-the-art optical devices and technology that meet functional needs

12. to have an accessible environment.

Consider whether these rights are unique to persons with low vision and whether they should guide your professional practice. You have learned the information provided by the many authors of this book, considered many of the issues facing people with low vision, and developed thoughts about what the future may hold. We, the editors, hope you will further the field of low vision—through research, administration, or direct services—and have the opportunity truly to empower the individuals you serve.

References
Appendix
Glossary
Resources
Index

REFERENCES

Aiex, N. K. (1987). Reading and the elderly. *Journal of Reading, 31,* 280–283.

Allan, J., & Erin, J. (1993 January). *The use of colored filters to enhance screen resolution for students with visual disabilities: A follow-up study.* Paper presented at the 1993 Conference of the Technology and Media, Division of the Council for Exceptional Children, Connecticut.

American Academy of Ophthalmology. (1992). *Policy statement: Unique competence of the ophthalmologist.* San Francisco: Author.

American Association of Retired Persons and the Administration of Aging. (1991). *A profile of older Americans.* American Association of Retired Persons.

American Foundation for the Blind. (1993). *AFB directory of services for blind and visually impaired persons in the United States and Canada* (24th ed.). New York: American Foundation for the Blind.

American Optical Corporation. (1959). *Elements of optics.* Southbridge, MA: Author.

American Optical Corporation. (1979). *Basic optical concepts.* Southbridge, MA: Author.

American Optical Corporation. (1986). *The human eye.* Southbridge, MA: Author.

American Optometric Association. (1989). *Policy statement: Definition of optometrist.* St. Louis: Author.

American Printing House for the Blind. (1995). *Annual report: June 1, 1994–June 30, 1995.* Louisville, KY: Author.

Apple, L., & Blasch, B. (1976). *Report of the workshop on low vision mobility* (Western Michigan University, Kalamazoo, November 3–5, 1975). Washington, DC: Veterans Administration, Department of Medicine and Surgery.

Apple, M. M., Apple, L. E., & Blasch, D. (1980). Low vision. In R. L. Welsch & B. B. Blasch (Eds.), *Foundations of orientation and mobility,* (pp. 187–223). New York: American Foundation for the Blind.

Applegate, W. B., Miller, S. T., Elam, J. T., Freeman, J. M., Wood, T. O., & Gettlefinger, T. C. (1987). Impact of cataract surgery with lens implantation on vision and physical function in elderly patients. *Journal of the American Medical Association, 257,* 1064–1066.

Ashcroft, S. C. (1963). A new era in education and a paradox in research for the visually limited. *Exceptional Children, 29,* 371–376.

Ashcroft, S. C., Halliday, C., & Barraga, N. C. (1965). *Study II: Effects of experimental teaching on the visual behavior of children educated as though they had no vision* (Office of Education Grant No. 32–52–01021–1034). Nashville, TN: George Peabody College for Teachers.

Attmore, M. (1990). *Career perspectives: Interviews with blind and visually impaired professionals.* New York: American Foundation for the Blind.

Bäckman, O., & Inde, K. (1976). *Low vision training.* Malmo, Sweden: Liberhemods.

Bailey, I. L. (1978, September). Specification of near-point performance. *Optometric Monthly,* 895–898.

Bailey, I. L., & Lovie, J. E. (1976). New design principles for visual acuity letter charts. *American Journal of Optometry and Physiological Optics, 53,* 740–745.

Baldasare, J., & Watson, G. (1986). Observations from the psychology of reading relevant to low vision research. In G. Woo (Ed.), *Low vision: Principles and applications* (pp. 272–287). New York: Springer-Verlag.

Ball, K., Owsley, C., & Beard, B. (1990). Clinical visual perimetry underestimates peripheral field problems in older adults. *Clinical Visual Sciences, 5,* 113–125.

Barraga, N. C. (1964). *Increased visual behavior in low vision children* (Research Series No. 13). New York: American Foundation for the Blind.

Barraga, N. C. (1970). *Teachers' guide for development of visual learning abilities and utilization of low vision.* Louisville, KY: American Printing House for the Blind.

Barraga, N. C. (1982). *Visual handicaps and learning* (2nd ed.). Austin, TX: Pro-Ed.

Barraga, N. C. (1986). Sensory perceptual development. In G. Scholl (Ed.), *Foundations of education for blind and visually handicapped children and youth: Theory and practice* (pp. 83–98). New York: American Foundation for the Blind.

Barraga, N. C., & Morris, J. E. (1980). *Program to develop efficiency in visual functioning.* Louisville, KY: American Printing House for the Blind.

Barron, C. (1991). Bioptic telescopic spectacles for motor vehicle driving. *Journal of the American Optometric Association, 62,* 37–41.

Beck, R., & Smith, C. (1988). *Neuro-ophthalmology: A problem-oriented approach.* Boston: Little, Brown.

Beliveau, M., & Smith, A. (Eds.). (1980). *The interdisciplinary approach to low vision rehabilitation.* Stillwater: Oklahoma State University, National Clearinghouse on Rehabilitation Information.

Beliveau, M., Yeadon, A., & Aston, S. (1993). *Innovative curriculum development research to develop inservice training curriculum for providers of long-term care to elderly blind/visually impaired.* Silver Spring, MD: NARIC.

Berg, R., Jose, R., & Carter, K. (1983). Distance training techniques. In R. T. Jose (Ed.), *Understanding low vision* (pp. 277–316). New York: American Foundation for the Blind.

Bier, N. (1970). *Correction of subnormal vision* (2nd ed.). London: Butterworths.

Bishop, V. (1971). *Teaching the visually limited child.* Springfield, IL: Charles C Thomas.

Bishop, V. (1988). Making choices in functional vision evaluations: "Noodles, needles, and haystacks." *Journal of Visual Impairment and Blindness, 82,* 94–99.

Bishop, V. (1991). Preschool visually impaired children: A demographic study. *Journal of Visual Impairment & Blindness, 85,* 69–74.

Blasch, B. B., & Apple, L. E. (1976). *Workshop on low vision mobility: Final report.* Washington, DC: Veterans Administration.

Bolles, R. N. (1995). *What color is your parachute?* Berkeley, CA: Ten Speed Press.

Bradfield, A. L., & Tucker, L. A. (1988). *Workplace visual functioning assessment for job modification and ac-commodation—State-of-the-art.* Mississippi State, MS: Rehabilitation Research and Training Center on Blindness and Low Vision.

Brady, F. B. (1979). *A singular view.* Oradell, N.J.: Medical Economics.

Bross, E., & White, C. W. (1986). Active and passive perceptual learning in the visually impaired. *Journal of Visual Impairment and Blindness, 80,* 528–531.

Brown, M. (1947). *Goodnight, moon.* New York: Harper-Collins.

Burns, P. C., & Roe, B. D. (1993). *Informal reading inventory* (4th ed.). Boston: Houghton Mifflin.

Burritt, O. (1916). President's report. In *Proceedings of the American Association of Instructors of the Blind* (pp. 9–13).

Bush, B. (1990, May 1). The quest for literacy. *American Way,* p. 143.

Calfee, R. (1994). Critical literacy: Reading and writing for a new millenium. In N. J. Ellsworth, C. N. Hedley, & A. N. Baratta (Eds.), *Literacy: A redefinition* (pp. 19–38). Hillsdale, NJ: Lawrence Erlbaum Associates.

Campbell, P. H. (1987). The integrated programming team: An approach for coordinating professionals of various disciplines in programs for students with severe and multiple handicaps. *Journal of the Association for Persons with Severe Handicaps, 12,* 107–116.

Carreiro, P., & Townsend, S. (1987). Routines: Understanding their power. In D. Frans (Ed.), *Teaching curriculum goals in routine environments: A manual for the instruction of multi-handicapped students* (pp. 1–4). Edmonton, Alberta: CONE Learning Systems.

Carroll, T. (1961). *Blindness: What it is, what it does, how to live with it.* Boston: Little, Brown.

Carter, K. (1983) Comprehensive preliminary assessments of low vision. In R. T. Jose (Ed.), *Understanding low vision* (pp. 85–104). New York: American Foundation for the Blind.

Carver, R. P. (1989). Silent reading rates in grade equivalents. *Journal of Reading Behavior, 21,* 155–166.

Cassin, B., Solomon, S., & Rubin, M. (1990). *Dictionary of eye terminology.* Gainesville, FL: Triad.

Caton, H. (Ed.). (1994). *Tools for selecting appropriate learning media.* Louisville, KY: American Printing House for the Blind.

Caton, H., Pester, E., & Bradley, E. J. (1982–83). *Patterns: The primary braille reading program.* Louisville, KY: American Printing House for the Blind.

Caton, H., Pester, E., & Bradley, E. J. (1987) *Patterns prebraille program.* Louisville, KY: American Printing House for the Blind.

Caton, H., Pester, E., & Bradley, E. J. (1990). *Read again: A braille program for adventitiously blinded print readers*. Louisville, KY: American Printing House for the Blind.

Charles, R., & Ritz, D. (1978). *Brother Ray, Ray Charles' own story*. New York: Warner Books.

Chiang, Y.-P., Bassi, L. J., & Javitt, J. C. (1992). Federal budgetary costs of blindness. *Milbank Quarterly, 70*, 319–340.

Cockburn, D. M. (1993). Ocular implications of systemic diseases in the elderly. In A. A. Rosenbloom & M. W. Morgan (Eds.), *Vision and aging* (2d ed.). Boston: Butterworth & Heinemann.

Colenbrander, A. (1977). Dimensions of visual performance (Low Vision Symposium, American Academy of Ophthalmology). *Transactions AAOO, 83*, 332–337.

Colenbrander, A. (1994). The functional vision score: A coordinated scoring system for visual impairments, disabilities and handicaps. In A. C. Kooijmans, P. L. Looijestijn, J. A. Welling, & G. J. van der Wildt (Eds.), *Low vision: Research and new developments in rehabilitation* (pp. 552–561). Amsterdam: IOS Press.

Corn, A. (1977). *Monocular mac*. New York: National Association for the Visually Handicapped.

Corn, A. L. (1980). *Development and assessment of an in-service training program for teachers of the visually handicapped: Optical aids in the classroom*. Unpublished doctoral dissertation, Teachers College, Columbia University.

Corn, A. (1983). Visual function: A theoretical model for individuals with low vision. *Journal of Visual Impairment and Blindness, 77*(8), 373–377.

Corn, A. (1990). Optical devices or large-type: Is there a debate? In A. W. Johnston & M. Lawrence (Eds.), *Low vision ahead II: Conference proceedings*. Kooyong, Australia: Association for the Blind.

Corn, A. L. (1994). Do persons with low vision have special rights? A challenge for service providers and an opportunity for consumers. In A. C. Kooinman, P. L. Looijestijn, & G. J. Van der Wilt (Eds.), *Studies in health, technology, and informatics: Low vision; Research and new developments in rehabilitation* (pp. 376–384). Oxford, England: IOS Press.

Corn, A. L., & Koenig, A. J. (1991). Least restrictive access to the visual environment. *Journal of Visual Impairment & Blindness, 85*, 195–197.

Corn, A. L., & Sacks, S. Z. (1994). The impact of nondriving on adults with visual impairments. *Journal of Visual Impairment & Blindness, 88*, 53–68.

Cowan, C., & Shepler, R. (1990). Teaching techniques for teaching young children to use low vision devices. *Journal of Vision Impairment and Blindness, 84*(9), 419–421.

Crews, J. E. (1991). Strategic planning and independent living for elders who are blind. *Journal of Visual Impairment & Blindness, 85*, 52–57.

Cummings, R., Whittaker, S., Watson, G., & Budd, J. (1985) Scanning characters and reading with a central scotoma. *American Journal of Optometry and Physiological Optics, 62*, 833–843.

Daugherty, K., & Moran, M. (1982). Neuropsychological, learning and developmental characteristics of the low vision child. *Journal of Visual Impairment & Blindness, 76*, 398–406.

Dickman, I. R. (1983). *Making life more livable: Simple adaptations for the homes of blind and visually impaired older people*. New York: American Foundation for the Blind.

Dodds, A. G. (1989). Motivation reconsidered: The importance of self-efficacy in rehabilitation. *British Journal of Visual Impairment, 7*, 11–15.

Dodds, A. G., Bailey, P., Pearson, A., & Yates, L. (1991). Psychological factors in acquired visual impairment. *Journal of Visual Impairment & Blindness, 85*, 306–310.

Duckworth, B. J. (1993). Adapting standardized academic tests in braille and large type. *Journal of Visual Impairment and Blindness, 87*, 405–407.

Eitan, S., Solomon, A., Lavie, V., Yoles, E., Hirschberg, D. L., Belkin, M., & Schwartz, M. (1994). Recovery of visual response of injured adult rat optic nerves treated with transglutaminase. *Science, 264*, 1764–1768.

Erhardt, R. (1989). *Erhardt developmental vision assessment*. Tucson, AZ: Therapy Skill Builders.

Espinola, O., & Croft, D. (1992). *Solutions: Access technology for people who are blind*. Boston: National Braille Press.

Fagerstrom, N. (1971). Administration and coordination of a training program in a low vision clinic. In E. J. Rex (Ed.), *Methods and procedures for training low vision skills*. Normal: Illinois State University.

Farrar, D. (1971). The visual examination, selection of low vision aids, and adaptive training. In E. J. Rex (Ed.), *Methods and procedures for training low vision skills*. Normal: Illinois State University.

Faye, E. E. (1970). *The low vision patient: Clinical experience with adults and children*. New York: Grune & Stratton.

Faye, E. E. (1984a). The effect of eye condition on functional vision. In E. Faye (Ed.), *Clinical low vision*, (2nd ed., pp. 172–189). Boston: Little, Brown.

Faye, E. E. (1984b). *Clinical low vision*. Boston: Little, Brown.

Feinbloom, W. (1931). Application of telescope spectacles to refraction. *American Journal of Optometry, 8*(5), 146–161.

Feinbloom, W. (1935). Introduction to the principles and practice of sub-normal vision correction. *Journal of the American Optometric Association, 6,* 3–18.

Ferraro, J., & Jose, R. T. (1983). Training programs for individuals with restricted fields. In R. T. Jose (Ed.), *Understanding low vision* (pp. 363–376). New York: American Foundation for the Blind.

Ferraro, S., & Ferraro, J. (1983). Establishing a training-instructional program. In R. T. Jose (Ed.), *Understanding low vision* (pp. 251–276). New York: American Foundation for the Blind.

Ferris, F. (1982). Senile macular degeneration: Review of epidemiologic features. *American Journal of Epidemiology, 118,* 132–151.

Ficke, S. C. (1985). *An orientation to the Older Americans Act* (rev. ed.). Washington, DC: National Association of State Units on Aging.

Flax, M. E. (1993). *Coping with low vision.* San Diego: Singular Publishing Group.

Fonda, G. (1955). Report on two hundred patients examined for correction of subnormal vision. *AMA Archives of Ophthalmology, 54,* 300–301.

Fonda, G. (1965). *Management of the patient with subnormal vision.* St. Louis: C. V. Mosby.

Fraunfelder, F. (1989). *Drug-induced ocular side effects and drug interactions* (3rd ed.). Philadelphia: Lea & Febiger.

Freeman, R. D., Goetz, E., Richards, D. P., & Groenveld, M. (1991). Defiers of negative prediction: A 14-year follow-up study of legally blind children. *Journal of Visual Impairment & Blindness, 85,* 365–370.

Gardner, L., & Corn, A. L. (1984). *Low vision: Topics of concern.* In G. T. Scholl (Ed.), *Quality services for blind and visually impaired students: Statements of position* (pp.). Reston, VA: ERIC Clearinghouse on Handicapped and Gifted Children.

Gardner, L., & Corn, A. L. (1991). *Low vision: Access to print: Statements of position* (pp. 6–8). Reston, VA: Division for the Visually Handicapped, Council for Exceptional Children.

Geisler, C. (1994). *Academic literacy and the nature of expertise: Reading, writing and knowing in academic philosophy.* Hillsdale, NJ: Lawrence Erlbaum Associates.

Genensky, S. M., Baran, P., Moshin, H. L., & Steingold, H. (1969). *A closed-circuit TV system for the visually handicapped* (Research Bulletin No. 19). New York: American Foundation for the Blind.

Genensky, S. M., Berry, S. H., Bikson, T. H., & Bikson, T. K. (1979). *Visual environmental adaptation problems of the partially sighted: Final report.* Santa Monica, CA: Santa Monica Hospital Medical Center, Center for the Partially Sighted.

Geruschat, D. (1980). Training with hand-held distance optical aids. In M. Beliveau & A. Smith (Eds.), *The interdisciplinary approach to low vision rehabilitation.* (RSA Grant No. 45-P8153512–01). Stillwater: Oklahoma State University, National Clearinghouse on Rehabilitation Information.

Geruschat, D. R., & De l'Aune, W. (1989). Reliability and validity of O & M instructor observations. *Journal of Visual Impairment & Blindness, 83,* 457–460.

Gibson, E. J. (1991). *An odyssey in learning and perception.* Cambridge, MA: MIT Press.

Ginsberg, A. P. (1984). A new contrast sensitivity vision test chart. *American Journal of Optometry, 61,* 403–407.

Gittinger, J., & Asdourian, G. (1988). *Manual of clinical problems in ophthalmology.* Boston: Little, Brown.

Goetz, L., & Gee, K. (1987). Functional vision programming: A model for teaching visual behaviors in natural contexts. In L. Goetz, D. Guess, & K. Stremel-Gampbell (Eds.), *Innovative program design for individuals with dual sensory impairments* (pp. 77–97). Baltimore: Paul H. Brookes Publishing Company.

Goldberg, S. (1991). *Ophthalmology made ridiculously simple.* Miami: Medmaster.

Goodlaw, E. (1991). Preventing cataracts and age-related maculaopathy. *Journal of Vision Rehabilitation, 5,* 1–8.

Goodrich, G. L. (1991). Low vision services in the VA: An "aging" trend. *Journal of Vision Rehabilitation, 5* (3), 11–17.

Goodrich, G. L., & Jose, R. T. (1993). *Low vision—The reference.* New York: The Lighthouse.

Goodrich, G. L., Mehr, E. B., & Darling, N. C. (1980). Parameters in the use of CCTV's and Optical Aids. *American Journal of Optometry and Physiological Optics, 57,* 881–892.

Graves, W. H., Maxson, J. H., & McCan, C. (1987). *Work environment visual demands protocol.* Mississippi State, MS: Rehabilitation Research and Training Center on Blindness and Low Vision.

Groenveld, M., Jan, J., & Leader, P. (1990). Observations on the habilitation of children with cortical visual impairment. *Journal of Visual Impairment & Blindness, 84,* 11–15.

Guess, D., Siegel-Causey, E., Roberts, S., Rues, J., Thompson, B., & Siegel-Causey, D. (1990). Assessment and analysis of behavior state and related variables among students with profoundly handicapping conditions. *Journal of the Association for Persons with Severe Handicaps, 15,* 211–230.

Guszak, F. J. (1985). *Diagnostic reading instruction in the elementary school* (3rd ed.). New York: Harper & Row.

Hall, A., & Bailey, I. (1989). A model for training vision functioning. *Journal of Visual Impairment and Blindness, 83*(8), 390–396.

Hall, A., Bailey, I., Kekelis, L., Raasch, T., & Goodrich, G. (1987). Retrospective survey to investigate use of distance magnifiers for travel. *Journal of Visual Impairment & Blindness, 81,* 418–423.

Hall, A. P., Sacks, S. Z., Dornbush, H., Raasch, T., & Kekelis, L. (1987). Evaluating patient success in a low vision clinic setting. *Journal of Vision Rehabilitation, 1,* 7–25.

Ham, W. T. (1983). Ocular hazards of light sources: Review of current knowledge. *Journal of Occupational Medicine, 25,* 101–103.

Hanninen, K. A. (1979). *Teaching the visually handicapped* (2nd ed.). Detroit: Blindess Publications.

Harley R., & Altmeyer, E. (1982). Cerebral palsy and associated visual defects. *Education of the Visually Handicapped, 14,* 41–49.

Hathaway, W. (1959). *Education and health of the partially seeing child* (rev. ed. by F. M. Foote, D. Bryan, & H. Gibbons). New York: Columbia University Press. (Original work published 1943)

Heinze (1986). Communication skills. In G. T. Scholl (Ed.), *Foundations of education for blind and visually handicapped children and youth: Theory and practice* (pp. 301–314). New York: American Foundation for the Blind.

Hellinger, G. (1967). Vision rehabilitation through low vision centers. *New outlook for the blind, 61,* 296–301.

Helmstetter, E., Murphy-Herd, M., Roberts, S., & Guess, D. (1984). *Individualized curriculum sequence and extended models for learners who are deaf and blind.* U.S. Department of Education Contract #300810357, University of Kansas Department of Special Education, Lawrence, KS.

Hobbs, N. (1965, October). *The professor and the student or the art of getting students into trouble.* Paper presented at the 48th annual convention of the American Council on Education, Washington, DC.

Holbrook, M. C., & Koenig, A. J. (1992). Teaching braille reading to students with low vision. *Journal of Visual Impairment and Blindness, 86,* 44–48.

Holcomb, J., & Goodrich, G. L. (1976). Eccentric viewing training. *Journal of the American Optometric Association, 47,* 1438–1443.

Holmes, R. B. (1967). *Training residual vision in adolescents educated previously as nonvisual.* Unpublished master's thesis, Illinois State University, Normal.

Huebner, K. M., Prickett, J. G., Welch, T. R., & Joffee, E. (Eds.). (1995). *Hand in hand: Essentials of communication and orientation and mobility for your students who are deaf-blind* (Vol. 1). New York: AFB Press.

Hyvärinen, L. (1985). Classification of visual impairment and disability. *Bulletin of the Society of Belgian Ophthalmology, 215,* 1–16.

Inde, K., & Bäckman, O. (1975). *Visual training with optical aids.* Malmo, Sweden: Hermods.

Industrial Home for the Blind. (1957). *Optical aids services—Survey on 500 cases—March 1953 to December 1955.* New York: Author.

Institute on Rehabilitation Issues. (1975). *Placement of the severely handicapped: A counselor's guide.* Institute, WV: Research and Training Center.

International Classification of Diseases, 9th Revision, Clinical Modification (ICD-9-CM). (1978). Ann Arbor, MI: Commission on Professional and Hospital Activities.

International Classification of Impairments, Disabilities and Handicaps. (1980). Geneva: World Health Organization.

Isenberg, S. (1989). *The eye in infancy.* Chicago: Year Book Medical.

Jackson, A., Silver, J., & Archer, D. (1986). An evaluation of follow-up systems in two low vision clinics in the United Kingdom. In G. Woo (Ed.), *Low vision: Principles and applications* (pp. 396–417). New York: Springer-Verlag.

Jackson, R. M. (1983). Early educational use of optical aids: A cautionary note. *Education of the Visually Handicapped, 15,* 20–29.

Jacobson, W. H. (1993). *The art and science of teaching orientation and mobility to persons with visual impairments.* New York: AFB Press.

Jahoda, G. (1993). *How can I do this, if I can't see what I'm doing?* Washington, DC: National Library Service for the Blind and Physically Handicapped.

Jan, J., & Groeneveld, M. (1993). Visual behaviors and adaptations associated with cortical and ocular impairment in children. *Journal of Visual Impairment & Blindness, 87,* 101–105.

Jan, J., Farrell, K., Wong, P. K., & McCormick, A. Q. (1986). Eye and head movements of visually impaired children. *Developmental Medicine and Child Neurology, 28,* 285–293.

Jan, J., Freeman, R. D., & Scott, E. P. (1977). *Visual impairment in children and adolescents.* New York: Grune & Stratton.

Johnson, C. A. (1976). Some physiological considerations for visual training. *Low Vision Abstracts, 2*(4), 1–3.

Johnson, G. (1995). Follow-up: Development of a national agenda for full employment. *Journal of Visual Impairment & Blindness, JVIB News Service, 89, (4),* 20–24.

Johnson, G., & Lefton, L. (Eds). (1981). Reading comprehension: Essential skills are not sufficient. In D. F. Fisher & C. W. Peters (Eds.), *Comprehension and the competent reader: Inter-specialty perceptions* (pp. 116–126). New York: Praeger.

Jose, R. T. (Ed.). (1983). *Understanding low vision.* New York: American Foundation for the Blind.

Jose, R. T. (1992). Low vision services. In A. L. Orr (Ed.), *Vision and aging: Crossroads for service delivery* (pp. 209–232). New York: American Foundation for the Blind.

Jose, R. T. (1994). Low vision certification proposal. *Journal of Vision Rehabilitation, 8,* 15.

Jose, R. T., & Smith, A. J. (1976). Increasing peripheral field awareness with fresnel prisms. *Optical Journal & Review of Optometry, 113*(12), 33–37.

Kahn, H. A. (1977). The Framingham Eye Study I: Outline and major prevalence findings. *American Journal of Epidemiology, 106,* 17–41.

Kahn, H. A., & Moorhead, H. B. (1973). *Statistics on blindness in the model reporting area 1969–1970* (Publication No. (NIH) 73–427). Washington, DC: U.S. Government Printing Office.

Kekelis, L., & Sacks, S. Z. (1992). The effects of visual impairment on children's social interactions in regular education programs. In S. Z. Sacks, L. Kekelis, & R. J. Gaylord-Ross (Eds.), *The development of social skills by blind and visually impaired students: Exploratory studies and strategies* (pp. 59–82). New York: American Foundation for the Blind.

Kelley, P., Wedding, J., & Smith J. (1992). *Medications used by students with visual and hearing impairments: Implications for teachers.* Presentation at the 70th Annual Convention of the Council for Exceptional Children, Baltimore.

Kendrick, D. (1993). *Jobs to be proud of.* New York: American Foundation for the Blind.

Kestenbaum, A. (1953). Reading glasses for patients with very poor vision. *American Journal of Ophthalmology, 36*(8), 1143–1144.

Kiester, E. (1990). *AIDS and vision loss.* New York: American Foundation for the Blind.

Kirchner, C., & Peterson, R. (1988). Employment: Selected characteristics. In C. Kirchner (Ed.), *Data on blindness and visual impairment in the U.S.* (2nd ed., pp. 169–177). New York: American Foundation for the Blind.

Kirscher, C., & Meissen, R. (1983) Reading speed under real and simulated visual impairment. *Journal of Visual Impairment & Blindness. 77,* 386–388.

Knowles, M. (1984). *Andragogy in action.* San Francisco: Jossey-Bass.

Knowlton, M., & Woo, I. (1989). Functional color vision deficits and performance of children on an educational task. *Education of the Visually Handicapped, 20*(4), 156–162.

Koenig, A. J. (1992). A framework for understanding the literacy of individuals with visual impairments. *Journal of Visual Impairment & Blindness, 86,* 277–284.

Koenig, A. J. (1996). Growing into literacy. In M. C. Holbrook, (Ed.), *Children with visual impairments: A parents' guide.* Bethesda, MD: Woodbine House.

Koenig, A. J., & Holbrook, M. C. (1989). Determining the reading medium for students with visual impairments: A diagnostic teaching approach. *Journal of Visual Impairment & Blindness, 83,* 296–302.

Koenig, A. J., & Holbrook, M. C. (1991). Determining the reading medium for visually impaired students via diagnostic teaching. *Journal of Visual Impairment and Blindness, 85,* 61–68.

Koenig, A. J., & Holbrook, M. C. (1993). *Learning media assessment of students with visual impairments: A resource guide for teachers.* Austin: Texas School for the Blind and Visually Impaired.

Koenig, A. J., & Holbrook, M. C. (1995). *Learning media assessment of students with visual impairments: A resource guide for teachers* (2nd ed.). Austin: Texas School for the Blind and Visually Impaired.

Koenig, A. J., & Ross, D. B. (1991). A procedure to evaluate the relative effectiveness of reading in large and regular print. *Journal of Visual Impairment and Blindness, 84*(5), 198–204.

Koenig, A. J., Layton, C. A., & Ross, D. B. (1992). The relative effectiveness of reading in large print and reading with low vision devices for students with low vision. *Journal of Visual Impairment & Blindness, 86,* 48–53.

Koestler, F. A. (1976). *The unseen minority: A social history of blindness in the United States.* New York: David McKay.

Kohler, I. (1964). The formation and transformation of the visual world. *Psychological Issues, 3*(4), 14–173.

Kozol, J. (1985). *Illiterate America.* Garden City, NY: Doubleday.

Langley, M. (1980). *Functional vision screening inventory for the multiple and severely handicapped.* Chicago: Stoelting.

Langley, M. (in press). *Potential assessment of visual efficiency.* Louisville, KY: American Printing House for the Blind.

Layton, C. A. (1994). Effects of repeated readings for increasing reading fluency in elementary students with low vision (Doctoral dissertation, Texas Tech University, 1993). *Dissertation Abstracts International, 55*(01), 70A.

Legge, G. E., Ross, J. A., Maxwell, K. T., & Luebker, A. (1989). Psychophysics of reading VII: Comprehension in normal and low vision. *Clinical Vision Sciences, 4,* 51–60.

Legge, G. E., Rubin, G, Pelli, D., & Schleske, M. (1985). Psychophysics of reading: Low vision. *Vision Research, 25,* 253–266.

Legge, G. E., Rubin, G. S., Pelli, D. G., Schleske, M. M., Luebker, A., & Ross, J. A. (1988). Understanding low vision reading. *Journal of Visual Impairment and Blindness, 82,* 54–58.

Levack, N. (1991). *Low vision: A resource guide with adaptations for students with visual impairments.* Austin: Texas School for the Blind and Visually Impaired.

Long, R. G. (1985). The relationship of visual behavior to mobility performance and beliefs in persons with low visions. *Dissertation Abstracts International, 47,* 501A. (University Microfilms No.).

Long, R. G., Reiser, J. J., & Hill, E. W. (1990). Mobility in individuals with moderate visual impairments. *Journal of Visual Impairment & Blindness, 84,*(3) 111–118.

Loshin, D. S. (1993). Futures in technology. In J. N. Erin, A. L. Corn, & V. E. Bishop (Eds.), *Low vision: Reflections of the past, visions of the future* (pp. 18–31). New York: AFB Press.

Loshin, D. S., & Juday, R. D. (1989). The programmable remapper: Clinical applications for patients with field defects. *Optometry & Vision Science, 66,* 389–395.

Loumiet, R., & Levack, N. (1993). *Independent living: A curriculum with adaptations for students with visual impairments* (2nd ed.). Austin: Texas School for the Blind and Visually Impaired.

Lowenfeld, B. (1973). Psychological considerations. In B. Lowenfeld (Ed.), *The visually handicapped child in school* (pp. 27–60). New York: John Day Company.

Lowenfeld, B., Abel, G. L., & Hatlen, P. H. (1969). *Blind children learn to read.* Springfield, IL: Charles C Thomas.

Ludwig, I., Luxton, L., & Attmore, M. (1988). *Creative recreation for blind and visually impaired adults.* New York: American Foundation for the Blind.

MacCuspre, P. A. (1992). The social acceptance and integration of visually impaired children in integrated settings. In S. Z. Sacks, L. Kekelis, & R. J. Gaylord-Ross (Eds.), *The development of social skills by blind and visually impaired students: Exploratory studies and strategies* (pp. 83–102). New York: American Foundation for the Blind.

Mancil, G. L. (1986). Evaluation of reading speed with four low vision aids. *American Journal of Optometry and Physiological Optics, 63,* 708–713.

Mancil, G. L. (1993). The delivery of vision care in non-traditional settings. In A. A. Rosenbloom & M. M. Morgan (Eds.) *Vision and aging* (2nd ed., pp. 403–423). Boston: Butterworth & Heinemann.

Mangold, S., & Mangold, P. (1989). Selecting the most appropriate primary literacy medium for students with functional vision. *Journal of Visual Impairment & Blindness, 83,* 294–296.

Maplesden, C. (1984). A subjective approach to eccentric viewing training. *Journal of Visual Impairment & Blindness, 78,* 5–7.

Massof, R. W., & Rickman, D. L. (1992). Obstacles encountered in the development of the low vision enhancement system. *Optometry & Vision Science, 69,* 32–41.

McCracken, R. (1967). The informal reading inventory as a means of improving instruction. In T. Barrett (Ed.), *The evaluation of children's reading.* Newark, NJ: International Reading Association.

McGillivray, R. (1994). Computer access evaluation for persons with low vision. *Aids and Appliances Review, 15,* 2–8.

McIllwaine, G. G., Bell, J. A., & Dutton, G. N. (1991). Low vision aids—Is our service cost effective? *Eye, 5,* 607–611.

McNeil, J. M. (1993). *Americans with disabilities: 1991–92: Data from the Survey of Income and Program Participation* (Current Population Reports, Series P-70, No. 33). Washington, DC: U.S. Bureau of the Census.

Mehr, E. B., & Freid, A. N. (1975). *Low vision care: Prescribing and counseling.* Chicago: Professional Press.

Mehr, E. B., & Mehr, H. M. (1969). Psychological factors in working with partially-sighted persons. *Journal of the American Optometric Association, 40*(8), 842–846.

Meredith, T. A. (1975). *The eye: Disease, diagnosis, and treatment.* Bowie, MD: Robert J. Brady.

Merriam Webster's collegiate dictionary (10th ed.). Springfield, MA: Merriam Webster.

Merry, R. V. (1933). *Problems in the education of visually handicapped children.* Cambridge, MA: Harvard University Press.

Miller, D. (1979). *Ophthalmology: The essentials.* New York: John Wiley and Sons.

Monbeck, M. E. (1973). *The meaning of blindness: Attitudes toward blindness and blind people.* Bloomington, IN: Indiana University Press.

Morgan, M. M. (1993). Normal age-related vision changes. In A. A. Rosenbloom & M. M. Morgan (Eds.), *Vision and aging* (2nd ed., pp. 178–199). Boston: Butterworth & Heinemann.

Morse, A. R., O'Connell, W., & Finkelstein, H. (1988). Assessing vision in nursing home residents. *Journal of Vision Rehabilitation, 2,* 1–10.

Morsink, C. V., Thomas, C. C., & Correa, V. I. (1991). *Interactive teaming: Consultation and collaboration in special programs.* Columbus, OH: Charles E. Merrill.

National Advisory Eye Council. (1993). *Vision research: A national plan, 1994–1998.* National Institutes of Health, National Eye Institute.

National Institute on Disability and Rehabilitation Research (1993) *Consensus statement: Protocols for choosing low vision devices, 1.* Washington, DC: U.S. Department of Education.

National Library Service for the Blind and Physically Handicapped. (1993). *Assistive devices for reading.* Washington, DC: Author.

National Society to Prevent Blindness. (1993). *Vision problems in the United States* (fact sheet). Schaumburg, IL: Author.

Neff, W. S. (1985). *Work and human behavior* (3rd ed.). New York: Aldine.

Nelson, K. A., & Dimitrova, E. (1993). Severe visual impairment in the United States and in each state, 1990. *Journal of Visual Impairment & Blindness, 87,* 80–85.

New NAEP report cites need for improved writing skills. (1994). *Reading Today, 12,* 36.

Newell, F. W. (1982). *Ophthalmology: Principles and concepts.* St. Louis: C.V. Mosby & Co.

Newell, F. W. (1992). *Ophthalmology: Principles and concepts* (7th ed.). St. Louis: Mosby Year Book.

Newell, S. W., & Walser, J. J. (1985). Nursing home glaucoma and acuity screening results in western Oklahoma. *Annals of Ophthalmology. 17,* 186–189.

Newsome, D. A., Swartz, M., Leone, N. C., Elston, R. C., & Miller, E. (1988). Oral zinc in macular degeneration. *Archives of Ophthalmology, 106,* 192–197.

Nietupski, J., & Hamrie-Nietupski, S. (1987). *An ecological approach to curriculum development.* In L. Goetz, D. Guess, & K. Stremel-Campbell (Eds.), *Innovative program design for individuals with dual sensory impairments* (pp. 225–253). Baltimore: Paul H. Brookes.

Nilsson, U. (1990). Visual rehabilitation with and without educational training in the use of optical aids and residual vision. A prospective study of patients with advanced age-related macular degeneration. *Clinical Vision Science, 6,* 3–10.

Nowakowski, R. W. (1994). *Primary low vision care.* East Norwalk, CT: Appleton & Lange.

Overbury, O., Greig, D., & West, M. (1982). The psychodynamics of low vision: A preliminary study. *Journal of Visual Impairment & Blindness, 76,* 101–104.

Owsley, C., Sloane, M., Ball, K., Roenker, D., & Bruni, J. (1991). Visual/cognitive correlates of vehicle accidents in older drivers. *Psychology and Aging, 63,* 403–415.

Parker, R. M., & Szymanski, E. M. (Eds.). (1992). *Rehabilitation counseling—Basics and beyond.* Austin, TX: Pro Ed.

Pavan-Langston, D. (1985). *Manual of ocular diagnosis and therapy.* Boston: Little, Brown.

Peli, E., Arend, L. E., & Timberlake, G. T. (1986). Computerized image enhancement for visually impaired people: New technology, new possibilities. *Journal of Visual Impairment & Blindness, 80,* 849–854.

Peli, E., Goldstein, R., Young, G., Tempe, C., & Buzney S. (1991). Image enhancement for the visually impaired: Simulation and experimental results. *Investigative Ophthalmology and Visual Science, 32,* 2337–2350.

Pelli, D. G., Robson, J. G., & Wilkins, A. J. (1988). The design of a new letter chart for measuring contrast sensitivity. *Clinical Vision Science, 2,* 187–189.

Ponchillia, P. E., & Ponchillia, S. V. (1996). *Foundations of rehabilitation teaching with persons who are blind or visually impaired.* New York: AFB Press.

Potts, A. M., Volk, D., & West, S. W. (1959). A television reader as a subnormal aid. *American Journal of Ophthalmology, 47,* 580–1.

Prentice, C. F., & Mehr, E. B. (1969). The typoscope of Prentice. *American Journal of Optometry & Archives of the American Academy of Optometry, 46,* 885–887.

Prevent Blindness America. (1994). *Vision problems in the U.S.* Schaumburg, IL: Author.

Quillman, R. D. (1980). *Low vision training manual.* Kalamazoo: Western Michigan University.

Quillman, R. D., & Goodrich, G. L. (1978–79). Low vision entering the 1980's. In *Blindness Annual* (pp. 36–50). Washington, DC: American Association of Workers for the Blind.

Rabby, R., & Croft, D. L. (1989). *Take charge: A strategic guide for blind job seekers.* Boston: National Braille Press.

Rainwater, C. (1971). *Light and color.* New York: Golden Press.

Rayner, K., & Bertera, J. (1979). Reading without a fovea. *Science, 206,* 468–469.

Ringgold, N. P. (1991). *Out of the corner of my eye: Living with vision loss in later life.* New York: American Foundation for the Blind.

Rodgin, M. von. (1910) Telescopic and microscopic spectacles. *Archiv. Soc. Am. Ophthal. Optom., 2,* (1–4) 237–243.

Roessing, L. J. (1980). *Minimum competencies for visually impaired students.* Unpublished manuscript, Fremont Unified School District, Fremont, CA.

Rosenberg, R. (1984). Light, glare and contrast in low vision care. In E. E. Faye (Ed.), *Clinical low vision* (pp. 197–212). Boston: Little, Brown.

Rosenbloom, A. A. (1966). Subnormal vision care: An analysis of clinic patients. *Proceedings of the Conference on Aid to the Visually Limited.* Washington, DC: American Optometric Association.

Rosenbloom, A. A. (1986). Care of the visually impaired elderly patient. In A. A. Rosenbloom & M. W. Morgan (Eds.), *Vision and aging: General and clinical perspectives* (pp. 337–348). New York: Professional Press Books.

Rosenbloom, A. A., & Goodrich, G. L. (1990). Visual rehabilitation: Historical perspectives—New challenges. In A. W. Johnston & M. Lawrence (Eds.). *Low vision ahead II: Conference proceedings.* Kooyong, Australia: Association for the Blind.

Rosenbloom, A. A., & Morgan, M. W. (1986). *Vision and aging: General and clinical perspectives.* New York: Professional Press Books.

Roy, T. (1985). Ocular syndromes and systemic diseases. Orlando, FL: Grune & Stratton.

Rubin, R. J. (1985). Private versus public responsibilities for long-term care. In: B. D. Dunlap (Ed.) *New federalism and long-term care for the elderly.* Millwood, VA: Center for Health Affairs.

Rusalem, H. R. (1972). *Coping with the unseen environment.* New York: Teachers College Press.

Salomone, P. R., & Paige, R. E. (1984). Employment problems and solutions: Perceptions of blind and visually impaired adults. *Vocational Guidance Quarterly, 33,* 147–156.

Samuels, S. J. (1979). The method of repeated readings. *Reading Teacher, 33,* 403–408.

Sanderson, G., Cumming, A., & Polkinghorne, P. (1986). A hospital rental system for low vision aids. *Australian and New Zealand Journal of Ophthalmology, 14,* 359–363.

Scadden, L. A. (1991). An overview of technology and visual impairment. *Technology and Disability, 1,* 11.

Schein, J. D. (1988). Acquired monocular disability. *Journal of Visual Impairment & Blindness, 82,* 279–281.

Schiff, W. (1980). *Perception: An applied approach.* Boston: Houghton Mifflin.

Schmidt, F. (1989). What jobs do blind and visually impaired people do? In F. Schmidt & G. Grace (Eds.), *Opening doors: Blind and visually impaired people and work* (pp. 9–22). Toronto: Canadian National Institute for the Blind.

Scholl, G. T. (Ed.). (1986). *Foundations of education for blind and visually handicapped children and youth: Theory and practice.* New York: American Foundation for the Blind.

Scott, R. A. (1969). *The making of blind men: A study of adult socialization.* New York: Russell Sage Foundation.

Sekuler, R., & Blake, R. (1990). *Perception* (2d ed.). New York: McGraw Hill.

Seligman, M. E. P. (1990). *Learned optimism.* New York: Alfred A. Knopf.

Shankweiler, D., & Liberman, I. Y. (1982). Misreading: A search for causes. In J. F. Davanagh, & I. G. Mat-

tingly, (Eds.), *Language by eye and ear* (pp. 293–317). Cambridge, MA: MIT Press.

Sharp, M., McNear, D., & Bousma, J. (1995). The development of a scale to facilitate reading mode decisions. *Journal of Visual Impairment and Blindness, 89,* 83–89.

Silver, J., & Thomsitt, J. (1977). Low-vision services in the United Kingdom. *Health Trends, 9.*

Skejskal, N., Zahn, J., & VonDollen, K. (1987). A questionnaire approach to success analysis of low vision patients. *Journal of Vision Rehabilitation, 1.*

Sloan, L. L. (1977). *Reading aids for the partially sighted: A systematic classification and procedure for prescribing.* Baltimore: Williams & Wilkins.

Sloan, L. L., & Habel, A. (1956). Reading aids for the partially blind: New methods of rating and prescribing optical aids. *American Journal of Ophthalmology, 42*(6), 863–872.

Smith, A. (1974). *Consider me seeing* (videotape). AN Department, Hillman Library, University of Pittsburgh, PA.

Smith, A. (1987). Low vision orientation and mobility: Strategies for assessing and enhancing visual efficiency in the environment. In C. Tee, W. Ng., G. Omar, & L. Fee (Eds.), *First Asia-Pacific seminar on low vision: Proceedings of the seminar* (pp. 77–91). Kuala Lumpur, Malaysia.

Smith, A. (1990). Mobility problems related to vision loss: Perceptions of mobility practitioners and persons with low vision. *Dissertation Abstracts International,* 9026646.

Smith, A., & Cote, Karen S. (1983). *Look at me. A resource manual for the development of residual vision in multiple impaired children.* Philadelphia: Pennsylvania College of Optometry Press.

Smith, A., & Geruschat, D. (1983). *Development and assessment of standard training protocols for the use of fresnel prisms of persons with peripheral field defects: Effects on independent travel and psychosocial adjustment. Final report.* (to the National Institute for Handicapped Research, Grant No. 12314136801A). Philadelphia: Low Vision Research and Training Center, Pennsylvania College of Optometry.

Smith, A., & O'Donnell, L. (1991). *Beyond arms reach: Enhancing distance vision.* Philadelphia: Pennsylvania College of Optometry Press.

Smith, A., De l'Aune, W., & Geruschat, D. (1992). Low vision mobility problems: Perceptions of O&M specialists and persons with low vision. *Journal of Visual Impairment & Blindness, 86,* 58–62.

Smith, M. (1984). *If blindness strikes: Don't strike out.* Springfield, IL: Charles C Thomas.

Snyder, L. H., Pyreck, J., & Smith, K. C. (1976). Vision and mental function of the elderly. *Gerontologist, 16,* 491–495.

Stanovich, K. E. (1980). Toward an interactive-compensatory model of individual differences in the development of reading fluency. *Reading Research Quarterly, 16*, 32–71.

Stein, H., Slatt, B., & Stein, R. (1992). *Ophthalmic terminology* (3rd ed.). St. Louis: Mosby Year Book.

Stein, J. C., & Gradle, H. (1977). Telescopic spectacles and magnifiers as aids to poor vision (repr. of 1924 ed.). *Transactions of the American Academy of Ophthalmology and Otolaryngology, 77*, 229–253.

Stevens, S. S. (1951). *Handbook of experimental psychology.* New York: John Wiley & Sons.

Straatsma, B. R., Foos, R. X., Horwitz, J., Gardner, K. M., & Pettit, T. H. (1985). Aging related cataract: Laboratory investigation and clinical management. *Annals of Internal Medicine, 102*, 82–92.

Stratton (1990). The principle of least restrictive materials. *Journal of Visual Impairment & Blindness, 84*, 3–5.

Sullivan, T. (1980). *You are special.* Milwaukee: Ideals Publishing.

Szlyk, J., Arditi, A., Coffey-Bucci, P., & Laderman, D. (1990). Self-report in functional assessment of low vision. *Journal of Visual Impairment & Blindness, 84*, 61–66.

Taylor, H. R., West, S. K., Rosenthal, F. S., Munoz, B., Newland, H. S., Abbey, H., & Emmett, E. A. (1988). Effect of ultraviolet radiation on cataract formation. *The New England Journal of Medicine, 319*, 1429–1433.

Thorndike, R. L. (1984). *Intelligence as information processing: The mind and the computer.* Bloomington, IN: Phi Delta Kappa.

Tielsch, J., Sommer, A., Witt, K., Katz, J., & Royall, R. (1990). Blindness and visual impairment in an American urban population: The Baltimore eye survey. *Archives of Ophthalmology, 108*, 286–290.

Tierney, R. J., Readence, J. E., Dishner, E. K. (1990). *Reading strategies and practices: A compendium* (3rd ed.). Boston: Allyn & Bacon.

Timberlake, G. .T., Mainster, M. A., Peli, E., Augliere, R. A., Essock, E. A., & Arend, L. E. (1986). Reading with a macular scotoma: Retinal location of scotoma and fixation area. *Investigative Ophthalmology and Visual Science, 27*, 1137–1147.

Troutman, M. (1992). *One is fun: Guidelines for better braille literacy.* Brantford, Ontario: Author.

Tuttle, D. (1984). *Self-esteem and adjusting with blindness.* Springfield, IL: Charles C Thomas.

U.S. Department of Labor. (1991). *Dictionary of occupational titles.* Washington, DC: U.S. Government Printing Office.

U.S. Department of Labor. (1994a). *Guide for occupational exploration.* Washington, DC: U.S. Government Printing Office.

U.S. Department of Labor. (1994b). *Occupational outlook handbook.* Washington, DC: U.S. Government Printing Office.

Utley, B., Goetz, L., Gee, K., Baldwin, M., & Sailor, W. (1981). *Vision assessment and program manual for severely handicapped and/or deaf-blind students* (Eric Document Reproduction Service No. ED 250–840.) Reston, VA: Council for Exceptional Children.

Vaughan, D. G., & Asbury, T. (1980). *General ophthalmology* (9th ed.). Los Altos, CA: Lange Medical Publications.

Vaughan, D. G., Asbury, T., & Riordan-Eva, P. (1992). *General ophthalmology* (13th ed.). Los Altos, CA: Lange Medical Publications.

Vaughan, D. G., Asbury, T., & Riordan-Eva, P. (1995). *General ophthalmology* (14th ed.) Norwalk, CT: Appleton & Lange.

Venezky, R. L. (1990). Definitions of literacy. In R. L. Venezky, D. A. Wagner, & B. S. Ciliberti (Eds.), *Toward a definition of literacy* (pp. 2–16). Newark, DE: International Reading Association.

Watson, G. R. (1980). Training with near and intermediate distance optical and nonoptical aids. In M. Beliveau & A. Smith (Eds.), *The interdisciplinary approach to low vision rehabilitation* (RSA grant No. 45-P8153512-01) Stillwater: Oklahoma State University, National Clearinghouse on Rehabilitation Information.

Watson, G. R., & Berg, R. V. (1983). Near training techniques. In R. T. Jose (Ed.), *Understanding Low Vision* (pp. 317–362). New York: American Foundation for the Blind.

Watson, G. R., Wright, V., De l'Aune, W., & Sweison, L. (1991). The rehabilitation of reading for low vision individuals with macular loss (final report to the National Institute on Disability and Rehabilitation Research). Silver Spring, MD: NARIC.

Watson, G. R., Wright, V., & De l'Aune, W. (1992). The efficacy of comprehension training and reading practice for print readers with macular loss. *Journal of Visual Impairment and Blindness, 86*, 37–43.

Wheatley, G. (1987). A follow-up study of optical low vision aid use and stressful life events. *Journal of Vision Rehabilitation, 1.*

Whittaker, S., Budd, J., & Cummings, R. (1988). Eccentric fixation with macular scotoma. *Investigative Ophthalmology and Visual Science, 29*, 268–278.

Wiener, W. R., & Luxton, L. (1994). The development of guidelines for university programs in rehabilitation teaching. *RE:view, 26*, 7–14.

Wiener, W. R., & Vopata, A. (1980). Suggested curriculum for distance vision training with optical aids. *Journal of Visual Impairment & Blindness, 74*, 49–56.

Wolff, P. (1959). Observations on newborn infants. In L. Stone, H. Smith, & L. Murphy (Eds.). *The competent infant* (pp. 257–272). New York: Basic Books.

World Health Organization. (1992). *Management of low vision in children: Report of a WHO consultation* (WHO Publication 93.27). Geneva: Author.

Wright, V., & Watson, G. R. (1995). *Learn to use your vision for reading workbook.* Lilburn, GA: Bear Consultants.

Yeadon, A. (1974). *Toward independence: The use of instructional objectives in teaching daily living skills to the blind.* New York: American Foundation for the Blind.

Yeadon, A. (1988). *International low vision directory.* Philadelphia: Institute for the Visually Impaired, Pennsylvania College of Optometry.

Younger, V., & Sardegna, J. (1991). *One way or another.* San Jose, CA: Sardegna Productions.

Younger, V., & Sardegna, J. (1994). *Guide to independence for the visually impaired and their families.* New York: Demos.

Visual Effects of Selected Syndromes and Diseases

Syndrome or Disease	Tear system	Lids	Eye muscles	Cornea	Aqueous	Iris	Choroid	Lens	Vitreous	Retina	Macula	Optic nerve	Anophthalmos	Microphthalmia	Colobomas	Corneal opacities (clouding)	Cataracts	Glaucoma	Photophobia	Iritis	Retinitis pigmentosa	Macular degeneration	Retinal detachment	Retinal tumors	Myopia	Astigmatism	Nystagmus	Strabismus	Ptosis	Optic atrophy	Ocular only	Mental retardation	Seizures	Cerebral palsy	Neurological disorders	Hearing impairment	Kidney dysfunction	Agenesis of corpus callosum	Muscle weakness	Progressive dysfunction	Skin differences	Vascular or heart dysfunction	Nasal/sinus dysfunction	Uro-genital differences	Vestibular dysfunction	Oral or facial anomalies	Growth differences	Bone differences	Secretory dysfunction	Systemic changes	Joint differences
	Part(s) of the Eye Involved															Ocular Disease or Disorder																Associated Disabilities																			
Aicardi syndrome										X		X			X																	X	X	X	X			X													
Alport's syndrome								X									X																			X	X														
Bassen-Kornzweig syndrome										X	X	X							X		X						X			X				X	X				X												
Batten-Mayou disease										X	X	X									X									X		X	X	X	X					X											
Best's disease										X	X											X									X																				
Bielschowsky-Jansky disease										X	X											X								X	X																				
Bourneville's disease (tuberous sclerbusis)										X														X								X	X		X		X				X	X									
Bowen's disease				X																											X																				
Chandler's syndrome						X												X																																	
CHARGE association						X								X	X	X	X	X									X	X	X	X		X				X						X	X	X	X	X					
Coat's disease						X																	X								X																				
Cogan's syndrome				X												X			X	X																X						X			X						
Cri-du-chat			X																						X			X		X		X										X				X					
Crouzon's syndrome			X									X															X	X		X																X					
De Grouchy's syndrome				X												X		X							X			X	X	X		X																			
De Morsier's disease (septo-optic dysplasia)											X	X															X																				X				
Down's syndrome			X					X		X							X								X		X	X				X			X							X				X					
Duane's syndrome			X																									X																		X					
Edward's syndrome (Trisomy 18)				X				X				X		X	X	X	X	X											X	X		X			X							X				X		X			
Fabry's disease				X				X		X						X																									X	X							X		
Galactosemia								X									X															X																			
Gaucher's disease				X							X					X					X													X							X									X	
Goldman-Favre syndrome									X	X											X				X																										
Grave's disease (hyperthyroidism)	X	X	X									X																																						X	

Syndrome/Disease	1	2	3	4	5	6	7	8	9	10	11	12	13	14	15	16	17	18	19	20	21	22	23	24	25	26	27	28	29	30
Hallerman-Streiff-Francoi's syndrome						X																					X		X	X
Hunter's syndrome	X					X											X			X	X	X	X		
Hurler's syndrome	X	X				X	X	X	X								X	X		X	X	X	X		X		X		X	X
Irvine-Gass syndrome				X	X				X																				
Laurence-Moon-Biedl syndrome				X	X								X				X			X	X				X
Lowe's syndrome		X		X	X	X	X	X					X	X	X		X	X							X
Marchesani's syndrome		X	X	X	X	X	X					X											X		
Marfan's syndrome	X	X		X	X	X	X	X	X			X				X	X			X	X		X	X
Mobius' disease	X				X			X	X				X											
Niemann-Pick disease		X		X	X	X	X				X		X	X				X	X					
Norrie's disease				X	X		X				X		X	X	X	X									
Paget's disease			X	X	X					X										X		X			
Patau's syndrome (Trisomy 13)	X	X	X	X	X	X	X	X	X			X	X	X	X	X				X		X			
Peter's anomaly	X	X		X	X	X		X			X	X				X			X			X		X	X
Posner-Schlossman syndrome	X	X		X	X	X				X														X	X
Refsum's disease				X	X	X					X	X	X				X			X		X		X	X
Rieger's syndrome	X	X		X	X				X																
Riley-Day syndrome	X	X	X	X	X	X	X		X				X	X						X		X			
Rubella syndrome	X	X		X	X	X		X	X			X	X	X		X	X		X	X		X		X	X
Scheie's syndrome		X		X	X	X		X			X	X	X				X			X		X		X	X
Stargardt-Behr's disease		X	X	X	X		X	X			X											X		
Stevens-Johnson syndrome	X	X	X	X	X				X				X	X	X	X				X	X
Still's disease	X	X	X	X	X	X	X			X							X			X	X
Sturge-Weber syndrome	X			X	X		X		X				X	X						X
Tay Sach's disease				X	X	X		X	X	X	X	X		X			X				X
Turner's syndrome	X			X	X	X		X	X			X		X			X			X	X			X	X
Usher's syndrome				X	X	X		X			X		X				X			X
Vogt-Spielmeyer disease				X	X	X		X			X				X		X	X		X	X
von Hippel-Lindau disease				X	X	X		X							X	X				X
von Recklinghausen's disease (eurofibromatosis)	X			X		X							X	X								X
Wilson's disease	X			X	X	X				X							X			X	X			X	X	X
Zellweger's disease	X			X	X	X	X	X		X	X	X	X				X	X							X	X

Sources: B. Cassin, S. Solomon, & M. Rubin, *Dictionary of Eye Terminology* (Gainesville, FL: Triad Publishing, 1990); J. Gittinger & G. Asdourian, *Manual of Clinical Problems in Ophthalmology* (Boston: Little, Brown and Company, 1988); S. Isenberg, *The Eye in Infancy* (Chicago: Yearbook Medical Publishers, 1989); F. Newell, *Ophthalmology: Principles and Concept*, 7th ed. (St. Louis: Mosby Year Book, 1992); D. Pavan-Langston, *Manual of Ocular Diagnosis and Therapy* (Boston: Little, Brown and Company, 1985); F. Roy, *Ocular Syndromes and Systemic Diseases* (Orlando, FL: Grune and Stratton, 1985); H. Stein, B. Slatt, & R. Stein, *Ophthalmic Terminology*, 3rd ed. (St. Louis: Mosby Year Book, 1992); D. G. Vaughan & T. Asbury, *General Ophthalmology*, 9th ed. (Los Altos, CA: Lange Medical Publications, 1980); D. G. Vaughan, T. Asbury, & P. Riordan-Eva, *General Ophthalmology*, 13th ed. (Norwalk, CT: Appleton & Lange, 1992).

Note: A syndrome is defined as a group of symptoms or defects that nearly always occur together and that may affect the whole body or any of its parts. The syndromes included in this table represent only a sampling of those that have an impact on the visual system but are conditions that professionals may encounter, particularly in children. It should also be noted that the conditions listed generally include characteristics that involve more than the visual system only and may have additional manifestations (Contributors: Virginia E. Bishop and Jane N. Erin).

GLOSSARY

Absorptive lenses Eyeglasses with lenses tinted to absorb much of the sun's light and prevent it from entering the eye; sunglasses.

Academic literacy Mastery of school-based reading and writing skills.

Accommodation The ability of the eye to maintain a clear focus as objects are moved closer to it by changing the shape of the lens.

Achromatopsia A congenital defect in or absence of cones, resulting in the inability to see color and reduced clear central vision.

Acquired/Adventitious Occurring or appearing later in life.

Age-related macular degeneration A condition associated with vascular diseases such as arteriosclerosis and stroke, in which central vision is gradually lost and acuity may decrease to 20/200 or less, but peripheral vision is usually retained. Also called Age-related maculopathy.

Albinism, Ocular The congenital absence of pigment in the iris and choroid that causes light sensitivity, nystagmus, and reduced acuity.

Albinism, oculocutaneous The congenital lack of pigment in the iris, choroid, hair, and skin that results in reduced acuity, light sensitivity, and nystagmus.

Amblyopia Reduced vision without observable changes in the structure of the eye, caused by eyes that are not straight or by a difference in the refractive error in the two eyes, sometimes called "lazy eye"; not correctable with lenses, since the brain's suppression is the cause.

Amsler grid A graphlike card used to determine central field losses, as in macular degeneration.

Angle of incidence The angle at which light strikes and exits a surface.

Angular magnification Increasing the apparent size of an object through the use of various lens systems, such as binoculars.

Aniridia A congenital malformation (usually incomplete) of the iris, accompanied by nystagmus, photophobia, reduced visual acuity, and often glaucoma.

Aniseikonia A condition in which each retina receives a different-size image because of different refractive errors in the two eyes.

Anisometropia Different refractive errors of at least 1 diopter in the two eyes.

Anophthalmia The congenital absence of the eyeball.

Anterior chamber The space between the iris and cornea inside the eye, filled with aqueous fluid.

Aphakia The absence of the lens, usually resulting from the removal of a cataract.

Aqueous The clear fluid in the space between the front of the vitreous and the back of the cornea, produced by the ciliary processes, that bathes the lens and nourishes the iris and inner surface of the cornea. Also called Aqueous humor.

Astigmatism A refractive error caused by a sphero-cylindrical curvature of the cornea; corrected with a cylindrical lens.

Augmentative visual cue An object, such as a light, that highlights another object to draw attention to it.

Bailey-Lovie Chart A distance visual acuity measurement chart in which the number of symbols in each row is the same and the spacing between symbols and rows are proportionate to the size of the symbol.

Binocular vision Vision that uses both eyes to form a fused image in the brain and results in three-dimensional vision.

Bioptic A miniature telescope mounted into a person's regular eyeglasses, positioned above or below the direct line of sight when facing forward, that is used for distance viewing.

Blepharitis An inflammation of the eyelids, accompanied by itching, redness, and swelling.

Blind spot See Scotoma.

Blink reflex A contraction of the eyelid muscles to close the lids that occurs spontaneously when there are sudden loud noises, bright lights, sneezing, or a perceived visual threat.

Canal of Schlemm A circular channel at the limbus that collects aqueous fluid from the anterior chamber and transmits it into the blood stream via the veins.

Cataracts A clouding of the lens, which may be congenital, traumatic, secondary to another visual impairment, or age related. When a cataract is surgically removed, an intraocular lens implant or contact lens or spectacle correction is necessary, to provide the refractive function of the absent lens.

Central scotoma Areas of diminished or absent vision that result in a "blind spot" in the center of the visual field.

Cerebrovascular accident (CVA) Stroke, or intracranial bleeding or infarctions.

Chorioretinitis An inflammation of the choroid and retina.

Choroid The vascular layer of the eye, between the sclera and retina, that nourishes the retina; part of the uveal tract.

Ciliary body Tissue inside the eye, composed of the ciliary processes and ciliary muscle; the former secretes aqueous, and the latter controls the shape of the lens.

Ciliary muscle A ring of muscle tissue in the ciliary body that expands or contracts to change the shape of the lens in accommodation.

Client assistance programs State-level resources to help individuals obtain appropriate services from rehabilitation agencies; rights assured under the Rehabilitation Act Amendments of 1984.

Clinical low vision evaluation A clinical evaluation to determine whether a person with low vision can benefit from optical devices, nonoptical devices, or adaptive techniques to enhance visual function.

Clinical low vision specialist An ophthalmologist or optometrist who specializes in low vision care.

Closed-circuit television system (CCTV) A device that provides electronic magnification by means of a video camera that projects the image onto a television monitor.

Cloze procedure A way of fostering growth in reading comprehension by replacing a given number of words in a reading selection with blanks; the student must guess at the words from context clues.

Coloboma Congenital cleft in some portion of the eye, caused by the improper fusion of tissue during gestation; may affect the optic nerve, ciliary body, choroid, iris, lens, or eyelid.

Color vision The perception of color as a result of the stimulation of specialized cone receptors in the retina.

Concave lens A lens that spreads out light rays and is used to correct for myopia. Also called Minus lens. See also Spherical lens.

Cone dystrophy The hereditary degeneration of cones, resulting in decreased vision and the lack of color perception.

Cones Specialized photoreceptor cells in the retina, primarily concentrated in the macular area, that are responsible for sharp vision and color perception.

Confrontation visual field testing A method for making a rough assessment of peripheral vision, which may suggest the need for more precise visual field testing.

Congenital Present at birth.

Conjunctiva A thin membrane lining the inner surface of the eyelid and part of the outer surface of the eyeball (not including the cornea).

Conjunctivitis An inflammation of the conjunctiva, viral, allergic, bacterial, or fungal. Some varieties are contagious, but others are not.

Contact lens A small plastic disc containing an optical correction, that is worn directly on the cornea as a substitute for eyeglasses.

Contrast sensitivity The ability to detect differences in grayness and background. Because more of the retina is used in discriminating contrast, it may be a better test of visual function, since it utilizes more than central visual acuity.

Convergence The movement, as an object approaches, of both eyes toward each other in an effort to maintain fusion of separate images.

Convex lens A lens that bends light rays inward and is used to correct for hyperopia. Also called Plus lens. See also Spherical lens.

Cornea The transparent tissue at the front of the eye that is curved to provide most of the eye's refractive power.

Corneal dystrophy A hereditary defect that causes the cornea to become cloudy; usually occurs later in life.

Critical Incidents Assessment A method of assessing mobility problems by observing actual mobility situations.

Critical literacy The use of higher-level cognitive ability to make the best use of functional literacy; includes problem solving, understanding, insight, and the capacity for action.

Critical viewing distance The distance at which an object can first be correctly identified.

Cryotherapy The use of intense cold (freezing) to treat retinal holes and to prevent the proliferation of blood vessels in retinopathy of prematurity.

Cylindrical lenses A lens whose shape is a segment of a cylinder, used to correct the refractive error in astigmatism.

Depth cues A visual perceptual concept in which nearer objects overlap those that are located at a distance.

Depth perception The overlapping of two slightly dissimilar images from the two eyes to give three-dimensional vision.

Diabetic retinopathy Range of retinal changes associated with long-standing diabetes; includes nonproliferative (early stages) and proliferative (when blood vessels grow abnormally and fibrous tissues form).

Diagnostic teaching The analysis of learning problems during lessons and targeted instruction to minimize or eliminate the problems.

Dichromatism A moderately severe defect in color vision, in which one of three types of color receptors is either absent or nonfunctioning; affects mostly males and is hereditary-sex linked.

Diopter The unit of measurement for the refractive power of a lens.

Diplopia Double vision resulting from the lack of fusion of the two images received by the two eyes.

Divergence The movement of the two eyes outward (away from each other) to maintain binocular vision.

Dynamic visual acuity The ability to discriminate and identify objects when the person is stationary and targets are moving and when both the person and the targets are moving.

Dynamic visual field The potential functional field range when a person moves through the environment.

Eccentric fixation The use of a portion of the retina that is not specialized for sharp vision when a portion of or the entire fovea has become nonfunctional. Also called Eccentric viewing.

Electronic magnification systems Machines that produce enlarged images, including closed-circuit televisions, computer systems, and low vision enhancement devices.

Emergent literacy The earliest phase in literacy learning, in which young children are actively engaged in experimenting with reading and writing and in gaining meaning from these activities.

Emmetropia A normal eye in which there is no refractive error.

Endophthalmitis An infection or inflammation inside the eye.

Enucleation Surgical removal of the eye.

Environmental adaptations-modifications Changes in the environment to maximize the use of vision.

Environmental manipulation Changing lighting, contrast, color, distance, and the size of objects in the environment to enhance visual functioning.

Electroretinogram (ERG) An electrophysiological test of retinal function; the wave forms show the function of rods, cones, and bipolar cells.

Esotropia A form of strabismus in which one or both eyes deviate inward; whereas esotropia is an observable condition, esophoria is the tendency to deviate inward.

Exotropia A form of strabismus in which one or both eyes deviate outward; exotropia is the observable condition, whereas exophoria is the tendency to deviate outward.

Extrinsic muscles The six muscles located on the outside of the eyeball but within the orbit that are responsible for turning the eye right, left, upward, or downward; also called the extraocular muscles.

Eyelids Structures that cover the front of the eyes to protect them, control the amount of light entering them, and distribute tears over the cornea.

Farnsworth panel D15 test A diagnostic test to determine type of color deficiency.

Field See Visual field.

Field expansion systems A variety of optical devices for individuals with reduced visual fields, including prism lenses, mirror magnifiers, and reverse telescopes.

Fixation Coordinated eye movements to enable an image to focus on the fovea.

Fixed pupil A pupil that does not respond to light by constricting.

Focal distance The distance between a lens and the point at which parallel light rays are brought to a focus.

Focal point The point at which parallel light rays are brought to a focus by a lens.

Fovea centralis An indentation in the center of the macula where the cones are concentrated, there are no blood vessels, and the clearest vision takes place.

Fresnel prisms A series of plastic prisms applied to regular eyeglass lenses that are used to correct eye deviations or to displace peripheral information onto areas of the retina.

Functional blindness Condition in which some useful vision may or may not be present but in which the individual uses tactile and auditory channels most effectively for learning.

Functional literacy The ability to apply reading and writing skills to practical tasks in everyday life.

Functional vision The ability to use vision in planning and performing a task.

Functional vision assessment An assessment of an individual's use of vision in a variety of tasks and settings, including measures of near and distance vision; visual fields; eye movements; and responses to specific environmental characteristics, such as light and color. The assessment report includes recommendations for instructional procedures, modifications-adaptations, and additional tests.

General learning media Instructional materials (globes, rulers, models, and charts) and teaching methods (demonstrations, verbal guidance, and lectures) to which modifications are made on the basis of visual need and learning style; literacy media are included in the broader context of learning media. See also, Literacy media.

Glare An annoying sensation produced by too much light in the visual field that can cause both discomfort and a reduction in visual acuity.

Glaucoma A condition characterized by an increase in intraocular pressure, visually associated with a buildup of aqueous fluid, that may cause damage to the nerves of the retina and the optic nerve and eventual visual field defects if left untreated.

Habilitation The education and development of children and youths with congenital or early-onset visual impairments, including the teaching of compensatory and visual efficiency skills as well as daily living skills.

Hand movements A method of measuring low vision when an individual cannot count fingers; the examiner notes the distance at which a waving hand can be perceived.

Hemianopsia A defect in either half of the visual field. Also called Hemianopia.

HOTV Test A visual acuity chart using irreversible letters; effective with preschool children who are able to match letters.

Hyperopia (farsightedness) A refractive error caused by an eyeball that is too short; corrected with a plus (convex) lens.

Hypertropia The upward deviation of one eye; hyperphoria is the tendency of one eye to turn upward.

Hypotropia The downward deviation of one eye; the least common of the eye deviations classified as strabismus.

Independent living skills Skills for performing daily tasks and managing personal needs; individuals with low vision often learn alternative or modified methods of performing these skills.

Index of refraction A measure of the refractive power of a substance, such as various types of lenses or glass or the ocular media of the eye.

Individualized Education Program (IEP) A written plan of instruction by a transdisciplinary educational team for a child who receives special education services that includes the student's present levels of educational performance, annual goals, short-term objectives, specific services needed, duration of services, evaluation, and related information. Under the Individuals with Disabilities Education Act (IDEA), each student receiving special services must have such a plan.

Individualized Written Rehabilitation Program (IWRP) A contract between a person with low vision and a rehabilitation agency that describes the services needed to achieve the person's employment objective.

Intake history A comprehensive case history that enables an examiner to understand an individual's visual problems and needs.

Interdisciplinary team Professionals from various disciplines who conduct and share the results of assessments and jointly plan instructional programs.

Intraocular lens (IOL) implant An artificial (plastic) lens that is inserted surgically when a cataract is removed to replace the function of the natural lens.

Iris The colored portion of the eye that expands or contracts to control the amount of light entering the eye.

Iritis An inflammation of the iris that may cause blurred vision, a constricted pupil, pain, and tearing; must be treated medically.

Ishihara color plates A series of patterns of colored dots used to identify color perception difficulties. The individual must distinguish colors to see numbers or trace a pathway.

Jaeger system A test of near vision using graded sizes of letters or numbers.

Keratitis Any of a wide variety of corneal infections, irritations, and inflammations.

Keratoconus A hereditary degenerative disease that is manifest in adolescence or later, in which the cornea thins and becomes cone shaped and vision is reduced.

Keratometer An instrument for measuring the curvature of the cornea that is used to measure astigmatism.

Keratopathy A defect in or disease of the cornea

Keratoscope A device used to examine the cornea.

Lacrimal system The apparatus for the production and drainage of tears; the lacrimal gland produces tears that are drained into the lacrimal sac, through the nasolacrimal duct and into the back of the nose.

Landolt "C" test A visual acuity chart with broken rings in Snellen sizes that are varied in position or direction.

Language Experience Approach (LEA) A reading instruction strategy that is based directly on a student's actual experiences.

LEA Symbols A distance acuity test depicting symbols (circle, house, apple, and square) that is used for testing a child's visual acuity.

Learning channel One or more of the primary senses (vision, hearing, or touch) that an individual uses most for learning.

Learning Media Assessment (LMA) A structured procedure that measures an individual's primary learning channel or channels, the best literacy medium, and the efficiency of that literacy medium.

Least restrictive materials Materials that are adapted only to the extent necessary to allow efficient learning.

Legal blindness Visual impairment in which distance visual acuity is 20/200 or less in the better eye after best correction with conventional lenses or visual field restriction is 20 degrees or less, often used as a criterion for determining eligibility for benefits or services in the United States.

Lens The transparent, biconvex structure within the eye that allows it to refract light rays, enabling them to focus on the retina; also, any transparent substance that can refract light in a predictable manner.

Light-absorptive lenses See Absorptive lenses.

Light-dark adaptation The ability of the eye to adjust to lighting conditions in a variety of situations.

Lighthouse Distance Acuity Chart A chart used to measure distance visual acuity at either 2 or 4 meters.

Lighthouse Flash Card Test A distance acuity test depicting symbols (house, apple, and umbrella) that is used for assessing a child's visual acuity.

Light perception The ability to discern the presence or absence of light, but not its source or direction.

Light projection The ability to discern the source or direction of light, but not enough vision to identify objects, people, shapes, or movements.

Limbus The junction of the cornea and the sclera.

Literacy The ability to read and write.

Literacy medium The form of the printed word (print or braille) that an individual uses to read and write.

Loupe A convex lens for magnifying that can be used in monocular or binocular forms, mounted in front of the eye, for viewing small objects at a very close distance.

Low vision A visual impairment after correction, but with the potential for use of available vision, with or without optical or nonoptical compensatory visual strategies, devices, and environmental modifications, to plan and perform daily tasks.

Low Vision Enhancement System (LVES) A head-borne device that electronically enlarges images seen at a distance.

Macula A small portion of the retina, with a concentration of cones for sharp central vision, that surrounds the fovea.

Macular degeneration Deterioration of central vision caused by a degeneration of the central retina.

Magnifiers A device to increase the size of an image through the use of lenses or lens systems; may be fixed focus (stand types, bar varieties) or variable focus (handheld).

Manual-bowl and computerized-bowl perimetry Devices used to test the central and peripheral field of vision.

Meniscus lens A spherical lens with a convex surface on one side and a concave surface on the other; the greater curve determines whether the lens is a "plus" or a "minus" lens.

Microphthalmia An abnormally small eyeball.

Microscopes A high-power convex lens that magnifies near-point objects. Usually mounted into eyeglasses and prescribed for one eye only.

Minus lens See Concave lens.

Monochromatism Poor or no color perception; the presence of only one type of retinal cone (cone monochromatism) or the absence of all cone function (rod monochromatism).

Monocular telescope A telescope that can be used in the preferred eye.

Monocularity The loss of vision in one eye due to injury or enucleation.

Motility, ocular Eye movement controlled by the extraocular muscles.

Multidisciplinary team Professionals from various disciplines who conduct separate assessments and provide individual services.

Myopia (nearsightedness) A refractive error resulting from an eyeball that is too long; corrected with a concave (minus) lens.

Neuropathy The reduced ability of a nerve or nerves to function, as in reduced tactile sensitivity in diabetic neuropathy.

No light perception (NLP) The total absence of vision.

Nonoptical devices Devices or modifications that do not involve optics, used to make visual information more accessible to individuals with low vision, such as book stands, trays, positioning-seating, modifications of illumination, and large print when indicated.

Nonparallel instruction Dual instruction in reading print and braille, with a greater emphasis on one or the other (usually on print reading).

Nystagmus An involuntary oscillation of the eyes, usually rhythmical and faster in one direction; may be side to side or up and down.

Occipital lobe The posterior part of the brain that is responsible for vision and visual perception; it includes the visual cortex, which is the cerebral end of the visual pathway.

Ocular media The four transparent layers of the eyes, specifically, the cornea, aqueous, lens, and vitreous.

Ophthalmologist A physician who specializes in the medical and surgical care of the eyes and is qualified to prescribe ocular medications and to perform surgery on the eyes. May also perform refractive and low vision work, including eye examinations and other vision services.

Optical device Any system of lenses that enhances visual function.

Optic atrophy The degeneration or malfunction of the optic nerve, characterized by a pale optic disk.

Optic chiasm The junction where the fibers coming from the nasal portion of the retina of each eye split off from their optic nerves and cross over to the opposite side to join fibers coming from the temporal portion of each retina from the opposite side.

Optic disk The point at which the nerve fibers from the inner layer of the retina becomes the optic nerve and exit the eye; the "blind spot" of the eye.

Optic nerve The sensory nerve of the eye that carries electrical impulses from the eye to the brain.

Optic nerve hypoplasia A congenitally small optic disk, usually surrounded by a light halo and representing a regression in growth during the prenatal period; may result in reduced visual acuity.

Optics The study of light, its ability to refract and reflect, and its behavior in lenses, prisms, mirrors, and the eye.

Optic tract Fibers of the optic nerve that extend beyond the optic chiasm.

Optokinetic drum A cylinder with vertical patterns of black lines that, when turned slowly, induces a kind of nystagmus; it measures the ability of the eye to perceive black bands of various widths, which corresponds to rough visual acuity measures, depending on the width of the bands. It is used with nonverbal individuals and young children, especially infants.

Optometrist A health care provider who specializes in refractive errors, prescribes eyeglasses or contact lenses, and diagnoses and manages conditions of the eye as regulated by state law.

Ora serrata The anterior edge of the retina, located just behind the ciliary body.

Orbits Two pyramidal cavities in the front of the skull that contain the eyeballs, eye muscles, and fatty cushioning layers, as well as nerves and blood vessels.

Orientation and mobility (O&M) instructor A professional who specializes in teaching travel skills to visually impaired persons, including the use of a cane, dog guide, or sophisticated electronic travel aids, as well as the sighted guide technique.

Orthoptics The techniques of treating problems in eye movement and coordination, binocular vision, and functional amblyopia through nonsurgical means, using lenses, prisms, or exercises; the orthoptist usually works under the supervision of an ophthalmologist.

Parallel instruction Dual instruction in print reading and braille, with equal emphasis on literacy in both media.

Pars plana The back portion of the ciliary body behind the limbus and between the ciliary processes and the ora serrata; the common site for the entrance of instruments used in vitrectomies.

Partial sight A term formerly often used to indicate visual acuity of 20/70 to 20/200 but also used to describe visual impairment in which usable vision is present.

Perceptual span The amount of information that an individual can decode and store in short-term memory in one fixation. The width is about 7–10 letters for a normal adult reader, but for a reader with low vision, the width may depend on the distance from the page and the intactness of the central visual field.

Phoria The tendency of the eyes to deviate, which is controlled by the brain's efforts to achieve binocular vision.

Phoropter A device used by eye care specialists to analyze the refractive error in persons with intact central vision using various lenses to determine which provide the best correction.

Photocoagulation The use of a laser to burn or destroy selected intraocular structures, such as intraocular tumors or abnormal blood vessels, and to create chorioretinal adhesions in retinal detachment surgery.

Photophobia Light sensitivity to an uncomfortable degree; usually symptomatic of other ocular disorders or diseases.

Photopic vision Clear vision under daylight conditions; involves the cones.

Photoreceptor cells Retinal cells (rods and cones) that convert light to electrical impulses that can be transmitted to the brain.

Phthisis bulbi A shrunken eyeball, usually a blind eye, that is the result of damage or disease.

Pigment epithelium A layer of cells between the retina and the choroid that has a nutritional function.

Plano lens A lens that is parallel on both sides (has no refractive power).

Plus lens See Convex lens.

Posterior chamber The space between the front of the vitreous and the back of the iris that is filled with aqueous fluid.

Preferential looking A means of testing the vision of nonverbal or preverbal children in which patterned stimuli are presented to the right or left, and the movement of the individual's eyes is noted.

Preferred distance The distance at which an individual is most comfortable in viewing an object.

Preferred visual field The location (in space) at which an individual seems to notice the most objects in the environment.

Presbyopia A decrease in accommodative power (focusing at near) caused by the increasing inelasticity of the lens-ciliary muscle mechanism that occurs approximately anytime after age 40.

Primary medium The literacy medium, whether print or braille, that will be used by an individual for gaining basic academic literacy skills.

Print Media Assessment Process (PMAP) A procedure for objectively assessing the relative effectiveness of reading in various print media.

Prism lenses Special triangle-shaped lenses that are incorporated into regular eyeglasses, to redirect the rays of light entering the eye, resulting in a realignment of the eyes or, in some cases, a shifting of images to permit binocular vision.

Projection magnification Increasing the size of an image to be viewed by the process of projection, such as by projecting the image of text onto a monitor.

Prosthesis An artificial eye.

Ptosis A drooping of the eyelid caused by paralysis or weak eyelid muscles; it may be congenital. Ptosis requires surgical correction if the droop interferes with vision.

Pupil The hole in the center of the iris through which light rays enter the back of the eye.

Pupillary reflex A reflexive constriction of the pupil when light stimuli are presented. Also called Pupillary responses.

Radial keratotomy A surgical procedure in which a series of deep radical cuts are made in the cornea to shorten the eye optically in order to reduce myopea.

Reading efficiency The rate at which a person can read a passage with at least 75 percent comprehension, using whatever medium is most comfortable.

Recession The surgical repositioning of an eye muscle to correct an eye deviation.

Refraction The bending of light rays as they pass through a substance. Also, the determination of the refractive errors of the eye and their correction with eyeglasses or contact lenses.

Refractive disorder Defects in the eye that cause visual acuity loss if uncorrected.

Refractive errors Conditions such as myopia, hyperopia, and astigmatism caused by corneal irregularities, in which parallel rays of light are not brought to a focus on the retina because of a defect in the shape of the eyball or the refractive media of the eye.

Rehabilitation The learning of skills impairment, including the relearning of vocational and daily living skills using adaptive equipment and techniques.

Rehabilitation counselor A professional trained to determine eligibility for rehabilitation and related services; provide counseling and guidance; coordinate job placement, follow-up, and postemployment services; and develop and implement Individualized Written Rehabilitation Programs (IWRPs).

Rehabilitation teacher A professional trained to teach the compensatory and adaptive skills that enable a visually impaired person to live and function independently.

Relative-distance magnification Increasing the size of an image on the retina by bringing the object to be viewed closer to the eyes.

Relative-size magnification Increasing the size of an image on the retina by increasing the size of an object to be viewed, such as with large print.

Resection To take a piece out of an ocular muscle to shorten it and correct an eye deviation.

Retina The inner sensory nerve layer next to the choroid that lines the posterior two-thirds of the eyeball. The retina reacts to light and transmits impulses to the brain.

Retinal detachment The separation of the retina from the underlying choroid, nearly always caused by a retinal tear. It usually requires surgical intervention to prevent loss of vision.

Retinal edema The swelling of the retina because of leaking blood vessels.

Retinitis pigmentosa A group of progressive, often hereditary, retinal degenerative diseases that are characterized by decreasing peripheral vision; some progress to tunnel vision, whereas others result in total blindness if the macula also becomes involved.

Retinoblastoma An intraocular malignant tumor of early childhood, often hereditary or caused by a mutated gene. Symptoms include redness, pain, inflammation, or gray or white pupil. Treatment options include chemotherapy, cryotherapy, radiation, and enucleation (surgical removal of the eye).

Retinoscopy The use of a hand-held light projected onto the pupil to measure the eye's refractive error by evaluating the behavior of the light reflected back from the retina.

Retinopathy of prematurity A series of retinal changes (formerly called retrolental fibroplasia), from mild to total retinal detachment, seen primarily in premature infants, that may be arrested at any stage. Believed to connected to the immature blood vessels in the eye and their reaction to oxygen, but may be primarily the result of prematurity with very low birthweight. Functional vision can range from near normal to total blindness.

Retrolental fibroplasia See Retinopathy of prematurity.

Rod monochromatism The absence of retinal cones or the presence of nonfunctional cones, resulting in the inability to distinguish color; characterized also by nystagmus, light sensitivity, and lowered visual acuity.

Rods Specialized retinal photoreceptor cells, that are located primarily in the peripheral retina, responsible for seeing form, shape, and movement and function best in low levels of illumination.

Saccadic eye movements Rapid eye movements in the same direction that are the most noticeable during reading, when there is a fixation and refixation on the perceptual span of letters.

Scanning Repetitive fixations that are required to look from one object to another.

Sclera The tough, white, opaque outer covering of the eye that protects the inner contents from most injuries.

Scleral buckle A procedure used for retinal detachment, in which a strap of preserved sclera or silicone rubber is surgically wrapped around the eyeball, and tightened to indent the sclera, forcing the retina into contact with the choroid and encouraging reattachment of the retina.

Scotoma A gap or blindspot in the visual field that may be caused by damage to the retina or visual pathways. Each eye contains one normal scotoma, corresponding to the location of the optic nerve head, which contains no photo-receptors.

Secondary medium A literacy medium that supplements print or will be developed later as a primary reading-writing medium; usually refers to braille when there is nonparallel literacy instruction.

Septo-optic dysplasia A severe form of optic nerve hypoplasia, in which the brain is also malformed. Endocrine deficiencies appear later as well.

Shape constancy The concept that objects remain the same shape, even though they may appear to change shape when viewed at different angles.

Size constancy The concept that objects remain the same size, even though they appear to be smaller when viewed from a distance.

Snellen Chart The traditional eye chart whose top line consists of the letter *E* and which is used in routine eye examinations.

Spherical lens A lens whose shape is a segment of a sphere. A convex (plus) lens is thicker in the center and is used to correct hyperopia; a concave (minus) lens is used to correct myopia. Other types of spherical lenses are biconvex (when both surfaces curve outward), plano-convex (a single-sided curve), biconcave (both surfaces curving inward), and plano-concave (when only one surface curves inward).

Static visual acuity The ability to discriminate and identify a variety of stationary targets when the viewer is stationary.

Static visual field The ability to describe the outermost objects seen in the stationary field of vision; the outer boundaries of the visual field.

Strabismus An extrinsic muscle imbalance that causes misalignment of the eyes; includes exotropia, esotropia, hypertropia, and hypotropia.

Sty An external infection of an eyelash follicle at the eyelid margin.

STYCAR Toy Test A text used to assess visual acuity in young children that requires a child to match a variety of small toys and utensils at a 10- and 20-foot distance; Snellen equivalents are obtainable.

Suspensory ligaments A circle of fine fibers (also called zonules) that are attached to the ciliary body, and hold the lens in position; they allow the lens to change shape in accommodation.

Sympathetic ophthalmia An inflammation of the uveal tract of an uninjured eye following a penetrating injury to the other eye.

Tangent screen perimetry A flexible technique for examining visual field with 30 degrees of fixation.

Teacher of students with visual impairments A specially trained and certified teacher who is qualified to teach special skills to students with visual impairments.

Telemicroscope A lens system in which an adaptation called a reading cap is used on a telescope to provide additional plus lens power to an existing system, transforming the telescope into a viewing device for intermediate distances.

Telescope A lens system that makes small objects appear closer and larger.

Threshold distance The distance at which an object can first be detected.

Trabecular meshwork A network at the angle of the iris and cornea that filters aqueous fluid as it leaves the anterior chamber. Interference with the flow of aqueous at the meshwork can lead to an elevation of intraocular pressure (glaucoma).

Tracing Visually following single or multiple stationary lines in the environment, such as hedge lines, roof lines, or baseboards.

Tracking Visually following a moving object.

Transdisciplinary team A group of professionals from many disciplines in which one team member acts as "primary programmer" and implements programs that have been designed by the other specialists based on their own assessments; sometimes, the "primary programmer also participates in or conducts the assessments, with the support and assistance of the other members of the team.

Trichromatism A condition in which all three kinds of retinal cones are present, but function is mildly impaired. A person with this condition is more likely to confuse colors than not to see them.

Tropia Marked deviations in the alignment of the eyes that cannot be controlled.

Tumbling E Test Another name for the Snellen Illiterate E chart that is used in testing visual acuity (central vision).

Tunnel vision Severe restriction of peripheral vision.

Uveal tract The vascular layer of the eye, composed of the choroid, ciliary body, and iris.

Uveitis An inflammation of any portion of the uveal tract.

Vision rehabilitation services The full range of clinical and instructional services related to the prescription and use of optical and nonoptical devices to maximize vision.

Vision skills instruction A program of instruction that encourages the use of visual skills, such as attending (fixating), tracking, shifting attention between objects, scanning, and reaching for objects.

Visual abilities The dimension of functional vision that includes visual acuity, visual fields, motility, brain function-control, and light-color perception.

Visual acuity The sharpness of vision with respect to the ability to distinguish detail, often measured as the eye's ability to distinguish the details and shapes of objects at a designated distance; involves central (macular) vision.

Visual clutter A combination of images and backgrounds that provides distracting details for some individuals who are unable to select a single object from its background (figure-ground difficulties).

Visual disability A visual impairment that causes a real or perceived disadvantage in performing specific tasks.

Visual discrimination The ability to perceive sufficient detail in an object (or letter or numeral) to identify it correctly.

Visual efficiency The extent to which available vision is used effectively.

Visual field The area that can be seen when looking straight ahead, measured in degrees from the fixation point. Also called Field of vision.

Visual functions The behaviors one employs using vision, such as shifting gaze or scanning an environment.

Visual impairment Any degree of vision loss that affects an individual's ability to perform the tasks of daily life, caused by a visual system that is not working properly or not formed correctly.

Visual perception The process of attaching meaning to a visual image.

Visual stimulation An instructional program that provides a rich and stimulating environment, thus encouraging the visual system to react and reinforcing visual functioning.

Visual training A systematic program of instruction, using direct and planned reinforcement procedures, that teaches a set of specific visual skills that would otherwise be acquired incidently. Specific skills include visual attending, visual examining, and visually guided motor behaviors.

Vitrectomy The surgical removal of the vitreous and its replacement with a saline solution.

Vitreous A transparent, clear, jelly-like substance that fills the back portion of the eye between the lens and the retina and it maintains the shape of the eyeball.

Work Environment Visual Demands (WEVD) Protocol An instrument that is sometimes used to analyze the visual demands of a job or work environment.

Working distance The distance between the eye and an object of regard, such as a page being read.

RESOURCES

An essential part of working with individuals with low vision is providing information about a wide variety of products and services they may require. Many of the devices needed by people who have low vision are not available in local stores. In addition, services available for persons with low vision differ considerably from place to place. Professionals should have information about products and services at their fingertips to direct appropriately the individuals with whom they work.

This resource guide, although by necessity not exhaustive, is a good place for professionals in the field of low vision to begin when looking for products or services needed for clients or for themselves. Although a complete listing of all sources of information and referral, products, and services is beyond the scope of this book, an effort was made to include some representative examples in all of the important product and service areas.

The first section, Sources of Information and Services, gives descriptive information on consumer organizations as well as a sampling of national organizations that provide information, consumer education materials, services, and referrals for services for individuals with low vision. A separate section lists organizations that focus on specific visual impairments. Also included in this section is a list of professional organizations of interest to low vision practitioners and a separate list of international organizations. The American Foundation for the Blind (AFB) acts as a national clearinghouse for information about blindness and visual impairment, operates a toll-free national hotline, and is a source of additional information. The AFB Technology Center ([212] 502-7642) is a repository of information about assistive technology.

The second section, Sources of Additional Information, includes a list of professional journals that provide invaluable information for professionals. In addition, a listing of available electronic information is provided. Sources of information on the Internet are proliferating but also change rapidly. This section provides information on what is available as of this writing. Readers should bear in mind that names and addresses in listings such as this one constantly change and should be verified.

A third section, Sources of Products and Services, is a guide to finding adaptive devices and services. Distributors of computer technology and electronic devices are listed first, followed by a list of distributors of optical devices for persons with low vision. These companies sell a wide variety of products that are useful to individuals with low vision and professionals who work with them. A separate list includes sources of catalogs and mail order distribution. The organizations and companies included here carry a wide variety of products, including independent living, health care, and recreation products; low vision devices; and communication aids. Low vision professionals might find it worthwhile to keep a number of catalogs from such distributors on hand.

More extensive listings can be found in the *Directory of Services for Blind and Visually Impaired Persons in the United States and Canada* published by AFB. The *Directory* also has listings of such useful services for low vision professionals as regional libraries for the blind and physically handicapped, talking book machine distributors, radio reading services, and phone-in newspapers.

SOURCES OF INFORMATION AND SERVICES

Consumer Organizations

American Council of the Blind
1155 15th Street, N.W., Suite 720
Washington, D.C. 20005
(202) 467-5081; (800) 424-8666
Promotes effective participation of blind people in all aspects of society. Provides information and referral, legal assistance, scholarships, advocacy, consultation, and program development assistance. Interest groups include the Deaf-Blind Committee and the Council of Citizens with Low Vision International. Publishes *The Braille Forum*.

Council of Citizens with Low Vision International
6511 26th Street West
Bradenton, FL 34207
(941) 742-5958; (800) 733-2258
FAX: (941) 755-9721
Promotes rights of partially sighted individuals to maximize use of their residual vision. Educates the public to the needs of visually impaired people. Informs persons with low vision of available services. Has support groups and chapters throughout the United States. Publishes *Vision Access*.

National Association for Parents of the Visually Impaired
P.O. Box 317
Watertown, MA 02272-0317
(800) 562-6265
FAX: (617) 972-7444
Provides support to parents and families of children and youth who have visual impairments. Operates a national clearinghouse for information, education, and referral. Publishes a newsletter, *Awareness*.

National Federation of the Blind
1800 Johnson Street
Baltimore, MD 21230
(410) 659-9314
FAX: (301) 685-5683
Strives to improve social and economic conditions of blind persons, evaluates and assists in establishing programs, and provides public education and scholarships. Interest groups include the Committee on the Concerns of the Deaf-Blind. Publishes *The Braille Monitor* and *Future Reflections*.

National Organizations

American Association of the Deaf-Blind
814 Thayer Avenue
Silver Spring, MD 20910
(301) 588-6545
FAX: (301) 588-8705
Promotes better opportunities and services for deaf-blind people and strives to ensure that a comprehensive, coordinated system of services is accessible to all deaf-blind people, enabling them to achieve their maximum potential through increased independence, productivity, and integration into the community. Publishes *The Deaf-Blind American*.

American Foundation for the Blind
11 Penn Plaza, Suite 300
New York, NY 10001
(212) 502-7600; (212) 502-7662 (TTY/TDD); (800) AFB-LINE
FAX: (212) 502-7777

E-mail:newyork@afb.org

Provides services to and acts as an information clearinghouse for people who are blind or visually impaired and their families, professionals, organizations, schools, and corporations. Stimulates research and mounts program initiatives to improve services to visually impaired persons; advocates for services and legislation, maintains the M.C. Migel Library and Information Center and the Helen Keller Archives; provides information and referral services; operates the National Technology Center and the Career and Technology Information Bank; produces videos and publishes books, pamphlets, the *Directory of Services for Blind and Visually Impaired Persons in the United States and Canada,* and the *Journal of Visual Impairment & Blindness.* Maintains the following offices throughout the country in addition to the headquarters office:

AFB Midwest
401 N. Michigan Avenue, Suite 308
Chicago, IL 60611
(312) 245-9961
FAX: (312) 245-9965

AFB Southeast
National Initiative on Literacy
100 Peachtree Street, Suite 620
Atlanta, GA 30303
(404) 525-2303
FAX: (404) 659-6957

AFB Southwest
260 Treadway Plaza
Exchange Park
Dallas, TX 75235
(214) 352-7222
FAX: (214) 352-3214

AFB West
111 Pine Street, Suite 725
San Francisco, CA 94111
(415) 392-4845
FAX: (415) 392-0383

Governmental Relations
1615 M Street, N.W., Suite 250

Washington, D.C. 20036
(202) 457-1487
FAX: (202) 457-1492

AFB Office
15 Mechanic Street, #3
Provincetown, MA 02657
(508) 487-5815
FAX: (508) 487-5815

American Printing House for the Blind
1839 Frankfort Avenue
Louisville, KY 40206
(502) 895-2405; (800) 223-1839
FAX: (502) 895-1509
Produces materials in braille and large print and on audiocassette; manufactures computer-access equipment, software and special educational devices for persons who are visually impaired; maintains an educational research and development program and a reference-catalog service providing information about volunteer-produced textbooks in accessible media.

Blinded Veterans Association
477 H Street, N.W.
Washington, D.C. 20001-2694
(202) 371-8880; (800) 669-7079
FAX: (202) 371-8258
Encourages and assists all blinded veterans to take advantage of rehabilitation and vocational training benefits, job placement assistance, and other aid from federal, state, and local resources by means of a field service program. Promotes extension of sound legislation and rehabilitation through liaison with other agencies. Through 38 regional groups and field service offices, operates a volunteer service program for blinded veterans in their communities and provides information and referral services.

Canadian National Institute for the Blind
1931 Bayview Avenue
Toronto, ON, M4G 3E8
Canada
(416) 480-7580
FAX: (416) 480-7677

Provides services to people who are blind or visually impaired through a network of divisional offices throughout Canada.

DB-LINK
The National Information Clearinghouse on Children Who Are Deaf-Blind
Northwestern Oregon State University
345 North Monmouth Avenue
Monmouth, OR 97361
(503) 838-8401; (800) 438-9376
(800) 854-7013 (TDD)
Identifies, coordinates, and disseminates information related to children ages 0-21 who are deaf-blind, including the following topics: early intervention; education; related medical, health, social, and recreational services; relevant legal issues; employment; independent living; and postsecondary education. A consortium of agencies comprise DB-LINK: American Foundation for the Blind, Helen Keller National Center for Deaf-Blind Youths and Adults, Perkins School for the Blind, and Teaching Research.

Hadley School for the Blind
700 Elm Street
Winnetka, IL 60093-0299
(708) 446-8111 (voice/TTY/TDD)
FAX: (708) 446-8153
Provides tuition-free home studies in academic studies as well as vocational and technical areas, personal enrichment, parent/child issues, compensatory rehabilitation education, and Bible study. Rehabilitation courses include topics such as braille abacus, and independent living without sight and hearing for adults who are deaf-blind.

Helen Keller National Center for Deaf-Blind Youths and Adults
111 Middle Neck Road
Sands Point, NY 11050-1299
(516) 944-8900 (voice/TDD)
(516) 944-8637 (TTY)
Through the national center and its 10 regional offices, provides diagnostic evaluations, comprehensive vocational and personal adjustment training, and job preparation and placement for people who are deaf-blind from every state and territory. Offers technical assistance and training to those who work with deaf-blind people. Publishes *The Nat-Cent News, National Parent Newsletter,* and *TAC Newsletter.*

National Accreditation Council for Agencies Serving the Blind and Visually Handicapped
15 East 40th Street
New York, NY 10016
(212) 683-5068
Administers program of standards development and accreditation programs, agencies and schools serving children and adults who are blind or visually impaired. Publishes standards available in print, braille, and cassette tape.

National Association for Visually Handicapped
22 West 21st Street
New York, NY 10010
(212) 889-3141
FAX: (212) 727-2931
Acts as an information clearinghouse and referral center regarding resources available to persons who are visually impaired.

National Council of Private Agencies of the Blind
Carroll Center for the Blind
770 Centre Street
Newton, MA 02158-2597
(617) 969-6200
Serves as an advocate concerning issues that relate to programs, operations, and funding affecting voluntary agencies serving blind and visually impaired persons. Acts as a unified voice in negotiating with federal and state agencies about fees and other matters concerning private agencies.

National Council of State Agencies for the Blind
1213 29th Street, N.W.
Washington, D.C. 20007
(202) 298-8468
Promotes communication among agencies involved in preventing blindness and offering services to severely visually impaired individuals.

National Eye Institute Information Center
National Institutes of Health
9000 Rockville Pike
Building 31, Room 6A03
Bethesda, MD 20892
(301) 496-5248; (301) 496-2234
Finances and conducts research on the eye and vision disorders; supports training of eye researchers; and publishes materials on visual impairment.

National Library Service for the Blind and Physically Handicapped
Library of Congress
1291 Taylor Street, N.W.
Washington, D.C. 20542
(202) 707-5100; (800) 424-8567
FAX: (202) 707-0712
Conducts a national program to distribute free braille and recorded materials of a general nature and braille music to individuals who are blind and who have physical disabilities. Provides reference information on all aspects of blindness and other physical disabilities that affect reading. Conducts national correspondence courses to train sighted persons as braille transcribers and blind persons as braille proofreaders. Provides talking book machines and cassette machines for disk records and cassette tapes. Selects, orders, and distributes materials through a network of 160 libraries nationwide that function as circulating centers, using the mails to serve readers. Materials mailed postage free.

Prevent Blindness America
500 East Remington Road
Schaumburg, IL 60173
(708) 843-2020; (800) 221-3004
FAX: (708) 843-8458
Conducts through a network of state affiliates a program of public and professional education, research, and industrial and community services to prevent blindness. Services include screening, vision testing, and dissemination of information on low-vision devices and clinics.

Recording for the Blind and Dyslexic
20 Roszel Road

Princeton, NJ 08540
(609) 452-0606; (800) 221-4792
FAX: (609) 987-8116
Lends recorded and computerized textbooks, library services, and other educational resources to people who cannot read standard print because of visual disorder or other disability. Maintains a lending library of recorded books and acts as a recording service for additional titles.

Rehabilitation Research and Training Center on Blindness and Low Vision
Mississippi State University
P.O. Drawer 6189
Mississippi State, MS 39762
(601) 325-2001; (800) 675-7782
FAX: (601) 325-8989
E-mail: rrtc@ra.msstate.edu
Provides in-service training and continuing education programs; offers graduate credit for vision specialists in vocational rehabilitation programs.

The Lighthouse Inc.
111 East 59th Street
New York, NY 10022
(212) 821-9200
Promotes vision rehabilitation services for all ages and maintains a wide variety of research and education programs. Through the Lighthouse National Center for Vision and Aging, the Lighthouse National Center for Vision and Child Development, Low vision Continuing Education, and the Research Institute, conducts research and demonstration projects; delivers technical assistance, consulting, and educational services regarding the needs of people who are blind or visually impaired; and maintains a toll-free information and resource service.

Organizations Related to Specific Visual Impairments

Achromatopsia Network
P.O. Box 214
Berkeley, CA 94701-0214
(510) 540-4700

Provides information about achromatopsia. Maintains support network for individuals with congenital achromatopsia and their families.

American Diabetes Association
1660 Duke Street
Alexandria, VA 22314
(703) 549-1500 x2342; (800) 232-3472
FAX: (703) 549-6995
Promotes knowledge of diabetes through public and professional education. Seeks to prevent and cure diabetes and to improve the lives of all people affected by diabetes. Provides services at the local level through over 800 chapters throughout the United States and 54 affiliates in all 50 states.

Association for Macular Diseases
210 East 64th Street
New York, NY 10021
(212) 605-3719
Provides information and education. Maintains support group for persons with macular degeneration. Funds eye bank devoted to research on macular degeneration.

Corneal Dystrophy Foundation
1926 Hidden Creek Drive
Kingwood, TX 77339
(713) 358-4227
Promotes public education about corneal dystrophy and supports research.

Foundation for Glaucoma Research
490 Post Street, Suite 830
San Francisco, CA 94102
(415) 986-3162
FAX: (415) 986-3763
Aims to eliminate blindness caused by glaucoma through the use of research and education. Informs professionals and public about glaucoma through publications, lectures, conferences. Maintains eye bank for glaucomatous tissue research.

Macular Degeneration, International
1968 W. Ina Road, #106
Tucson, AZ 85741
(520) 797-2525 (Fax and Tel.)

Serves persons with juvenile or age-related macular degeneration and supports research on finding the causes and treatments of macular degeneration.

Myopia International Research Foundation
1265 Broadway, Room 608
New York, NY 10001
(212) 684-2777
Promotes research into the causes, treatment, and prevention of progressive myopia. Launched the Myopia International Research Network to promote worldwide coordinated scientific research on myopia by doctors and interested patients.

National Marfan Foundation
382 Main Street
Port Washington, NY 11050
(516) 883-8712; (800) 862-7236
FAX: (516) 883-8712
Disseminates information about Marfan syndrome to patients, family members, and physicians; provides means for patients and relatives to share experiences and support; fosters research and public education.

NOAH (National Organization for Albinism and Hypopigmentation)
1530 Locust Street, No. 29
Philadelphia, PA 19102-4415
(215) 545-2322; (800) 473-2310
Provides information on albinism and hypopigmentation; provides peer support; sponsors conferences on the subject; publishes a newsletter regularly. Has network of state chapters. Founding member of Albinism World Alliance.

The Foundation Fighting Blindness
Executive Plaza 1, Suite 800
11350 McCormick Road
Hunt Valley, MD 21031-1014
(410) 785-1414; (410) 785-9687 (TTY/TDD); (800) 683-5555
FAX: (410) 771-9470
Supports research on the cause, prevention, and treatment of retinitis pigmentosa allied inherited retinal degenerations. Holds regional and na-

tional workshops for volunteers and professionals.

Professional Organizations

American Academy of Ophthalmology
655 Beach Street
P.O. Box 7424
San Francisco, CA 94120-7424
(415) 561-8500
Promotes continuing education for ophthalmologists and quality care in ophthalmology. Publishes informational material for professionals and the public. Sponsors the National Eye Care Project to give free eye care to elderly persons.

American Academy of Optometry
4330 East West Highway, Suite 1117
Bethesda, MD 20814-4408
(301) 718-6500
Promotes excellence in standards of optometric practice. Fosters research and knowledge dissemination. Conducts annual meeting. Publishes *Optometry and Vision Sciences* and a quarterly newsletter.

American Optometric Association
243 North Lindberg Boulevard
St. Louis, MO 63141
(314) 991-4100
FAX: (314) 991-4101
Improves the quality of vision care through promoting high standards, continuing education, information dissemination, and professional involvement. Conducts conferences; operates placement service; maintains optometric museum and library; also maintains Virginia office.

Association for Education and Rehabilitation of the Blind and Visually Impaired
206 North Washington Street, Suite 320
Alexandria, VA 22314
(703) 548-1884
FAX: (703) 683-2926
Promotes all phases of education and work for people of all ages who are blind and visually impaired, strives to expand their opportunities to take a contributory place in society, and disseminates information. Certifies rehabilitation teachers, orientation and mobility specialists, and classroom teachers. Subgroups include Division 7, Low Vision. Publishes *RE:view, AER Report, Job Exchange Monthly,* and *RT News,* a quarterly newsletter.

Council for Exceptional Children Division on Visual Impairment
1920 Association Drive
Reston, VA 22091-1589
(703) 620-3660; (800) 845-6232
(703) 620-3660 (voice and TDD)
The largest international professional organization for individuals serving children with disabilities and children who are gifted. CEC has 17 specialized divisions. Primary activities include advocating for appropriate government policies; setting professional standards; providing continuing professional development; and assisting professionals to obtain conditions and resources necessary for effective professional practice. Publishes numerous related materials, journals, and newsletters.

Organizations of International Activity

International Council for Education of People with Visual Impairment (ICEVI)
4 Taman Jesselton
10450 Penang
Malaysia
Promotes educational opportunities for children and adults with visual impairment throughout the world.

International Society of Low Vision Research and Rehabilitation
VISIO
Amersfoortsestraatweg 180
1272 RR Huizen
The Netherlands
02159-8-57-11
Stimulates scientific research in the areas of low vision and rehabilitation of people with low vi-

sion and promotes the exchange of information. Publishes *Journal of Videology*.

SOURCES OF ADDITIONAL INFORMATION

Journals

Journal of Videology
International Society of Low Vision Research and Rehabilitation
VISIO
Amersfoortsestraatweg 180
1272 RR Huizen
The Netherlands
02159-8-57-11

Journal of Visual Impairment & Blindness
American Foundation for the Blind
11 Penn Plaza, Suite 300
New York, NY 10001
(212) 502-7648; (800) AFB-LINE (800 232-5463)
FAX: (212) 502-7774

RE:view
Heldref Publications
Helen Dwight Reed Educational Foundation
1319 18th Street, N.W.
Washington, D.C. 20036
(202) 296-5149

The Journal of Vision Rehabilitation
Media Periodicals Division
Trozzolo Resources, Inc.
1102 Grand, 23rd Floor
Kansas City, MO 64106
(800) 347-2665
FAX: (816) 842-8188

Online Resources

Accessible Web
http://www.gsa.gov/coca/wwwcode.html
Host organization: General Services Administration.
Content: Accessible web design.

Apple Disability Access
http://www.apple.com/disability.welcome.html
Content: Disability information.

ATRC
http://www.utirc.utoronto.ca/adtech/welcomelb/html
Host organization: Adaptive Technology Resource Centre, Toronto University.
Content: Issues related to accessibility.

Berkeley Access
http://access.berksys.com/
Host organization: Berkeley Systems.
Content: Access to graphical user interfaces by blind people.

CALL
http://call-centre.cog.sci.ed.ac.uk/callhome
Host organization: Communication Aids for Language and Learning Centre, University of Edinburgh.
Content: Research and developments in communication and writing aids in associated techniques.

Center for Assistive Technology
http://cosmos.ot.buffalo.edu/aztech/html
Host organization: University of Buffalo.

Cost 219
http://www.nta.no/cost219/frontpage.html
Content: Information about the European COST 219 project on future telecommunication and teleinformatic facilities for disabled and elderly people.

Disability Mall
http://disability.com
Host organization: Evan Kemp Associates, Inc.
Content: Commercial site about disability and disability products.

DO-IT
http://weber.u.washington.edu/-doit/
Host organization: University of Washington DO-IT program.

EASI

http://www.rit.edu.-easi/easiem/html

Host organization: Equal Access to Software and Information project.

Content: Projects and documents regarding accessibility. Also contains a list of resources (Internet servers) that give documents in electronic format.

IBM

http://www.austin.ibm.com/pspino/snshome/hmtl

Content: Information about IBM products for people with a disability. Freeware can be downloaded.

MedWeb

http://www.cc.emory.edu/whscl/medweb.disabled.html

Content: List of servers concerning disability and some articles and databases.

MoBic

http://www.cs.uni-magdeburg.del-mobic

Host organization: Tide MoBIC project.

Content: Orientation and navigation system for blind persons.

MOSAIC

http://bucky.aa.uic.edu/#george

Host organization: National Center for Supercomputing Applications, University of Illinois.

Content: Overview of access methods to the Worldwide Web by disability and by platform operating system.

NIDRR

http://www.ed.gov

Host organization: National Institute on Disability and Rehabilitation Research.

O&M Project

http://ccwf.cc.utexas.edu/-jshouman/OandM/

Host organization: University of Texas.

Pandora

http://pandora.inescn.pt/

Content: Information about technology and disability.

Rehabilitation Information System

http://www.icdi.wvu.edu

Host organization: West Virginia RRTC.

SDRU

http://phoenix.herts.ac.uk/psydocs.sdru/index.html

Host organization: Sensory disabilities research unit at University of Hertfordshire.

Content: Evaluation of technological developments for people with sensory disabilities.

Trace Center

http://trace.wisc.edu

Host organization: University of Wisconsin

VAESS

http://www.shef.ac.uk/uni/projects/vaess

Host organization: Tide VAESS project.

Content: Voices, attitudes, and emotions in speech synthesis.

Windows Access

http://ucunix.edu/-hamilt/wintip31.html

Content: Low vision guide to using Windows 3.1

World Friends

http://hale.ssd.k12.wa.us/tony.www/world-friends.html

Content: Listing of magazines available on the Internet, directed at students with disabilities.

SOURCES OF PRODUCTS AND SERVICES

Distributors of Computer Technology and Electronic Devices

Acrontech International

5500 Main Street

Williamsville, NY 14221

(716) 854-3814

AI Squared

P.O. Box 669

Manchester Center, VT 05255

(802) 362-3612
E-mail:zoomtext@aisquared.com

Ann Morris Enterprises
890 Fams Court
East Meadow, NY 11554
(516) 292-9232

Arkenstone
1390 Borregas Avenue
Sunnyvale, CA 94089
(408) 752-2200; (800) 444-4443
FAX: (408) 745-6739

Artic Technologies
55 Park Street
Troy, MI 48083
(810) 588-7370

Arts Computer Products
145 Tremont Street, Suite 407
Boston, MA 02111
(617) 482-8248

Berkeley Systems
2095 Rose Street
Berkeley, CA 94709
(510) 883-6280
FAX (510) 849-9426
http://access.berksys.com

Carolyn's
P.O. Box 14577
Bradenton, FL 34208
(800) 648-2266
FAX: (813) 761-8306

Celexx Trading Company
2535 Seminole
Detroit, MI 48214
(800) 886-3269

Coburn Optical Industries
4606 S. Garnett Road, Suite 200
Tulsa, OK 74146
(800) 262-8761; (918) 665-1815

C TECH
130 Pascack Road
Pearl River, NY 10965
(914) 735-7907

Data Transforms
616 Washington Street
Denver, CO 80203
(303) 832-1501

E-Z Reader
1408 N. Westshore Boulevard, Suite 506
Tampa, FL 33607
(813) 286-2816

Finally Software
4000 MacArthur Boulevard, Suite 3000
Newport Beach, CA 92663
(714) 854-4434

4X
P.O. Box 555
Millwood, NY 10546
(914) 762-3555
FAX (914) 944-0605

Gracefully Yours
12527 Ulmerton Road
Largo, FL 34644
(800) 331-2211

Hexagon Products
P.O. Box 1295
Park Ridge, IL 60068-7295
(708) 692-3355
E-mail: 76064.1776@compuserve.com
http://ourworld.compuserve.com
homepages/hexacon

HumanWare
6245 King Road
Loomis, CA 95650
(916) 652-7253; (800) 722-3393
FAX: (916) 652-7296

Innoventions
5921 S. Middlefield Road

Suite 102
Littleton, CO 80123-2877
(800) 854-6554

LS&S Group
P.O. Box 673
Northbrook, IL 60065
(708) 498-9777; (800) 468-4789

Magnisight
P.O. Box 2653
Colorado Springs, CO 80901
(800) 753-4767

Maxi-Aids
42 Executive Boulevard
P.O. Box 3290
Farmingdale, NY 11735
(516) 752-0521; (800) 522-6294

Mentor O&O
3000 Longwater Drive
Norwell, MA 02061
(800) 992-7557

Microsystems Software
600 Worcester Road
Framingham, MA 01701
(800) 828-2600
FAX (508) 626-8515
http://www.microsys.com

Okay Vision-Aide Corporation
14811 Myford
Tustin, CA 92680
(800) 325-4488
(714) 669-1081

Optelec USA
6 Lyberty Way
P.O. Box 729
Westford, MA 01886
(508) 392-0707; (800) 828-1056
FAX: (508) 692-6073

Overseer Electronic Visual Aids
6826 Logan Avenue, South
Richfield, MN 55423
(612) 866-7606

Pelco Sales, Inc.
300 West Pontiac Way
Clovis, CA 93612-5699
(800) 421-1146; (800) 537-1991 (CA)

Read EZ Reader
P.O. Box 433
9780 Hope Acres Road
White Plains, MD 20695-0433
(301) 932-6565
FAX (301) 934-4365

Seeing Technologies
7074 Brooklyn Road
Minneapolis, MN 55429
(800) 462-3738

SkiSoft
1644 Massachusetts Avenue
Suite 79
Lexington, MA 02173
(617) 863-1876
infor@skisoft.com
http://www.skisoft.com

Sunburst Communications
39 Washington Avenue, Box 30
Peasantville, NY 10570-9970
(800) 431-1934; (800) 221-9971

Talking and Visual Aids
8136 Appoline
Detroit, MI 48228
(313) 935-1266

TeleSensory Corporation
455 North Bernardo
P.O. Box 7455
Mountain View, CA 94039-7455
(415) 960-0920; (800) 227-8418; (800) 345-2256
FAX: (415) 969-9064
http://www.telesensory.com/indext.htm

Turbo Power
3109 Scotts Valley Drive, Suite 122
Scotts Vallet, CA 95066
(408) 438-8608

Typewriting Institute for the Handicapped
3102 W. Augusta Avenue
Phoenix, AZ 85051
(602) 939-5344

Visionware
Distributed by Optelec, Inc.
6 Lyberty Way
P.O. Box 729
Westford, MA 01886
(508) 392-0707; (800) 828-1056
FAX: (508) 692-6073

Visual Solutions
1918 Washington, Street
P.O. Box 2338
Davenport, IA 52809
(319) 355-3706; (319) 322-5778

Washington Computer Services
2601 North Shore Road
Bellingham, WA 98226
(206) 734-8248

Worthington Data Solutions
417-A Ingalls Street
Santa Cruz, CA 95060
(408) 458-9938

Distributors of Optical Devices

Bausch and Lomb
P.O. Box 743
Rochester, NY 14603
(716) 338-6000; (800) 628-9543

Beecher Research Company
906 Morse Avenue
Schaumburg, IL 60193
(708) 893-0187; (800) 934-8765

Charles Nusinov & Sons
6635 Belair Road
Baltimore, MD 21206
(301) 254-6659

Cleveland Society for the Blind
Sight Center Aids and Appliances
1909 East 101 Street
Cleveland, OH 44106
(216) 791-8118 X226

Corning Medical Optics, MP 21-2
North American Optical
Corning
Corning, NY 14831
(607) 974-7417; FAX: (607) 974-7088

Data Display Systems
2240 Colby Avenue
Los Angeles, CA 90064-1593
(213) 879-0966

Designs for Vision
760 Koehler Avenue
Ronkonkoma, NY 11779
(516) 585-3404; (800) 345-4009
FAX: (516) 585-3404

Eschenbach Optik of America
904 Ethan Allen Highway
Ridgefield, CT 06877
(203) 438-7471

Foley's Low Vision Aids
1357 E. David Road
Kettering, OH 45429
(513) 294-2433

Hal-Hen Company
35-53 24th Street, P.O. Box 6077
Long Island City, NY 11106-9990
(718) 392-6020

Keeler Instruments
456 Parkway
Broomall, PA 19008
(215) 353-4350; (800) 523-5620
FAX: (215) 353-7814

Low Vision Devices
540 E. Horatio Avenue
Maitland, FL 32751
(407) 628-3133

McLeod Optical
100 Jefferson Park Road
Warwick, RI 02888
(401) 487-3000

New Concepts Marketing
P.O. Box 261
Port Richey, FL 34673-0261
(813) 842-3231

Night Vision Aid Distributors
1401 Royal Avenue, 4th Floor
Baltimore, MD 21217
(301) 225-9400; (800) 638-2300; (301) 225-9409
(TDD)

NoIR Medical Technologies
P.O. Box 159
South Lyon, MI 48178
(800) 521-9746

Phillip Barton-Vision Systems
3911 York Lane
Bowie, MD 20715
(301) 262-3665

Selsi Importing Company
40 Veterans Boulevard
P.O. Box 497
Carlstadt, NJ 07072
(201) 935-0388; (212) 473-4451

Stocker & Yale, Inc.
138 Brimbal Avenue
Beverly, MA 01915
(508) 927-3940

Sources of Catalogs and Mail Order Distribution

American Printing House for the Blind
1839 Frankfort Avenue
P.O. Box 6085

Louisville, KY 40206-0085
(502) 895-2405; (800) 223-1839
FAX: (502) 895-1509

American Thermoform Corporation
2311 Travers Avenue
City of Commerce, CA 90040
(213) 723-9021

Ann Morris Enterprises
890 Fams Court
East Meadow, NY 11554
(516) 292-9232

Exceptional Teaching Aids
20102 Woodbine Avenue
Castro Valley, CA 94546
(415) 582-4859; (800) 549-6999

Guild for the Blind
180 North Michigan, Suite 170
Chicago, IL 60601-7643
(312) 236-8569
FAX: (312) 236-8128

Horizons for the Blind
16A Meadowdale Center
Carpentersville, IL 60110
(708) 836-1400; (800) 318-2000
FAX: (708) 836-1443

Independent Living Aids
27 East Mall
Plainview, NY 11803
(516) 752-8080
(800) 537-2118
FAX: (516) 752-3135

Lighthouse Low Vision Products
36-20 Northern Boulevard
Long Island City, NY 11101
(800) 829-0500; (800) 334-5497
FAX: (718) 786-5620

LS&S Group
P.O. Box 673
Northbrook, IL 60065
(708) 498-9777; (800) 468-4789

Maxi-Aids
42 Executive Boulevard
P.O. Box 3290
Farmingdale, NY 11735
(516) 752-0521; (800) 522-6294

Science Products
P.O. Box 888
Southeastern, PA 19399
(800) 888-7400; (800) 222-2148
FAX: (215) 296-0488

INDEX

Photo Credits